HANDBOOK OF POSITIVE EMOTIONS

Handbook of Positive Emotions

Edited by

Michele M. Tugade
Michelle N. Shiota
Leslie D. Kirby

Foreword by Barbara L. Fredrickson

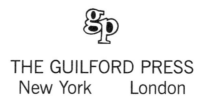

THE GUILFORD PRESS
New York   London

© 2014 The Guilford Press
A Division of Guilford Publications, Inc.
72 Spring Street, New York, NY 10012
www.guilford.com

Printed in the United States of America

This book is printed on acid-free paper.

Last digit is print number: 9   8   7   6   5   4   3   2   1

Library of Congress Cataloging-in-Publication Data

Handbook of positive emotions / edited by Michele M. Tugade, Michelle N. Shiota,
Leslie D. Kirby.
    pages cm
    Includes bibliographical references and index.
    ISBN 978-1-4625-1397-0 (hardcover)
    1. Positive psychology. 2. Emotions. I. Tugade, Michele M.   II. Shiota,
Michelle N.   III. Kirby, Leslie D. (Leslie Deneen)
    BF204.6.H356 2014
    152.4—dc23
                                                            2013043129

About the Editors

Michele M. Tugade, PhD, is Associate Professor in the Department of Psychology at Vassar College, where she directs the Emotions and Psychophysiology Laboratory. Her research focuses on the function of positive emotions in the coping process, the mechanisms that promote resilience in the face of stress and adversity, and emotion-related processes associated with health and well-being. Dr. Tugade received a Ruth L. Kirschstein National Research Service Award from the National Institute of Mental Health and is an elected member of the International Society for Research on Emotions.

Michelle N. Shiota, PhD, is Associate Professor of Psychology at Arizona State University, where she directs the Shiota Psychophysiology Lab for Affective Testing. Her research and publications focus on positive emotion, positive reappraisal, aging and emotion, and emotion in close relationships. Dr. Shiota is an associate editor of the American Psychological Association journal *Emotion* and coauthor of the textbook *Emotion*. She is an elected member of the Society for Experimental Social Psychology.

Leslie D. Kirby, PhD, is Research Assistant Professor and Senior Lecturer in Psychology at Vanderbilt University, where she codirects the Discrete Emotions and Appraisal Lab. Her research focuses on human emotions from the perspective of appraisal theory, with a particular interest in the differential motivational functions served by various positive emotions. Dr. Kirby received a Ruth L. Kirschstein National Research Service Award from the National Institute of Mental Health and is an elected member of the International Society for Research on Emotions.

Contributors

Anthony H. Ahrens, PhD, Department of Psychology, American University, Washington, DC

R. Toby Amoss, PhD, Department of Psychology, Georgia State University, Atlanta, Georgia

Lisa Feldman Barrett, PhD, Department of Psychology, Northeastern University, Boston, Massachusetts

Chelsea Boccagno, BA, Department of Psychology, Vassar College, Poughkeepsie, New York

Jeffrey S. Burgdorf, PhD, Department of Biomedical Engineering, Northwestern University, Evanston, Illinois

Belinda Campos, PhD, Department of Chicano/Latino Studies, University of California, Irvine, Irvine, California

Jennifer S. Cheavens, PhD, Department of Psychology, Ohio State University, Columbus, Ohio

Joey T. Cheng, PhD, University of British Columbia, Vancouver, British Columbia, Canada

Paul Condon, MA, Department of Psychology, Northeastern University, Boston, Massachusetts

Stéphane Côté, PhD, Rotman School of Management, University of Toronto, Toronto, Ontario, Canada

Alexander F. Danvers, BA, Department of Psychology, Arizona State University, Tempe, Arizona

David DeSteno, PhD, Department of Psychology, Northeastern University, Boston, Massachusetts

Hillary C. Devlin, BA, Department of Psychology, Yale University, New Haven, Connecticut

Lisa M. Diamond, PhD, Department of Psychology, University of Utah, Salt Lake City, Utah

John T. Dombrowski, MA, Department of Psychology, College of William and Mary, Williamsburg, Virginia

Sunny J. Dutra, MS, MPhil, Department of Psychology, Yale University, New Haven, Connecticut

Phoebe C. Ellsworth, PhD, Department of Psychology, University of Michigan, Ann Arbor, Michigan

Courtney N. Forbes, BA, Teach for America, New York, New York

Barbara L. Fredrickson, PhD, Department of Psychology, University of North Carolina at Chapel Hill, Chapel Hill, North Carolina

Philip A. Gable, PhD, Department of Psychology, University of Alabama, Tuscaloosa, Alabama

Shelly L. Gable, PhD, Department of Psychology, University of California, Santa Barbara, Santa Barbara, California

Devon N. Gangi, BA, Department of Psychology, University of Miami, Coral Gables, Florida

Gian C. Gonzaga, PhD, Gestalt Research, Santa Monica, California

Vladas Griskevicius, PhD, Department of Marketing, Carlson School of Management, University of Minnesota, Minneapolis, Minnesota

June Gruber, PhD, Department of Psychology, Yale University, New Haven, Connecticut

Lauren N. Hardy, MA, Department of Psychology, DePaul University, Chicago, Illinois

Eddie Harmon-Jones, PhD, School of Psychology, University of New South Wales, Sydney, Australia

Aleena C. Hay, MS, Department of Psychology, Yale University, New Haven, Connecticut

Dacher Keltner, PhD, Department of Psychology, University of California, Berkeley, Berkeley, California

Leslie D. Kirby, PhD, Department of Psychology, Vanderbilt University, Nashville, Tennessee

Sylvia D. Kreibig, PhD, Department of Psychology, Stanford University, Stanford, California

Janxin Leu, PhD, Department of Psychology, University of Washington, Seattle, Washington

Kimberly M. Livingstone, PhD, Department of Psychology, Northeastern University, Boston, Massachusetts

Corinna E. Löckenhoff, PhD, Department of Human Development, Cornell University, Ithaca, New York

Sonja Lyubomirsky, PhD, Department of Psychology, University of California, Riverside, Riverside, California

Jason P. Martens, MA, Department of Psychology, University of British Columbia, Vancouver, British Columbia, Canada

Nicole M. McDonald, PhD, Child Study Center, Yale School of Medicine, New Haven, Connecticut

Daniel S. Messinger, PhD, Departments of Psychology and Pediatrics, University of Miami, Coral Gables, Florida

Joseph A. Mikels, PhD, Department of Psychology, DePaul University, Chicago, Illinois

Chelsea Mitamura, MS, Department of Psychology, University of Wisconsin–Madison, Madison, Wisconsin

Jannay Morrow, PhD, Department of Psychology, Vassar College, Poughkeepsie, New York

Joseph R. Moskal, PhD, Department of Biomedical Engineering, Northwestern University, Evanston, Illinois

Judith Tedlie Moskowitz, PhD, MPH, Osher Center for Integrative Medicine, Department of Medicine, University of California, San Francisco, San Francisco, California

S. Katherine Nelson, MA, Department of Psychology, University of California, Riverside, Riverside, California

Samantha L. Neufeld, PhD, Department of Psychology, Arizona State University, Tempe, Arizona

Michael J. Owren, PhD, Department of Psychology, Emory University, Atlanta, Georgia

Jaak Panksepp, PhD, Department of Veterinary and Comparative Anatomy, College of Veterinary Medicine, Washington State University, Pullman, Washington

Carly K. Peterson, PhD, Minneapolis VA Health Care System, Minneapolis, Minnesota

Tom F. Price, PhD, School of Psychology, University of New South Wales, Sydney, Australia

Andrew E. Reed, PhD, Department of Psychology, Stanford University, Stanford, California

Lorie A. Ritschel, PhD, Department of Psychiatry and Behavioral Sciences, Emory University School of Medicine, Atlanta, Georgia

Laura R. Saslow, PhD, Osher Center for Integrative Medicine, University of California, San Francisco, San Francisco, California

Disa A. Sauter, PhD, Social Psychology Program, University of Amsterdam, Amsterdam, The Netherlands

Michelle N. Shiota, PhD, Department of Psychology, Arizona State University, Tempe, Arizona

Craig A. Smith, PhD, Department of Psychology and Human Development, Vanderbilt University, Nashville, Tennessee

Sanjay Srivastava, PhD, Department of Psychology, University of Oregon, Eugene, Oregon

Jennifer E. Stellar, PhD, Department of Psychology, University of California, Berkeley, Berkeley, California

Todd M. Thrash, PhD, Department of Psychology, College of William and Mary, Williamsburg, Virginia

Eddie M. W. Tong, PhD, Faculty of Arts and Sciences, National University of Singapore, Singapore

Jessica L. Tracy, PhD, Department of Psychology, University of British Columbia, Vancouver, British Columbia, Canada

Michele M. Tugade, PhD, Department of Psychology, Vassar College, Poughkeepsie, New York

Piercarlo Valdesolo, PhD, Department of Psychology, Claremont McKenna College, Claremont, California

Aaron C. Weidman, MA, Department of Psychology, University of British Columbia, Vancouver, British Columbia, Canada

Christine D. Wilson-Mendenhall, PhD, Department of Psychology, Northeastern University, Boston, Massachusetts

Claire I. Yee, BA, Department of Psychology, Arizona State University, Tempe, Arizona

Jennifer Yih, MS, Department of Psychology and Human Development, Vanderbilt University, Nashville, Tennessee

Foreword

Handbook of Positive Emotions draws together a richly diverse set of scholarly perspectives on the contemporary science of pleasant affective states. Readers will encounter herein leading-edge theory and research that promises to challenge them to appreciate positive emotions with greater nuance and greater attunement to context and supporting values.

The *Handbook* will serve as an invaluable resource for scholars across generations who are interested in the science of positive emotions. With its 27 chapters, the sheer size of this volume exemplifies how much this area of affective science has matured over the past decade. We now know, for example, that positive emotions have a much more complex narrative than was previously assumed. Part of what makes this volume distinctive is that it shines a light on the important nuances between specific positive emotions. Scholars interested in understanding the richness of select positive emotions will find much to savor in the *Handbook*, as the emotions of happiness, pride, love, compassion, gratitude, challenge, hope, awe, elevation, and inspiration are all explored. The book also integrates new insights regarding the social and biological facets of positive emotions, including state-of-the-science theoretical viewpoints and debates. In addition, contributors raise thoughtful discussions about automatic and controlled processes of positive emotion activation, the role of cultural norms in positive affective experience, and positive emotions across different contexts and populations.

This volume presents well-balanced viewpoints that push the field beyond a discussion of the hedonic value of positive emotions. The chapters reveal that positive emotions have both "good" and "bad" attributes. Collectively, the contributors provide a comprehensive view of the complexity of positive emotions in both form and function as they broaden and build upon the foundations set by earlier empirical and theoretical work. As the authors demonstrate, positive emotions are associated with a host of benefits to health, well-being, social relationships, and decision making. Importantly, the story of positive emotions does not end there, as several costs associated with positive emotional experience are identified as well. Positive emotions can go awry, for instance, depending on the contexts in which they are experienced, the goals that they are intended to serve, and the individual differences that their expression and activation confer.

As with all academic disciplines, the range of perspectives and viewpoints adds to the wisdom of a field. The *Handbook* showcases this wisdom by presenting the most current topics and areas of theoretical debate to date, systematically reconstructing and evaluating various positions. After reading through the chapters, readers will come away with the feeling that they have examined a particular theoretical debate from nearly every possible angle. Each contributor offers the gift of making complex concepts accessible. Readers will also discover countless new avenues for research in these pages, because each chapter concludes with a discussion of possible future directions in multiple areas of inquiry.

My hope is that readers will come away from their engagement with the *Handbook* inspired to take an active part in the conduct, dissemination, and/or application of the science of positive emotions. With continued wars and civil unrest, economic and educational challenges, and pressing environmental concerns, our local and global communities need the fruits of this rapidly growing area of scientific inquiry now more than ever.

BARBARA L. FREDRICKSON, PhD
University of North Carolina at Chapel Hill

Contents

Part III. Social Perspectives and Individual Differences

Part IV. Select Positive Emotions

Part V. Outcomes of Positive Emotions

Introduction

Michele M. Tugade
Michelle N. Shiota
Leslie D. Kirby

After decades of neglect, psychological research on positive emotions has burgeoned within the past 20 years. Indeed, important theoretical and empirical advances have made positive emotion an especially flourishing area of research. Offering a comprehensive survey of current literature, ideas, and practices, the *Handbook of Positive Emotions* aims to serve as a central resource for scholars, providing a rich overview of the state of this young but growing field.

The field of positive emotions is expanding at a rapid pace, with advances in the literature accumulating almost daily. It can be challenging to keep abreast of these new developments as they continue to emerge. Unfortunately, it is commonplace for researchers who address diverse questions throughout the field to work independently of one another, with limited cross-pollination of ideas or integration of findings that represent different theoretical perspectives. At this point, it is time to take a step back and review the products of the extensive, if somewhat scattered, theoretical and empirical work on positive emotion. The broader perspective to be gained by this endeavor can support a new wave of large-scale theory development, raising questions for the next decades of positive emotion science to address.

The *Handbook of Positive Emotions* is intended to help promote this integrative effort. This interdisciplinary volume brings together researchers from a wide range of perspectives on positive emotion, and presents the major themes guiding their research. One distinctive feature of this volume is that, for several chapters, the editors brought together teams of coauthors who had not previously collaborated with one another, and encouraged them to integrate their approaches. Although this was a challenging process, rich discussions among the authors often ensued, and the fruits of these discussions enhanced the perspectives offered by the chapters. In other chapters, authors were asked to reach beyond their individual programs of research to cover a variety of perspectives and/or a wide body of relevant empirical work, again with an eye to integration. In a number of these chapters, the authors propose a new way of thinking about existing research that has powerful implications for future directions in the field. Ultimately, the *Handbook* offers an overview of the existing science of positive emotions that is both comprehensive and forward-thinking, including detailed summaries of well-established perspectives, as well as chapters offering an expanded range of views on a given topic. In all, this volume provides a detailed view of the main themes and controversies surrounding the field. In what follows, we provide a short preview of the five central themes in the *Handbook of Positive Emotions*.

Part I: Theoretical Foundations

In Part I: *Theoretical Foundations*, contributors review the most prominent theories concerning positive emotions in the field today. The volume opens with Smith, Tong, and Ellsworth (Chapter 1), who examine the differentiation of positive emotions through the lens of cognitive appraisal theory, which theory posits that emotions are elicited on the basis of a meaning analysis (cognitive appraisal) along several dimensions (e.g., personal relevance, agency, certainty, control) that evaluates the relevance of one's circumstances for personal well-being. Smith and colleagues argue that there is considerably more differentiation among positive emotions than is allowed for in many theoretical perspectives, and discuss the distinctive properties of several benefit-related emotions (happiness, pride, gratitude) and opportunity-related emotions (interest, challenge/determination, hope). For each, they consider the appraisals hypothesized to elicit the emotion and discuss how these appraisals are related to the motivational functions the emotion is believed to serve. They close their chapter by discussing several emotions currently not well captured by appraisal theory (affection, compassion, awe, and tranquility), and consider ways in which appraisal theory might be developed further in order to account better for the full range of positive emotions.

In Chapter 2, Tugade, Devlin, and Fredrickson review the broaden-and-build the-ory, which proposes that positive emotions function to broaden one's thoughts and actions, and as a consequence, help to build personal, cognitive, social, and coping-related resources for the future. This chapter first reviews recent advances and empirical support for the model. The authors then consider possible mechanisms that might explain the broadening and building functions of positive emotions. Toward this aim, a dual-process model is discussed, which focuses on the interplay between conscious and nonconscious mechanisms of positive emotion activation to promote resilience. The authors close the chapter by discussing new areas of inquiry in research on automatic and controlled processes of positive emotion.

Shiota (Chapter 3) then takes an evolutionary approach to the study of positive emotions. She first asks what it means to apply an evolutionary perspective to the study of emotions, considering implications for theory building and empirical research. She then provides a comprehensive review and integration of various theoretical perspectives on the adaptive functions of positive affect and emotions, and illustrates how an evolutionary analysis of positive emotions can provide a unifying framework. Finally, she emphasizes important caveats in taking an evolutionary perspective in the study positive emotions and discusses potential strategies for researchers to implement as a way of addressing these issues. She closes the chapter by recommending topics for future studies in this rich and vibrant area of research.

Condon, Wilson-Mendenhall, and Barrett (Chapter 4) consider the implications of "atypical positive emotions," such as pleasant fear or unpleasant happiness. They review their theoretical approach, the conceptual act theory, which posits that emotions are based on psychological constructions that emerge from the categorization of ongoing (and continually modified) valence and arousal in the body and brain. According to this theory, at a given moment in time, people label their current feeling of affect (or core affect), using their stored knowledge of emotions. Condon and colleagues discuss the temporal dynamics of affective experience, showing how a "negative" emotion such as fear can shift to become a more pleasant experience (what they call "pleasant fear"). This chapter pushes the boundaries of what may "count" as a positive emotion, which has broad implications for theory and research on positive emotions.

In the final chapter of this section, Livingstone and Srivastava (Chapter 5) take a personality perspective to discuss individual differences in positive emotionality. In their review of the literature, they first examine the links between personality traits and positive emotional experience and expression. They argue that although the trait approach is a cornerstone in the field of personality psychology, the scope of this discipline goes beyond broad, stable dispositions to include within-person processes that are context-sensitive. To demonstrate the breadth of the field, they review two areas of personality research that have explored individual differences in such contextualized processes: *motivation* and the *self-regulation* of positive emotions, including processes that people use to generate, modulate, and alter positive emotions.

Part II: Biology of Positive Emotion

Within Part II: *Biology of Positive Emotion*, authors discuss the neurobiological (human and nonhuman), autonomic, vocal/acoustic, facial, and other sensory aspects of positive emotional experience and communication. In Chapter 6, Harmon-Jones, Price, Gable, and Peterson review the literature on neurobiological processes associated with approach motivation. They review theory and research on asymmetrical frontal cortical activity and its relationship with affective valence (positive vs. negative) and motivational direction (approach vs. avoidance). They consider implications of research finding that the "negative" emotion of anger shares many properties with positive emotions, including a strong association with approach motivation. They then review research suggesting that positive affective states varying in approach motivational intensity may differentially influence a variety of important cognitive processes (e.g., attentional scope, cognitive categorization).

In Chapter 7, Burgdorf, Panksepp, and Moskal review key issues and core findings in research on the neuroscience of positive emotion in nonhuman animals. They emphasize that animal neuroscience can play an important role in studying the neural substrates of emotion, offering greater ability to manipulate brain activity experimentally and to observe the effects on behavior than is generally possible with humans. They also acknowledge the problem of identifying animal behaviors that can serve as valid indicators of positive emotion and offer an example of how this problem might be approached. They then summarize evidence on the neural underpinnings of two main classes of positive emotion—appetitive/high-approach positive emotion and sensory pleasure—and briefly address three other neurobehavioral systems in animals that may be analogues to human positive emotions.

In Chapter 8, Kreibig examines the interplay between autonomic nervous system responding and positive emotions, presenting an affective psychophysiology approach to identifying meaningful categories of positive emotion states. Her analysis offers a new twist on the topic, emphasizing the evolution of positive emotion episodes over time as the dynamics of a situation change, as well as the implications of different kinds of emotion-eliciting situations.

The final two chapters in this section turn to the expressive aspects of positive emotions. In Chapter 9, Owren and Amoss focus on laughter, arguing that this signal is ubiquitous yet remarkably diverse. They analyze the acoustic properties of laughter, highlighting its variability and idiosyncrasies. After reviewing several perspectives on its possible functions, the authors propose a unifying framework in which laughter serves a core social bonding function, associating laugher with the experience of positive affect in others' minds. Chapter 10 (Sauter, McDonald, Gangi, and Messinger) broadens the scope, providing a comprehensive and integrative review of research on nonverbal signals of positive emotion in the voice (including prosody), the body (including touch, gestures, and posture), and the face (including smiles of different positive emotions, and nonverbal cues beyond smiles). A lifespan development approach is one distinctive feature of this chapter. Each chapter in this section closes with a discussion of limitations in the existing literature, as well as proposals for future research.

Part III: Social Perspectives and Individual Differences

In Part III: *Social Perspectives and Individual Differences*, chapters focus on the social contexts and consequences of positive emotions, as well as individual differences in the tendency to experience positive emotions, and outcomes associated with positive emotional traits. In Chapter 11, Valdesolo and DeSteno consider the implications of positive emotions for social cognition, with a particular emphasis on *intertemporal choice*—decisions in which short- and long-term outcomes are pitted against each other. Their new perspective ultimately highlights a key way in which positive emotions may enhance an individual's social value and support cooperative relationships with others. In Chapter 12, Yee, Gonzaga, and Gable also emphasize social functions of positive emotions, emphasizing their roles in the formation, growth, and maintenance of close relationships. The authors note that several major theories emphasizing intra-individual functions of positive emotions have clear analogues in terms of processes in close relationships, and they offer empirical evidence supporting the analogy in each case.

In Chapter 13, Mitamura, Leu, Campos, Boccagno, and Tugade consider the broader social context of positive emotions, contrasting cultural norms for positive emotion in individualistic Western cultures with norms in Asian and Latino cultures. Prominent theories of cultural factors likely to shape positive emotion are briefly reviewed, followed by evidence on the ways in which culture shapes positive emotion experience, meaning, expression, regulation, and functional consequences.

Chapters 14 and 15 both turn to the issues of individual differences in positive emotion. In Chapter 14, Kirby, Tugade, Morrow, Ahrens, and Smith consider the implications of individual differences in the ability to differentiate among experiences of positive emotion. They argue that the ability to differentiate subjectively the experience of positive emotions is associated with well-being. In making this case, they discuss how the ability to differentiate among positive emotions is related to, but distinct from, other emotion-relevant individual differences, including alexithymia and emotional intelligence. In addition, they describe and present initial data using a new individual-difference measure of the ability to differentiate positive emotional experience. Finally Mikels, Reed, Hardy, and Löckenhoff (Chapter 15) offer a lifespan development approach, pointing to evidence suggesting that positive emotion remains stable or even increases well into old age. They consider theories that might account for this trajectory, emphasizing the role of underlying emotion regulatory mechanisms in producing the "positivity effect," and exploring practical implications of these mechanisms for older adults' functioning in the context of relationships, decision making, and physical health.

Part IV: Select Positive Emotions

Part IV: *Select Positive Emotions* showcases the causes and consequences, structure, and experience of specific positive emotion constructs that have empirical grounding in the current literature. In the chapter on *happiness,* Nelson and Lyubomirsky (Chapter 16) begin by discussing what happiness is, since definitions can vary tremendously across researchers with different theoretical and empirical backgrounds. They then review evidence from intervention studies demonstrating that despite the stability of happiness in most people over time, happiness can in fact be increased (i.e., mood/emotions and life satisfaction), albeit not in the ways most people expect. Ultimately, they argue that there are multiple routes to happiness (and increases in happiness). These vary across individuals, situations, and time, and future research should determine what specific positive actions are going to be most effective for specific individuals in specific situations at specific times.

Chapter 17 (Tracy, Weidman, Cheng, and Martens), presents *pride* as a complex emotion, related to the attainment and maintenance of social status, that is distinct from some other positive emotions in that its effects on well-being, mental health, and relationships are not unambiguously positive. They trace the historical evolution of the concept of pride, as well as research on expressions of pride, developmental trajectories in pride, and the neuroscience of pride. One key issue that emerges from their research is that in its evolution, pride seems to have been multifaceted. They make a case for two separate facets of pride, each with distinctive properties and functions. "Authentic" pride is related to genuine accomplishments and the subsequent confidence that comes from those accomplishments. "Hubristic" pride, on the other hand, is more related to arrogance.

The next three chapters cover other-focused positive emotions, critical for supporting intimate relationships and harmonious group living. In Chapter 18, Diamond reviews the extensive contemporary research on the nature, dynamics, and underlying biology of *romantic love*. She discusses love as a complex emotion-motivation system. She considers whether love is better thought of as emotion in its own right, or as a context for the experience of a multitude of other emotions. She argues that regardless of conceptualization, romantic love has implications for and impacts not only our intimate relationships but also our broader social functioning and overall well-being.

Stellar and Keltner (Chapter 19) offer a rich overview and analysis of *compassion*, which has the fundamental drive "to care for the weak" and "not to harm others." They describe compassion as a discrete emotion, but as part of a family of other-focused emotions including empathy, sympathy, and pity. They analyze the crucial antecedents of compassion—suffering that is relevant in some way to the individual perceiving the suffering, the perceiver's belief about the deservedness of the suffering, and finally, an appraisal of the sufferer's ability to cope. They then discuss the evolutionary significance, as well as properties, of compassion (facial expressions, touch, voice, autonomic nervous system activity, and the neuroscience of compassion). Ultimately, they make a strong case for compassion as a discrete positive emotion and point out key areas for future research, such as exploring the roles between the sufferer and the observer.

The chapter on *gratitude* (Ahrens and Forbes, Chapter 20) considers empirical research on the relation of dispositional gratitude to physical and mental health, the effects of interventions to increase feelings of gratitude, and the role of gratitude in interpersonal relationships. They then discuss the utility of exploring different subtypes of gratitude, which are distinct in their antecedent appraisals and their action tendencies.

The remaining chapters in Part IV focus on positive emotions in the context of what can be, rather than what is. In Chapter 21, Shiota, Thrash, Danvers, and Dombrowski make a case for the adaptive significance of self-transcending positive emotional experiences, including awe, elevation, and inspiration. For each of these emotions, the authors provide a theoretical definition of the construct, followed by a discussion of empirical evidence in support of these theories. *Awe* involves perceived vastness and need for accommodation. Much of the empirical work on awe has focused on the role of awe in cognition, perception, and self-concept. *Elevation* is described as a warm, uplifting feeling when witnessing acts of goodwill toward others. Feeling elevated has important implications for prosocial behavior and cooperation. Finally, *inspiration* is a subjective psychological state that involves transcendence, evocation, and approach motivation, and can promote creativity, productivity, and well-being. So much of positive emotion research has involved self-focused emotions. This chapter is important for demonstrating the richness of positive emotional experience, by placing attention on that which is greater than the self.

Next, we include a chapter on *challenge*, an emotion that motivates persistence in the face of goal obstacles, thus playing an important role in the pursuit of mastery and gain. In this chapter, Kirby, Morrow, and Yih (Chapter 22) note how challenge has an interesting appraisal structure for a positive emotion. In challenge, unlike most positive emotions, one does not currently have what one wants; however, one believes that one is able to attain it. This motivates the individual to strive toward the goal. The authors also discuss the importance of state-level challenge in the development of traits such as grit and resilience, and explore applications of challenge research that demonstrate the importance of this positive emotion in personal and professional domains.

The final chapter in this section reviews the classic components of *hope* theory—agency and pathways—and discusses the unique properties of hope as a positive emotion. The authors also address the importance of hope in achievement situations, cognitive domains, and health contexts (Cheavens and Ritschel, Chapter 23).

Part V: Outcomes of Positive Emotions

This final section of the *Handbook*, Part V: *Outcomes of Positive Emotions*, may be especially useful for scholars interested in the health and clinical applications of positive emotion science, as well as issues relating positive emotions to organizations and marketing. In the first chapter in this section, which addresses the health consequences of positive emotions, Moskowitz and Saslow (Chapter 24) review substantial evidence linking positive emotions to a broad range of health-related outcomes, including cardiovascular functioning, immune responding, morbidity, and mortality. The authors eloquently discuss new directions in stress and coping research, with studies showing that positive emotions can co-occur with negative emotions, even in the most dire circumstances, and contribute to beneficial outcomes in physical health. Importantly, the authors discuss how, as with any growing, multidisciplinary literature, some inconsistencies and shortcomings can arise. Moskowitz and Saslow close with a discussion of potential psychological, biological, and behavioral pathways by which positive affect and related constructs may impact health, and they offer recommendations to help move the field forward.

The next chapter asks the opposing question, "Can positive emotions actually be bad for us?" While some disorders involve deficits in positive emotion, others may involve dysfunctionally high levels of positive emotions. Gruber, Dutra, Hay, and Devlin (Chapter 25) explore the nature of positive emotion disturbance across a variety of disorders including bipolar disorder and major depressive disorder (MDD). The authors discuss three processes of positive emotion that may be important for understanding positive emotion disturbance, including emotional *reactivity* to positive stimuli, the *anticipation* of positive cues, and the *regulation* of positive emotion. The authors review the interpersonal consequences of bipolar

disorder and MDD, and offer directions for future research that investigates "the boundary conditions of how and in what manner positive emotion can go awry" (p. 442).

We shift gears in the next two chapters to investigate the role of positive emotion in organizational settings. In Chapter 26, Côté discusses the important roles that positive emotions play in motivation, team building, and effective communication at the organizational level. He reviews a substantial literature on the *intra*personal consequences of positive emotions in organizations, with a focus on judgment and decision-making processes, job satisfaction and performance, creativity, and cooperation. Next, he reviews the *inter*personal consequences of positive emotional display with respect to leadership and negotiations, highlighting the importance of authenticity. At the group level of analysis, the overall positive affective tone is discussed as an important marker of workplace success. Côté suggests that future research on discrete positive emotions is necessary to further our knowledge about when positive emotions help and when they impede success in the workplace.

Finally, Neufeld and Griskevicius (Chapter 27) focus on the role of positive emotions in marketing and social influence. The authors begin by thoroughly reviewing and synthesizing important themes from classic theories of affect. Next, they discuss important empirical evidence on a host of mechanisms through which positive emotion affect people's responses to social influence, such as information processing, evaluation and judgment, and risk and variety seeking. In their final section, Neufeld and Grisevicius discuss complicating factors in this line of research. They offer suggestions for how researchers may advance the literature in marketing and social influence by considering positive emotions in cultural contexts (examining the persuasive power of emotions across cultures), health settings (exploring messaging and framing), and groups (investigating prosocial behavior).

Final Remarks

We hope that the chapters in the *Handbook of Positive Emotions* will help to set an agenda for future research in this important and rapidly growing field. Each chapter is offered by one or more leading researchers in their area of expertise, and showcases up-to-date theory and research, with a discussion of important future directions. The *Handbook* provides a well-balanced perspective on positive emotions science, providing readers with a thorough overview of current topics and areas of theoretical debate. We encourage readers to analyze both the promises and limitations of positive emotions research with a critical eye, considering what the future of positive emotions research may have in store. With such information, readers can draw their own conclusions and take part in the ongoing debates in the field.

PART I

Theoretical Foundations

CHAPTER 1

The Differentiation of Positive Emotional Experience as Viewed through the Lens of Appraisal Theory

Craig A. Smith
Eddie M. W. Tong
Phoebe C. Ellsworth

What is the nature of positive emotional experience? Is there a variety of positive emotions with distinctive feelings and motivational tendencies, such as joy, pride, and gratitude, as some theory (e.g., Frijda, 1986; Roseman, 2001; Smith 1991) and people's subjective experience tend to suggest? Or is positive emotional experience relatively undifferentiated, primarily represented by various forms of happiness, and serving fairly nonspecific adaptational functions as both basic emotion theory (e.g., Ekman, 1984; Izard, 1977; Tomkins, 1962), and some contemporary positive psychological theory (e.g., Fredrickson, 1998, 2001) would lead one to expect?

Certainly, scholars of emotion have long emphasized negative over positive emotional experience, and an examination of emotion theories leads one to expect very little differentiation among positive emotions. For instance, Darwin (1872/1965) devoted separate chapters to suffering, grief, reflection/ill temper, anger, disgust/contempt, fear/surprise, and shame, but only one to unequivocally positive emotions (joy/high spirits, love, tender feelings, and devotion). Surprise is included in the chapter on fear, and pride in the chapter on contempt. Basic emotion theorists have generally followed this lopsided emphasis on negative emotions. Tomkins (1962) and Izard (1977) proposed interest and surprise (an ambiguously positive emotion) in addition to joy, along with six negative emotions. Plutchik (1980) proposed joy, trust, and anticipation, which resembled hope. Ekman, Sorenson, and Friesen's (1969) groundbreaking study of cross-cultural recognition of facial expressions included four negative emotions, surprise (which was confused with fear in the only preliterate sample), and only one positive emotion, happiness. These were regarded as the canonical six basic emotions for decades to follow: happiness, sadness, fear, anger, disgust, and surprise.

More recently, Fredrickson (1998, 2001) has directed attention to positive emotional experience through her broaden-and-build model of positive emotion. However, the focus of this model is on properties of positive emotion in general, and the distinctive properties and motivational urges of different positive emotions are explicitly downplayed (e.g., Fredrickson, 2001, p. 219). For example, a chapter written in support of the broaden-and-build framework is titled "Gratitude (Like Other Positive Emotions) Broadens and Builds" (Fredrickson, 2004).

However, such theorizing seems to fly in the face of common experience, in which we seem capable of experiencing a broad range of distinct positive emotions accompanied by urges to act in fairly specific ways. Thus, the urge to express appreciation to someone else in gratitude seems very different than the urge to call attention to oneself and show off in pride, and both these urges seem distinct from the urge to relax and savor one's circumstances in contentment.

In this chapter we take on the issue of the differentiation of positive emotional experience, viewing it from our perspective as appraisal theorists. We argue that although positive emotional experience may be less differentiated than negative emotional experience, there is still a fair bit of differentiation to be found.

We first discuss appraisal theory, some of its key assumptions, and why it represents a powerful perspective for examining emotional differentiation. We then draw on the theory to discuss, somewhat generally, the nature of positive emotional experience, including what our use of the term "positive" does and does not encompass. Then, after briefly reviewing some of the existing evidence for the differentiation of positive emotional experience in general, we briefly and somewhat speculatively consider the likely motivational properties and appraisals associated with 10 different positive emotions (happiness, pride, gratitude, interest, hope, challenge/determination, affection, compassion, awe, and tranquility).

Why Appraisal Theory?

Appraisal theory provides a powerful theoretical lens for examining emotional differentiation. As in most contemporary approaches to emotion (e.g., Ekman, 1984; Frijda, 1986; Izard, 1977; Plutchik, 1980), emotions are viewed as largely adaptive responses to the perceived environmental demands confronting an individual, with emotion viewed, in part, as a signal system that serves important adaptational functions (e.g., Frijda & Swagerman, 1987; Simon, 1966). Different emotions are elicited by circumstances having different types of adaptational relevance. The emotional response serves as a compelling signal to call the person's attention to his or her circumstances, while the distinctive feeling conveys considerable information about the nature of those circumstances. The motivational urges and physiological activities associated with the emotion motivate and physically prepare the person to respond. For example, in fear, the subjective feeling alerts the person to a potentially dangerous situation, and the associated motivational urges and physiological changes promote heightened vigilance while preparing the person potentially to flee. Notably, there is considerable coherence across the various aspects of the emotional response. Each distinctive emotion serves a fairly distinct adaptational function (fear motivates caution and avoidance of harm) that is most applicable in a particular range of circumstances (circumstances involving threat or danger), and when called forth under those circumstances, the components of the emotional response—the subjective feeling state, the physiological changes (heightened attention and autonomic activation), and motivational urges (to attend carefully, and possibly to flee)—are all organized in support of that adaptational function.

A key puzzle raised in this general perspective is how the emotion system "knows" what to signal. That is, how does the system detect that the person is facing a threat that warrants fear, or a loss that calls for sadness, or a success that deserves joy? The solution to this puzzle is complicated by the fact that there are large individual differences in how people respond to very similar sets of circumstances. An anxiety-inducing threat to one person might be an exciting challenge to another, and of little consequence to a third. It is seldom the case that the adaptational significance of a particular set of circumstances is determined by the circumstances alone. Instead, this significance is defined by considering those circumstances in light of the individual's unique configuration of needs, goals, abilities, and beliefs (e.g., Roseman & Smith, 2001; Smith & Lazarus, 1990). Appraisal theory was developed to take on this puzzle, and to provide an account of how emotions might be elicited in this context-dependent manner.

The central premise of appraisal theory is that, rather than being evoked by circumstances directly, emotions are evoked in response to a meaning analysis, or "appraisal," in which the adaptive implications of the circumstances for the individual are evaluated in relation to her or his own current needs, goals and abilities, with different evaluations leading to different emotional responses (Roseman & Smith, 2001; Smith & Ellsworth, 1985). The idea that evaluations of the environment are central to emotions is not unique to appraisal theory. Philosophers (Aristotle, Spinoza, Descartes, Hume, and Sartre) and psychologists (James, Stumpf, Schachter, Russell, and Barrett) have proposed similar ideas. What is distinctive about contemporary appraisal theories is that they have not just argued vaguely that the interpretation of environmental circumstances determines the emotional response, but have attempted to define the perceptions of the particular aspects of the situation that are most important for emotions and their differentiation. Thus, appraisal theorists have developed and tested specific models that describe both the major issues that are evaluated in appraisal (often referred to as components or dimensions of appraisal, such as personal relevance, agency, and control; see below), and the specific outcomes of those evaluations that differentially elicit a broad range of emotions (to describe the appraisal patterns underlying the elicitation of happiness vs. sadness vs. anger, etc.; e.g., Roseman, 2001; Scherer, 2001; Smith & Ellsworth, 1985; Smith & Lazarus, 1990).

The efforts to develop these models have often been informed by a careful consideration of the adaptational functions thought to be served by the various emotions. For instance, rather than simply ask which appraisals evoke a particular emotion, such as happiness, appraisal theorists have tended to ask about both the adaptational value of happiness and the appraisals that identify a set of circumstances in which happiness is adaptive. Consequently, many appraisal

models tend to go beyond describing the appraisals hypothesized to elicit the various emotions, to describing the adaptational functions believed to be served by the emotions, as well as how the appraisals relate to those functions (e.g., Ellsworth & Smith, 1988b; Roseman, 2001; Smith, 1991; Smith & Ellsworth, 1985).

We believe that this integrated approach carries considerable theoretical power for describing the differentiation of emotional experience, including positive emotional experience. To date, a number of distinct but overlapping appraisal models have been proposed (for a review, see Ellsworth & Scherer, 2003), and the available data indicate that they provide a good accounting of a broad range of emotional experience (e.g., Ellsworth & Smith, 1988b; Frijda, Kuipers, & ter Schure, 1989; Roseman, 1991; Smith & Ellsworth, 1985). As with emotion research in general, this work has focused primarily on the differentiation of negative emotion. However, as we review below, the differentiation of positive emotional experience has not been entirely neglected. First, however, we describe the appraisals we discuss in this chapter, which are common to most appraisal theories (see, Ellsworth & Scherer, 2003).

Novelty or Change

To start an emotional episode, something attracts the perceiver's attention, which may (or may not) turn out to be significant. This has been called the "gateway" to emotion (Ellsworth, 1991), and further appraisals are quickly generated, refining and defining the emotion. If the event is appraised as insignificant for the perceiver's concerns, the organism returns to baseline and no specific emotion develops.

Motivational or Personal Relevance

A key determinant as to whether, and how strongly, an emotion will be elicited is how personally relevant, or important, to one's concerns the circumstances are perceived as being. If the situation does not meaningfully touch upon one's concerns, little or no emotion will result, but if one's concerns are strongly implicated, strong emotions are likely. As a general rule, rather than differentiating among different emotional states, appraisals of personal relevance contribute to the intensity of the resulting emotion, with greater perceived relevance producing stronger emotional reactions (Ellsworth & Scherer, 2003; Smith & Lazarus, 1990).

Motivational Congruence or Goal Conduciveness

Another fundamental dimension of appraisal is the degree to which one's circumstances are evaluated as consistent or inconsistent with one's goals. This appraisal tends to be closely related to the valence of the emotional reaction, with appraisals of goal conduciveness generally producing subjectively pleasant emotions, and appraisals of nonconduciveness generally producing unpleasant ones. Thus, it is tempting to classify emotions associated with appraisals of goal conduciveness as "positive emotions" and emotions associated with appraisals of nonconduciveness as "negative emotions." However, we believe that such a classification is overly simplistic and caution against it.

Closely related, but distinct from goal conduciveness, is an appraisal dimension reflecting the *intrinsic pleasantness* of the stimulus situation, discussed by a number of appraisal theorists (Frijda, 1986; Scherer, 1984; Smith & Ellsworth, 1985). Some stimuli, such as sunny days and music (Smith & Ellsworth, 1985), are inherently pleasant, and instantly perceived as things to be approached or savored, whereas others, including bad smells and pain, are inherently unpleasant, and perceived as things to be avoided or rejected. All else being equal, intrinsically pleasant stimuli yield appraisals of goal conduciveness, but this is not always the case. Inherently pleasant stimuli can be motivationally incongruent (e.g., the smell of freshly baked cookies for someone on a strict diet), and inherently unpleasant stimuli can be motivationally congruent (e.g., when a runner in training "goes for the burn"; Lazarus & Smith, 1988).

Certainty

Sometimes there is no question about what is happening or what will happen, but sometimes it is hard to understand what is happening or to predict what will happen next, and the perceiver feels uncertain. Closely related to certainty, a somewhat distinctive appraisal in some models (e.g., Smith, 1991; Smith & Lazarus, 1990) concerns *future expectancy*—an evaluation as to whether, for any reason, the situation is expected to improve or to get worse.

Agency

The perceiver sees that the stimulus event was caused by the self, some other person, or circumstances beyond anyone's control. This component of appraisal is seen as being important in providing a target for the person's subsequent coping efforts. In some schemes, this component is conceptualized as an attribution of causal agency (Roseman, 1984, 2001; Scherer, 2001), whereas in others, it has been somewhat more narrowly defined as an evaluation of responsibility or accountability (e.g., Smith & Lazarus, 1990).

Control

The person feels more or less able to cope with what is happening, or control what will happen next. This appraisal component is typically seen as influential in shaping the person's efforts to cope with the situation, with appraisals of high control leading to motivation to persevere, and appraisals of low control leading to motivation to give up and disengage from the situation.

Whenever an appraisal changes, the emotional experience changes. As more appraisals are made, the emotional experience becomes more differentiated, moving, for example, from feeling bad to anger, to righteous indignation. Combinations of these appraisals can account for a wide variety of emotional experiences, more than those covered by basic emotion theories, but probably not all. Our short list of appraisals can account for the branches of the tree, but probably not all the twigs.

And, it should be noted, many appraisal theorists would argue that there exists a multitude of twigs. These theorists are skeptical of the idea of discrete, basic emotions, instead believing that emotional experience can vary continuously. They conceptualize each of the appraisals as a continuous variable, and argue that a change in evaluation along any of the appraisal dimensions results in a change in emotional experience. There is a potentially infinite number of emotional states, some corresponding to words that exist in the language, such as fear, sorrow, or *schadenfreude*, but also many that do not. For example, as a person's appraisal of his or her ability to control a threatening situation increases, his or her emotional experience may change from negative to positive, from fear to hope to challenge, with nameless intermediate feelings along the way (Ellsworth & Scherer, 2003; Frijda, 1986). There may be as many positively toned as negatively toned emotional experiences, but, at least in English, there are fewer words for positive emotions (Averill, 1980).

At the same time, appraisal theorists also believe that emotion categories are significant, in that they correspond to common reactions to certain types of appraised situations that call for particular responses. Emotional reactions often center around one or more of these adaptationally meaningful appraised situations but can transform themselves as the situation unfolds and the appraisals change with it. Thus, although keeping in mind the continuous nature of emotional experience, there is still considerable value to examining the properties—the adaptational functions, appraisals, and behavioral urges—associated with the major categories of emotional experience. Examining such categories has often been the approach that appraisal theorists have taken in their empirical investigations, and it is the approach that we take here in our survey of positive emotions.

In the 1980s, when appraisal theories were first introduced, the differentiation of positive emotions had generally been neglected in research on emotion. Although the first major study of appraisal theory examined more positive emotions than were included in most contemporary research (Smith & Ellsworth, 1985), the differentiation of positive emotions was not a major goal of the research, and it is quite possible that the appraisals most important for distinguishing among positive emotions are somewhat different from the appraisals most important for distinguishing among emotions in

general. Before we address this question, however, we must consider what is meant by "positive emotion."

What Do We Mean by "Positive" Emotion?

Defining "positive" emotions is probably at least as difficult as defining emotion itself—a topic that has been debated vigorously for decades with no clear resolution in sight! Accordingly, we do not presume to present a definitive definition of positive emotion here; however, we consider three possible defining characteristics that are commonly suggested as distinguishing characteristics of positive emotions—that they are adaptive, that they involve approach or appetitive motivation (Watson & Tellegen, 1985), and that they feel good (have pleasant valence).

We reject the idea that serving adaptive functions is what defines emotions as "positive." We would argue that *all* emotions, even the most unpleasant emotions (e.g., sadness or guilt) serve important adaptive functions. We would also argue that *any* emotion can, and often does, arise under circumstances in which it has deleterious, maladaptive effects. Thus, for instance, sadness motivates one to seek help or to disengage from a hopeless situation, so that one can reengage in something else (e.g., Klinger, 1975; Smith & Lazarus, 1990). At the same time, any emotional response can be maladaptive under certain circumstances, especially if it results from a misappraisal of a situation (e.g., when anger is evoked in response to an innocent behavior). In the case of pride, considered a positive emotion in Western cultures, deleterious consequences are so common that it has been characterized as one of the "seven deadly sins," and a well-known aphorism counsels that "pride goeth before a fall" (from Proverbs 16:18). In our view, all emotions serve adaptive functions, albeit imperfectly. Thus, looking to the adaptive consequences of an emotional experience is of no help in attempting to distinguish positive from negative emotions.

A second possible definition is that positive emotions involve an approach motivation, while negative emotions are focused on avoidance. As argued by Watson and Tellegen (1985), negative emotions often seem to function in service of self-protection. That is, negative emotions typically serve to alert the person to avoid potential harms (e.g., as in disgust or fear; Lazarus, 1991), or to help ameliorate the consequences of actual, realized harms (as in anger, sadness, or guilt; Lazarus, 1991). In contrast, positive emotions often serve more appetitive functions, either alerting the person to as yet unrealized gains (opportunities, as in challenge/determination; Kirby, Morrow, & Yih, Chapter 22, this volume) and motivating him or her to achieve them, or rewarding and reinforcing actual, realized gains (benefits, as in happiness, pride, and gratitude; Smith, 1991). This distinction is not perfect because, as we discuss below, some positive emotions, such as tranquility, seem to involve little appetitive motivation, and at least one classically negative emotion, anger, seems to be associated with considerable approach (and possibly appetitive) motivation (e.g., Carver & Harmon-Jones, 2009).

In a similar manner, there is no denying that most positive emotions "feel good," and this is true even for emotions such as challenge/determination, in which a desired goal is being pursued but has not yet been achieved. Conversely, most negative emotions are quite unpleasant to experience. However, exceptions for both positive and negative emotions abound. As in thrill rides, people often actively seek out and enjoy intense fear experiences under certain controlled conditions, and even the experience of intense sadness can be quite cathartic, such as when one has a "good cry." Conversely, challenge/determination can be quite unpleasant subjectively, when tinged with worry or dread, and compassion for another can involve strong negative feelings in response to the other's plight. Not all instances of emotions with a negative label (e.g., fear) are necessarily unpleasant, nor are all instances of emotions with a positive label pleasant; within any category wide variation is possible (for a related view on atypical emotions, see Condon, Wilson-Mendenhall, & Barrett, Chapter 4, this volume).

In summary, although we do not have a perfect way to differentiate positive from negative emotional experience, we argue that much differentiation can be captured by the idea that negative emotions often are ones that subjectively feel bad and often serve self-protective motivational functions, whereas positive emotions are often ones that subjectively feel good and often serve more appetitive motivational functions. Clearly there are emotional states that provide exceptions to these characterizations, and we believe that such states are highly interesting.

Appraisal-Based Evidence of Differentiation among Positive Emotions

Although not specifically focused on positive emotions, appraisal theory has given some attention to positive emotional experience from the very beginning. Magda Arnold (1960), the first to use the term "appraisal," proposed that the appraisal of environmental changes as beneficial or harmful is fundamental. From an evolutionary point of view, it is important for the organism to be sensitive and responsive to opportunities as well as to threats. Richard Lazarus (e.g., Lazarus, Kanner, & Folkman, 1980), who further developed the idea of appraisal and its role in the elicitation and differentiation of emotion, placed particular emphasis on the positive emotions, arguing that they promote exploration as well as motivation for mastery and achievement, and that they also provide occasions to build and renew one's resources. His theory was in many ways a precursor to the broaden-and-build perspective (Fredrickson, 2001), and he urged researchers to devote more attention to the study of positive emotions (Lazarus et al., 1980). A number of more detailed appraisal models emerged in the mid-1980s (Frijda, 1986; Roseman, 1991; Scherer, 1984; Smith & Ellsworth, 1985), and each featured some positive differentiation. For instance, Nico Frijda (1986), in the first full-length development of appraisal theory, discussed joy, interest, sexual desire, love, compassion, tenderness, pride, contentment, and a sense of challenge, and argued for their importance in promoting adaptive behaviors such as exploration, social bonding, learning and mastery, recuperation, and of course the sine qua non of survival—reproduction. More recently, with the rise of positive psychology, researchers have begun detailed explorations of a number of positive emotions, including pride (Tracy & Robins, 2007), interest (Silvia, 2005), gratitude (Emmons &

McCullough, 2003), awe (Keltner & Haidt, 2003), contentment (Fredrickson, 1998), and compassion (Goetz, Keltner, & Simon-Thomas, 2010).

In the first major empirical research on appraisal theory, Smith and Ellsworth (1985) included nine negative emotions and six positive emotions, including surprise, which was seen as positive by their sample. The five other positive emotions were happiness, pride, hope, interest, and challenge. Considerable differentiation among the appraisal patterns characteristic of these six emotions was observed. For instance, happiness and pride were seen as very pleasant, with little or no effort required, and were characterized by both a relatively high sense of certainty and a desire to attend to the situation. The main difference between them was that proud people felt more strongly than happy people that they were responsible for the favorable event. Hope and challenge were less unequivocally positive and involved more effort, particularly challenge. Challenge involved both a strong motivation to exert oneself and a strong sense of personal agency that was not shared by hope. Hope and challenge shared with interest a strong need to attend to the situation. Hope and surprise were the only positive emotions that involved a sense of uncertainty.

In a follow-up study Ellsworth and Smith (1988b) examined the appraisals associated with positive emotions more closely. They asked participants to describe pleasant past experiences characterized by various combinations of the appraisals of effort, agency, and certainty. Participants then rated their appraisals and 24 different emotions, 10 negative and 14 positive. Ellsworth and Smith found evidence for 10 distinct positive emotions. Of these, seven were predicted: tranquility, playfulness, surprise, challenge, interest, sympathy, and relief. Love, friendliness, and gratitude were not differentiated from each other: All involved perceptions of another person as the cause of the pleasant event. Of course, this does not mean that these three emotions are identical—it is likely that they differ in other appraisals that were not assessed in the study. Oddly, hope and pride also occurred together. The authors hypothesized that this may have been due to the failure of the method to capture changes in emotion over time: For the

same event, for example, being accepted to a good college, participants may have remembered both their feeling of hope before they heard the good news and their feeling of pride afterwards. The final pleasant emotion was a generalized happiness, which was highly correlated with all of the other positive emotions.

Although Ellsworth and Smith (1988b) found distinctive appraisal patterns for the positive emotions, they also found considerably more overlap—reports of several different positive emotions for the same event—than in a parallel study of negative emotions (Ellsworth & Smith, 1988a). Pleasant emotional experience was less differentiated than unpleasant experience. Several scholars have suggested that negative emotions are often aroused by emergencies, situations that require an immediate appropriate response. Thus, the emotional response must be specific and precisely tailored to the situation in order to motivate the particular behavior necessary for survival—fight or flight, for example. Although noticing and taking advantage of opportunities is also important for survival, an opportunity is rarely a crisis, so precise emotional differentiation may be less necessary. Nonetheless, Ellsworth and Smith (1988b) found that pleasant emotions were considerably more differentiated than is reflected in most emotion taxonomies.

In summary, this early research suggested that positive emotions are probably less differentiated than negative emotions, but much more differentiated than had been presumed by previous theorists. In the rest of this chapter we build on this initial work to take into account more recent work on particular positive emotions, and to somewhat speculatively consider, from an appraisal perspective, the distinctive properties of 10 different positive emotions: happiness, pride, gratitude, interest, challenge/determination, hope, affection, compassion, awe, and tranquility.

In examining these 10 emotions, we are not attempting to be comprehensive. We are certain that there are numerous other positive emotional states with distinctive properties. Nor do we claim to have identified and considered the "most important" positive emotional states. Some we include because they have received considerable attention from appraisal and other emotions theorists, and seem to be well captured by existing appraisal models. Others we include because they seem to be important emotions that are *not* well captured by current appraisal models, and thus represent challenges that might spark some theoretical growth. In combination, however, we believe that an examination of these 10 emotions makes a powerful case for both the idea that there is considerable differentiation of positive emotional experience and the corresponding motivations, and the idea that appraisal theory provides a powerful lens for examining this differentiation.

With regard to the second idea, one of the themes we hope the reader will appreciate is that, for each emotion we consider, there is considerable coherence among the adaptational functions hypothesized to be served by the emotion, the appraisals hypothesized to elicit the emotion, and the motivational urges, or action tendencies, that help shape the behaviors the person performs. It is this coherence among the various facets of the emotional response that we believe appraisal theory is especially well poised to highlight.

Happiness, Pride, and Gratitude: Benefit-Related Emotions

Happiness

We consider each of the first three emotions we describe to be "benefit-related," in that each arises under conditions associated with some sort of success, or benefit, in which people appraise their circumstances both as being relevant to their concerns and (largely) as desired. Of the three, happiness is the most general, overarching response, and these two appraisals may be all that are required to elicit this emotion. Thus, happiness seems to be a fairly general response to positive circumstances. That happiness can be a fairly general response to positive events was noted by Weiner (1985) in his attributional model of emotions, and was also captured by Ellsworth and Smith (1988b) when they titled their early examination of the differentiation of positive emotions "Shades of Joy." The generality of happiness is reflected in the broad range of circumstances that can evoke it, which include both intrapersonal events (e.g., good academic grades; Storm &

Storm, 1987) and interpersonal ones (e.g., interaction with loved ones; Berenbaum, 2002), and both current and future events (e.g., Lazarus 1991). Given the broad range of circumstances that can evoke it, it is little wonder that people have a tendency to simply say they feel "happy" (or just "good") in response to positive events, even when they are also experiencing other positive emotions.

The motivational urges, or action tendencies, most strongly associated with happiness are to celebrate and to savor the moment (Smith & Kirby, 2010). This is consistent with proposals that a key function of happiness, through its highly pleasant hedonic state, is to reward/reinforce success (e.g., Smith, 1991; Smith & Lazarus, 1990), so that the efforts leading to the success are more likely to be repeated in the future. Notably, with motivational urges to savor and celebrate, happiness does not particularly motivate one immediately to persevere in achieving a pending goal; as we review below, other emotions serve this function. Rather, happiness is evoked by the successful attainment of a goal. In line with this idea, as an outcome of perceived success, happiness can also signal that one can down-regulate effort related to this goal and can channel resources to other goals (Martin, 2001).

Considerable evidence suggests that people who are happy tend to be cursory and schematic in their information-processing strategies (e.g., Bodenhausen, Kramer, & Susser, 1994; Forgas, 1998), which is consistent with happiness being a celebratory emotion but suggests a potential downside to happiness. Although happy individuals can be good analytic thinkers when properly motivated (e.g., Wegener, Petty, & Smith, 1995), happiness may not be an advantageous emotional state when careful analysis is required. On the other hand, some evidence suggests that happiness can increase creative, out-of-the-box thinking (Fredrickson & Branigan, 2005).

Pride

Like happiness, pride is a benefit-related emotion that arises in response to a success; thus, like happiness, it is evoked by appraisals that the situation is both personally relevant and goal conducive. However, pride is more specialized than happiness and involves a further appraisal of personal agency (e.g., Smith, 1991). The person takes credit for bringing about the desired situation; thus, pride serves as a reinforcer of personal accomplishment. Consistent with this function, the motivational urges most strongly associated with pride are to reward the self, and to show off (Smith & Kirby, 2010). Thus, more specifically than happiness, pride reinforces success in a way that encourages the person to develop a positive view of the self, and to gain confidence in his or her abilities (e.g., Lazarus, 1991; Mascolo & Fischer, 1995; Tracy & Robins, 2004). In this sense, pride likely plays an important role in building personal resources in the sense discussed by Fredrickson (1998, 2001) in her broaden-and-build theory. The confidence achieved through pride can help to sustain perseverance, leading to mastery in the face of adversity in the future (see our discussion of challenge/determination, below; Williams & DeSteno, 2008).

Pride, however, does have a dark side because confidence can shade into overconfidence, and one's positive sense of self can escalate into a sense of superiority and entitlement (e.g., Shiota, Campos, Keltner, & Hertenstein, 2004). When this happens, not only might the egotism lead to interpersonal difficulties, as the person is seen by others as obnoxious and unreasonable, but the overconfidence can set up failure in the face of a true challenge if the person overestimates his or her abilities and fails to make the preparations necessary for success (e.g., by not studying for an exam).

These two faces of pride, the self-enhancing, accomplishment-promoting side, and the overinflating, potentially self-destructive side, have led to proposals that there are two distinct forms of pride: authentic pride, which is associated with prosocial traits and positive self-esteem, and hubristic pride, which is associated with narcissistic traits and emotional vulnerability (e.g., Tracy & Robins, 2004, 2007; Tracy, Weidman, Cheng, & Martens, Chapter 17, this volume). Given the available evidence, we cannot tell whether these two faces of pride represent distinct pride-related emotions, or a single emotion whose elicitation is in one case based on a fairly accurate appraisal of one's success and one's contributions to it, but in the other is based on a misappraisal of self-worth and influence. Regardless, we believe that the dynamics of pride, including a clearer articulation of when and under what conditions pride will be elicited and function more authentically versus hubristically, are well worth examining further.

Finally, we note that it is quite possible, and even common, for one to experience pride in another person's achievement (e.g., Neumann, Steinhäuser, & Roeder, 2009). We do not believe that such pride is fundamentally different from personal pride. We believe that it reflects a set of interpersonal processes—in this case, the human ability to identify with other individuals, and to adopt their concerns as one's own—that appraisal theory has not yet fully confronted at a theoretical level (see, e.g., Smith, David, & Kirby, 2006). This is an issue we discuss further in our consideration of affection and compassion.

Gratitude

Gratitude is a third benefit-related emotion that is evoked, like happiness and pride, when the person appraises the situation as one in which a need or desire is fulfilled. However, in direct contrast with pride, there is an appraisal of external rather than internal agency. Thus, gratitude arises when a beneficial situation is seen as having been brought about, at least in part, by external influences. Often the external influence is another person (the "benefactor"), but it also can reflect impersonal factors (e.g., fate, God, and even chance; e.g., Wood, Froh, & Geraghty, 2010). The action tendency most strongly associated with gratitude (Smith & Kirby, 2010; Watkins, Scheer, Ovnicek, & Kolts, 2006) is to act in a prosocial manner, and more specifically, to thank or in some way repay the benefactor, which serves the adaptational function of reinforcing the benefactor's beneficence.

This function has long been seen as socially important. Adam Smith (1790/1976) argued that gratitude enables a society to function even when the economic incentives for prosocial behavior are absent. Gratitude has been theorized to elicit altruism (Trivers, 1971), reciprocity (Gouldner, 1960), and a general prosocial orientation (Schwartz,

1967). It has also been argued that gratitude can function to uplift not just the well-being of the benefactor but also that of people in general (e.g., Bartlett & DeSteno, 2006); hence, gratitude often serves to strengthen social relationships (e.g., Algoe, Haidt, & Gable, 2008; Fredrickson, 2004). Thus gratitude seems to function as a very important thread in our social fabric.

The frequent experience of gratitude may also yield significant intrapersonal benefits. As reviewed by Ahrens and Forbes (Chapter 20, this volume), training oneself to recognize the generosity and good in one's environment by keeping a daily gratitude journal, in which one makes note of specific events that happened during the day about which one is grateful, can result in a wide range of positive outcomes, including improvements in physical health and psychological well-being.

Nonetheless, gratitude can come at a price. Feelings of gratitude often carry with them a sense of indebtedness and obligation that can be quite unpleasant (Watkins et al., 2006), especially if the person feels unable to repay the perceived debt. In such cases, gratitude can lead to anxiety, distress, and guilt. Sometimes people may not solicit or accept help, even when they need it, in order to avoid the sense of obligation that gratitude can bring.

Interest, Challenge/Determination, and Hope: Opportunity-Related Emotions

Interest

In its rudimentary forms, interest may have the simplest appraisal structure of all the emotions. Mere novelty or change in one's circumstances can be sufficient to evoke initial interest, as in the orienting response (Sokolov, 1963). For more sustained interest, little more than uncertainty about the circumstances and their implications is likely required, although appraised personal relevance may well heighten the interest. The action tendency associated with interest, although it may be more of a reflexive response than a tendency, is to attend to whatever is eliciting the interest, be it an external event or internal thoughts.

Perhaps because the eliciting appraisals are so simple and not necessarily valenced, and because novelty and relevance are present in most emotion-eliciting situations, not all psychologists consider interest an emotion (e.g., Lazarus, 1991). However, those who do see it as a "knowledge emotion" or as an "epistemology-based emotion" that serves to focus attention on an unknown or complex object and to activate the necessary cognitive effort to understand it (e.g., Ellsworth & Smith, 1988b; Silvia, 2001, 2008). It is because interest, with its associated attentional activity, provides a fundamental basis for learning that we have classified it here as an "opportunity-based" emotion, along with challenge/determination and hope.

However, interest is distinct from these emotions in several ways. First, interest is involved in most emotional encounters. The primary exceptions to this are emotions such as disgust, in which the motivational urge is to direct attention away from the emotion-eliciting situation, or emotions such as boredom or tranquility, which differ from most emotions because they are characterized by appraisals of low personal relevance (Smith, 1991). Second, we consider interest, when it is experienced without other emotions, to be a positive emotion both because it is somewhat appetitive, in that it motivates attention that leads to learning and knowledge acquisition, and because, taken by itself, it seems to feel good. However, theoretically, appraisals of goal conduciveness do not appear to play a direct role in its elicitation (e.g., Turner & Silvia, 2006); thus, interest is just as likely to be present in highly negative situations evoking additional emotions such as fear and anger as it is in positive situations involving happiness, pride, and challenge.

Although long-neglected in emotion research, recent research has begun to focus on interest, and to elucidate the factors that evoke and sustain it. For instance, in line with its proposed relation to appraisals of personal relevance, people are more likely to show interest for objects that are important to them (Connelly, 2011; Ellsworth & Smith, 1988b). Moreover, Silvia and his colleagues (2005, 2008; Turner & Silvia, 2006) found evidence that interest is stronger when the target object is seen as novel or complex, but as something within one's ability to understand (which they called "high novelty-complexity" and "high coping potential," respectively). This observation highlights the dimensional rather than the categorical nature of emotion, in that, at some point, with increasing appraisals of control or coping potential, interest will shade into feelings of challenge/determination, which we consider next.

Challenge/Determination

According to Smith (1991; Smith & Lazarus, 1990), the appraisals evoking challenge/determination are ones of "effortful optimism"—the evaluation that things are not currently as desired, but that with effort they could be. This evaluation combines appraisals of personal relevance and some form of goal inconsistency with appraisals of high control or coping potential. Consistent with this appraisal, the motivational urges most closely associated with this emotion are to persevere and to stay focused (Smith & Kirby, 2010). This is highly consistent with the adaptational function proposed for challenge, which is to motivate perseverance, even under conditions of adversity, in a way that promotes mastery and growth.

That challenge involves appraisals of motive inconsistency makes it distinctive from the other positive emotions considered so far, and, according to Smith and Kirby (2011), makes this emotion "stress-related." However, as noted by Smith and Lazarus (1990), in terms of Selye's (1974) seminal conceptualization of stress, challenge/determination represents a form of positive stress, or "eustress," rather than a more negative form of stress, which Selye labeled as "distress." The positive nature of the stress in challenge/determination is reflected in our identifying this emotion as an "opportunity-related" emotion.

The appraisal of high control/coping potential associated with challenge/determination is what distinguishes it from most negative, stress-related emotions. This appraisal combines with the perceived goal-discrepancy to define the situation as an opportunity where, with effort, one can fulfill one's desires and achieve the as yet unmet goal (e.g., Kirby et al., Chapter 22, this volume; Smith, 1991; Smith & Kirby, 2011). If coping potential is less certain or seen as not quite being up to the task demands, the situation is seen as more threatening, and challenge can shade into anxiety (e.g., Blascovich & Mendes, 2000), and if the coping ability is appraised as very low, such that the goal is seen as unattainable, sadness/resignation is evoked, and the person is motivated to give up and disengage from the goal.

By being the motivational engine of accomplishment and personal growth, challenge/determination represents a vital emotion to human functioning. However, it is not without its liabilities. If appraisals of high coping ability are unrealistic, the emotion can promote failure by motivating the person to take on a difficult task or opportunity that is actually out of reach. If the situation is dangerous, it can promote bodily harm and even death. In such circumstances, a more adaptive response would be to disengage from the situation if possible and invest one's resources in something else.

Hope

In many ways, hope is similar to challenge/determination, in that it orients a person toward attaining an as yet unrealized goal, and, like challenge, is an opportunity-based emotion. Empirically, measures of hope and challenge have often been found to be highly correlated, and have sometimes been combined to measure "hope-challenge" (e.g., Smith & Kirby, 2009). However, we believe that a strong case can be made for there being important distinctions between these states.

Like challenge/determination, the eliciting appraisals for hope include both personal relevance and some sort of goal incongruence; thus, hope, too, is a stress-related emotion. However, whereas high levels of appraised control/coping potential are fairly definitive for challenge/determination, this appraisal does not appear to be necessary for hope. Instead, all that seems to be required is the expectation, even if uncertain, that somehow, regardless of personal agency, things could work out and the goal might be achieved. Thus, instead of being elicited and maintained by appraisals of "effortful optimism," all that is required for hope is mere "optimism" (Smith, 1991). The main motivational function of hope is to keep a person committed to an uncertain goal instead of abandoning it (Lazarus, 1991; Lazarus et al., 1980).

The ability of hope to sustain commitment in the face of extreme adversity is very important to human functioning. Hope may help foster commitment to difficult social causes, for which change may require decades of persistent effort, and it may also be crucial for fostering relatively high levels of functioning and subjective well-being in the face of chronic, incurable, or even terminal health conditions (e.g., Taylor, Kemeny, Reed, Bower, & Gruenewald, 2000). At the same time, the ability of hope to sustain commitment to extremely difficult causes is a double-edged sword. Although beneficial under certain conditions, under others hope can be harmful because it can prevent one from disengaging from a truly hopeless cause and investing elsewhere, which among other things, can lead to severe depression (e.g., Klinger, 1975). Clearly, hope's contributions to both positive and negative functioning warrant further study (for a review of hope research, see Cheavens & Ritschel, Chapter 23, this volume).

Emotions Presenting Theoretical Challenges to Appraisal Theory: Affection, Compassion, Awe, and Tranquility

Affection

Love is truly a many-splendored thing. Love subsumes a wide variety of emotional states, so that one could make a strong case for the differentiation of positive emotional experience merely by considering love in its various forms: romantic love, platonic love, and parental love, to name a few. Considering each of these types of love is well beyond the scope of this chapter. However, almost all these forms share the affective quality of *affection*, the liking one person has for another person, on which we focus here.

Affection presents important puzzles to appraisal theory in at least two different ways. First, the appraisal pattern associated with it is not well captured by existing models. The focus is on another person; thus, other agency may be perceived; however, the relevant appraisal seems to be more about the existence and characteristics of the other person rather than his or her agency in doing a particular thing. Personal relevance is clearly involved, as is goal conduciveness. However, the goal or motive in affection seems different than in other emotions because rather than being concrete it may often be diffuse, often representing little more than wanting to be with, or in a close relationship with, another.

The motivational functions associated with affection clearly revolve around forming and continuing social relationships (e.g., Shiota et al., 2004), ranging from romantic and familial relationships crucial to reproduction and childrearing, to friendships that are important in the formation of social networks and conducting cooperative activities.

It is this important role that affection plays in interpersonal bonding that provides its second puzzle for appraisal theory. As noted in our discussion of pride, affection, and the pair-bonding it promotes, enables the individual to extend his or her self-definition to encompass important others in his or her social environment, including spouses, children, and close friends, among others (e.g., Aron, Aron, Tudor, & Nelson, 1991; Smith et al., 2006). Through this expanded definition of self, appraisal of personal well-being, which often seems self-centered, can be highly social. However, the processes leading to such expanded definitions of self or self-interest, and the social nature of appraisal and the resulting emotions, are currently not well captured by appraisal theory. In our view, better capturing these more social aspects of appraisal and emotion represents an extremely important agenda for future research.

Compassion

The study of compassion should clearly be on this agenda. As an emotion that motivates us to become invested in the plight of another person experiencing misfortune and to help him or her, compassion is important in defining our very humanity. As such, compassion appears to be important to our survival, and we admire it in others. For instance, as Goetz and colleagues (2010) noted, the offspring of compassionate caregivers are more likely to survive; compassionate individuals are more sought after as mating partners; and compassionate people are more likely to find supportive social networks

However, compassion is an emotion that appraisal theory is currently ill-equipped to handle. In compassion we often become emotionally involved even though personal relevance is low, and often it arises around individuals we may only know casually, if at all; thus, it is not limited to those we include in our definition of personal self-interest. There is clearly motive inconsistency involved in the situation, but often the compassionate person's own motives are not particularly involved in this inconsistency.

Existing research has identified some of the situational factors that increase the likelihood of a compassionate response: Someone who is sensitive to the needs of others is especially likely to be compassionate (Cassell, 2002); feeling a sense of connectedness to the victim, such as seeing the victim as being similar to the self (e.g., Valdesolo & DeSteno, 2011), increases the likelihood of a compassionate response, as does the perception that the victim does not deserve to suffer (Cassell, 2002). However, these attributes do not correspond well to the appraisal components included in contemporary models, as described earlier. Thus, compassion stands as a strong challenge for the future development of appraisal theory (for a review of compassion research, see Stellar & Keltner, Chapter 19, this volume).

Finally, given the definition of "positive emotion" as emotion that feels good, compassion may not be a positive emotion at all. It is certainly a socially desirable emotion, but the actual feeling is often akin to distress.

Awe

In a number of respects, awe is similar to interest: The stimulus situation that evokes it commands attention, and two of the main action tendencies associated with awe are to seek information and to reflect on the situation (another is to savor the moment; Smith & Kirby, 2010). However, the experience of awe is clearly something more than the experience of interest.

Awe is a common response to artistic works, scientific discovery, natural wonders, religious experiences, and sweeping political changes. The things that elicit awe tend to be unusual, perceptually or conceptually complex, and rich in information (Keltner & Haidt, 2003), the same sort of stimulus properties that tend to evoke sustained interest. In addition, they almost always seem to be external to the self (Shiota, Keltner, & Mossman, 2007), which implies that some form of external agency is involved. Like interest, awe does not appear to be strongly valenced, and appraisals of goal conduciveness are not centrally involved in its elicitation, although the experience of awe usually seems to be subjectively pleasant (Shiota et al., 2007).

However, the truly distinctive features of awe do not seem to be well captured by the components included in existing appraisal models. In awe there seems to be a perception that one is small or insignificant, the belief that there exists something greater than the self, a lower focus on mundane concerns, and a sense of connection with the world (Shiota et al., 2007; Shiota, Thrash, Danvers, & Dombrowski, Chapter 21, this volume). According to Keltner and Haidt (2003), objects evoking awe are often perceived as vast and complicated, in that they seem to go beyond one's ordinary expectations, knowledge, and understanding.

The adaptive significance of awe is not well understood, but Keltner and Haidt (2003) posit that awe motivates the person to seek a better understanding of the awe-inspiring object because there is a recognition that it in some way extends beyond ones current frame of reference. This reevaluation often results in the person accommodating to the object by substantially revising his or her expectations, knowledge, and understanding. Emotion researchers have only relatively recently turned their attention to awe, which clearly merits further study. A deeper theoretical understanding of awe and its motivational functions will likely result in significant accommodations to appraisal theory and emotion theory more generally.

Tranquility

Tranquility presents an interesting challenge to emotion theory in general, although for appraisal theory of the four theoretically challenging emotions we are considering, it is the one accounted for most readily. Our inclusion of tranquility as an emotion is predicated on the assumption, shared by a number of emotion theories (e.g., Izard, 1977), that the person is always in some emotional state, and that the absence of arousal is as much an emotional state as a high level of arousal. Tranquility is somewhat unique among emotions, in that it is evoked in situations appraised as having low personal relevance (boredom is likely another such emotion, but one that is more negatively valenced). The appraisals leading to tranquility are that one's circumstances are largely in line with ones goals and that nothing needs to be done right now (Ellsworth & Smith, 1988b). The motivational urges most strongly associated with this state are to clear one's mind and to relax (Smith & Kirby, 2010). Subjectively, the state is pleasant and involves a sense that all is well with the world. In a term used by Lazarus and colleagues (1980), tranquility functions as a "breather." It motivates the person to take a break from contending with the vicissitudes of life. This gives the person the opportunity to recuperate from the stresses and strains of life.

Although the appraisal pattern associated with tranquility is readily accommodated by appraisal theory, accepting tranquility and its adaptational functions as being truly emotional requires a theoretical reorientation toward emotion. In particular, one must reject, or at least substantially modify, a somewhat classic view that argues that emotions represent emergency reactions to highly relevant adaptational situations, involving high levels of physiological arousal. This classic view of emotions has clearly contributed to the bias in emotion theory toward negative emotions. Conversely, changing one's perspective on emotion to embrace tranquility as an emotion helps to open the door to appreciating the richness and complexity of positive emotion.

Conclusions

From this review, we hope that two conclusions are evident. First, although positive emotional experience may not be as differentiated as negative emotional experience, it is still highly differentiated. As our review indicates, a number of distinctive positive emotional states serve a variety of adaptational functions, including rewarding success, encouraging perseverance, sustaining engagement, promoting pair-bonding, promoting social responsibility, and more—functions that are clearly vital to human functioning. Second, due to its principled and integrated consideration of the various components of emotional experience (e.g., emotion-eliciting appraisals, physiological responses, motivational tendencies, and adaptational functions), appraisal theory provides an especially powerful theoretical lens for exploring this emotional differentiation. At the same time, several of the distinctive emotional states we have examined, not to mention others that we have not considered, present interesting theoretical challenges to appraisal theory. Thus, the use of appraisal theory to explore the differentiation of positive emotional experience promises not only to enrich our understanding of human emotions in important ways but also to promote the continued development of appraisal theory as a powerful perspective for studying emotion.

References

Algoe, S. B., Haidt, J., & Gable, S. L. (2008). Beyond reciprocity: Gratitude and relationships in everyday life. *Emotion, 8,* 425–429.

Arnold, M. B. (1960). *Emotion and personality.* New York: Columbia University Press.

Aron, A., Aron, E. N., Tudor, M., & Nelson, G. (1991). Close relationships as including other in the self. *Journal of Personality and Social Psychology, 60,* 241–253.

Averill, J. R. (1980). On the paucity of positive emotions. In K. R. Blankstein, P. Pliner, & J. Polivy (Eds.), *Advances in the study of communication and affect: Vol. 6. Assessment and modification of emotional behavior* (pp. 7–45). New York: Plenum Press.

Bartlett, M. Y., & DeSteno, D. (2006). Gratitude and prosocial behavior: Helping when it costs you. *Psychological Science, 17,* 319–325.

Berenbaum, H. (2002). Varieties of joy-related pleasurable activities and feelings. *Cognition and Emotion, 4,* 473–494.

Blascovich, J., & Mendes, W. B. (2000). Challenge and threat appraisals: The role of affective cues. In J. P. Forgas (Ed.), *Feeling and thinking: The role of affect in social cognition* (pp. 59–82). Cambridge, UK: Cambridge University Press.

Bodenhausen, G. V., Kramer, G. P., & Susser, K. (1994). Happiness and stereotypic thinking in social judgment. *Journal of Personality and Social Psychology, 66,* 621–632.

Carver, C. S., & Harmon-Jones, E. (2009). Anger is an approach-related affect: Evidence and implications. *Psychological Bulletin, 135,* 183–204.

Cassell, E. J. (2002). Compassion. In C. R. Snyder & S. J. Lopez (Eds.), *Handbook of positive psychology* (pp. 434–445). New York: Oxford University Press.

Connelley, D. A. (2011). Applying Silvia's model of interest to academic text: Is there a third appraisal? *Learning and Individual Differences, 21,* 624–628.

Darwin, C. (1965). *The expression of the emotions in man and animals.* Chicago: University of Chicago Press. (Original work published 1872)

Ekman, P. (1984). Expression and the nature of emotion. In K. R. Scherer & P. Ekman (Eds.), *Approaches to emotion* (pp. 319–343). Hillsdale, NJ: Erlbaum.

Ekman, P., Sorenson, E. R., & Friesen, W. V. (1969). Pan-cultural elements in facial displays of emotions. *Science, 164,* 86–88.

Ellsworth, P. C. (1991). Some implications of cognitive appraisal theories of emotion. In K. T. Strongman (Ed.), *International review of studies of emotion* (Vol. 1, pp. 143–161). New York: Wiley.

Ellsworth, P. C., & Scherer, K. R. (2003). Appraisal processes in emotion. In R. J. Davidson, K. R. Scherer, & H. H. Goldsmith (Eds.), *Handbook of affective sciences* (pp. 572–595). New York: Oxford University Press.

Ellsworth, P. C., & Smith, C. A. (1988a). From appraisal to emotion: Differences among unpleasant feelings. *Motivation and Emotion, 12,* 271–302.

Ellsworth, P. C., & Smith, C. A. (1988b). Shades of joy: Patterns of appraisal differentiating pleasant emotions. *Cognition and Emotion, 2,* 301–331.

Emmons, R. A., & McCullough, M. E. (2003). Counting blessings versus burdens: An experimental investigation of gratitude and subjective well-being in daily life. *Journal of Personality and Social Psychology, 84,* 112–127.

Forgas, J. P. (1998). On being happy and mistaken: Mood effects on the fundamental attribution error. *Journal of Personality and Social Psychology, 75,* 318–331.

Fredrickson, B. L. (1998). What good are positive emotions? *Review of General Psychology, 2,* 300–319.

Fredrickson, B. L. (2001). The role of positive emotions in positive psychology: The broaden and build theory of positive emotions. *American Psychologist, 56,* 218–226.

Fredrickson, B. L. (2004). Gratitude (like other positive emotions) broadens and builds. In R. A. Emmons & M. E. McCullough (Eds.), *The psychology of gratitude* (pp. 145–166). New York: Oxford University Press.

Fredrickson, B. L., & Branigan, C. (2005). Positive emotions broaden the scope of attention and thought-action repertoires. *Cognition and Emotion, 19,* 313–332.

Frijda, N. H. (1986). *The emotions.* Cambridge, UK: Cambridge University Press.

Frijda, N. H., Kuipers, P., & ter Schure, E. (1989). Relations among emotion, appraisal, and emotion action readiness. *Journal of Personality and Social Psychology, 57,* 212–228.

Frijda, N. H., & Swagerman, J. (1987). Can computers feel?: Theory and design of an emotional system. *Cognition and Emotion, 1,* 235–257

Goetz, J. L., Keltner, D., & Simon-Thomas, E. (2010). Compassion: An evolutionary analysis and empirical review. *Psychological Bulletin, 136,* 351–374.

Gouldner, A. W. (1960). The norm of reciprocity: A preliminary statement. *American Sociological Review, 25,* 161–178.

Izard, C. E. (1977). *Human emotions.* New York: Plenum Press.

Keltner, D., & Haidt, J. (2003). Approaching awe, a moral, spiritual, and aesthetic emotion. *Cognition and Emotion, 17,* 297–314.

Klinger, E. (1975). Consequences of commitment to and disengagement from incentives. *Psychological Review, 82,* 1–25.

Lazarus, R. S. (1991). *Emotion and adaptation.* New York: Oxford University Press.

Lazarus, R. S., Kanner, A. D., & Folkman, S. (1980). Emotions: A cognitive phenomenological analysis. In R. Plutchik & H. Kellerman (Eds.), *Theories of emotion* (pp. 189–217). New York: Academic Press.

Lazarus, R. S., & Smith, C. A. (1988). Knowledge and appraisal in the cognition–emotion relationship. *Cognition and Emotion, 2,* 281–300.

Martin, L. L. (2001). Mood as input: A configural view of mood effects. In L. L. Martin & G. L. Clore (Eds.), *Theories of mood and cognition: A users guide* (pp. 135–157). Mahwah, NJ: Erlbaum.

Mascolo, M. F., & Fischer, K. W. (1995). Developmental transformations in appraisals for pride, guilt and shame. In J. P. Tangney & K. W. Fischer (Eds.), *Self-conscious emotions: The psychology of shame, guilt, embarrassment, and pride* (pp. 64–113). New York: Guilford Press.

Neumann, R., Steinhäuser, N., & Roeder, U. R. (2009). How self-construal shapes emotion: Cultural differences in the feeling of pride. *Social Cognition, 27,* 327–337.

Plutchik, R. (1980). *Emotion: A psychoevolutionary synthesis.* New York: Harper & Row.

Roseman, I. J. (1984). Cognitive determinants of emotions: A structural theory. In P. Shaver (Ed.), *Review of personality and social psychology* (Vol. 5, pp. 11–36). Beverly Hills, CA: Sage.

Roseman, I. J. (1991). Appraisal determinants of discrete emotions. *Cognition and Emotion, 5,* 161–200.

Roseman, I. J. (2001). A model of appraisal in the emotion system: Integrating theory, research, and applications. In K. R. Scherer, A. Schorr, & T. Johnstone (Eds.), *Appraisal processes in emotion: Theory, methods, research* (pp. 68–91). New York: Oxford University Press.

Roseman, I. J., & Smith, C. A. (2001). Appraisal theory: Overview, assumptions, varieties, controversies. In K. R. Scherer, A. Schorr, & T. Johnstone (Eds.), *Appraisal processes in emotion: Theory, methods, research* (pp. 3–19). New York: Oxford University Press.

Scherer, K. R. (1984). On the nature and function of emotion: A component process approach. In K. R. Scherer & P. Ekman (Eds.), *Approaches to emotion* (pp. 293–317). Hillsdale, NJ: Erlbaum.

Scherer, K. (2001). Appraisal considered as a process of multilevel sequential checking. In K. R. Scherer, A. Schorr, & T. Johnstone (Eds.), *Appraisal processes in emotion: Theory, methods, research* (pp. 3–19). New York: Oxford University Press.

Schwartz, B. (1967). The social psychology of the gift. *American Journal of Sociology, 73,* 1–11.

Selye, H. (1974). *Stress without distress.* Philadelphia: Lippincott.

Shiota, M. N., Campos, B., Keltner, D., & Hertenstein, M. (2004). Positive emotion and the regulation of interpersonal relationships. In P. Phillipot & R. Feldman (Eds.), *Emotion regulation* (pp. 127–156). Mahwah, NJ: Erlbaum.

Shiota, M. N., Keltner, D., & Mossman, A. (2007). The nature of awe: Elicitors, appraisals, and effects on self-concept. *Cognition and Emotion, 21,* 944–963.

Silvia, P. J. (2001). Interest and interests: The psychology of constructive capriciousness. *Review of General Psychology, 5,* 270–290.

Silvia, P. J. (2005). What is interesting?: Exploring the appraisal structure of interest. *Emotion, 5,* 89–102.

Silvia, P. (2008). Appraisal components and emotion traits: Examining the appraisal basis of trait curiosity. *Cognition and Emotion, 22,* 94–113.

Simon, H. A. (1966). Motivational and emotional controls of cognition. *Psychological Review, 74,* 29–39.

Smith, A. (1976). *The theory of moral sentiments* (6th ed.). Indianapolis, IN: Liberty Classics. (Original work published 1790)

Smith, C. A. (1991). The self, appraisal, and coping. In C. R. Snyder & D. R. Forsyth (Eds.), *Handbook of social and clinical psychology: The health perspective* (pp. 116–137). New York: Pergamon.

Smith, C. A., David, B., & Kirby, L. D. (2006). Emotion-eliciting appraisals of social situations. In J. P. Forgas (Ed.), *Affect in social thinking and behavior* (pp. 85–101). New York: Psychology Press.

Smith, C. A., & Ellsworth, P. C. (1985). Patterns of cognitive appraisal in emotion. *Journal of Personality and Social Psychology, 48,* 813–838.

Smith, C. A., & Kirby, L. D. (2009). Relational antecedents of appraised problem-focused coping potential and its associated emotions. *Cognition and Emotion, 23,* 481–503.

Smith, C. A., & Kirby, L. D. (2010, January). *Pleasure is complicated: On the differentiation of positive emotional experience.* Paper presented at the 11th Annual Meeting of the Society of Personality and Social Psychology, Las Vegas, NV.

Smith, C. A., & Kirby, L. D. (2011). The role of appraisal and emotion in coping and adaptation. In R. J. Contrada & A. Baum (Eds.), *Handbook of stress science: Biology, psychology, and health* (pp. 195–208). New York: Springer.

Smith, C. A., & Lazarus, R. S. (1990). Emotion and adaptation. In L. A. Pervin (Ed.), *Handbook of personality: Theory and research* (pp. 609–637). New York: Guilford Press.

Sokolov, J. N. (1963). *Perception and the conditioned reflex.* Oxford, UK: Pergamon.

Storm, C., & Storm, T. (1987) . A taxonomic study of the vocabulary of emotions. *Journal of Personality and Social Psychology, 53,* 805–816.

Taylor, S. E., Kemeny, M. E., Reed, G. M., Bower, J. E., & Gruenewald, T. L. (2000). Psychological resources, positive illusions, and health. *American Psychologist, 55,* 99–109.

Tomkins, S. S. (1962). *Affect, imagery, consciousness: Vol. 1. The positive affects.* New York: Springer-Verlag.

Tracy, J. L., & Robins, R. W. (2004). Putting the self into self-conscious emotions: A theoretical model. *Psychological Inquiry, 15,* 103–125.

Tracy, J. L., & Robins, R. W. (2007). The psychological structure of pride: A tale of two facets. *Journal of Personality and Social Psychology, 92,* 506–525.

Trivers, R. L. (1971). The evolution of reciprocal altruism. *Quarterly Review of Biology, 46,* 35–57.

Turner, S. A., Jr., & Silvia, P. J. (2006). Must interesting things be pleasant?: A test of competing appraisal structures. *Emotion, 6,* 670–674.

Valdesolo, P., & DeSteno, D. (2011). Synchrony and the social tuning of compassion. *Emotion, 11,* 262–266.

Watkins, P. C., Scheer, J., Ovnicek, M., & Kolts, R. (2006). The debt of gratitude: Dissociating gratitude and indebtedness. *Cognition and Emotion, 20,* 217–241.

Watson, D., & Tellegen, A. (1985). Toward a consensual structure of mood. *Psychological Bulletin, 98,* 219–235.

Wegener, D. T., Petty, R. E., & Smith, S. M. (1995). Positive mood can increase or decrease message scrutiny: The hedonic contingency view of mood and message processing. *Journal of Personality and Social Psychology, 69,* 5–15.

Weiner, B. (1985). An attributional theory of achievement motivation and emotion. *Psychological Review, 92,* 548–573.

Williams, L. A., & DeSteno, D. (2008). Pride and perseverance: The motivational role of pride. *Journal of Personality and Social Psychology, 94,* 1007–1017.

Wood, A. M., Froh, J. J., & Geraghty, A. W. A. (2010). Gratitude and well-being: A review and theoretical integration. *Clinical Psychology Review, 30,* 890–905.

CHAPTER 2

■ ■ ■ ■ ■ ■ ■ ■

Infusing Positive Emotions into Life

The Broaden-and-Build Theory and a Dual-Process Model of Resilience

Michele M. Tugade
Hillary C. Devlin
Barbara L. Fredrickson

Positive emotions are infused into our lives in various ways. We may actively cultivate feelings of joy by seeking the company of our best friend when we are feeling disheartened or sad; we may tell a funny joke to ease the tension when feeling angry; or we may take a deep breath of tranquility when feeling anxious or fearful. The very act of harnessing positive emotions in the midst of negative feelings has been shown to foster resilience (Tugade & Fredrickson, 2004, 2007). Understandably, however, it can be difficult to "put a smile on one's face" or "look on the bright side" when one feels the sting of rejection or the bite of criticism. Indeed, it may not always be easy or even appropriate to conjure up feelings of positivity when feeling sad, angry, anxious, or fearful. Are there circumstances that ease the process by which positive emotions are infused in negative situations?

Our central aim in this chapter is to review the many ways that positive emotions can fuel resilience in the face of stress. The principles of the broaden-and-build theory of positive emotions (Fredrickson, 1998, 2001) are reviewed as a platform for discussing recent advancements in resilience research.

Then, we discuss a dual-process model of resilience (Tugade, 2011) that examines both automatic and controlled processes of positive emotion elicitation in the midst of stress. Finally, we present the empirical evidence to support the dual-process model and discuss future directions in this area of research.

The Broaden-and-Build Theory

The broaden-and-build theory details the unique adaptive function of positive emotions (Fredrickson, 1998, 2001). From an evolutionary standpoint, positive emotions signal safety, cueing an individual that it is fine to roam and explore one's environment or sit quietly still without the threat of harm. The broaden-and-build theory of positive emotions was proposed to account for the unique effects of positive versus negative emotions that could not be explained by existing theories of emotions. For example, according to numerous theories (Frijda, 1986; Lazarus, 1991; Levenson, 1994), negative emotions were viewed as inciting specific behavioral action tendencies. Fear fueled the urge to escape, whereas anger provoked the urge to attack, and so on. From an evolutionary perspective, the specific action tendencies paired with discrete emotions functioned to ensure survival. Each discrete emotion had a specific action tendency, and consequently, served an adaptive function. Yet, unlike negative emotions such as fear and anger, the specific action tendencies of positive emotions were less specified. Indeed, rather than encouraging specific behavioral action, positive emotions, in some cases, seemed to call forth behavioral *inaction*. For example, joy was theorized to incite *aimless activation,* and contentment was said to generate *inactivity* (Frijda, 1986). Such vagueness and lack of specificity led to the proposal that positive emotions may, in fact, serve functions quite distinct from negative emotions. But if not to act to enhance immediate survival, what, if any, function did positive emotions serve?

According to the broaden-and-build theory, rather than fueling specific action tendencies, positive emotions appear to activate broadened and expansive thought–action tendencies. Positive emotions both broaden our thinking (by expanding our attention, facilitating flexible thinking, decision making, and creativity). These experiences in turn accumulate and compound, thereby allowing for growth in a number domains: psychological (e.g., flourishing, mindfulness), social (e.g., social connections), and physical (e.g., heart rate indices such as vagal tone) (Fredrickson, Cohn, Coffey, Pek, & Finkel, 2008; Kok et al., 2013). The consequence, then, is more expansive thinking and greater breadth of action that helps one to build personal resources (e.g., cognitive, social, intellectual, and coping resources). These new resources, in turn, would have increased the odds that human ancestors survived subsequent threats to life and limb.

Positive emotions also have an "undoing" function. The undoing hypothesis provides a valuable framework for understanding the important role of positive emotions in the coping process (Fredrickson & Levenson, 1998; Levenson, 1988). Research and theory indicate that negative emotions such as fear, anger, or anxiety have an alarm function; they produce sympathetic arousal that physiologically prepares the body to fight or to flee. In contrast, research shows that positive emotions such as contentment, joy, or

interest, have a quieting function; they dismantle the sympathetic arousal generated by negative emotions, helping to bring physiological reactivity back to levels in effect prior to the onset of the stressor (Fredrickson & Levenson, 1998; Fredrickson, Mancuso, Branigan, & Tugade, 2000; Tugade & Fredrickson, 2004).

Empirical research provides support for the undoing hypothesis, which predicts that those who experience positive emotions on the heels of a high-activation negative emotion will show the fastest cardiovascular recovery from the stressor. In one experimental paradigm, researchers first experimentally induce negative emotion. Immediately afterwards, positive emotions are experimentally induced, often via the presentation of emotionally evocative films. The undoing hypothesis has been tested by measuring the time elapsed from the start of the randomly assigned film (to elicit joy, contentment, sadness, or neutrality) until the cardiovascular reactions induced by negative emotion returns to baseline levels. In three independent samples, participants who experienced positive emotions (joy and contentment) exhibited faster cardiovascular recovery than those who experienced neutrality, and faster than those who experienced sadness, which exhibited the most protracted recovery (Fredrickson & Levenson, 1998; Fredrickson et al., 2000). These findings indicate that positive emotions have the unique ability to speed physiological recovery from lingering negative emotional arousal. While the precise cognitive and physiological mechanisms of the undoing effect remain unknown, the broaden-and-build theory suggests that broadening at the cognitive level may mediate undoing at the cardiovascular level. Phenomenologically, positive emotions may help people place the events in their lives in a broader context, lessening the resonance of any particular negative event.

The response patterns supported by both the undoing hypothesis and the broaden-and-build theory indicate that positive emotions give individuals the momentary pause necessary to restore lost resources after experiencing stress. In this way, positive emotions give individuals short "breathers" from stressful experiences (Lazarus & Folkman, 1984), allowing them the opportunity to replenish cognitive and energetic resources that may have been depleted by a stressful situation. That positive emotions can restore depleted resources is important for understanding the role of positive emotions in the coping process. We now turn to theory and research indicating that experiencing positive emotions alongside negative emotions can promote psychological and physiological resilience.

Positive Emotions Fuel Resilience

"Resilience" has been defined as the ability to bounce back from negative experiences and exhibit flexible adaptation in the face of ever-changing demands over the life course (Block & Block, 1980; Block & Kremen, 1996; Lazarus, 1993). Prior research has uncovered that one underlying mechanism of a resilient response is the experience of positive emotions in the face of stress. Such positive emotions have been found to aid in speeding the physiological recovery from negative life events (e.g., Conway, Tugade, Catalino, & Fredrickson, 2013; Tugade, 2011; Tugade & Fredrickson, 2004, 2007; Tugade, Fredrickson, & Barrett, 2004).

Research has shown that there are individual differences in the ability to harness positive emotions, using them to one's benefit in the face of a stressful event. Given the evidence showing that positive emotions indeed produce beneficial outcomes in the coping process (e.g., Folkman & Moskowitz, 2000a, 2000b; Fredrickson, 2000), certain individuals appear to have a greater tendency to draw on positive emotions in times of stress, intuitively understanding and using positive emotions to their advantage. Our research has shown that this tendency may be characteristic of psychologically resilient people (Tugade & Fredrickson, 2004; Tugade et al., 2004). If highly resilient individuals are theorized to rebound efficiently in the face of stressful experiences, then this ability to recover from stress should be reflected physiologically as well. To test this hypothesis, we identified individuals with low and high resilience based on self-reported responses to the ego-resiliency scale (Block & Kremen, 1996). We then experimentally induced experiences of anxiety by asking individuals with low and high

resilience to prepare a speech to be delivered in front of a video camera for evaluation (in fact, no participants actually delivered their prepared speeches). As expected, the speech preparation instructions induced cardiovascular arousal as well as subjective reports of anxiety as intended, with no differences between individuals with low and high resilience. Differences in trait resilience, however, emerged in two important ways. First, individuals with high (vs. low resilience) were more likely to report experiencing positive emotions, such as interest, alongside their self-reported anxiety. Second, highly resilient participants evidenced faster cardiovascular recovery from the arousal generated by the anxiety-inducing task, reflecting the ability to physiologically "bounce back" from stress. Mediational analyses revealed that the experience of positive emotions contributed, in part, to highly resilient participants' abilities to achieve efficient emotion regulation, demonstrated by accelerated cardiovascular recovery from negative emotional arousal. These findings indicate that highly resilient individuals are characterized by use of positive emotions to cope with stress (Tugade & Fredrickson, 2004; Tugade et al., 2004).

Other research has shown that trait resilient people use positive emotions to cope with large-scale sources of stress, such as a national tragedy. Fredrickson, Tugade, Waugh, and Larkin (2003) examined whether trait resilience predicts the accrual of psychological resources following a national crisis, such as the September 11, 2001, terrorist attacks. Specifically, precrisis trait resilience predicted a greater frequency of positive emotional experiences (e.g., love, gratitude) after the terrorist attacks. The presence of these positive emotions in the midst the stress in turn predicted a greater accumulation of postcrisis psychological resources (e.g., optimism, tranquility, life satisfaction) in the weeks that followed.

The ability of trait-resilient people to down-regulate distress is evident throughout the lifespan. One study of older adults found that trait resilience predicted less emotional reactivity and an enhanced recovery in the face of various stressors (Ong, Bergeman, Bisconti, & Wallace, 2006). Resilient individuals appeared to be more effective in regulating their negative emotions and exhibited greater emotional recovery on the day following a stressful event. These findings emerged in a sample of elderly widows coping with the loss of a spouse, as well as a general older adult population coping with an assortment of everyday stressors.

Dual-Process Model of Resilience

The research outlined thus far provide a compelling case for the important role of positive emotions when coping with stress, and raise an important question that warrants further investigation—namely, what processes trigger positive emotions in the face of negative life events? Tugade (2011) proposed a dual-process model of resilience, which asserts that there are two unique, yet complementary pathways through which positive emotions can be activated during times of stress. These include the controlled, response-focused processing of positive emotion activation, which has been the primary focus of prior resilience research, and the relatively unexplored pathway of automatic positive emotion processing.

Dual-process theories are prevalent in social and personality psychology (Barrett, Tugade, & Engle, 2004; Chaiken & Trope, 1999). The central tenet in these theories is that thoughts, feelings, and behaviors are driven by two separate though complementary processes: automatic and controlled. Automatic and controlled processes are characterized by four important qualities (Bargh, 1994): *awareness* (whether you are consciously aware that a process is happening), *efficiency* (the extent to which you expend cognitive or attentional resources), *intention* (whether you see yourself as having agency in your thoughts, feelings, or behavior), and *control* (whether you are able to modify the behavior in any way). Dual-process theories can be applied to resilience by examining how positive affect is generated via automatic or controlled processes in the service of managing stress.

Controlled Processes of Resilience

Much of the previous work on resilience has examined the role of controlled processes of positive affect activation in the face of stress. Controlled processes are characterized by a conscious or deliberate cultivation of positive emotions to aid in coping. For example, research shows that people who cultivate humor in times of stress can accrue benefits to coping.

Generating Humor to Cope

Humor is a positive emotional reaction that involves noticing something incongruous with one's expectations and results in a feeling of pleasure (Martens, 2004). The ability to see, access, and share humor involves an ability and willingness to see things from a different perspective and to laugh at oneself (Critchey, 2002). In this way, humor has been viewed as an important factor for combating the unfavorable elements of stressful circumstances. Guiding people toward generating humor has been found to be therapeutically beneficial (Baker, 1993; Martens, 2004; Prerost, 1989).

Research indicates that individual differences in trait resilience predict the ability to harness the beneficial effects of positive emotions when coping with negative emotional experiences. For instance, resilient individuals have been described as happy and energetic people who frequently use humor as a coping strategy (e.g., Werner & Smith, 1992; Wolin & Wolin, 1993), which has been shown to help people cope effectively with stressful circumstances (e.g., Martin & Lefcourt, 1983; Nezu, Nezu, & Blissett, 1988). Likewise, Masten, Best, and Garmezy (1990) have found that resilient children under high stress exhibit higher scores on humor generation than less resilient children facing equally high levels of stress. These findings demonstrate that coping with the use of humor, a strategy associated with positive emotions, allows resilient people to reduce stress and restore perspective, as well as remain engaging to others, thereby maintaining positive social support networks (Kumpfer, 1999).

How does humor facilitate coping? One explanation focuses on the active cultivation of positive emotion. Samson and Gross (2012) differentiated between positive (good-spirited) humor and negative (mean-spirited) humor to investigate which humor style facilitates coping. Indeed, their research found that positive (vs. negative) humor increases positive emotional experiences and decreases negative emotional experiences. In line with previous theorizing, it appears that humor may allow people to appreciate situations from different perspectives, and that having an alternative perspective provides an opportunity for clarity and insight (Lefcourt et al., 1995; Vaillant, 2000). Thus, generating positive humor can allow individuals to see the situation from alternative perspectives that may be more desirable (Samson & Gross, 2012), and can be enhanced during stress in the service of coping and social goals (Giuilani, McRae, & Gross, 2008).

Mindfulness

"Mindfulness," a cognitive state of intentional sustained attention (toward one's inner or outer experience), is a strategy with the potential to increase resilience. Mindfulness is most commonly defined as a state of awareness that is oriented in the present moment and performed nonjudgmentally and with acceptance (Keng, Smoski, & Robins, 2011). Mounting research indicates that mindfulness is associated with adaptive coping strategies and enhanced coping efficacy. Specifically, notable strategies with which mindfulness is frequently associated include stress approach skills (i.e., cognitively and emotionally taking on a stressor and actively working toward resolving it, as opposed to avoidant strategies in which the stressful situation is ignored—an approach that is ineffective in the long term; Weinstein, Brown, & Ryan, 2009); positive reappraisal (i.e., reinterpreting a negative event or emotion as positive; Garland, Gaylord, & Frederickson, 2011; and controlled or reduced emotional reactivity to aversive stimuli (Farb et al., 2010). Research further reveals that mindfulness heightens positive affect and reduces not only psychological distress (e.g., rumination, anxiety, anger) (Keng, Smoski, & Robins, 2011; Robins, Keng, Ekblad, & Brantley, 2012) but also physical pain (Schutze, Rees, Preece, & Schutze, 2010). From a physiological standpoint, mindfulness has even been shown to alter autonomic nervous system functioning by, specifically, reducing cortisol and increasing parasympathetic nervous system activity (Greeson, 2009).

Mindfulness-based stress reduction (MBSR; Kabat-Zinn, 2005) involves techniques that cultivate greater awareness of the mind and body. In one study, novice meditators who were trained in MBSR techniques over the course of 8 weeks evidenced greater left-hemispheric brain activation, a region consistently shown to be associated with positive affect (Davidson, Jackson, & Kalin, 2000). Another meditation practice, loving-kindness meditation (LKM), involves actively cultivating positive emotions in order to learn about the nature of one's emotional experiences. In a field study, Fredrickson and her colleagues (2008) trained working adults to practice LKM in their daily lives over the course of 9 weeks. Findings indicated that those who practiced LKM evidenced increased daily experiences of positive emotions, which in turn helped to build personal resources, including resilience. Together, these findings indicate that meditation may at first be a deliberative practice; however, over time, the emotional and bodily awareness that result from meditation may produce increases in daily positive emotion, which in turn may interrupt the stressor before it fully unfolds, and help to buffer against future stressors.

Capitalization

Sharing good news with loved ones may be another way that people to cope with stress (Tugade & Frederickson, 2007). "Capitalization," or the act of sharing personal positive events, is a conscious, interpersonal process that cultivates positive emotions through a social exchange (Gable, Reis, Impett, & Asher, 2004; Langston, 1994). Various intrapersonal outcomes have been found to result from the act of sharing good news with others. The process is thought to promote savoring, and it allows the individual to derive further benefits from a prior positive event by increasing memorability and marking its significance (Bryant, 2003; Gable et al., 2004). Furthermore, capitalization has been found to build various resources that can benefit the individual. Specifically, sharing one's own positive news with others predicts increases in positive emotion (e.g., pride), subjective well-being, life satisfaction, self-esteem, and an "open-minded broadened mental focus" (e.g., Gable & Reis, 2010; Gable et al., 2004). It has also been linked to decreases in negative affect and loneliness (Gable & Reis, 2010).

Meaning Making

Another important controlled process of positive emotion that has been found to generate numerous benefits is meaning making, through which an individual finds sources of meaning within a negative life event. Specifically, Folkman and Moskowitz (2000a) have identified three "meaning-making" pathways that each facilitates experiences of positive emotions amid hardship. These pathways include (1) positive reappraisal, or identifying positive aspects within the difficult situation, (2) problem-focused coping, or direct attempts to manage the stressor, and (3) infusing ordinary events with meaning, which involves identifying positive meaning within seemingly everyday occurrences, both planned (e.g., getting together with friends) and unexpected (e.g., a minor compliment). These different forms of meaning making all engender a host of notable benefits that facilitate effective coping. For example, Folkman and Moskowitz have found that the infusion of ordinary events with meaning provides many psychological benefits, including an often-needed lift in one's spirits. Folkman (1997) also suggested that this act might foster positive outcomes involving social support, hope, and attitudes toward the self.

Benefit Finding

Benefit finding and benefit reminding are coping strategies also characterized by finding positive meaning amid hardship (Affleck & Tennen, 1996; Tennen & Affleck, 1999). Substantial evidence indicates that this form of meaning making is linked to decreased depression, increased social support and physical activity (Littlewood, Vanable, Carey, & Blair, 2008), a sense of meaningfulness (Thompson, 1991), psychological adjustment (Taylor, Lichtman, & Wood, 1984), and greater physical health outcomes (Affleck, Tennen, Croog, & Levine, 1987). Furthermore, benefit finding also appears to exert its positive effects in areas outside of the health realm. For example, it has been linked to increased feelings of forgiveness after an interpersonal transgression (McCullough, Root, & Cohen, 2006), and writing about the benefits of a traumatic event appears to foster feelings of resolve and decreased bitterness (King & Miner, 2000).

Automatic Processes of Resilience

Automatic processes are distinguishable from controlled processes in several ways. A process is described as automatic if it is *unintentional, effortless,* and *uncontrollable,* occurring outside of the individual's conscious awareness, whereas controlled processes are *deliberate, controllable,* and *effortful,* operating within the bounds of conscious detection (Bargh, 1994).

Often, through the incorporation of subliminally presented valenced stimuli, previous research has shown that numerous processes can be largely automatized, including emotion regulation (Mauss, Bunge, & Gross, 2007; Williams, Bargh, Nocera, & Gray, 2009); assigning hedonic valence (pleasant–unpleasant; Handley & Lassiter, 2002), computing the relevance or value of an environmental cue (Cacioppo & Gardner, 1999; Hunt, Ishigami, & Klein, 2006), and goal pursuit (Bargh & Chartrand, 1999; Gollwitzer & Bargh, 2005). Notwithstanding, it is unlikely that a given response is either *exclusively* automatic or controlled, but that a continuum of automatization better represents emotion regulation (Bargh & Williams, 2007; Barrett, Mesquita, Oschner, & Gross, 2007; Mauss, Bunge, & Gross, 2007). In line with dual-process theories of mind, automatic and controlled processes run in concert to contribute to behavior (Barrett et al., 2004).

As we reviewed earlier, controlled processes of positive affect activation, such as meaning making, provide many valuable benefits in managing stressors that persist over the long term (e.g., chronic illness, bereavement) (Bonanno & Keltner, 2007; Folkman, 1997; Lechner, Carver, Antoni, Weaver, & Phillips, 2006). It seems possible, however, that this process may be less efficient—and perhaps even costly—in the face of immediate short-term stressors (Tugade, 2011). When a crisis occurs suddenly or unexpectedly (e.g., heart attack, natural disaster), controlled processes of positive emotion may be inefficient because the individual needs to devote his or her attention and resources to more pressing concerns. Therefore, the dual-process model of resilience proposes that another pathway of resilience (i.e., the automatic activation of positive emotion) may free resources when individuals face short-term stressors and crises.

The automatic activation of positive emotion is ubiquitous in everyday life, which makes it a ripe topic for further investigation. Automatic processes are also known as bottom-up processes because they are often stimulus-driven. For example, people may be confronted with an unexpected emotion elicitor (e.g., a snake in their path; a pleasant dessert) that may activate an emotional response outside of immediate conscious awareness. Automatic processes of positive emotion can be activated in several ways, which we detail in the next sections.

Nonconscious Priming

Automatic processes include positive emotions being activated unconsciously or with very little deliberate effort (Tugade, 2011). Commonly, these emotional experiences can occur as a result of a sensory experience activated by an aspect of one's surroundings. For example, the warmth of sunshine on a summer day can elicit feelings of joy, and the scent of the ocean can rekindle a memory of a relaxing vacation. These examples illustrate automatic activations of positive emotion that involve minimal conscious effort and may even occur without any awareness of what generated the positive feelings.

Implicit Goals

Another way to understand the automatic processes of resilience is to investigate goals for coping that can be automatically initiated and enacted outside of one's conscious awareness (Bargh, 1989). Research on automatic emotion regulation shows that it is possible for an implicit goal to alter one's emotional experience in a given situation automatically. For instance, one may have an implicit goal to hold back one's tears whenever a situation elicits sadness. This automatic emotion regulation goal can occur without the individual making a conscious decision to do so, without expending attentional or physiological resources, and without deliberate control (Mauss, Cook, & Gross, 2007). Thus, emotion regulation

strategies can indeed be automatically activated in the service of minimizing stressful experiences. These automatically activated strategies have minimal costs for individuals and can therefore produce positive outcomes for psychological well-being (Mauss, Cook, & Gross, 2007; Williams et al., 2009).

Frequency of Activation

Automatic processes of positive affect can also develop over time through the repeated use of a well-practiced coping strategy (Tugade, 2011). In this way, automatic and controlled processes work hand-in-hand. The controlled processes of positive affect can become automatized, much like processes associated with behavioral learning. When an individual has frequent, consistent pairings of a specific stimulus and an internal process, activation of that process (e.g., thinking about pleasant memories) becomes automatic when one detects the stimulus with which it was repeatedly paired (e.g., saying good-bye at the airport) (Bargh & Chartrand, 1999). This allows for the automatization of behavior or affect that has worked successfully for an individual.

It has been posited that a controlled process of emotion regulation (e.g., meaning making) can become automatic if it is frequently employed, and eventually, may no longer require any conscious effort in its use (Gyurak, Gross, & Etkin, 2011). This interplay of automatic and controlled processes illustrates their complementary nature, and the dual-process model of resilience has proposed that both pathways can be involved in a resilient response (Tugade, 2011).

Accessibility

Even more subtly, some automatic processes of positive emotion may not involve any changes in emotional state at all, but rather may merely heighten one's accessibility of emotion. As Robinson (2007) explains, chronic accessibility is one's "preparedness to recognize stimuli of a given type" (p. 227). In prior research, accessibility of different categories (e.g., older adults) has been successfully increased through the use of nonconscious primes (Bargh, Chen, & Burrows, 1996). During such tasks, participants are supraliminally exposed to a concept (e.g., through embedded words in a scrambled sentences task), and this prime can heighten their accessibility to a category without any awareness that this process is taking place (Bargh, Gollwitzer, Lee-Chai, Barndollar, & Trötschel, 2001; Epley & Gilovich, 1999; Srull & Wyer, 1979) Accessibility to emotional knowledge has been successfully primed in past research, and this method serves to increase cognitive accessibility to affective concepts without influencing one's current emotional state (Innes-Ker & Niedenthal, 2002; Silvia, Phillips, Baumgaertner, & Maschauer, 2006).

Costs and Benefits of Automatic and Controlled Processes

Are there costs and benefits associated with dual processes of emotion? Much of the benefits of automatic regulation are inherent in its definition. Because automatic regulation does not require deliberate action, it frees up cognitive and physiological resources for use elsewhere (Mauss, Cook, & Gross, 2007; Williams et al., 2009). Lack of effort makes automatized regulation more adaptive for coping when deliberate strategies are difficult, while expedited activation lends itself to a faster response immediately following the detection of environmental triggers.

Existing research supports the distinctness of automatic and controlled processes in both their physiological and response elicitation. Indeed, studies show that distinct neural pathways exist to coordinate explicitly and implicitly elicited responses to emotional stimuli (Barrett et al., 2007; Ellenbogen, Schwartzman, Stewart, & Walker, 2006; Morris et al., 1996), supporting the assertion that automatic regulation enables a faster response because it bypasses cortical structures. Finally, automatic elicitation of anxiety associates more reliably with cortisol levels than do controlled processes (Ellenbogen et al., 2006), implicating automatic regulation as an effective tool in motivating the body to action, while its unintentionality lends efficiency in sustaining a response with minimal effort or cognitive constraint.

Meanwhile, controlled regulation of emotions affords an individual the ability to assess his or her coping alternatives and elect the most favorable choice. It allows for executive processes such as cognitive reappraisal (Gross, 2002), benefit finding (Affleck & Tennen, 1996; Tennen & Affleck, 1999), and positive meaning making in the midst of stressful situations (Folkman & Moskowitz, 2000a, 2000b). Deliberate processes can give an individual the time to consider behavioral options for navigating through his or her social and emotional world. Indeed, research shows that considering benefits in chronic stress allows one to find coherence in disruptive life events, to persist with coping goals while maintaining positivity, and to reorder life priorities (Folkman & Moskowitz, 2000a, 2000b). Thus, when faced with chronic stressors that persist over time, controlled regulation may confer important coping advantages for individuals.

In the midst of an immediate short-term stressor, however, effortful regulation is associated with increased cognitive load, making it less efficient in the face of other processing demands (Bargh, 1989; Mauss, Bunge, & Gross, 2007). Given the involvement of cortical structures, controlled regulation does not allow for the fast response that automatic regulation offers. The effort to cultivate positive emotions can itself be taxing, particularly for individuals coping with an ongoing illness or the diagnosis of a serious disease (Moskowitz, Wrubel, Acree, & Folkman, 2001, as cited in Moskowitz & Epel, 2006). Research and theory indicate that when coping with a long-term stressor (e.g., long-term caregiving; grieving the loss of a loved one), it may be beneficial to use strategies that initially alleviate the stressor (e.g., automatic regulation), and later, after affective equilibrium has been achieved, to then engage in more deliberative strategies (e.g., meaning making, instrumental coping) (cf. Folkman & Moskowitz, 2004; Stroebe & Schut, 1999).

It is through these processes that we can best envision the costs and benefits of automatic and controlled processing outside of what is inherent from their definitions. Aside from speed and flexible attention allocation, a significant difference between automatic and controlled regulation is evident in freed-up cognitive and physiological resources to support coping efforts. When conscious attempts at coping are difficult, automatically activated positive emotions can be useful in supplementing more deliberate regulation strategies to increase the possibility of successful coping. In addition, previous research indicates that automatic regulation may be useful for resilience in response to immediate, short-term stressors, whereas the controlled activation of positive emotion may have advantages in response to chronic, long-term stressors.

The Accessibility of Positive Emotions and Coping: A Preliminary Study

The dual-process model of resilience (Tugade, 2011) proposes that resilience involves an interplay between automatic and controlled processes of positive emotion. Research shows that finding positive meaning in negative circumstances is associated with physical and psychological health benefits (e.g., Folkman & Moskowitz, 2000b). This deliberate coping strategy may be costly, however, due to the conscious effort involved in cultivating positive emotions during times of stress.

In one study, we examined the effect of automatically activating positive (vs. neutral, negative) affect on coping. More specifically, we investigated whether making positive emotion accessible would facilitate positive meaning finding under stressful circumstances. We reasoned that the automatic activation of positive affect can disrupt the trajectory of a stress response, freeing up resources to cope with a distressing situation.

Participants were college undergraduates recruited through an online participant pool, and they were compensated with partial course credit for their participation. The participant sample ($N = 167$) comprised 66% females and 34% males, with a mean age of 18.53 ($SD = 0.84$). Participants completed all tasks and questionnaires on a computer in a laboratory.

Positive and Negative Affect

Participants first completed the Positive and Negative Affect Schedule (PANAS; Watson, Clark, & Tellegen, 1988), which provided a baseline assessment of current mood. This measure provided a list of 14 positive emotions (e.g., calm, excited, proud) and 10 neg-ative emotions (e.g., anxious, angry, guilty). Participants were asked to report the degree to which they were currently experiencing each emotion on a 7-point Likert scale (1 = *not at all*; 7 = *a great deal*).

Stress Induction

Participants were experimentally induced to experience anxiety via a mental imagery task. They listened to an audio recording of the following vignette via headphones:

> You have a lot of schoolwork to do and too little time to get it all done. You are just looking over all the work you have to complete this week. You have two tests and a big paper due, all of which you haven't even started yet. You feel completely overwhelmed.

Participants were told to imagine this scenario vividly and reflect on how they would feel in this situation. After the visualization, they reported the degree to which they experienced five discrete negative emotions (e.g., anxiety, anger) in response to the scenario. Participants reported significant increases in anxiety, shame, guilt, anger, and sadness after the stressful mental imagery, as compared to their baseline reports of these emotions (all p's < .001), suggesting that this manipulation was effective in inducing stress of all participants in our sample.

Affect Accessibility Manipulation

Immediately after the stress induction, participants completed a scrambled sentences task that served as a nonconscious prime to increase emotion accessibility. Each participant was randomly assigned to one of the three emotion accessibility conditions (i.e., positive, neutral, or negative). Participants were provided with 20 sentences that each contained a string of five words (e.g., *pleasant the she bricks stacked*), and were instructed to form a grammatically correct sentence using four of the five words (e.g., *she stacked the bricks*). Embedded in each item was a term associated with positive affect (e.g., "pleasant," "smile"), negative affect (e.g., "fright," "cry"), or neutrality (e.g., "glanced," "degree"), depending on the participant's randomly assigned emotion accessibility condition. This scrambled sentences task has been used in prior research to activate accessibility to different categories nonconsciously, such as stereotypes, goal orientations, conformity, and emotion (Bargh et al., 1996, 2001; Epley & Gilovich, 1999; Innes-Ker & Niedenthal, 2002; Srull & Wyer, 1979).

Positive-Meaning Scale

Immediately after completing the emotion accessibility task, participants completed a brief self-report scale to assess ability to find positive meaning in a stressor. Participants were asked to recall the stressful academic scenario they had visualized earlier and indicate the degree to which they could find positive meaning in this event. Ability to find positive meaning was assessed through two self-report items from the Moos (1988) Coping Responses Inventory: "Did you think about how much worse things could be?" and "Did you think that you are much better off than other people?") rated on a 7-point scale from 1 (*not at all*) to 7 (*a great deal*). To quantify finding positive meaning, an aggregate index of positive meaning was created for each participant by computing the mean of the scores of the two items (alpha = .86). Responses of *not applicable* were considered missing.

Positive Meaning Writing Task

Participants were then asked to write freely about the ways they could find positive meaning in the stressor. The instructions read:

> Think back to the scenario you imagined earlier, during the mental visualization task (about schoolwork). There are different ways that people approach a situation like this. One way is to try to find positive meaning in the situation. We would like you to try this approach and write down your thoughts in the box below. Just let your thoughts run freely.

They were told that they could write as much as they liked in response to this prompt. After the writing task, participants completed another assessment of current mood using the PANAS (Watson et al., 1988), then completed a series of individual-differences measures.

Individual-Differences Measures

Ego-Resiliency Scale

This scale includes 14 items (e.g., "I quickly get over and recover from being startled") rated on a 4-point scale (1 = *does not apply at all*, 4 = *applies very strongly*) to assess trait psychological resiliency, or one's ability to adapt to stress and negative life events (Block & Kremen, 1996).

COPE Inventory

This Brief COPE scale includes 28 items rated on a 4-point scale (1 = *not at all*, 4 = *a lot*) to assess the use of different coping strategies in response to stress (e.g., acceptance, self-distraction, positive reframing) (Carver, Scheier, & Weintraub, 1989). We were particularly interested in the Positive Reframing subscale, which included two items: "I tried to see it in a different light, to make it seem more positive" and "I looked for something good in what was happening."

Tolerance of Ambiguity

This scale assesses how an individual copes with ambiguous information (Norton, 1975). Participants indicate the degree to which they agree with 16 statements (e.g., "What we are used to is always preferable to what is unfamiliar") on a 7-point scale from 1 (*strongly disagree*) to 7 (*strongly agree*).

Results

We hypothesized that positive affect accessibility would facilitate positive meaning making in the midst of stress. An analysis of variance (ANOVA), with emotion accessibility as the independent variable (positive, neutral, negative) and the Positive Meaning-Making Scale as the dependent variable was run to assess group differences in ability to find positive meaning in the academic stressor. As predicted, the accessibility of positive (vs. neutral or negative) affect facilitated participants' abilities to find positive meaning in the stressful event, $F(2, 166) = 6.49$, $p < .01$. Planned contrasts revealed that those in the positive accessibility group were significantly more likely than both the neutral and negative groups to find positive meaning in the stressful situation they had experienced ($p < .0001$). These results persisted, even when we controlled for the individual-differences measures of trait resilience, $F(1, 163) = 6.23$, $p < .05$; tolerance of ambiguity, $F(1, 163) = 6.30$, $p < .05$; and positing–reframing coping style, $F(1, 162) = 6.86$, $p < .05$.

Discussion

Our aim in the preliminary study was to investigate whether positive affect accessibility would facilitate positive meaning making in the midst of a stressful circumstance. Because of the cognitive effort often required in stress, positive meaning making can be difficult in the midst of an immediate, short-term stressor (Tugade, 2011). In line with our predictions, findings from the present research indicated that one underlying mechanism of resilience is positive emotion accessibility. Having positive emotions accessible can facilitate one's abilities to use positive emotions to cope with stress.

There are limitations in the current research that should be noted. The present study involved a college-age sample comprised almost entirely of young adults. This raises the question of possible age differences in the outcomes of these automatically activated processes. For instance, research on the positivity effect shows that as one ages, automatic processes of coping are more likely to be enacted (Carstensen & Mikels, 2005). For instance, older (vs. younger) adults quickly shift attention away from negative stimuli to positive emotional stimuli (Isaacowitz, Wadlinger, Goren, & Wilson, 2006a, 2006b; Mather & Carstensen, 2005). If automatically activated coping comes more naturally for older individuals, a prime as subtle as heightened emotion accessibility may be more effective in easing positive meaning making for younger individuals. Future research should address how moderator variables, such as age, might have an impact on one's responsiveness to various positive emotion interventions.

Additionally, this study examined ability to find positive meaning within an imagined stressor rather than a naturally occuring negative life event. This method benefited us in multiple ways. Most importantly, it allowed us to control the content and severity of the stressor across all of the participants. It is possible, however, that while positive emotion accessibility was powerful enough to facilitate meaning-making abilities in response to this imagined stressor, it may not be powerful enough to exert these effects in the face of actual negative experiences that are significantly impacting an individual's life. Other methodologies, such as experience sampling, that allow for the examination of coping as it unfolds in daily life would be particularly valuable in addressing this question in future research.

Last, our primary measure of meaning-making ability asked participants to self-report on their perceived ability to find meaning within the stressor. It seems plausible that positive emotion accessibility may have led to a greater orientation toward positivity overall, and that participants in the positive accessibility condition were therefore more likely to perceive themselves more favorably on any given domain—regardless of their actual coping response. It will be important in future studies to investigate whether positive emotion accessibility facilitates the use of other positive coping strategies (e.g., humor generation, mindfulness, social capitalization) beyond mere self-reported perceptions of these skills.

Conclusions and Future Directions

We have reviewed theory and research illuminating the interplay of automatic and controlled processes of positive emotion that underlie resilience. There is no shortage of actively generated strategies to increase positive emotions in the service of coping. These strategies have been found to be valuable in managing long-term stressors such as illness and trauma (e.g., Bonanno & Keltner, 1997; Folkman & Moskowitz, 2000b). Although highly effective, these strategies may be difficult to generate in the midst of a highly stressful experience due to a depletion of resources that accompany distress.

There are a number of new directions to take in this line of research. Future studies should investigate the different ways that positive emotions may be generated via automatic and controlled processing under times of stress. In particular, we feel it is important to gain greater understanding of the automatic processes of positive emotion. While there is a substantial existing body of work examining controlled processes of emotion, there is still a dearth of research investigating automatic processing. In their dual-process framework of emotion regulation, Gyurak and colleagues (2011) outline several implicit emotion regulation processes that have all received little attention in the literature to date, and urge researchers to pursue further this worthy topic.

From an indiviudal-differences perspective, the study of emotion accessiblity can reveal information about who has greater ease in generating positive emotions to cope with stress. Indiviudals who are exposed to more positive emotions, for example, may have these emotions easily accessible to them. Future studies could examine the different environmental and situational contexts that engender positive emotions.

One possible strategy for increasing positive emotion accessibility includes surrounding oneself in an environment that frequently activates positive emotion and may help an individual to then cope more efficiently when stressors arise. Additionally, it has been suggested that well-practiced coping strategies may become automatic if repeatedly activated over time (Tugade, 2011). If an individual makes a conscious effort to use controlled processes of positive emotion in daily life, he or she may then be well equipped to utilize these coping strategies when they are needed most—in times of stress. Furthermore, if an individual consistently responds to stress by recruiting a particular coping strategy, this continual pairing of the stressor and coping strategy may also facilitate automaticity.

It is also important to address whether there are individual-difference variables that impact the effectiveness of coping strategies across individuals. For example, might it be maladaptive to encourage an individual to adopt strategies that do not match his or her natural coping tendencies? Research by Tamir (2005) has revealed that the effectiveness of a particular emotion induction (e.g., happiness, worry) can be impacted by perceptions about the utility of that emotion. This notion is also supported by recent work suggesting that the effectiveness of a controlled emotion regulation process (i.e., cognitive reappraisal) is impacted by one's implicit valuation of that coping strategy (Hopp, Troy, & Mauss, 2011).

Summary

The research reported in this chapter suggests that strategies eliciting positive emotions are important for establishing beneficial coping outcomes, especially for resilient individuals. Resilient people may initially use positive emotions strategically while coping with a stressful situation, actively cultivating positive emotions to down-regulate distress. To the extent that this same strategy is enacted over time, the conscious strategy can become automatized (Bargh & Chartrand, 1999). Using positive emotions to cope, then, may be likened to mastering a skill. With repeated practice, the skill becomes automatic, requiring only minimal attention or cognitive effort. These benefits of positive emotions can be valuable for coping in the short run and can also have long-lasting benefits for an individual.

References

Affleck, G., & Tennen, H. (1996). Construing benefits from adversity: Adaptational significance and dispositional underpinnings. *Journal of Personality, 64*(4), 899–922.

Affleck, G., Tennen, H., Croog, S., & Levine, S. (1987). Causal attribution, perceived benefits, and morbidity after a heart attack: An 8-year study. *Journal of Consulting and Clinical Psychology, 55*(1), 29–35.

Baker, R. (1993). Some reflections on humour in psychoanalysis. *International Journal of Psychoanalysis, 74*(5), 951–960.

Bargh, J. A. (1989). Conditional automaticity: Varieties of automatic influence on social perception and cognition. In J. S. Bargh & J. A. Uleman (Eds.), *Unintended thought* (pp. 3–51). New York: Guilford Press.

Bargh, J. A. (1994). The Four Horsemen of automaticity: Awareness, efficiency, intention, and control in social cognition. In R. S. Wyer, Jr. & T. K. Srull (Eds.), *Handbook of social cognition* (2nd ed., pp. 1–40). Hillsdale, NJ: Erlbaum.

Bargh, J. A., & Chartrand, T. L. (1999). The unbearable automaticity of being. *American Psychologist, 54*(7), 462–479.

Bargh, J. A., Chen, M., & Burrows, L. (1996). Automaticity of social behavior: Direct effects of trait construct and stereotype activation on action. *Journal of Personality and Social Psychology, 71*(2), 230–244.

Bargh, J. A., Gollwitzer, P. M., Lee-Chai, A., Barndollar, K., & Trötschel, R. (2001). The automated will: Nonconscious activation and pursuit of behavioral goals. *Journal of Personality and Social Psychology, 81*(6), 1014–1027.

Bargh, J. A., & Williams, L. E. (2007). The nonconscious regulation of emotion. In J. J. Gross (Ed.), *Handbook of emotion regulation* (pp. 429–445). New York: Guilford Press.

Barrett, L. F., Mesquita, B., Ochsner, K. N., & Gross, J. J. (2007). The experience of emotion. *Annual Review of Psychology, 58*, 373–403.

Barrett, L. F., Tugade, M. M., & Engle, R. W. (2004). Individual differences in working memory capacity and dual-process theories of the mind. *Psychological Bulletin, 130*(4), 553–573.

Block, J., & Kremen, A. M. (1996). IQ and ego-resiliency: Conceptual and empirical connections and separateness. *Journal of Personality and Social Psychology, 70*, 349–361.

Block, J. H., & Block, J. (1980). The role of ego-control and ego resiliency in the organization of behavior. In W.A. Collins (Ed.), *Minnesota Symposium on Child Psychology* (Vol. 13, pp. 39–101). Hillsdale, NJ: Erlbaum.

Bonanno, G. A., & Keltner, D. (1997). Facial expressions of emotion and the course of conjugal bereavement. *Journal of Abnormal Psychology, 106*(1), 126–137.

Bryant, F. B. (2003). Savoring Beliefs Inventory (SBI): A scale for measuring beliefs about savouring. *Journal of Mental Health, 12*, 175–196.

Cacioppo, J. T., & Gardner, W. L. (1999). Emotion. *Annual Review of Psychology, 50*, 191–214.

Carstensen, L. L., & Mikels, J. A. (2005). At the intersection of emotion and cognition: Aging and the positivity effect. *Current Directions in Psychological Science, 14*(3), 117–121.

Carver, C. S., Scheier, M. F., & Weintraub, J. K. (1989). Assessing coping strategies: A theoretically based approach. *Journal of Personality and Social Psychology, 56*(2), 267–283.

Chaiken, S., & Trope, Y. (Eds.). (1999). *Dual-process theories in social psychology*. New York: Guilford Press.

Conway, A. M., Tugade, M. M., Catalino, L. I., & Fredrickson, B. L. (2013). The broaden-and-build theory of positive emotions: Form, function, and mechanisms. In S. David, I. Boniwell, & A. Conley Ayers (Eds.), *Oxford handbook of happiness: Psychological approaches to happiness* (pp. 17–34). Oxford, UK: Oxford University Press.

Critchey, S. (2002). *On humour*. New York: Routledge.

Davidson, R. J., Jackson, D. C., & Kalin, N. H. (2000). Emotion, plasticity, context, and regulation: Perspectives from affective neuroscience. *Psychological Bulletin, 126*, 890–909.

Ellenbogen, M. A., Schwartzman, A. E., Stewart, J., & Walker, C. (2006). Automatic and effortful emotional information processing regulates different aspects of the stress response. *Psychoneuroendocrinology, 31*(3), 373–387.

Epley, N., & Gilovich, T. (1999). Just going along: Nonconscious priming and conformity to social pressure. *Journal of Experimental Social Psychology, 35*, 578–589.

Farb, N. A. S., Anderson, A. K., Mayberg, H., Bean, J., McKeon, D., & Segal, Z. V. (2010). Minding one's emotions: Mindfulness training alters the neural expression of sadness. *Emotion, 10*, 25–33.

Folkman, S. (1997). Positive psychological states and coping with severe stress. *Social Science and Medicine, 45*(8), 1207–1221.

Folkman, S., & Moskowitz, J. T. (2000a). Positive affect and the other side of coping. *American Psychologist, 55*(6), 647–654.

Folkman, S., & Moskowitz, J. T. (2000b). Stress, positive emotion, and coping. *Current Directions in Psychological Science, 9*, 115–118.

Folkman, S., & Moskowitz, J. T. (2004). Coping: Pitfalls and promise. *Annual Review of Psychology, 55*, 745–774.

Fredrickson, B. L. (1998). What good are positive emotions? *Review of General Psychology, 2*(3), 300–319.

Fredrickson, B. L. (2000). Cultivating positive emotions to optimize health and well-being. *Prevention and Treatment, 3*. Retrieved from *www.unc.edu/peplab/publications/Fredrickson_2000_Prev&Trmt.pdf.*

Fredrickson, B. L. (2001). The role of positive emotions in positive psychology: The broaden-and-build theory of positive emotions. *American Psychologist, 56*(3), 218–226.

Fredrickson, B. L., Cohn, M. A., Coffey, K. A.,

Pek, J., & Finkel, S. M. (2008). Open hearts build lives: Positive emotions, induced through loving-kindness meditation, build consequential personal resources. *Journal of Personality and Social Psychology, 95*, 1045–1062.

Fredrickson, B. L., & Levenson, R. W. (1998). Positive emotions speed recovery from the cardiovascular sequelae of negative emotions. *Cognition and Emotion, 12*(2), 191–220.

Fredrickson, B. L., Mancuso, R. A., Branigan, C., & Tugade, M. M. (2000). The undoing effect of positive emotions. *Motivation and Emotion, 24*(4), 237–258.

Fredrickson, B. L., Tugade, M. M., Waugh, C. E., & Larkin, G. (2003). What good are positive emotions in crises?: A prospective study of resilience and emotions following the terrorist attacks on the United States on September 11th, 2001. *Journal of Personality and Social Psychology, 84*, 365–376.

Frijda, N. H. (1986). *The emotions.* Cambridge, UK: Cambridge University Press.

Gable, S. L., & Reis, H. T. (2010). Good news!: Capitalizing on positive events in an interpersonal context. In M. P. Zanna (Ed.), *Advances in experimental social psychology* (Vol. 42, pp. 198–257). New York: Elsevier.

Gable, S. L., Reis, H. T., Impett, E., & Asher, E. R. (2004). What do you do when things go right?: The intrapersonal and interpersonal benefits of sharing positive events. *Journal of Personality and Social Psychology, 87*, 228–245.

Garland, E. L., Gaylord, S. A., & Fredrickson, B. L. (2011). Positive reappraisal coping mediates the stress-reductive effect of mindfulness: An upward spiral process. *Mindfulness, 2*, 59–67.

Giuliani, N. R., McRae, K., & Gross, J. J. (2008). The up- and down-regulation of amusement: Experiential, behavioral, and autonomic consequences. *Emotion, 8*(5), 714–719.

Gollwitzer, P. M., & Bargh, J. A. (2005). Automaticity in goal pursuit. In A. J. Elliot & C. S. Dweck (Eds.), *Handbook of competence and motivation* (pp. 624–646). New York: Guilford Press.

Greeson, J. M. (2009). Mindfulness Research Update. *Complementary Health Practice Review, 14*, 10–18.

Gross, J. J. (2002). Emotion regulation: Affective, cognitive, and social consequences. *Psychophysiology, 39*(3), 281–291.

Gyurak, A., Gross, J. J., & Etkin, A. (2011). Explicit and implicit emotion regulation: A dual-process framework. *Cognition and Emotion, 25*(3), 400–412.

Handley, I. M., & Lassiter, G. D. (2002). Mood and information processing: When happy and sad look the same. *Motivation and Emotion, 26*(3), 223–255.

Hopp, H., Troy, A. S., & Mauss, I. B. (2011). The unconscious pursuit of emotion regulation: Implications for psychological health. *Cognition and Emotion, 25*(3), 532–545.

Hunt, A. R., Ishigami, Y., & Klein, R. M. (2006). Eye movements, not hypercompatible mappings, are critical for eliminating the cost of task set reconfiguration. *Psychonomic Bulletin and Review, 13*(5), 923–927.

Innes-Ker, A., & Niedenthal, P. M. (2002). Emotion concepts and emotional states in social judgment and categorization. *Journal of Personality and Social Psychology, 83*(4), 804–816.

Isaacowitz, D. M., Wadlinger, H. A., Goren, D., & Wilson, H. R. (2006a). Is there an age-related positivity effect in visual attention?: A comparison of two methodologies. *Emotion, 6*(3), 511–516.

Isaacowitz, D. M., Wadlinger, H. A., Goren, D., & Wilson, H. R. (2006b). Selective preference in visual fixation away from negative images in old age?: An eye-tracking study. *Psychology and Aging, 21*(1), 40–48.

Kabat-Zinn, J. (2005). *Coming to our senses: Healing ourselves and the world through mindfulness.* New York: Hyperion.

Keng, S. L., Smoski, M. J., Robins, C. J. (2011). Effects of mindfulness on psychological health: A review of empirical studies. *Clinical Psychology Review, 31*, 1041–1056.

King, L. A., & Miner, K. N. (2000). Writing about the perceived benefits of traumatic events: Implications for physical health. *Personality and Social Psychology Bulletin, 26*(2), 220–230.

Kok, B. E., Coffey, K. A., Cohn, M. A., Catalino, L. I., Vacharkulksemsuk, T., Algoe, S. B., et al. (2013). How positive emotions build physical health: Perceived positive social connections account for the upward spiral between positive emotions and vagal tone. *Psychological Science, 24*(7), 1123–1132.

Kumpfer, K. L. (1999). Outcome measures of interventions in the study of children of substance-abusing parents. *Pediatrics, 103*, 1128–1144.

Langston, C. A. (1994). Capitalizing on and coping with daily-life events: Expressive responses to positive events. *Journal of Personality and Social Psychology, 67*, 1112–1125.

Lazarus, R. S. (1991). *Emotion and adaptation.* New York: Oxford University Press.

Lazarus, R. S. (1993). Coping theory and research: Past, present, and future. *Psychosomatic Medicine, 55*, 234–247.

Lazarus, R. S., & Folkman, S. (1984). *Stress, appraisal, and coping.* New York: Springer.

Lechner, S. C., Carver, C. S., Antoni, M. H., Weaver, K. E., & Phillips, K. M. (2006). Curvilinear associations between benefit finding and psychosocial adjustment to breast cancer. *Journal of Consulting and Clinical Psychology, 74*(5), 828–840.

Lefcourt, H. M., Davidson, K., Shepherd, R., Phillips, M., Prkahin, K., & Mills, D. (1995). Perspective-taking humor: Accounting for stress moderation. *Journal of Social and Clinical Psychology, 14*(4), 373–391.

Levenson, R. W. (1988). Emotion and the autonomic nervous system: A prospectus for research on autonomic specificity. In H. L. Wagner (Ed.), *Social psychophysiology and emotion: Theory and clinical applications* (pp. 17–42). Chichester, UK: Wiley.

Levenson, R. W. (1994). Human emotions: A functional view. In P. Ekman & R. Davidson (Eds.), *The nature of emotion: Fundamental questions* (pp. 123–126). New York: Oxford University Press.

Littlewood, R. A., Vanable, P. A., Carey, M. P., & Blair, D. C. (2008). The association of benefit finding to psychosocial and health behavior adaptation among HIV+ men and women. *Journal of Behavioral Medicine, 31*(2), 145–155.

Martens, W. H. J. (2004). Therapeutic use of humor in anti-social personalities. *Journal of Contemporary Psychotherapy, 34*, 351–361.

Martin, R. A., & Lefcourt, H. M. (1983). Sense of humor as a moderator of the relation between stressors and moods. *Journal of Personality and Social Psychology, 45*(6), 1313–1324.

Masten, A. S., Best, K. M., & Garmezy, N. (1990). Resilience and development: Contributions from the study of children who overcome adversity. *Development and Psychopathology, 2*(4), 425–444.

Mather, M., & Carstensen, L. L. (2005). Aging and motivated cognition: The positivity effect in attention and memory. *Trends in Cognitive Sciences, 9*(10), 496–502.

Mauss, I. B., Bunge, S. A., & Gross, J. J. (2007). Automatic emotion regulation. *Social and Personality Psychology Compass, 1*, 146–167.

Mauss, I. B., Cook, C. L., & Gross, J. J. (2007). Automatic emotion regulation during anger provocation. *Journal of Experimental Social Psychology, 43*(5), 698–711.

McCullough, M. E., Root, L. M., & Cohen, A. D. (2006). Writing about the benefits of an interpersonal transgression facilitates forgiveness. *Journal of Consulting and Clinical Psychology, 74*(5), 887–897.

Moos, R. H. (1988). *The Coping Responses Inventory manual.* Palo Alto, CA: Social Ecology Laboratory, Stanford University and Department of Veterans Affairs Medical Center.

Morris, J. S., Frith, C. D., Perrett, D. I., Rowland, D., Young, A. W., Calder, A. J., et al. (1996). A differential neural response in the human amygdala to fearful and happy facial expressions. *Nature, 383*, 812–815.

Moskowitz, J. T., Epel, E. S. (2006). Benefit finding and diurnal cortisol slope in maternal caregivers: A moderating role for positive emotion. *Journal of Positive Psychology, 1*, 83–92.

Moskowitz, J. T., Wrubel, J., Acree, M., & Folkman, S. (2001, June). *When positive emotions are not positive.* Paper presented at the annual meeting of the American Psychological Association, San Francisco.

Nezu, A. M., Nezu, C. M., & Blissett, S. E. (1988). Sense of humor as a moderator of the relation between stressful events and psychological distress: A prospective analysis. *Journal of Personality and Social Psychology, 54*(3), 520–525.

Norton, R. W. (1975). Measurement of ambiguity tolerance. *Journal of Personality Assessment, 39*, 607–619.

Ong, A. D., Bergeman, C. S., Bisconti, T. L., & Wallace, K. A. (2006). Psychological resilience, positive emotions, and successful adaptation to stress in later life. *Journal of Personality and Social Psychology, 91*(4), 730–749.

Prerost, F. J. (1989). Intervening during crises of life transitions: Promoting a sense of humor as a stress moderator. *Counseling Psychology Quarterly, 2*(4), 475–480.

Robins, C. J., Keng, S. L., Ekblad, A., & Brantley, J. (2012). Effects of mindfulness-based stress reduction on emotional experience and expression: A randomized controlled trial. *Journal of Clinical Psychology, 68*, 1–15.

Robinson, M. D. (2007). Personality, affective processing, and self-regulation: Toward process-based views of extraversion, neuroticism, and agreeableness. *Social and Personality Psychology Compass, 1*, 223–235.

Samson, A. C., & Gross, J. J. (2012). Humour as emotion regulation: The differential consequences of negative versus positive humor. *Cognition and Emotion, 26*(2), 375–384.

Schutze, R., Rees, C., Preece, M., & Schutze, M. (2010). Low mindfulness predicts pain catastrophizing in fear-avoidance model of chronic pain, *Pain, 148*, 120–127.

Silvia, P. J., Phillips, A. G., Baumgaertner, M. K., & Maschauer, E. L. (2006). Emotion concepts and self-focused attention: Exploring parallel effects of emotional states and emotional knowledge. *Motivation and Emotion, 30*, 229–235.

Srull, T. K., & Wyer, R. S. (1979). The role of category accessibility in the interpretation of information about persons: Some determinants and implications. *Journal of Personality and Social Psychology, 37*(10), 1660–1672.

Stroebe, M. S., & Schut, H. (1999). The dual process model of coping with bereavement: Rationale and description. *Death Studies, 23*, 197–224.

Tamir, M. (2005). Don't worry, be happy?: Neuroticism, trait-consistent affect regulation, and performance. *Journal of Personality and Social Psychology, 89*, 449–461.

Taylor, S. E., Lichtman, R. R., & Wood, J. V. (1984). Attributions, beliefs in control, and adjustment to breast cancer. *Journal of Personality and Social Psychology, 46*, 489–502.

Tennen, H., & Affleck, G. (1999). Finding benefits in adversity. In C. R. Snyder (Ed.), *Coping: The psychology of what works* (pp. 279–304). New York: Oxford University Press.

Thompson, S. C. (1991). The search for meaning following a stroke. *Basic and Applied Social Psychology, 12*, 81–96.

Tugade, M. M. (2011). Positive emotions and coping: Examining dual-process models of resilience. In S. Folkman (Ed.), *Oxford handbook of stress, health, and coping* (pp. 186–199). New York: Oxford University Press.

Tugade, M. M., & Fredrickson, B. L. (2004). Resilient individuals use positive emotions to bounce back from negative emotional experiences. *Journal of Personality and Social Psychology, 86*(2), 320–333.

Tugade, M. M., & Fredrickson, B. L. (2007). Regulation of positive emotions: Emotion regulation strategies that promote resilience. *Journal of Happiness Studies, 8*(3), 311–333.

Tugade, M. M., Fredrickson, B. L., & Barrett, L. F. (2004). Psychological resilience and positiveemotional granularity: Examining the benefits of positive emotions on coping and health. *Journal of Personality, 72*, 1161–1190.

Vaillant, G. E. (2000). Adaptive mental mechanisms: Their role in a positive psychology. *American Psychologist, 55*, 89–98.

Watson, D., Clark, L. A., & Tellegen, A. (1988). Development and validation of brief measures of positives and negative affect: The PANAS scales. *Journal of Personality and Social Psychology, 54*(6), 1063–1070.

Weinstein, N., Brown, K. W., & Ryan, R. M. (2009). A multi-method examination of the effects of mindfulness on stress attribution, coping, and emotional well-being. *Journal of Research in Personality, 43*, 374–385.

Werner, E. E., & Smith, R. S. (1992). *Overcoming the odds: High-risk children from birth to adulthood.* Ithaca, NY: Cornell University Press.

Williams, L. E., Bargh, J. A., Nocera, C. C., & Gray, J. R. (2009). The unconscious regulation of emotion: Nonconscious reappraisal goals modulate emotional reactivity. *Emotion, 9*, 847–854.

Wolin, S. J., & Wolin, S. (1993). *The resilient self.* New York: Villard Books.

CHAPTER 3

■ ■ ■ ■ ■ ■ ■ ■ ■

The Evolutionary Perspective in Positive Emotion Research

Michelle N. Shiota

The histories of emotion science and of evolutionary theory are closely intertwined. After publishing *On the Origin of Species* in 1859, Darwin engaged in several years of collaborative research on emotional expression; the resulting book, *The Expression of the Emotions in Man and Animals* (1872/1965), was one of two that applied his new theory of natural selection to the understanding of human behavior. Early to mid-20th-century social science largely emphasized the social construction of human behavior rather than evolutionary origins. Nonetheless, the notion of emotions as adaptations would reemerge from time to time. William James's (1884) answer to the question "What Is an Emotion?" emphasized the functional and instinctive nature of emotional responding, and Walter Cannon (1929) went on to identify the branch of the peripheral nervous system mediating "fight–flight" responses in mammalian fear and rage.

In the 1960s and 1970s, the emerging sociobiology movement showed new interest in evolutionary perspectives on human behavior (e.g., Hamilton, 1964; Trivers, 1971; Wilson, 1975). This trend was accompanied by a new wave of theorizing about emotions as adaptations, led by Sylvan Tomkins (1962, 1963) and Robert Plutchik

(1980), among others. By the early 1970s, studies documenting high levels of cross-cultural agreement on the meaning of several "prototype" emotional expressions, conducted by two independent research teams (Ekman, 1971; Izard, 1977), provided the first strong evidence that some aspects of emotion might be part of an inherited human nature. Although debate continues over which aspects of emotion are innate rather than psychologically/socially constructed, about the adaptive function(s) of emotion, and about the nature of emotion itself, there is widespread agreement among researchers that human affect is fundamentally a product of natural selection (e.g., Ekman, 1992; Frijda, 1988; Lazarus, 1991; Nesse & Ellsworth, 2009; Russell, 2003; Scherer, 2009; Tooby & Cosmides, 2008).

Ironically, the emphasis on emotion as adaptation, combined with a tendency to equate "selection pressure" with mortal threat, led to decades of focus on negative emotion and neglect of positive emotion. Groundbreaking cross-cultural studies of several aspects of emotion included a single positive state among several negative emotions (e.g., Ekman et al., 1987; Levenson, Ekman, Heider, & Friesen, 1992; Scherer, 1997), and most research has followed this lead. Fortunately, the 21st century has brought the science of positive emotion to life. Researchers have advanced multiple theories of the adaptive significance of positive emotion, and these theories generated a surge of empirical science. The aims of this chapter are to articulate what it means to apply an evolutionary perspective to emotion research; to summarize several theories of the adaptive significance of positive emotion and sample the research linked to these theories; and to discuss potential pitfalls, as well as promising future directions in positive emotion research, guided by an evolutionary perspective.

What *Is* an Evolutionary Perspective on Emotion?

The basic principles of evolution are commonly misunderstood even among well-educated people (National Science Board, 2000), yet modern evolutionary theory relies on a few fairly simple premises (Lewin & Foley, 2004). First, individual members of a species differ from each other in many ways, and some of these differences are inherited by offspring from their parents. Darwin did not know what a "gene" was, as the structure of DNA was not discovered by Watson and Crick until 1953. However, it is now clear that genetic variability is one important basis for individual differences in physical and behavioral traits, and while shared environment and learning certainly account for some continuity between parents and offspring, genes are an important mechanism as well. Genetic variability arises in the first place because genes must be copied before they can be passed down to offspring via eggs and sperm, and the copying process sometimes introduces errors, or *mutations*.

The second key principle is that of natural selection. Some mutations create gene variants, or *alleles*, whose effects on *phenotype* (observable traits) lead on average to higher rates of reproduction than alternative alleles. Since genes are passed down from parents to offspring, such alleles will, of necessity, be more common in the next generation. Alleles that lead on average to lower rates of reproduction will become less common. Genetic traits are not inherently adaptive or maladaptive, but they become so by virtue

of their interaction with fitness-relevant features of the environment, or "selection pressures." Moreover, traits are not adaptive or otherwise in isolation, but in concert with other traits. Thus, natural selection tends to produce coherence among traits rather than conflict. For example, the availability of food high up in trees and competition for food closer to the ground are the presumed selection pressures behind the giraffe's long neck (Cameron & du Toit, 2007), but this elongation in turn required extensive modification of the skeleton, joints, skin, and cardiovascular system, as well as increasing the adaptive value of a complex visual system (Pellow, 2001). As a result, natural selection is considered by many to be the only viable explanation for complex, integrated functional design in species-typical morphology and behavior (Tooby & Cosmides, 2005).

Selection pressures are most commonly defined in terms of direct implications for individual survival and reproduction. For humans, however, one's ingroup is an extremely important part of the environment, presenting a number of additional selection pressures. Humans are "ultrasocial," unique in the extent to which we cooperate with unrelated or loosely related conspecifics in the basic matters of life—acquiring food, building shelter, protecting ourselves and our kin, and raising offspring (Campbell, 1983). While the extent of this interdependence might be somewhat disguised in modern urban society, an ostracized individual in the hunter–gatherer tribal life that characterized early humans would have found his or her fitness severely compromised, and isolation has striking health consequences even now (Hawkley & Cacioppo, 2010). As we see below, the idea that emotions may serve social as well as intraindividual functions, supporting the intimate, collaborative, and reciprocal relationships on which human fitness depends, may be particularly important in understanding the adaptive functions of positive emotion (Shiota, Campos, Keltner, & Hertenstein, 2004).

Finally, this process, aggregated over many generations, explains how a single, chance mutation and the traits produced by it can spread through a population to become species-typical. While chance events that kill or aid large segments of a population at random can also cause striking changes in population genetics (i.e., random drift), such events do not necessarily move the population as a whole in a direction that is adaptive or coherent.

Given these principles, theorists have found it easy to conceptualize negative emotions as evolved, coordinated cognitive–physiological–behavioral responses to the environment (e.g., Ekman, 1992; Lazarus, 1991; Levenson, 1999). Predators, toxins, and untrustworthy conspecifics are uncontroversial mammalian adaptive problems. Complex yet coherent instincts that promoted escape from the first ("fear"), avoidance of the second ("disgust"), and retaliation against the third ("anger") would clearly have been adaptive. This approach guides emotion research in a number of important ways. It leads to a tendency to define emotion constructs in terms of the adaptive problems emotions are thought to solve, and the specific environmental selection pressures that those problems entail (Tooby & Cosmides, 2008). While U.S. researchers have tended to rely on convenient, English-language labels for emotion constructs (Russell, 1991), the emphasis is not necessarily on the colloquial meaning of these labels. Rather, the emphasis is on adaptive problems and the physiological, cognitive, and behavioral aspects of well-designed solutions to those problems. This approach offers a hypothesis-generation strategy that has led to a tremendous amount of solid empirical science.

An evolutionary approach also heightens the importance of two sources of evidence: cross-cultural data and comparative research with nonhuman animals. Evolved mechanisms such as emotions would presumably be species-typical, reflecting adaptive problems that go deep into our evolutionary past (e.g., predation, altricial offspring). This leads to an expectation of continuity across cultures and even species. The assumption that shared genes must manifest in universal morphology and behavior is not at all necessary, as ecological, cultural, and situational contexts can alter gene expression in profound ways, in addition to their effects via learning (e.g., Carroll, 2005; Roseman, 2011; Shweder & Sullivan, 1993). Nonetheless, evidence that some aspect of emotion plays out in similar ways across cultures is often used to argue that that aspect of emotion is innate, and such research has offered crucial support for the general notion of emotion as adaptation (e.g., Ekman et al., 1987; Levenson et al., 1992; Russell, Lewicka, & Niit, 1989; Scherer, 1997; Tracy & Robins, 2008; Tsai, Levenson, & Carstensen, 2000). Evidence that supports theorized interactions between evolved emotion mechanisms and specific environmental features in predicting cultural or situational variability in emotional responding, though now rare, can be just as useful in this regard (Bracha, 2004; Roseman, 2011).

If the adaptive problem giving rise to an emotional trait was encountered by the shared ancestors of humans and other animals, then the trait is likely to be shared as well. Complex adaptations of our mammalian ancestors are unlikely to have disappeared in humans, unless later environmental changes actually rendered them maladaptive (Lewin & Foley, 2004). This presumption opens the door to comparative research on emotion with nonhuman animals—especially other mammals. This approach has been both fruitful and controversial. Neuroscience techniques that are currently impracticable in humans can be used to study laboratory animals, and have led to tremendous gains in our understanding of the neural bases of apparently emotional behavior (e.g., Berridge & Kringelbach, 2008; Carter, DeVries, & Getz, 1995; Knutson, Burgdorf, & Panksepp, 2002; Panksepp, 1998; Phelps & LeDoux, 2005; Van der Vegt et al., 2003). However, some have argued that the dramatic changes in cortical structure and connectivity that accompanied human evolution make the assumption of homology untenable (e.g., Barrett, 2006). A compromise between these two camps may involve taking a cautious approach to applying animal neuroscience to humans, using the former as a basis for hypothesis-driven research with the latter (e.g., Phelps & LeDoux, 2005), and generating hypotheses about interactions between ancient mammalian emotional response circuits and more recently evolved human cognitive capabilities.

As a theoretical perspective, evolutionary theory lends itself well to the understanding of emotion and is extremely useful for generating hypotheses. Unfortunately, early theorists may have taken the phrase "survival of the fittest" a bit too literally. Adaptive problems are not limited to immediate threats to life and limb. It is the total lifetime fitness consequences of a mutation and its associated traits that determine adaptiveness (Cosmides & Tooby, 2000); opportunities to enhance fitness are just as important as threats in this regard, and traits that help us take advantage of such opportunities are just as adaptive as those that help us escape mortal danger (Kenrick & Shiota, 2008; Tooby & Cosmides, 2008). Theories of positive emotion tend to emphasize this aspect of functionality.

The Adaptive Functions of Positive Emotion(s): Multiple Theories

As noted earlier, the major psychological theories of emotion all consider human affect to be adaptive in the evolutionary sense (e.g., Ekman, 1992; Frijda, 1988; Lazarus, 1991; Nesse & Ellsworth, 2009; Russell, 2003; Scherer, 2009; Tooby & Cosmides, 2008). Different researchers emphasize different aspects of emotional responding in their articulation of function, however, and their specific theories drive different kinds of research. While discrete emotion theorists are typically the most explicit about the presumed role of natural selection in emotional responding, it is important to recognize the role evolutionary thinking has played in other theories of positive emotion as well.

Core Affect and the Signal Value of Affect Valence

The circumplex model posits that the universal affect system in humans comprises two mechanisms—one that computes valence on a continuous, negative-to-positive dimension, and another that registers the individual's current state of arousal (Russell, 2003). At any point in time an individual will be somewhere in the resulting two-dimensional space; this location is "core affect." A key feature that distinguishes core affect theory from the perspectives discussed below is its emphasis on *internal feeling state* as the functional aspect of emotion, rather than physiological and behavioral responses to events in the environment.

In this case, the focus is on the signal value of subjective affect valence and implications for how information is processed (Russell, 2003). When we feel good, it is our mind's cue that all is well and we should proceed along trusted paths. When we feel bad, it is a cue that something has gone wrong and we should think and act cautiously. Classic research suggests that people tend to evaluate their environment in ways that are congruent with the valence of their affect—wearing "rose-colored glasses" when mood is positive but more critical lenses when mood is negative (see Pham, 2007, for a review). Experimentally elicited positive mood improves people's judgments of consumer products (e.g., Gorn, Goldberg, & Basu, 1993), weak persuasive arguments (e.g., Bless, Bohner, Schwarz, & Strack, 1990), advertisements (e.g., Murry & Dacin, 1996), and political candidates (e.g., Isbell & Wyer, 1999), among a variety of other targets. According to the affect infusion model (Forgas, 1995), this effect is not limited to situations where people are unmotivated or unable to think systematically about their judgments, and thus rely on simple heuristics. Rather, systematic information processing may infuse current mood even more deeply into judgment processes via selective, affect-congruent attention to different aspects of the target and memory for relevant information, resulting in effects on judgment and decision making that outlast the mood itself.

Positive mood can influence not only the direction of judgment but also which cognitive processes are used to interpret new information. When we feel good, we tend to go with whatever process or response is dominant at the time. Often this involves relying on a simple heuristic for judgment, such as a stereotype (e.g., Bodenhausen, Kramer, & Süsser, 1994), event script (Bless et al., 1996), the fundamental attribution error (Forgas, 1998), or the mood congruency effect described earlier (Forgas, 1995). However, if a situation primes an alternate default setting (e.g., counterstereotypic thoughts), then positive affect will keep the person moving in that cognitive direction (e.g., Huntsinger, Clore, & Bar-Anan, 2010; Huntsinger, Isbell, & Clore, 2012; Huntsinger, Sinclair, Dunn, & Clore, 2010). Across all of these lines of evidence, the implication is that positive affect tells us "keep doing what you're doing," whatever that may be.

Behavioral Activation/Approach Motivation

Although threats to fitness are highly salient, the environment also presents many important opportunities to enhance fitness, such as food, water, shelter, and important relationship partners. Just as avoidance is a globally adaptive response to threats, fitness-relevant opportunities must generally be approached. An early proponent of this theory was Jeffrey Gray (1982), who suggested that the neural foundations of mammalian motivation comprises two key systems— one for behavioral activation in the face of anticipated reward, and another for behavioral inhibition in the face of likely threat or punishment. This theory has given rise to a strong body of research that bridges personality psychology, neuroscience, and behavior. At the trait level, self-report measures of dispositional reward and threat sensitivity are largely orthogonal to each other, and differentially predict emotional responding to experimental situations involving punishment and reward (Carver & White, 1994).

At the neural level, a dopaminergic circuit including the nucleus accumbens, ventral tegmental area, amygdala, and areas of the prefrontal cortex has been found to mediate reward–approach behavior in laboratory mammals, as well as the subjective experience of reward anticipation in humans (O'Doherty, 2004). The roots of this circuit are truly ancient, as dopaminergic pathways have been found to mediate the pursuit of food even in worms (Sawin, Ranganathan, & Horvitz, 2000). This circuit is activated by a wide range of reward types, including foods, drugs, video games, physically attractive people, babies, humor, and peak moments in music (e.g., Bartels & Zeki, 2004; Blood & Zatorre, 2001; Glocker et al., 2009; Kampe, Frith, Dolan, & Frith, 2002; Koepp et al., 1998; Mobbs, Grecius, Abdel-Azim, Menon, & Reiss, 2003; O'Doherty, 2004; Small, Zatorre, Dagher, Evans, & Jones-Gotman, 2001). The prefrontal parts of this circuit may be lateralized, as studies have consistently found that greater relative activation in the left frontal cortex relative to the right is associated with stronger trait behavioral activation and positive affect, as well as experimentally elicited positive affect (Davidson, 2004; Harmon-Jones, 2003). In contrast, greater relative activation on the right is associated with most negative-valence emotions. In an interesting exception to this rule, anger shows a lateralization profile similar to that for positive emotion, suggesting that anger is inherently an approach-motivation state despite its negative subjective valence (Carver & Harmon-Jones, 2009; Coan & Allen, 2003; Harmon-Jones & Allen, 1998). In its essence, this theory posits that the core of positive emotion involves a common mechanism for approaching a wide range of fitness-relevant opportunities (see Harmon-Jones, Price, Gable, & Peterson, Chapter 6, this volume, for a more detailed discussion of approach motivation).

The Broaden-and-Build Model

The broaden-and-build model (Fredrickson, 1998, 2001; presented in detail by Tugade, Devlin, & Fredrickson, Chapter 2, this volume) also posits that positive emotions help people develop fitness-critical resources. However, the focus of this theory is less on acquisition of specific, immediate rewards, and more on long-term implications of positive affect for how we approach the environment as a whole. According to this model, positive emotion triggers a host of cognitive changes that broaden the scope of one's attention to the environment, promote open-minded and creative information processing, and facilitate building long-term material, cognitive, and social resources.

The tenets of the broaden-and-build model are supported by considerable research. Experimentally elicited positive affect has been found to enhance creativity (Isen, Daubman, & Nowicki, 1987), as well as to facilitate a global, big-picture attentional focus rather than a local, detail-oriented focus (Fredrickson & Branigan, 2005). Positive emotions appear to broaden our attention to the social as well as material environment, eliminating the own-race bias in ability to recognize specific faces that is typically observed (Johnson & Fredrickson, 2005). Most important for the model, several studies support the role of positive emotions in an "upward spiral" in which positive emotions lead to increased personal resources (including social support and physical health) and more effective coping, which in turn lead to yet more positive affect, higher well-being, and resilience in the face of stressful events (e.g., Fredrickson, Cohn, Coffey, Pek, & Finkel, 2008; Fredrickson & Joiner, 2002; Tugade & Fredrickson, 2004; Tugade, Fredrickson, & Barrett, 2004). This suggests that, as the theory predicts, positive emotions have implications for fitness that go beyond the acquisition of immediately available rewards.

Functionally "Discrete" Positive Emotions

The theories summarized earlier all address adaptive functions of positive affect or emotions as a class. Others have noted the importance of differentiating several specific kinds of fitness-relevant opportunities presented by the environment, and well-designed solutions to these adaptive problems, in generating hypotheses about positive emotional responding (e.g., Fredrickson, 1998; Kenrick & Shiota, 2008; Shiota, Keltner, Campos, Oveis, & Hertenstein, 2013; Tooby & Cosmides, 2008). This approach conceptualizes emotions as coherent packages of cognitive, perceptual, physiological, motivational, and behavioral responses that work together to address specific adaptive problems, possibly under the guidance of a "superordinate program" coordinating these multiple components (e.g., Levenson, 1999; Tooby & Cosmides, 2008). Specific emotion constructs are defined not in terms of modern-day emotion vocabulary but in terms of the specific adaptive problem each emotion is thought to solve.

While this approach draws heavily on the "basic" emotion theory that has often been contrasted with valence-focused theories, the two are not incompatible. Evolution tends to tinker with existing mechanisms when addressing a new adaptive problem, rather than designing a new mechanism from scratch (Jacob, 1977). As noted earlier, evidence suggests that an ancient dopaminergic circuit was the original mechanism for approaching food—the most basic opportunity (O'Doherty, 2004; Sawin et al., 2000). New adaptive opportunities created a need for offshoots of the original mechanism, and these offshoots appear to involve neural mechanisms that interact with rather than replace the dopaminergic reward system (Shiota et al., 2013). Thus, evolution is most likely to have produced a phylogenetic tree of the positive emotions themselves, in which functionally distinct emotions can be thought of as "prototypes without sharp boundaries" rather than categorically distinct modules (Nesse & Ellsworth, 2009, p. 131).

To the extent that positive emotion prototypes should have evolved to address different kinds of adaptive opportunities, theoretical definitions of these prototypes can generate solid hypotheses about overlap and differentiation among different varieties of positive emotion (Campos et al., 2013). One example of a positive emotion taxonomy generated by this approach is summarized in Table 3.1.

The first two constructs address opportunities to acquire basic material resources and "digest" those resources once they have been consumed. At its simplest level, *anticipatory enthusiasm* is thought to address the problem of acquiring food—especially food that is elusive, distant, or trying to escape (i.e., prey). Although food is the prototypical elic-

TABLE 3.1. A Taxonomy of Functionally Discrete Positive Emotions

Emotion	Adaptive opportunity and function
Enthusiasm	Acquire food, other material resources
Contentment	Rest in safety to digest, encode route to success
Sexual desire	Attract high-quality mate
Nurturant love	Nurture altricial offspring, vulnerable kin
Attachment love	Elicit others' nurturance and care
Pride	Increase status among conspecifics
Amusement	Develop flexible, complex cognitive-behavioral repertoire (i.e., "play")
Awe	Accommodate new information from environment

itor of enthusiasm, incentive cues of other kinds of rewards may elicit the same response (O'Doherty, 2004; Panksepp, 1998). Pursuing prey requires intense physical effort, and recent research finds that anticipation of reward (as in a "lottery" game) elicits comprehensive sympathetic nervous system responding across alpha-adrenergic, beta-adrenergic, and cholinergic mechanisms that would support this effort (Shiota, Neufeld, Yeung, Moser, & Perea, 2011). Cognitively, anticipatory enthusiasm promotes narrowed attentional focus, presumably on the reward, as well as increased reliance on heuristics and internal knowledge structures in processing new information (e.g., Gable & Harmon-Jones, 2008; Griskevicius, Shiota, & Neufeld, 2010). Behaviorally, enthusiasm has been found to increase financial risk-taking behavior (Li, Neufeld, Griskevicius, Shiota, & Kenrick, 2013).

Once a reward has been acquired and consumed, that experience must be "digested" in two senses (Fredrickson, 1998). First, food must literally be digested, which requires a period of physical rest in a safe place. Second, the actions that led to success should be carefully encoded, increasing the chance of success in the future. The emotion *contentment* is elicited by the fulfillment of basic physical needs (Berenbaum, 2002; Ellsworth & Smith, 1988), and evidence suggests that it does promote these functions. Experimentally elicited contentment involves comprehensive sympathetic nervous system withdrawal and increased parasympathetic influence, both of which would aid in digestion (Kreibig, 2010). Contentment also selectively increases the desirability of home-enhancing consumer products—an effect mediated by the desire to be in a safe and comfortable place (Griskevicius, Shiota, & Nowlis, 2010). The cognitive aspect of digestion is supported by research with laboratory animals; in one study, rats that had just found and consumed a food treat in a maze showed a sequence of hippocampal place cell firing that was the reverse of the sequence during the search itself, suggesting heightened encoding of the successful pathway to reward (Foster & Wilson, 2006).

Other positive emotions are thought to support our intimate relationships with mates, offspring, kin, and other important social partners. Bowlby (1969) differenti-ated among three behavioral programs—sex, caregiving, and attachment—that correspond to three positive emotion constructs involving "love" (see also Shaver, Morgan, & Wu, 1996). *Sexual desire* addresses the opportunity to attract and pursue a high-quality mate. The autonomic physiology of sexual arousal is well established, with high levels of parasympathetic influence on vasculature serving the genitalia and low levels of sympathetic activation in the early stages, but with increasing sympathetic activation as arousal increases (Rowland, 2006). Sexual desire is conveyed through expressive signals distinct from those of romantic love, including lip licks, lip wipes, and tongue protrusions (Gonzaga, Turner, Keltner, Campos, & Altemus, 2006). Sexual desire also promotes subtle behaviors that are thought to attract mates. In men, mating motive activation leads to increases in conspicuous consumption and risk taking, as well as decreases in loss aversion (Baker & Maner, 2008; Griskevicius et al., 2007; Li, Kenrick, Griskevicius, & Neuberg, 2012). In women, mating motive activation promotes public (but not private) helping, conveying high agreeableness and social support (Griskevicius et al., 2007).

The opportunity to raise altricial offspring, who are extremely vulnerable long after birth, requires a quite different solution—*nurturant love*. Although offspring and young kin are prototypical elicitors of this emotion, it can also be elicited by others showing morphological and behavioral "cuteness," including vulnerable adult humans and baby nonhuman animals (Lorenz, 1971). Effective nurturance requires vigilance against threat, as well as active caregiving behavior (Hrdy, 1999). Effects of nurturant love on physiology and behavior are consistent with this theoretical definition. College-age participants viewing photographs of baby animals show a profile of increased heart rate and decreased blood pressure that somewhat resembles the "challenge" profile identified in studies of coping (Shiota et al., 2011). Cognitive effects of nurturant love, including more critical evaluation of weak persuasive messages and reduced financial risk taking (Griskevicius, Shiota, & Neufeld, 2010; Li et al., 2013) suggest a bias toward vigilance and caution. It is unclear whether the adaptive problem of one's own vulnerability (especially in early childhood) and the solutions to that problem are sufficiently different from those of nurturant love to necessitate a separate construct, but one has been proposed—*attachment love*. Attachment love and nurturant love appear to share many physiological features (Feldman, Weller, Zagoory-Sharon, & Levine, 2007; Panksepp, 1998; Shiota et al., 2011). Implications for cognition may be quite different, however. Whereas attachment love promotes heuristic-based social cognition, nurturant love promotes more critical thinking (Griskevicius, Shiota, & Neufeld, 2010). More research is needed to assess the extent of overlap and differentiation among these three constructs.

Hierarchical social structures offer another kind of opportunity, the opportunity to acquire social status. In laboratory mammals and humans, dominance promotes increased reward consumption, greater risk taking, and a general increase in behavioral activation (e.g., Davis, Krause, Melhorn, Sakai, & Benoit, 2009; Galinsky, Gruenfeld, & Magee, 2003), increasing access to a wide range of fitness-relevant resources. *Pride* is thought to promote dominant behavior when one has accomplished a valued goal, taking advantage of status-related opportunities (Tracy & Robins, 2007; Williams & DeSteno, 2009). The behavioral expression of pride is well documented and includes the postural expansion associated with dominance in many group-living mammals (Tracy & Robins, 2007). Experimentally elicited pride also leads to increased desirability of public display products (e.g., expensive watches), an effect mediated by the desire to draw attention to oneself (Griskevicius, Shiota, & Nowlis, 2010).

The last two constructs in the taxonomy address problems related to learning. Mammalian predation, foraging, and self-defense all involve complex and unpredictable fitness-critical situations in which the organism must be able to choose quickly from a range of behavioral options to enact a flexible, yet well-rehearsed, response; innate fixed-action patterns will not suffice. Mammalian play—practicing "nonserious" variants of complex functional behaviors—allows developing individuals to rehearse important skills while also encouraging innovation (Pellegrini, Dupuis,

& Smith, 2007; Pellegrini & Smith, 2005; Smith, 1982). In humans, play can be physical (e.g., rough-and-tumble; "tag"; sports), social (e.g., role playing, teasing), and/or cognitive (e.g., puzzles, word play, humor). Also, ultraaltricial humans continue to play throughout their lives, whereas play behavior is limited to juveniles in most other mammals.

Although the term *amusement* as used by researchers typically refers to humor, it can be applied more broadly to the positive emotion that facilitates play (e.g., Griskevicius, Shiota, & Neufeld, 2010; Shiota et al., 2011). Consistent with this conceptual definition, the primate "play face" (open-mouth Duchenne smile with "dropped" jaw and relaxed neck muscles) observed during play in nonhuman primates, human infants, and preschool children is identical to the amusement expression displayed by adults (Campos et al., 2013; Dickson, Walker, & Fogel, 1997; Preuschoft & van Hooff, 1997; Sarra & Otta, 2001). Amusement is also communicated easily by tone of voice, independent of semantic content (Sauter & Scott, 2007; Simon-Thomas, Keltner, Sauter, Sinicropi-Yao, & Abramson, 2009). Behaviorally, experimentally elicited amusement promotes creativity and financial risk-taking, as well as increased use of heuristics in processing persuasive messages (Griskevicius, Shiota, & Neufeld, 2010; Isen et al., 1987; Li et al., 2013), all of which are consistent with a nonserious, risk-tolerant yet playful approach to the situation at hand.

Finally, humans have a cognitive capacity that may be unique—the ability to form abstract mental representations of the world, or "schemas." Cognitive schemas allow humans to access and operate on a database of internalized conceptual knowledge that goes far beyond learned behavioral routines and mapping of space. Stimuli that are novel, complex, and inconsistent with one's current worldview offer an opportunity to expand that database. However, taking advantage of that opportunity requires interruption of ongoing behavior, as well as physiological and cognitive shifts that promote accommodative cognition (Keltner & Haidt, 2003). The emotion *awe* is thought to promote this set of responses (Keltner & Haidt, 2003; Shiota, Keltner, & Mossman, 2007). Experimentally elicited awe is accompanied by strong withdrawal of sympathetic nervous system influence on the heart, consistent with an increase in intake of information from the environment (Shiota et al., 2011; see also Bradley, 2009). Posed awe expressions are quite different from those of most other positive emotions, and do not include the smile thought to emphasize affiliative intent (Campos et al., 2013). Cognitive effects of awe are also different from many other positive emotions, including reduced reliance on heuristics in processing persuasive messages (Griskevicius, Shiota, & Neufeld, 2010), and on internal event scripts in processing new stories (i.e., "going out to dinner"; Danvers & Shiota, 2012).

Component-Process Model

Scherer's (2009) component-process model (CPM) of emotion differs greatly from the "discrete" emotion approach in terms of the neural mechanisms thought to underlie emotional experience. The CPM posits that variation in emotional experience results not from selective activation of categorically discrete basic emotion programs, but rather from different profiles of emotional responding that result from several sequential "stimulus evaluation checks" and the output of each check in terms of physiological responding, facial expression, cognitive changes, and so forth. This model has not been applied extensively to research on positive emotions. However, researchers have recently begun to apply CPM principles to predicting and understanding why different positive emotions might have different implications for a variety of domains. For example, Tiedens and Linton (2001) have proposed that appraisals of low versus high certainty about an eliciting situation account for differential effects of positive emotions on the use of heuristics in persuasive message processing. This approach builds on a longer history of using the CPM appraisal dimensions to predict differential implications of various negative emotions (e.g., Han, Lerner, & Keltner, 2007; Keltner, Ellsworth, & Edwards, 1993; Lerner & Keltner, 2001; Lerner & Tiedens, 2006), as well as to explain the morphological elements of facial expressions of negative emotion (e.g., Scherer, 1992).

While the CPM predicts a more continuous and multidimensional structure of positive emotion space than discrete emotion models, Scherer (2009) has also noted that humans may be biologically prepared to experience cross-culturally "modal" points in emotion space that reflect particular, recurring adaptive problems. At this point, the hypotheses of discrete emotion models and the CPM may begin to converge. In practice, research driven by the CPM sometimes adopts study designs that look quite similar to those testing discrete emotion approaches (e.g., Banse & Scherer, 1996; Scherer, 1997). However, the CPM also promotes research asking a somewhat different question, which is whether the specific pattern of effects of various emotions on some outcome can be explained in terms of continuous appraisal dimensions reflected in the stimulus evaluation checks. While this approach has been applied to positive emotion infrequently so far, the positive emotions offer a strong opportunity to test CPM predictions using a whole "new" set of emotion constructs.

Conclusions, Caveats, and Future Directions

Evolutionary perspectives have powerfully shaped the young and rapidly developing field of positive emotion. Although theories of positive emotion vary in how explicitly they invoke adaptive function in deriving hypotheses, every major perspective does emphasize functionality at some level of analysis. The theoretical perspectives discussed earlier are by no means mutually exclusive. Some theories are embedded within others (e.g., discrete emotion theories of positive emotion draw heavily upon approach-motivation evidence and theory), whereas others address different adaptive problems and aspects of functionality (e.g., dimensional approaches address the adaptive implications of subjective feelings, whereas other approaches focus more on adaptiveness of physiological and behavioral responding). Recent models of emotion are beginning to integrate the tenets and empirical data associated with several of these theories (e.g., Nesse & Ellsworth, 2009; Shiota et al., 2013). Importantly, the very youth of positive emotion science offers an opportunity to those who seek to test structural theories of emotion such as the dimensional models, discrete emotion models, and the CPM. These structural models, originally developed to account for patterns of data observed among negative emotions, could now be applied in an a priori manner to the study of positive emotion constructs. Which model (if any) accounts best for patterns of responding across a wide range of positive emotions is an empirical question that has yet to be answered.

While adopting an evolutionary perspective offers many advantages, some caveats are also in order. Evolutionary thinking tends to promote a strong focus on adaptations (traits selected for directly via natural selection), but evolution produces far more in the way of "exaptations" (adaptations adopted for a new purpose to address a new adaptive problem) and "spandrels" or by-products (traits that have no adaptive significance, or even negative significance, that became species-typical only due to shared genetic origin with an actual adaptation) than adaptations themselves (Buss, Haselton, Shackelford, Bleske, & Wakefield, 1998). One example of this reasoning might be: "People seem to have a universal positive response to kittens and puppies, so love of baby animals must be adaptive." This tendency is exacerbated by the ease of post hoc reasoning about evolutionary origins, especially in the domain of emotion (e.g., "Maybe we love baby animals because once grown, these animals support our welfare"). There are a number of ways to help us avoid this problem (Tooby & Cosmides, 2005). One is to theorize forward from adaptive problems, rather than backward from already documented (or glaringly obvious) traits. Another strategy is to look for situational moderators that alter how adaptive mechanisms will be expressed, but would not be predicted by other theoretical approaches. Yet another strategy involves documenting theory-consistent mediators of observed processes, while ruling out mediators predicted by other theoretical approaches. Finally, researchers should always consider the possibility that some response is actually an exaptation of some prior trait. For example, the possibility that awe is an exaptation of a phylogenetically older emotion state is plausible given its apparent restriction to the human experience, and it raises a number of research questions that are interesting in their own right (see Shiota, Thrash, Danvers, & Dombrowski, Chapter 21, this volume, for a more detailed discussion).

The naturalistic fallacy (that what is evolved is morally justified or right) is also an ongoing concern in interpreting findings generated by an evolutionary approach. This problem is more one of application of research than the research itself, but the two are not always easy to separate. In the positive emotion domain the naturalistic fallacy may not seem especially worrisome because the adaptations at stake are generally pleasant, prosocial, and desirable. However, there are exceptions. Our powerful emotional response to anticipated reward is clearly important for motivation and fitness, yet it also causes profound human distress in the form of addiction to chemical and behavioral dopamine agonists (alcohol, cocaine, amphetamines, sex, food, gambling, etc.). Propensity for addiction may indeed be part of "human nature," but that hardly makes it desirable or right. In these situations an understanding of the evolutionary origins of some trait can help predict specific details of the environmental features that activate or inhibit it, and these details are useful in designing strong interventions.

Finally, a well-applied evolutionary perspective requires that researchers have a strong understanding of the selection pressures in play while some trait was undergoing natural selection. Unfortunately, psychologists too often assume that the "EEA" (Environment of Evolutionary Adaptedness) for human traits is equal to the African savannah some 100,000 years ago, where the human species is thought to have reached its current form. The EEA is not a specific time or place in history (Tooby & Cosmides, 2005). Rather, the EEA must be defined with respect to the specific adaptation in question and the environment experienced by the population while selection for that adaptation was in progress. This has a number of implications for emotion research. First, the EEA for traits shared with other animals must be defined with a theory of the phylogenetic origin of the trait, combined with an informed understanding of the selection pressures experienced by the relevant population at the time. Second, comparative research should be applied to humans only when it is consistent with our phylogenetic history. Third, human evolution introduced new cognitive mechanisms that should be presumed to interact with any older emotion systems in complex ways. Theories of human emotion that are grounded in animal behavior and neuroscience should aim to account for the implications of human cognition for the modern expression of emotional nature.

These caveats notwithstanding, an evolutionary perspective offers great opportunity for understanding this relatively neglected half of our emotional nature. Theories of positive emotion encourage an emphasis on both subtle cognitive outcomes and overt behaviors (e.g., Forgas, 1995; Fredrickson, 2001; Shiota et al., 2013), opening the door to studies of implicit cognition, as well as conscious judgment and decision-making. Evolutionary theories of emotion can address nature–nurture interactions and support an emphasis on emotions as algorithms for responding adaptively to complex situations, addressing the richness and variability of emotional life, as well as its origins (e.g., Bracha, 2004; Roseman, 2011; Shweder & Sullivan, 1993). For too long, psychologists have emphasized the undesirable side of "human nature"; an evolutionary perspective on positive emotion can help to correct this imbalance.

References

Baker, M. D., & Maner, J. K. (2008). Risk-taking as a situationally sensitive male mating strategy. *Evolution and Human Behavior, 29*(6), 391–395.

Banse, R., & Scherer, K. R. (1996). Acoustic profiles in vocal emotion expression. *Journal of Personality and Social Psychology, 70*(3), 614–636.

Barrett, L. F. (2006). Are emotions natural kinds? *Perspectives on Psychological Science, 1*(1), 28–58.

Bartels, A., & Zeki, S. (2004). The neural correlates of maternal and romantic love. *NeuroImage, 21*, 1155–1166.

Berenbaum, H. (2002). Varieties of joy-related pleasurable activities and feelings. *Cognition and Emotion, 16*(4), 473–494.

Berridge, K. C., & Kringelbach, M. L. (2008). Affective neuroscience of pleasure: Reward in humans and animals. *Psychopharmacology, 199*(3), 457–480.

Bless, H., Bohner, G., Schwarz, N., & Strack, F. (1990). Mood and persuasion: A cognitive response analysis. *Personality and Social Psychology Bulletin, 16*(2), 331–345.

Bless, H., Clore, G. L., Schwarz, N., Golisano, V., Rabe, C., & Wölk, M. (1996). Mood and the use of scripts: Does a happy mood really lead to mindlessness? *Journal of Personality and Social Psychology, 71*(4), 665.

Blood, A. J., & Zatorre, R. J. (2001). Intensely pleasurable responses to music correlate with activity in brain regions implicated in reward and emotion. *Proceedings of the National Academy of Sciences, 98*, 11818–11823.

Bodenhausen, G. V., Kramer, G. P., & Süsser, K. (1994). Happiness and stereotypic thinking in social judgment. *Journal of Personality and Social Psychology, 66*, 621–632.

Bowlby, J. (1969). *Attachment: Vol. 1. Attachment and loss.* New York: Basic Books.

Bracha, H. S. (2004). Freeze, flight, fight, fright, faint: Adaptationist perspectives on the acute stress response spectrum. *CNS Spectrums, 9*(9), 679–685.

Bradley, M. M. (2009). Natural selective attention: Orienting and emotion. *Psychophysiology, 46*(1), 1–11.

Buss, D. M., Haselton, M. G., Shackelford, T. K., Bleske, A. L., & Wakefield, J. C. (1998). Adaptations, exaptations, and spandrels. *American Psychologist, 53*(5), 533–548.

Cameron, E. Z., & du Toit, J. T. (2007). Winning by a neck: Tall giraffes avoid competing with shorter browsers. *American Naturalist, 169*(1), 130–135.

Campbell, D. T. (1983). The two distinct routes beyond kin selection to ultrasociality: Implications for the humanities and social sciences. In D. Bridgeman (Ed.), *The nature of prosocial development: Theories and strategies* (pp. 11–39). New York: Academic Press.

Campos, B., Shiota, M. N., Keltner, D., Gonzaga, G. C., Goetz, J., & Shin, M. (2013). What is shared, what is different?: Core relational themes and expressive displays of eight positive emotions. *Cognition and Emotion, 27*(1), 37–52.

Cannon, W. B. (1929). *Bodily changes in pain, hunger, fear, and rage.* Oxford, UK: Appleton.

Carroll, S. B. (2005). *Endless forms most beautiful: The new science of evo devo.* New York: Norton.

Carter, C. S., DeVries, A. C., & Getz, L. L. (1995). Physiological substrates of mammalian monogamy: The prairie vole model. *Neuroscience and Biobehavioral Reviews, 19*(2), 303–314.

Carver, C. S., & Harmon-Jones, E. (2009). Anger is an approach-related affect: Evidence and implications. *Psychological Bulletin, 135*(2), 183–204.

Carver, C. S., & White, T. L. (1994). Behavioral inhibition, behavioral activation, and affective responses to impending reward and punishment: The BIS/BAS scales. *Journal of Personality and Social Psychology, 67*, 319–333.

Coan, J. A., & Allen, J. J. B. (2003). Frontal EEG asymmetry and the behavioral activation and inhibition systems. *Psychophysiology, 40*(1), 106–114.

Cosmides, L., & Tooby, J. (2000). Evolutionary psychology and the emotions. In M. Lewis & J. M. Haviland-Jones (Eds.), *Handbook of emotions* (2nd ed.). New York: Guilford Press.

Danvers, A., & Shiota, M. N. (2012). [Awe reduces reliance on event schemas in processing new stories]. Unpublished raw data, Arizona State University.

Darwin, C. (1965). Selections from *The Expression of the Emotions in Man and Animals.* Chicago: University of Chicago Press. (Original work published 1872)

Davidson, R. J. (2004). What does the prefrontal cortex "do" in affect: Perspectives on frontal EEG asymmetry research. *Biological Psychology, 67*, 219–233.

Davis, J. F., Krause, E. G., Melhorn, S. J., Sakai, R. R., & Benoit, S. C. (2009). Dominant rats are natural risk takers and display increased motivation for food reward. *Neuroscience, 162*(1), 23–30.

Dickson, K. L., Walker, H., & Fogel, A. (1997). The relationship between smile type and play type during parent–infant play. *Developmental Psychology, 33*(6), 925–933.

Ekman, P. (1971). Universals and cultural differences in facial expressions of emotion. In J. Cole (Ed.), *Nebraska Symposium on Motivation* (Vol. 19, pp. 207–283). Lincoln: University of Nebraska Press.

Ekman, P. (1992). An argument for basic emotions. *Cognition and Emotion, 6*, 169–200.

Ekman, P., Friesen, W. V., O'Sullivan, M., Chan, A., Diacoyanni-Tarlatzis, I., Heider, K., et al. (1987). Universals and cultural differences in the judgments of facial expressions of emotion. *Journal of Personality and Social Psychology, 51*, 712–717.

Ellsworth, P. C., & Smith, C. A. (1988). Shades of joy: Patterns of appraisal differentiating pleasant emotions. *Cognition and Emotion, 2*, 301–331.

Feldman, R., Weller, A., Zagoory-Sharon, O., & Levine, A. (2007). Evidence for a neuroendocrinological foundation of human affiliation: Plasma oxytocin levels across pregnancy and the postpartum period predict mother–infant bonding. *Psychological Science, 18*(11), 965–970.

Forgas, J. P. (1995). Mood and judgment: The affect infusion model. *Psychological Bulletin, 117*(1), 39–66.

Forgas, J. P. (1998). On being happy and mistaken: Mood effects on the fundamental attribution error. *Journal of Personality and Social Psychology, 75*(2), 318–331.

Foster, D. J., & Wilson, M. A. (2006). Reverse replay of behavioural sequences in hippocampal place cells during the awake state. *Nature, 440*, 680–683.

Fredrickson, B. L. (1998). What good are positive emotions? *Review of General Psychology, 2*, 300–319.

Fredrickson, B. L. (2001). The role of positive emotions in positive psychology: The broaden-and-build theory of positive emotions. *American Psychologist, 56*, 218–226.

Fredrickson, B. L., & Branigan, C. (2005). Positive emotions broaden the scope of attention and build thought–action repertoires. *Cognition and Emotion, 19*, 313–332.

Fredrickson, B. L., Cohn, M. A., Coffey, K. A., Pek, J., & Finkel, S. M. (2008). Open hearts build lives: Positive emotions, induced through loving-kindness mediation, build consequential personal resources. *Journal of Personality and Social Psychology, 95*(5), 1045–1062.

Fredrickson, B. L., & Joiner, T. (2002). Positive emotions trigger upward spirals toward emotional well-being. *Psychological Science, 13*(2), 172–175.

Frijda, N. H. (1988). The laws of emotion. *American Psychologist, 43*(5), 349–358.

Galinsky, A. D., Gruenfeld, D. H., & Magee,

J. C. (2003). From power to action. *Journal of Personality and Social Psychology, 85*(3), 453–466.

Gable, P. S., & Harmon-Jones, E. (2008). Approach-motivated positive affect reduces breadth of attention. *Psychological Science, 19*(5), 476–482.

Glocker, M. L., Langleben, D. D., Ruparel, K., Loughead, J. W., Valdez, J. N., Griffin, M. D., et al. (2009). Baby schema modulates the brain reward system in nulliparous women. *Proceedings of the National Academy of Sciences, 106*(22), 9115–9119.

Gonzaga, G. C., Turner, R. A., Keltner, D., Campos, B., & Altemus, M. (2006). Romantic love and sexual desire in close relationships. *Emotion, 6*(2), 163–179.

Gorn, G., Goldberg, M., & Basu, K. (1993). Mood, awareness and product evaluation. *Journal of Consumer Psychology, 2,* 237–256.

Gray, J. A. (1982). *The neuropsychology of anxiety: An enquiry into the functions of the septo-hippocampal system.* Oxford, UK: Oxford University Press.

Griskevicius, V., Shiota, M. N., & Neufeld, S. L. (2010). Influence of different positive emotions on persuasion processing: A functional evolutionary approach. *Emotion, 10,* 190–206.

Griskevicius, V., Shiota, M. N., & Nowlis, S. M. (2010). The many shades of rose-colored glasses: Discrete positive emotions and product perception. *Journal of Consumer Research, 37*(2), 238–250.

Griskevicius, V., Tybur, J. M., Sundie, J. M., Cialdini, R. B., Miller, G. F., & Kenrick, D. T. (2007). Blatant benevolence and conspicuous consumption: When romantic motives elicit strategic costly signals. *Journal of Personality and Social Psychology, 93*(1), 85–102.

Hamilton, W. D. (1964). The genetical evolution of social behavior. *Journal of Theoretical Biology, 7*(1), 1–16.

Han, S., Lerner, J. S., & Keltner, D. (2007). Feelings and consumer decision making: The appraisal-tendency framework. *Journal of Consumer Psychology, 17*(3), 158–168.

Harmon-Jones, E. (2003). Clarifying the emotive functions of asymmetrical frontal cortical activity. *Psychophysiology, 40,* 838–848.

Harmon-Jones, E., & Allen, J. J. B. (1998). Anger and frontal brain activity: EEG asymmetry consistent with approach motivation despite negative valence. *Journal of Personality and Social Psychology, 74,* 1310–1316.

Hawkley, L. C., & Cacioppo, J. T. (2010). Loneliness matters: A theoretical and empirical review of consequences and mechanisms. *Annals of Behavioral Medicine, 40*(2), 218–227.

Hrdy, S. B. (1999). *Mother Nature: Maternal instincts and how they shape the human species.* New York: Pantheon.

Huntsinger, J. R., Clore, G. L., & Bar-Anan, Y. (2010). Mood and global–local focus: Priming a local focus reverses the link between mood and global–local processing. *Emotion, 10*(5), 722–726.

Huntsinger, J. R., Isbell, L. M., & Clore, G. L. (2012). Sometimes happy people focus on the trees and sad people focus on the forest: Context-dependent effects of mood in impression formation. *Personality and Social Psychology Bulletin, 38*(2), 220–232.

Huntsinger, J. R., Sinclair, S., Dunn, E., & Clore, G. L. (2010). Affective regulation of stereotype activation: It's the (accessible) thought that counts. *Personality and Social Psychology Bulletin, 36*(4), 564–577.

Isbell, L. M., & Wyer, R. S., Jr. (1999). Correcting for mood-induced bias in the evaluation of political candidates: The roles of intrinsic and extrinsic motivation. *Personality and Social Psychology Bulletin, 25*(2), 237–249.

Isen, A. M., Daubman, K. A., & Nowicki, G. P. (1987). Positive affect facilitates creative problem solving. *Journal of Personality and Social Psychology, 52,* 1122–1131.

Izard, C. E. (1977). *Human emotions.* New York: Plenum Press.

Jacob, F. (1977). Evolution and tinkering. *Science, 196,* 1161–1166.

James, W. (1884). What is an emotion? *Mind, 9,* 188–205.

Johnson, K. J., & Fredrickson, B. L. (2005). "We all look the same to me": Positive emotions eliminate the own-race bias in face recognition. *Psychological Science, 16*(11), 875–881.

Kampe, K. K., Frith, C. D., Dolan, R. J., & Frith, U. (2002). Reward value of attractiveness and gaze. *Nature, 413,* 589–590.

Keltner, D., Ellsworth, P. C., & Edwards, K. (1993). Beyond simple pessimism: Effects of sadness and anger on social perception. *Journal of Personality and Social Psychology, 64*(5), 740–752.

Keltner, D., & Haidt, J. (2003). Approaching awe: A moral, spiritual, and aesthetic emotion. *Cognition and Emotion, 17,* 297–314.

Kenrick, D. T., & Shiota, M. N. (2008). Approach and avoidance motivation(s): An evolutionary perspective. In A. J. Elliot (Ed.), *Handbook of approach and avoidance motivation* (pp. 273–288). Mahwah, NJ: Erlbaum.

Knutson, B., Burgdorf, J., & Panksepp, J. (2002). Ultrasonic vocalizations as indices of affective states in rats. *Psychological Bulletin, 128*(6), 961–977.

Koepp, M. J., Gunn, R. N., Lawrence, A. D., Cunningham, V. J., Dagher, A., Jones, T., et al. (1998). Evidence for striatal dopamine release during a video game. *Nature, 393,* 266–268.

Kreibig, S. D. (2010). Autonomic nervous system activity in emotion: A review. *Biological Psychology, 84*(3), 394–421.

Lazarus, R. S. (1991). *Emotion and adaptation.* New York: Oxford University Press.

Lerner, J. S., & Keltner, D. (2001). Fear, anger, and risk. *Journal of Personality and Social Psychology, 81*(1), 146–159.

Lerner, J. S., & Tiedens, L. Z. (2006). Portrait of the angry decision maker: How appraisal tendencies shape anger's influence on cognition. *Journal of Behavioral Decision Making, 19*(2), 115–137.

Levenson, R. W. (1999). The intrapersonal functions of emotion. *Cognition and Emotion, 13,* 481–504.

Levenson, R. W., Ekman, P., Heider, K., & Friesen, W. V. (1992). Emotion and autonomic nervous system activity in the Minangkabau of West Sumatra. *Journal of Personality and Social Psychology, 62,* 972–988.

Lewin, R. & Foley, R. (2004). *Principles of human evolution.* Malden, MA: Blackwell Science.

Li, Y. J., Kenrick, D. T., Griskevicius, V., & Neuberg, S. L. (2012). Economic decision biases and fundamental motivations: How mating and self-protection alter loss aversion. *Journal of Personality and Social Psychology, 102*(3), 550–561.

Li, Y. J., Neufeld, S. L., Griskevicius, V., Shiota, M. N., & Kenrick, D. T. (2013). *Chancy or chary?: Discrete positive emotions differentially shift risk-taking preference.* Manuscript in preparation.

Lorenz, K. (1971). *Studies in animal and human behaviour* (Vol. 2) (R. Martin, Trans.). Cambridge, MA: Harvard University Press.

Mobbs, D., Grecius, M. D., Abdel-Azim, E., Menon, V., & Reiss, A. L. (2003). Humor modulates the mesolimbic reward centers. *Neuron, 40,* 1041–1048.

Murry, J. P., & Dacin, P. A. (1996), Cognitive moderators of negative emotion effects: Implications for understanding media-context. *Journal of Consumer Research, 22,* 439–447.

National Science Board. (2000). *Science and Engineering indicators 2000 (NSB-00-1).* Washington, DC: U.S. Government Printing Office.

Nesse, R. M., & Ellsworth, P. C. (2009). Evolution, emotions, and emotional disorders. *American Psychologist, 64*(2), 129–139.

O'Doherty, J. P. (2004). Reward representations and reward-related learning in the human brain: Insights from neuroimaging. *Current Opinion in Neurobiology, 14*(6), 769–776.

Panksepp, J. (1998). *Affective neuroscience: The foundations of human and animal emotions.* New York: Oxford University Press.

Pellegrini, A. D., Dupuis, D., & Smith, P. K. (2007). Play in evolution and development. *Developmental Review, 27,* 261–276.

Pellegrini, A. D., & Smith, P. K. (Eds.). (2005). *The nature of play: Great apes and humans.* New York: Guilford Press.

Pellow, R. A. (2001). Giraffe and okapi. In D. MacDonald (Ed.), *The encyclopedia of mammals* (2nd ed.). Oxford, UK: Oxford University Press.

Pham, M. T. (2007). Emotion and rationality: A critical review and interpretation of empirical evidence. *Review of General Psychology, 11*(2), 155–178.

Phelps, E. A., & LeDoux, J. E. (2005). Contributions of the amygdala to emotion processing: From animal models to human behavior. *Neuron, 48*(2), 175–187.

Plutchik, R. (1980). *Emotion: A psychoevolutionary synthesis.* New York: Harper & Row.

Preuschoft, S., & van Hooff, J. A. R. A. M. (1997). The social function of "smile" and "laughter": Variations across primate species and societies. In U. Segerstrale & P. Molnar (Eds.), *Nonverbal communication: Where nature meets culture* (pp. 171–190). Mahwah, NJ: Erlbaum.

Roseman, I. (2011). Emotional behaviors, emotivational goals, emotion strategies: Multiple levels of organization integrate variable and consistent responses. *Emotion Review, 3*(4), 434–443.

Rowland, D. L. (2006). The psychobiology of sexual arousal and response: Physical and psychological factors that control our sexual response. In R. D. McAnulty & M. M. Burnette (Eds.), *Sex and sexuality: Vol. 2. Sexual function and dysfunction* (pp. 37–65). Westport, CT: Praeger.

Russell, J. A. (1991). Culture and the categorization of emotions. *Psychological Bulletin, 110*(3), 426–450.

Russell, J. A. (2003). Core affect and the psychological construction of emotion. *Psychological Review, 110,* 145–172.

Russell, J. A., Lewicka, M., & Niit, T. (1989). A cross-cultural study of a circumplex model of affect. *Journal of Personality and Social Psychology, 57*(5), 848–856.

Sarra, S., & Otta, E. (2001). Different types of smiles and laughter in preschool children. *Psychological Reports, 89,* 547–558.

Sauter, D. A., & Scott, S. K. (2007). More than one kind of happiness: Can we recognize vocal expressions of different positive states. *Motivation and Emotion, 31*(3), 192–199.

Sawin, E. R., Ranganathan, R., & Horvitz, H. R. (2000). *C. elegans* locomotory rate is modulated by the environment through a dopaminergic pathway and by experience through a serotonergic pathway. *Neuron, 26*(3), 619–631.

Scherer, K. R. (1992). What does facial expression express? In K. T. Strongman (Ed.), *International review of studies on emotion* (Vol. 2, pp. 139–165). New York: Wiley.

Scherer, K. R. (1997). The role of culture in emotion-antecedent appraisal. *Journal of Personality and Social Psychology, 73*(5), 902–922.

Scherer, K. R. (2009). The dynamic architecture of emotion: Evidence for the component process model. *Cognition and Emotion, 23*(7), 1307–1351.

Shaver, P. R., Morgan, H. J., & Wu, S. (1996). Is "love" a basic emotion? *Personal Relationships, 3*(1), 81–96.

Shiota, M. N., Campos, B., Keltner, D., & Hertenstein, M. J. (2004). Positive emotion and the regulation of interpersonal relationships. In P. Philippot & R.S. Feldman (Eds.), *The regulation of emotion* (pp. 127–155). Mahwah, NJ: Erlbaum.

Shiota, M. N., Keltner, D., Campos, B., Oveis, C., & Hertenstein, M. (2013). *Beyond happiness: Toward a science of discrete positive emotions.* Manuscript submitted for publication.

Shiota, M. N., Keltner, D., & Mossman, A. (2007). The nature of awe: Elicitors, appraisals, and effects on self-concept. *Cognition and Emotion, 21*(5), 944–963.

Shiota, M. N., Neufeld, S. L., Yeung, W. H., Moser, S. E., & Perea, E. F. (2011). Feeling good: Autonomic nervous system responding in five positive emotions. *Emotion, 11*(6), 1368–1378.

Shweder, R. A., & Sullivan, M. A. (1993). Cultural psychology: Who needs it? *Annual Review of Psychology, 44,* 497–523.

Simon-Thomas, E. R., Keltner, D. J., Sauter, D., Sinicropi-Yao, L., & Abramson, A. (2009). The voice conveys specific emotions: Evidence from vocal burst displays. *Emotion, 9*(6), 838–846.

Small, D. M., Zatorre, R. J., Dagher, A., Evans, A. C., & Jones-Gotman, M. (2001). Changes in brain activity related to eating chocolate: From pleasure to aversion. *Brain, 124,* 1720–1733.

Smith, P. K. (1982). Does play matter?: Functional and evolutionary aspects of animal and human play. *Behavioral and Brain Sciences, 5*(1), 139–184.

Tiedens, L. Z., & Linton, S. (2001). Judgment under emotional certainty and uncertainty: The effects of specific emotions on information processing. *Journal of Personality and Social Psychology, 81*(6), 973–988.

Tomkins, S. S. (1962). *Affect, imagery, and consciousness: Vol. 1. The positive affects.* New York: Springer.

Tomkins, S. S. (1963). *Affect, imagery, and consciousness: Vol. 2. The negative affects.* New York: Springer.

Tooby, J., & Cosmides, L. (2005). Conceptual foundations of evolutionary psychology. In D. M. Buss (Ed.), *The handbook of evolutionary psychology* (pp. 5–67). Hoboken, NJ: Wiley.

Tooby, J., & Cosmides, L. (2008). The evolutionary psychology of the emotions and their relationship to internal regulatory variables. In M. Lewis, J. M. Haviland-Jones, & L. F. Barrett (Eds.), *Handbook of emotions* (3rd ed., pp. 114–137). New York,: Guilford Press.

Tracy, J. L., & Robins, R. W. (2007). The prototypical pride expression: Development of a nonverbal behavior coding system. *Emotion, 7,* 789–801.

Tracy, J. L., & Robins, R. W. (2008). The nonverbal expression of pride: Evidence for cross-cultural recognition. *Journal of Personality and Social Psychology, 94*(3), 516–530.

Trivers, R. L. (1971). The evolution of reciprocal altruism. *Quarterly Review of Biology, 46*(1), 35–57.

Tsai, J. L., Levenson, R. W., & Carstensen, L. L. (2000). Autonomic, subjective, and expressive responses to emotional films in older and younger Chinese Americans and European Americans. *Psychology and Aging, 15*(4), 684–693.

Tugade, M. M., & Fredrickson, B. L. (2004). Resilient individuals use positive emotions to bounce back from negative emotional experiences. *Journal of Personality and Social Psychology, 86*(2), 320–333.

Tugade, M. M., Fredrickson, B. L., & Barrett, L. F. (2004). Psychological resilience and positive emotional granularity: Examining the benefits of positive emotions on coping and health. *Journal of Personality, 72*(6), 1161–1190.

Van der Vegt, B. J., Lieuwes, N., van de Wall, E. H., Kato, K., Moya-Albiol, L., Martínez-Sanchis, S., et al. (2003). Activation of serotonergic neurotransmission during the performance of aggressive behavior in rats. *Behavioral Neuroscience, 117*(4), 667–674.

Williams, L. A., & DeSteno, D. (2008). Pride and perseverance: The motivational role of pride. *Journal of Personality and Social Psychology, 94,* 1007–1017.

Wilson, E. O. (1975). *Sociobiology: The new synthesis.* Cambridge, MA: Harvard University Press.

CHAPTER 4

What Is a Positive Emotion?

The Psychological Construction of Pleasant Fear and Unpleasant Happiness

Paul Condon
Christine D. Wilson-Mendenhall
Lisa Feldman Barrett

Imagine yourself in the following scenarios:

> You are sitting stiffly in a roller coaster car, creeping up one click at a time. You reach the peak of the hill and are suddenly whizzing downwards. Your heart is pounding and your stomach drops as crisp air blasts your face. You *delight* in the uncontrollable *rush* dipping and swirling high above the ground. You feel an *invigorating fear.*

> You are walking down the hall, trying to get to a meeting on time. You run into a difficult colleague and end a tense exchange with a biting remark. Your *stomach tightens* the moment the last sarcastic jab escapes your lips. The *cutting retort echoes poisonously* in your head as your colleague *sulks* away. You feel a *disturbing happiness.*[1]

Humans partition the world into categories. In most scientific models of emotion, *fear, disgust,* and *sadness* are categorized as unpleasant or "negative" emotions; *gratitude, joy,* and *pride* are categorized as pleasant or "positive" emotions.[2] But human experience is more complex and varied.

There are times when negative emotions such as *fear* can feel pleasant (e.g., riding a roller coaster), and positive emotions such as *happiness* can feel unpleasant (e.g., after successfully verbalizing a retort at a difficult person). These examples appear to violate traditional scientific and colloquial understandings of emotion, but they are common in everyday life.

From a cognitive science perspective, it is not surprising to find instances of pleasant fear or unpleasant happiness. Research on concepts and categorization has demonstrated that some instances of a category are more typical, or better examples of the category, than others (see Figure 4.1; Barsalou, 1985; Rosch & Mervis, 1975). For example, apple and orange are more typical instances of the category *fruit* than coconut and olive (Rosch & Mervis, 1975). Likewise, fury and rage are more typical instances of the category *anger* than impatience and resentment (Russell & Fehr, 1994).[3] Categories have a graded structure, which means members of the category have varying degrees of typicality. Some members of a category are less

Fruit TYPICAL **Fear**

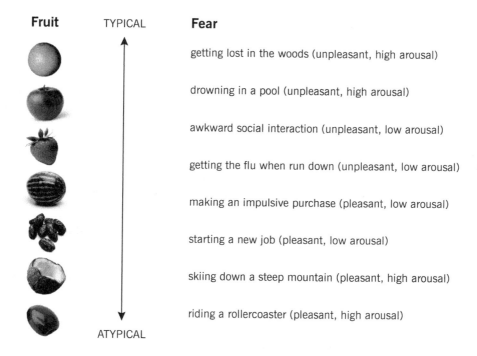

getting lost in the woods (unpleasant, high arousal)

drowning in a pool (unpleasant, high arousal)

awkward social interaction (unpleasant, low arousal)

getting the flu when run down (unpleasant, low arousal)

making an impulsive purchase (pleasant, low arousal)

starting a new job (pleasant, low arousal)

skiing down a steep mountain (pleasant, high arousal)

riding a rollercoaster (pleasant, high arousal)

ATYPICAL

FIGURE 4.1. Items considered typical are rated as good examples of a category. Apples are more typical examples than olives of the category *fruit* (Rosch & Mervis, 1975). Based on the organization of emotion concepts typically found in the affective circumplex (e.g., Russell & Barrett, 1999), unpleasant experiences are more typical examples than pleasant experiences of the category *fear* (situations appear with predicted variations in typicality; Wilson-Mendenhall, Barrett, & Barsalou, 2013a).

typical, or atypical, of the category. The pleasant fear of riding a roller coaster is an atypical example of the categories *positive emotion* and *fear*.

In this chapter, we consider atypical emotions—categories of negative emotion, such as *fear*, which feel pleasant, and categories of positive emotion, such as *happiness*, which feel unpleasant—and focus on the consequences for the study of positive emotion. We first describe our theoretical approach, the conceptual act theory, which emphasizes that variety exists *within* emotion categories (e.g., instances of fear differ from each other). This model defines emotions as psychological constructions that emerge from the categorization of ongoing affective variations of arousal and valence in the body and brain. Next, we discuss the cognitive science literature on concepts and categorization, and explore the notion of typicality. We then discuss a novel approach to concepts called "situated conceptualiza-

tion," which is based on grounded cognition and employed by the Conceptual Act Theory to understand emotion. We then present recent empirical research that demonstrates the reality of atypical emotion experience. In conclusion, we consider how the exploration of atypical emotion may further positive emotion theory and research.

A Psychological Construction Perspective

The construct of atypical emotion contradicts the traditional emotion models that dominated affective science during the 20th century. "Basic emotion" theorists, for example, sought evidence for the universality of six emotion categories: anger, fear, sadness, disgust, joy, and surprise (e.g., Buck, 1999; Davis, 1992; Ekman, 1972; Izard, 1993; LeDoux, 2000; Levenson, 1994; McDougall, 1908/1921; Panksepp, 1998; Tomkins, 1962, 1963). These emotions were considered universal because it was thought that everyone experienced them and they always looked and felt the same, and as a result could be universally recognized by their signs, for example, through facial expressions. Each emotion was thought to manifest from a specific neural network in the brain, with coherent response patterns in autonomic physiology, behavior, and subjective experience (e.g., Ekman, 1972; Izard, 1971; Panksepp, 1998; Tomkins, 1962, 1963). The devotion of a neural network to anger, for example, suggests that anger will always look the same, feel the same, and produce the same actions (barring other processes like "display rules"; e.g., Matsumoto, 1990). Basic emotion theory, therefore, precludes the possibility of atypical emotions. Appraisal models, which also motivated emotion research in the 20th century, assume that patterns of cognitive evaluations produce emotions. In this view, a person's cognitive interpretation of a situation causes different emotions. The experience of being cut off by the driver of another car in busy traffic, for example, could result in anger or fear: Evaluating the other's actions as intentional and conflicting with one's own goal produces anger, whereas evaluating the incident as a threat to one's own life produces fear. Appraisal models allow for great heterogeneity in emotional responding, in principle (e.g., Ellsworth & Scherer, 2003; Frijda, 1986; Scherer, 2009; Smith & Ellsworth, 1985), but these models tend to focus on singular patterns of responding that correspond to the six basic types (cf. Barrett, 2009b). Elsewhere these models have been referred to as "the modal model" (Barrett, Ochsner, & Gross, 2007) or "the natural kinds" model of emotion (Barrett, 2006a).

The empirical evidence to date fails to support the existence of these modal emotion types, however, and points to a more varied and complex emotional life (even when the eliciting conditions are experimentally designed to produce these types). Several literature and meta-analytic reviews have converged on the conclusion that emotions do not correspond with consistent and specific signatures for each emotion category in the brain, peripheral nervous system, voice, or facial expressions (e.g., reviews in chronological order: Duffy, 1934; Hunt, 1941; Mandler, 1975; Ortony & Turner,

1990; Turner & Ortony, 1992; Cacioppo, Berntson, Larsen, Poehlmann, & Ito, 2000; Russell, 2003; Russell, Bachorowski, & Fernandez-Dols, 2003; Barrett, 2006a; Barrett, Lindquist, et al., 2007; Kagan, 2007; Mauss & Robinson, 2009; Barrett, 2011; Lindquist, Wager, Kober, Bliss-Moreau, & Barrett, 2012). Although the modal model still has its advocates (e.g., Ekman & Cordaro, 2011; Panksepp & Watt, 2011; Roseman, 2011; Scherer, 2009; Shariff & Tracy, 2011), alternative psychological construction approaches to emotion have gained substantial empirical support.

Psychological construction models of emotion offer a theoretical position for making a priori predictions about the experience of atypical emotion. Psychological construction models date back to the beginning of psychological science (Gendron & Barrett, 2009) but are not as well known as "basic emotion" and "appraisal" models. Our own version of psychological construction, the Conceptual Act Theory,[4] posits that emotions are not unique mental states, but rather emerge from psychological processes that are not specifically dedicated to emotion. The psychological processes that construct emotion also construct phenomena of the mind that are usually considered nonemotional, for example, *memories, cognitions*, and *perceptions*. Thus, emotions are not realized in dedicated neural circuits or networks but rather are constructed through the interaction of the networks responsible for more basic psychological mechanisms. In this chapter, we focus on two mechanisms that together produce the emergent state of atypical and typical emotions: core affect and conceptualization.

"Core affect" is a state of pleasure or displeasure with some degree of arousal. It is constantly changing based on how homeostatic shifts in the body are represented in the brain (based on how the actual visceral sensory inputs are integrated with prior experience; Barrett, 2006b, 2006c; Russell, 2003; Russell & Barrett, 1999). These homeostatic shifts can occur as a person perceives an object and predicts the best course of action (Barrett & Bar, 2009) because of lack of sleep, or because of glucose depletion or inflammatory processes. Core affect is often described as a basic evaluative process that is performed by the brain; people think that evaluation is a process that contributes to emotion. But evaluation might just be another name for what emotions are. The fact that core affect contributes to the process of valuation does not mean that the brain is performing an ongoing evaluative process that produces changes in core affect. Rather, as emotions unfold, a person's core affective state typically shifts, which means that affect is an important ingredient of emotion. Objects in the world are considered pleasant or unpleasant as a function of their ability to alter core affect. Because scientists can reliably measure core affect, it serves as a neurophysiological barometer of how a person's internal state is becoming linked with the external world (Barrett & Bliss-Moreau, 2009). Physical changes that make up core affect are necessary but not sufficient for an emotion, however. Affective changes must be related to the situation at hand to make a meaningful whole.

A "situation," by definition, includes internal changes in the body and mind, as well as external events in the environment. In an emotion, bodily changes and events in the world are knit together in a conceptualization of a situated affective response. Conceptual interpretation of a situation creates a unified, meaningful representation of subjective experience, cognition, and the body in context (Barsalou, 1999, 2003, 2005; Wilson-Mendenhall, Barrett, Simmons, & Barsalou, 2011). As people experience a situation, they categorize the agents, objects, setting, behaviors, events, properties, relations, bodily states, core affect, mental states, and so forth, that are present (Barsalou, 1999, 2003, 2005; Wilson-Mendenhall et al., 2011). As patterns of brain activity occur across multiple modalities (sensation, perception, action, core affect, attention, etc.), the brain uses prior experience in these modalities, in the form of conceptual knowledge, to conceptualize the current situation. People develop concepts for emotions (e.g., *anger, fear, pride*) as they do many other aspects of experience that are concrete (e.g., *car, chair, apple, trumpet*) or abstract (e.g., *gossip, truth, science, meeting*). When a pattern of activity is similar to an instance of an emotion stored in memory (including the context), the information stored in that instance becomes active to guide behavior. When this occurs, it often shifts core affect, perceptual construal, actions, executive functioning, and so on, because the concept

produces inferences about how the body and mind should respond in the situation (based on prior knowledge). The conceptualization functions as a prediction for appropriate action. This often occurs without awareness, although it is possible to shift conceptualizations consciously. Through conceptualization, bodily changes become tied to events in the external world as a coherent (and often complex) aspect of experience. Affect becomes conceptualized in relation to the immediate situation and produces an emergent state that is an atypical or typical emotion.

Unlike the "basic emotion" and "appraisal" approaches to emotion, the conceptual act theory makes precise predictions about heterogeneity within emotion categories (Barrett, 2009b, 2013). The conceptual act theory, through its emphasis on conceptualization, explains how and why different instances of the same emotion category might feel and look nothing alike. Different patterns of brain activity, or instances, include situational context and become associated with one emotion category. In turn, each emotion category is represented by many instances across diverse contexts. The heterogeneity within an emotion category is extremely important because it allows humans to tailor actions to the situation. One would respond differently during the thrilling fear of a roller-coaster ride compared with the terrorizing fear of driving an uncontrollable car. Although riding a giant roller coaster and driving a dysfunctional car both elicit fear, those fears feel and look very different from one another. In summary, the conceptual act theory defines an emotion as a conceptual act involving the relation of bodily changes to external events. Thus, the science of concepts proves important to this model and makes clear predictions about the existence of atypical emotions. We next discuss the nature of concepts as understood in cognitive science.

Concepts

Concepts make human activity meaningful from the mundane to the complex, from the individual to the social, and, in relation to emotion, concepts render affective changes in the body and brain meaningful. Concepts enable humans to integrate incoming information, categorize novel experiences based on their similarity to past experience, and make predictions about how to act. Consider what it means to have a concept for *apple*. The concept *apple* allows a person to discern an apple from another fruit, such as a tomato. The ability to store the concept *apple* in long-term memory allows a person to make such distinctions automatically. Furthermore, activation of the concept *apple* across contexts can lead to different behaviors, such as eating an apple for lunch or bobbing for an apple at a carnival. Thus, concepts have adaptive function. Likewise, the activation of emotion concepts such as *anger* or *surprise* creates the perception of these emotions in the affective changes within the self and in others (Barrett, 2012; Barrett, Mesquita, & Gendron, 2011). Emotion concepts make affective changes in the body meaningful, guide action, allow communication about one's state to another, and influence another's mental state and actions (Barrett, 2012). Although the importance of conceptualization is undisputed, the *nature* of concepts and how they are instantiated via cognitive processes has been debated for centuries (Murphy, 2002).

Aristotle was the first to argue that concepts are rooted in a definition, and philosophers who followed agreed that definitions were the appropriate way to assign category membership (Murphy, 2002). The complicated nature of concepts is made apparent, however, exactly when attempting to define one. In a famous argument, the philosopher Ludwig Wittgenstein (1953) demonstrated that activities categorized as a *game* fail to conform to any specific definition. No conceptual core captures every instance that falls into the category *game* and excludes every instance that does not fall in the category *game*. The elements of a game, such as play, competition, or sport, all fail to define *game* because activities referred to as *game* do not include all of these elements, and sporting activities that are not considered games (e.g., hunting) often do. Even attempts to define concrete concepts, such as *chair*, fail to encompass all the different objects that could be categorized as a chair, and likewise fail to exclude instances that are non-chairs. There is no conceptual core, such as "four legs with a back" that allows one to discriminate chairs from another piece of furniture,

such as a couch or stool. Definitions also fail to include atypical cases such as a car seat, which does not have four legs, and fail to exclude nonmembers of the category, such as a dog, which does have four legs and a back. Concepts have also eluded definition in the realm of emotion (although basic emotion theories essentially propose definitions for emotions). *Love*, for example, has been the target of definitional attempts by philosophers and psychologists for many years, yet no consensus ever emerged (Fehr & Russell, 1991). In summary, the search for necessary and sufficient conditions for inclusion in a conceptual category fails; definitions fail to include all instances of a category and fail to exclude nonmembers of a category (Murphy, 2002).

The argument that concepts are represented as definitions has fallen out of favor both in cognitive science (Murphy, 2002) and as an approach to emotion concepts (Niedenthal, 2008; Russell, 1991). This approach has since been dubbed the classical view of concepts (Murphy, 2002). Two theses of the classical view, in particular, demonstrate why definitions are not useful as representations of concepts. The classical view assumes that every object is either in or not in the category of interest, leaving no room for in-between cases. The classical view also precludes distinction between category members; anything that meets the definition of the category is just as good a category member as anything else. Any two objects that meet the requirements of a definition are equally good examples of the category, and any two objects that do not fit the definition are equally bad members of the category. This assumption suggests that the fear of driving a dysfunctional car on a busy highway and the fear of riding a roller coaster in a theme park are equally good examples of the category *fear*, whereas situations that constitute any other emotion are equally bad examples of *fear*. The classical view does not distinguish typical from atypical members of a category.

The empirical data examining mental representation of concepts have proven the classical view incorrect. Research in the 1970s largely derailed the classical view by demonstrating that people do not rely on definitions in their cognitive representation of categories. Rosch and colleagues (Rosch, 1975;

Rosch & Mervis, 1975) found evidence for typicality effects by asking people to rate how good an example various members (e.g., oriole, penguin) were of the category (e.g., *bird*). Participants rated examples such as *robin* and *oriole* as very typical, but other examples, such as *penguin* and *ostrich*, as atypical. With respect to emotions, participants rated *maternal love* and *friendship* as better examples of *love* than *patriotic love* or *love of work* (Fehr & Russell, 1991). Participants also rated *fury* as a better example of the category *anger* than *impatience* (Russell & Fehr, 1994). According to the classical view, however, a robin and a penguin are equally good examples of *bird* and maternal love and patriotic love are equally good examples of *love*. It is quite clear that people do not subscribe to this view.

Objects can be close to a prototype (i.e., the ideal or best example of a given category), moderately close, or atypical (i.e., not very close).[5] Cases that are equally distant from the prototypes of two different categories are considered borderline for each category. This variation in typicality among members of a category is consequential for many reasons. In general, when a task requires someone to relate an item to a category, the item's typicality influences performance (Murphy, 2002). When learning artificial categories, people learn typical items before atypical ones, and they learn categories more quickly when they learn typical items first (Rosch, Simpson, & Miller, 1976). Finally, typical items are also more useful for inferences about category members (Rips, 1975). Similar effects have been found with emotion concepts. Participants who read narratives about various gratitude experiences reported that narratives containing central, compared to peripheral, features would induce greater feelings of gratitude among the protagonist (Lambert, Graham, & Fincham, 2009). For the emotion categories *love* and *anger*, typicality predicted how awkward a sentence appeared when a subtype was substituted for the category in a sentence (Fehr & Russell, 1991; Russell & Fehr, 1994). For example, the sentence "*Romantic love* has to be worked at and strived for to be truly achieved" was rated as less awkward than "*Infatuation* has to be worked at and strived for to be truly achieved." Typicality also predicted participants' ability to recall

statements about an emotional experience of *compassionate love* (Fehr & Sprecher, 2009). Thus, typicality influences a range of judgments about instances of an emotion category.

The ubiquity of typicality across all categories raises questions about what causes variation in typicality. Why is *olive* considered an atypical instance of the category *fruit*, whereas *apple* is considered typical? Why is the *pleasant fear* of riding a roller-coaster atypical, compared with the *unpleasant fear* of running for one's life? Rosch and Mervis provided the first explanation for typicality effects: Items are typical when they have high *family resemblance* with other members of the category (Rosch & Mervis, 1975), which means that a given item shares a high number of properties with other members of the category. Typical items tend to share properties with other category members but tend not to share properties with category nonmembers. This view explains why commonly encountered examples of a category are not necessarily typical examples of the category. Chickens are fairly common birds, for example, but they do not have common bird properties (e.g., ability to fly) (Rosch & Mervis, 1975). Likewise, the pleasant fear of risk taking or riding a roller-coaster might be a common experience, but pleasant fear does not share many properties with other members of the *fear* category. In particular, *pleasant fear* does not share the valence attribute with instances of fear that are unpleasant. Variations in arousal may also predict typicality of emotion experiences (e.g., *low arousal fear* of an awkward social interaction). The family resemblance view predicts that pleasant fear and low arousal fear are atypical emotions, and that these instances will be more similar to other categories (e.g., excitement).

Other factors beyond family resemblance cause variation in typicality. Three possible determinants of graded structure of concepts received attention: *central tendency, ideals,* and *frequency of instantiation* (Barsalou, 1985). An object's central tendency is similar to its family resemblance but encompasses any kind of central tendency information (average, median, or modal values on dimensions; highly probable properties; etc.). "Familiarity" refers to a person's subjective estimate of how often he or she has experienced an entity across all contexts, whereas frequency of instantiation is the same person's subjective estimate of how often he or she has experienced an object as a member of a *particular category*. Barsalou (1985) suggested that frequency of instantiation is more important than familiarity in determining typicality. "Ideals" are characteristics that objects should have to best serve a goal associated with their category. Barsalou proposed, for example, the ideal for *foods to eat on a diet* is *zero calories*. The fewer calories an object has, the better it serves the goal associated with the category (i.e., *losing weight*). Objects with decreasing numbers of calories become increasingly good examples, and are therefore more typical of the category *foods to eat on a diet*. If a person's goal is *thrill seeking*, then pleasant fear may become a typical instance of fear (ideals are probably a major reason that people believe in basic emotions, an issue we raise below). The typicality of a given instance is dynamic and will fluctuate depending on context.

Different factors can influence typicality depending on the type of category in question. Whereas central tendency and familiarity determine typicality in common taxonomic categories (categories that have a structured hierarchy, e.g., in biology: kingdom, phylum, class, order, family, genus, species), ideals are more likely to determine typicality in goal-derived categories (e.g., *foods not to eat on a diet, things to take from one's home during a fire*) (Barsalou, 1985). To test the hypothesis that ideals predict typicality better than central tendency or frequency of instantiation for goal-derived categories, prior work examined the correlation of central tendency, ideals, and frequency of instantiation with typicality ratings for various objects (Barsalou, 1985). Participants generated instances of various categories (e.g., *birthday presents, clothes to wear in the snow, birds, fruit*) and judged them on questions that assessed (1) the instance's similarity to the category's central tendency, (2) the instance's similarity to ideals related to the goals served by the category, and (3) subjective estimates of how often the instance occurred as a member of the category. For example, a participant might have generated the instance "penguin" for the category *bird*, a taxonomic category, and the instance "necktie" for the category

birthday presents, a goal-derived category. The participant then made ratings, such as "How good an example is 'penguin' of the category *bird*?" (typicality); "How frequently does 'penguin' appear as a member the category *bird*?" (frequency of instantiation); and "*How colorful is a* 'penguin'?" or "*How thoughtful is the gift of a* 'necktie'?" (ideals). Family resemblance (central tendency) scores were calculated from a series of similarity judgments comparing all possible pairs of the generated instances (e.g., "*How similar are penguin and oriole?*"). Taxonomic and goal-derived categories differed in determinants of typicality. For common taxonomic categories (e.g., *bird*), central tendency accounted for the greatest amount of unique variance, although ideals and frequency also accounted for a significant amount of variance in typicality. For goal-derived categories (e.g., *clothes to wear in the snow*), ideals and frequency independently predicted variance in typicality, but central tendency did not. Thus, the factors that determine typicality depend on the nature of the category.

Ideals also causally determine variance in typicality ratings. An experimental study investigated the typicality of ideal instances of two novel categories that comprised different people (Barsalou, 1985). In one category, all members *jogged*. In another category, all members *read the newspaper*. Different members of each category performed their respective activities daily, weekly, or monthly. These categories were learned under two different conditions. In a *related dimension condition*, half of the participants were told that the category defined by jogging was *physical education teachers*, while the category defined by reading the newspaper was *current events teachers*. In an *unrelated dimension condition*, participants believed that Q *programmers* comprised a category of people who jogged while Z *programmers* comprised a category of people who read the newspapers. After learning these categories, participants were asked to rate how good an example of the category an individual person was (e.g., "How good of an example is John Davis of the category *physical education teacher*?"). As predicted, the rate at which each person performed the key activity (jogging, reading the newspaper) determined the typicality of that person for the category only in the *related dimension category*, not the *unrelated dimension category*. This makes sense because those people were the ideals represented by the category (i.e., people who jog daily are considered typical examples of physical education teachers, whereas people who jog less are considered atypical examples of physical education teachers). Thus, ideals determined typicality when defining dimensions of the category were related to participants' stereotypes for the category. Central tendency had a greater influence on typicality ratings when subjects did not have ideals for the categories (because jogging and reading the newspaper have little relation to the ideals of programming different computer languages).

The variables that determine typicality may also differ depending on the person's mindset or expertise with the categories and objects at hand. Tree experts relied on ideals, whereas novices relied on familiarity, for example, when rating the typicality of trees (Lynch, Coley, & Medin, 2000). The extent to which trees fulfilled the ideal dimensions of *height* and *weediness* correlated with experts' typicality ratings of the trees; however, familiarity was the sole predictor of typicality for tree novices. The influence of knowledge or mindset would likely generalize to typicality judgments of emotion categories. If one's ideal dimension for *positive emotion* includes *bring about desirable consequences*, then states such as compassion and gratitude might be rated as the most typical positive emotions. The focus on downstream consequences, for example, represents the rubric for analyzing mental states in the Abhidharma, a Buddhist compendium of mental states (Dreyfus, 2002; Dreyfus & Thompson, 2007). Empirical analysis of the emotion concept *gratitude* also provided indirect evidence for typicality effects depending on knowledge (i.e., differences between ordinary people and researchers) (Lambert et al., 2009). Ordinary people include generalized gratitude (e.g., feeling grateful for one's stock in life) among their emotion concepts. Emotion researchers, however, limit their definitions of gratitude to those experiences that result from specific benefits given by another person. Lambert and colleagues (2009) suggested that narrow definitions benefit empirical research through the ability to examine correlates and consequences of gratitude. In this example, benefit-triggered gratitude is related to the ideal *states conducive to laboratory study*.

Summary

The classical view of concepts failed because it did not predict the continuum of typicality that category members exhibit. The classical view, for example, does not distinguish between pleasant and unpleasant fear, and suggests that these experiences are equally good examples of the *fear* category. Despite this knowledge about the varied instances within categories, scientists have relentlessly pursued the typical or ideal instances of emotion experiences. Instances of each basic emotion category (i.e., fear, anger, sadness, disgust, joy, surprise) are the ideals of those categories. These are the instances that most people consider the clearest cases of emotion that necessarily have all of the component parts (Russell, 2003; Russell & Barrett, 1999). The ideal fear experience, for example, is one that motivates fleeing or fighting behavior upon encountering a threat in the environment (such as a bear or snake) and is accompanied by a very specific facial expression (i.e., widened eyes, open mouth) and physiological profile (e.g., increased heart rate, blood pressure, and skin conductance). Ideal episodes are quite rare in everyday life, however, and fear experiences and expressions are much more varied. In general, the ideal of a category is not the one that is most frequently encountered, but the one that maximally achieves the goal that the category is organized around (Baraslou, 1985, 2003). On the other hand, atypical experiences of emotion categories might be quite common in everyday life. We next turn to a situated view of concepts and discuss how emotions can be understood as conceptual acts situated in an environment. This perspective provides the theoretical basis for studying atypical emotions.

Situated Conceptualization

In a situated view of concepts, the situational context is integrated with the representation of a concept. This has been called "situated conceptualization" (Barsalou, 2003, 2005,

2008), which means that concepts are rooted in an environmental context and typically include a setting, agents, objects, behaviors, events, and internal states, each represented by relevant concepts. Representations of concepts are flexible across situations, and widely varying sets of background concepts contextualize them in each situation. The representation of *apple*, for example, exists within a network of background concepts representing elements of the entire situation. A given representation of *apple* includes concepts for a setting (e.g., *grocery store, orchard, classroom, dinner table*), concepts for internal features of the body and mind (e.g., *feeling satiated, craving*), and events (e.g., *buying, picking, eating*). Just as there are different types of apples, so too there are different situated conceptualizations of different apples. The varied environmental and social situations in which an instance of a category can occur illuminate the variety of experiences within one category.

Situated conceptualizations explain representations of abstract concepts as well. Abstract concepts refer to an entire situation, not just part of one. *Game*, for example, is represented as a situated conceptualization. *Game* integrates an agent, other people, objects, competing or collaborating, a goal, and so forth (cf. Wilson-Mendenhall, Simmons, et al., 2013). Abstract concepts such as *game* involve relational structures that integrate and organize information in situated conceptualizations. For each situation to which the category *game* applies, there will be different situated conceptualizations, with some being more typical than others. Thus, a situated conceptualization view can accommodate the various instances in which an abstract concept occurs. So too, emotions are abstract concepts that can be represented as situated conceptualizations, with some conceptualizations being more typical than others.

Emotions as Situated Conceptualizations

The conceptual act theory postulates that emotions are situated conceptualizations that function to give meaning to affective changes in the body and brain, guide behavior, allow communication, and aid social influence (Barrett, 2006b, 2012). Across the lifespan, people experience many of the same situations on several occasions. Knowledge about these situations becomes entrenched in memory, thereby supporting skilled performance in the same situations and novel ones that are similar. Situated conceptualizations represent this knowledge of repeated situations. Over time, patterns of perceptual symbols and simulations across modalities automatically trigger the situated conceptualizations for some activity. The first time a child experiences a core affective state of high arousal and displeasure combined with information conveyed by his or her caretakers and culture, he or she might learn that the experience is fear. As environmental and psychological situations are encountered and repeated over time, experiences become associated with the word "fear," and the individual develops situated conceptualizations of fear and uses this knowledge to guide responding in similar and novel situations. A situated conceptualization triggers when a complex simulation becomes active across modalities (Barsalou, 1999, 2003, 2005). These processes often occur without awareness—the brain always categorizes and conceptualizes experience to guide a response (Barsalou, 1999).

An emotion concept such as *fear* or *happiness* is represented across a number of modality-specific systems and includes a subjective phenomenological feeling, a representation of the events that led up to the emotion, features in the environment attended to, a relationship to an event or person, probabilistic behaviors that follow, and any other objects or dimensions of experience in the environment. In heightened states of core affect, people automatically and effortlessly categorize their state using conceptual knowledge about emotion (Barrett, 2006b). The conceptualization of an emotion state can also produce heightened core affect if other aspects of the situation trigger the conceptualization first. The activation of conceptual knowledge of *fear*, for example, determines when core affect will be experienced as fear rather than anger or excitement (Lindquist & Barrett, 2008a). Simulating an experience of *fear* in one's mind, absent of physical events in the environment, can also cause shifts in core affect.

The construct of situated conceptualization addresses two central predictions about emotion that stem from the Conceptual Act

Theory. First, because situations can vary, a single emotion category will include a range of situated conceptualizations. This means there is potential for considerable variability of experience within one emotion category. Consider *sadness*. After a short night of sleep, someone might wade through a crowded cafe to obtain a cup of coffee, only to realize that he forgot his wallet at the office, thereby activating a relevant situated conceptualization for sadness. The person's core affect shifts into a highly unpleasant state and might encourage him to give up the pursuit for coffee and opt for rest. The situated conceptualization may engage attention to focus on the lack of energy and thereby recruit a compensatory strategy to rest, which could replenish energy for more productive work at a later time. During this evolving process, the chatter of colleagues or supervisors and other information in the environment (e.g., a stack of papers, a list of e-mails) may be construed as overwhelming and taxing. As a result, core affect might shift into feelings of strong negative valence, which initially encourage retreat from normal activity and decrease arousal significantly, but then motivate subsequent actions, such as searching memory and environment for resources to restore one's affective state or gain new resources. Analogously, if someone reflects on losing a loved one, a relevant situated conceptualization for sadness in this situation becomes active. During this evolving process, one may interpret memories as knowledge that there can never be another interaction. When sharing this situation with a mutual friend, however, the person may celebrate and tribute the lost other; as a result, one's core affective state may shift into feelings of pleasant valence (for similar descriptions of situated conceptualizations for *fear*, see Wilson-Mendenhall et al., 2011). Both experiences may evoke *sadness*, but the phenomenal experience, the core affective state, and the behavioral outcomes during the emotional experience may differ. The first includes a sense of desperation, whereas the other includes a sense of longing. In one situation, one may wish to end the pursuit for coffee and opt for rest; in the other, one may wish to celebrate or pay tribute to the loved one. Within an emotion category, a number of situations with different contexts will name the same emotion but

look, feel, and change behavior in different ways.

The second prediction of the conceptual act theory that stems from the situated conceptualization approach is that an instance of any emotion category can be pleasant or unpleasant. That is, the valence within a category, such as *fear*, is variable. The valence of an emotional experience is determined by core affect, which is pleasant or unpleasant, and functions as a critical feature of any emotion concept that is activated as part of the situated conceptualization. Perhaps the most well-known organization of emotion categories—within the affective circumplex structured by valence and arousal—is driven by prototypical episodes (Russell & Barrett, 1999). Prototypical *fear* experiences, for example, are unpleasant and highly arousing: the alarm of an animal poised to attack, the terror of being held at gunpoint, the panic of losing control of a car. Nonetheless, atypical *fear* experiences are sometimes pleasant: the scary thrill of zipping downward on a roller-coaster, the nervous exhilaration of performing before a crowd, one's apprehensive vivacity before competing in a sporting event. Consider parallel examples for *happiness*. Typical *happiness* experiences are pleasant and arousing: the glowing gratification of scoring high on a test, the warm delight of spending time with loved ones during a holiday, the sunny cheerfulness that a long-awaited vacation brings. Nonetheless, atypical happiness experiences are sometimes unpleasant: the exhausting relief of finishing a time-consuming project, the freeing reprieve of friend's comforting words when distressed, the uneasy goodbyes when moving away for a dream job. In these cases, the feeling of happiness appears to shift valence upward (toward pleasant), but it is a relative shift that tends to make the feeling tone simply less unpleasant. Thus, as situated experiences develop for the concepts *fear, anger, gratitude*, and *joy* over time, there is an expansion of emotional experiences, some pleasant and others unpleasant, that fall into each category.

The construct of an atypical emotion raises questions about the trajectory of affective experience during a particular emotional episode. In this view (and consistent with other constructionist views; e.g., Kirkland & Cunningham, 2012), various elements of situated conceptualizations change dynamically across time. A person's experience of *fear*, for example, may dynamically shift as an emotional episode unfolds. For example, core affect may change as an emotional episode unfolds, shifting as different elements of the situated conceptualization unfold, foregrounded or backgrounded by attention. When elements of a situation are similar to a situated conceptualization of an emotion in memory, this situated conceptualization becomes active, but it is dynamically changing. A situated conceptualization for sadness may become active when one thinks about a loved one who passed away during a holiday. This is not a static process, however; the affective trajectory (including other facets of the situation) are dynamically changing. As one initially thinks about the loved one who passed away, core affect shifts to unpleasant, but when a specific memory of the loved one laughing during a funny tradition arises, the core affect may shift to pleasant. Core affect is shifting as conceptualization of the elements in the situation occurs, which could produce atypical emotion experiences such as pleasant sadness. When a complex emotion is learned, it appears that the situated conceptualization that becomes entrenched in memory is capturing a trajectory across time, which includes the way elements of the situation are changing.

For atypical emotions, it appears that slight changes in how facets of the situation are being conceptualized (perhaps due to attentional focus) may easily change the emotion concept that becomes active to guide interpretation of the situation (i.e., it is more likely that the situation could be conceptualized as different emotions). In this way, the situations in which atypical emotions are grounded often seem more ambiguous. The pleasant experience of riding a roller coaster, for example, can be conceptualized as an atypical instance of *pleasant fear* or a typical instance of *excitement*, depending on the how elements of the situation are conceptualized. The ability to conceptualize a situation flexibly may also underscore various forms of emotion regulation (see Barrett, Wilson-Mendenhall, & Barsalou, 2014). Of course, these points are theoretical conjectures and await empirical investigation.

A long-standing debate in affective science concerns whether pleasant and unpleasant affect vary along one continuous bipolar dimension (i.e., pleasant to unpleasant affect) or along two separate and independent dimensions, one each for pleasant and unpleasant affect (e.g., Cacioppo, Gardner, & Berntson, 1997, 1999; Larsen, McGraw, & Cacioppo, 2001; Larsen & Stastny, 2011; Nowlis & Nowlis, 1956; Russell & Carroll, 1999). The existence of two unipolar dimensions suggests that mixed emotions result from an amalgam of multiple conceptualizations of the same situation. Rather, a bipolar dimension precludes the possibility of mixed emotions and leads one to consider the possibility of atypical emotions. This debate about "mixed emotions" versus "atypical emotions" can be resolved by considering the fact that a person cannot be aware of two scenes, or objects, or percepts within the same modality at exactly the same moment in time (as illustrated by a Necker cube, Gestalt images such as the young lady/old lady ambiguous figure, and incongruent inputs into two eyes in studies of binocular rivalry). Conscious experience can move at great speed (estimated at 100–150 milliseconds per conscious moment; Edelman & Tononi, 2000; Gray, 2004), so that pleasant and unpleasant experiences can come in and out of focus quickly, like different perceptions of a Necker cube. Research that limits the time window to momentary experience does not find dialectic representations at single moments (Miyamoto, Uchida, & Ellsworth, 2010; Scollon, Diener, Oishi, & Biswas-Diener, 2005; Yik, Russell, & Barrett, 1999). Thus, it is unlikely that pleasure and displeasure co-occur in real time, although people can quickly shift from one experience to another and summarize all of the contents in working memory (Barrett, Mesquita, Ochsner, & Gross, 2007). The same argument can be made about emotional complexity, or feeling more than one emotion at once (Charles, 2005).

Summary

The situated conceptualization view of emotion differs from other theories of emotion. Whereas the "modal model" or "natural kinds" views suggest that evolved mechanisms such as affect programs (i.e., basic emotion theories) or cognitive appraisals (i.e., appraisal theories) produce the prototypical or ideal instances of emotion categories, the conceptual act theory emphasizes basic ingredients (i.e., core affect and conceptualization) as the mechanisms that produce an emergent state of emotion. This theory argues that evolution resulted in these basic ingredients rather than specific mechanisms dedicated to each discrete emotion category. While some appraisal models do acknowledge heterogeneity (e.g., Clore & Ortony, 2008; Ellsworth & Scherer, 2003; Frijda, 1986; Scherer, 2009), most of the "modal models" of emotion downplay the importance of variation within one category (cf. Barrett, 2009b). The conceptual act theory is unique in emphasizing the variation in experience within one category. Of greatest import, the emphasis on atypical emotions offers a dynamic theoretical basis for better understanding complex and apparently ambiguous emotional states.

Empirical Investigations of Atypical Emotions

Atypical Fear, Sadness, and Happiness and Their Neural Correlates

Because so little work has addressed the atypical instances of emotion, a first step is to investigate whether people are familiar with such experiences, and whether they find laboratory examples compelling. As part of a larger study, Wilson-Mendenhall, Barrett, and Barsalou (2013a) examined typical and atypical instances of fear, sadness, and happiness. They defined typical emotional experiences as fear, sadness, or happiness that evoked the valence that has been used for classification within the affective circumplex (i.e., unpleasant fear, unpleasant sadness, pleasant happiness). They defined atypical emotional experiences as instances of fear, sadness, or happiness that were opposite in valence to the typical examples, that is, pleasant fear, pleasant sadness, and unpleasant happiness. Table 4.1 presents an example atypical and typical scenario for each emotion category. Participants listened to auditorily presented typical and atypical scenarios designed to induce familiar, vivid experiences of fear, sadness, or happiness (Wilson-Mendenhall et al., 2013a). They were encouraged to

TABLE 4.1. Example Atypical and Typical Scenarios

Atypical scenarios

You are jogging onto the soccer field, your cleats digging into the firm ground. *You hear a booming voice welcome the crowd to the state championship.* You jump in place to shake off the restlessness in your stomach. Looking around at your team, a rushing excitement deepens your competitive fire. *You feel an energizing fear.*

You are standing on your college quad, dressed in a smart looking cap and gown. *You listen for the graduation decree and upon hearing it fling your cap upward.* Following energetic classmates, you sweat lightly as you march away a graduate. You catch a friend's eye and flashback to your delightfully lively freshman dorm. *You feel a spirited sadness.*

You are walking down the hall, trying to get to a meeting on time. *You run into a difficult colleague and end a tense exchange with a biting remark.* Your stomach tightens the moment the last sarcastic jab escapes your lips. The cutting retort echoes poisonously in your head as your colleague sulks away. *You feel a disturbing happiness.*

Typical scenarios

You are walking to your car alone, the city parking deck dimly lit. *You hear an explosive bang and see a man running with a pointed gun.* You quickly drop behind a car and attempt to control your shallow breathing. You try to dismiss the horrendous vision of what will happen if he finds you. *You feel a perilous fear.*

You are walking into a friend's house, dropping by to return a movie. *You witness your significant other in an intimate embrace with your friend.* Your stomach is nauseated, the shocking infidelity settling into your body. Your mind is spinning trying to understand the terrible betrayal of trust. *You feel a devastating sadness.*

You are performing a challenging piano solo, your fingers working the keys. *You finish the piece and receive thunderous applause as you rise.* You bend at the waist into a deep bow and sense your heart thumping rapidly. Glowing with satisfaction, you continue to feed off the crowd's energy. *You feel a proud happiness.*

Note. Scenarios also systematically varied in arousal. For comparison, all the examples shown here are high arousal. From Wilson-Mendenhall, Barrett, and Barsalou (2013). Copyright 2013 by C. D. Wilson-Mendenhall, L. F. Barrett, and L. W. Barsalou. Adapted by permission.

immerse themselves in each scenario as they listened with eyes closed, and experience the scenario as if it were actually happening to them, in as much vivid detail as possible. Participants tended to rate both the typical and atypical instances of each emotion as familiar and relatively easy to immerse oneself in (i.e., "being there" immersed in the feeling). Although it might come as a surprise that atypical instances were not rated as relatively less familiar than typical instances, typicality is often not driven by frequency or familiarity (see the earlier discussion of typicality determinants). Chicken is an atypical instance of the category bird, for example, but chickens are familiar birds to most people (Rosch, 1975). In a similar fashion, the thrill of riding a roller-coaster may be an atypical instance of fear, but it is a familiar experience for most people. Because this initial evidence suggests that atypical scenarios are familiar and compelling, it highlights the importance of studying the variability within emotion categories.

Psychological construction approaches predict that tremendous variety in emotional life exists because coordinated and interacting neural systems produce countless possible emotional experiences (Barrett, 2009a, 2009b, 2013). Consistent with this view, recent meta-analyses of emotion experience implicate many of the anatomically inspired, large-scale networks robustly identified in resting state data (Kober et al., 2008; Lindquist et al., 2012). Little is known, however, about how these distributed networks function to produce the variety of emotions that people routinely experience in the real world. Because typicality is an important dimension for characterizing variability in emotional experience, Wilson-Mendenhall and colleagues (2013a) investigated whether this within-category factor predicts neural activity in large-scale brain networks.

To compare the underlying neural processes engaged during atypical versus typical emotional experiences, the relative differences in activity within specific large-scale networks were examined for atypical versus typical instances of fear, sadness, and happiness (collapsed across the three categories). Wilson-Mendenhall and colleagues (2013a) predicted and found that atypical instances (vs. typical instances) were associated with heightened activity in the "default mode" network (Buckner, Andrews-Hanna, & Schacter, 2008) as participants immersed themselves in the scenarios. As Figure 4.2A illustrates, reliably greater activity was observed in the core midline default network hubs, medial prefrontal cortex and posterior cingulate, and also in other network regions, including dorsomedial prefrontal cortex, left temporal pole, and bilateral posterior superior temporal sulcus (STS)/temporal–parietal junction (TPJ). These regions map onto what has recently been distinguished as a subsystem of the default network that is robustly active during mental state inference and social cognition (Andrews-Hanna, Reidler, Sepulcre, Poulin, & Buckner, 2010). Modern psychological construction theories emphasize this network's role in conceptualizing affective states to produce situated emotions (e.g., Barrett, 2006b, 2012; Barrett & Satpute, 2013). Recent meta-analyses support this view, showing consistent activity in the default network during emotional experiences (Kober et al., 2008; Lindquist et al., 2012). Furthermore, social cognition research has repeatedly demonstrated default network involvement in the social inference and contextual grounding that supports self-projection into a situation (Andrews-Hanna et al., 2010; Bar, 2007; Buckner & Carroll, 2007; Harrison et al., 2008; Mitchell, 2009). Significantly greater activity in the "default" network during scenario immersion suggests that the situations evoking atypical emotional experiences require greater social inference and contextual grounding as the self-relevant emotional experience is being constructed.

Furthermore, Wilson-Mendenhall and colleagues (2013a) predicted and found that atypical (vs. typical) instances were associated with heightened activity in the salience network when participants were asked to rate the pleasantness or unpleasantness of their emotional experiences when immersed in each scenario. "Salience" refers to the process by which highly processed sensory information is integrated with visceral, autonomic, and hedonic information to inform decision making (Menon & Uddin, 2010; Seeley et al., 2007). Because valence is the prominent feature that makes the instance atypical, it was hypothesized that focusing on the affective feeling would place greater demands on integrating shifting body sig-

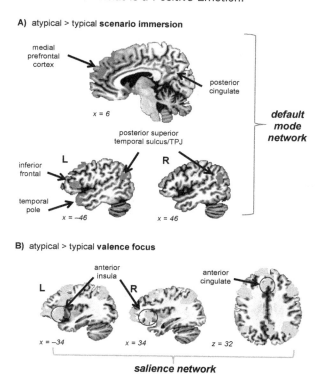

FIGURE 4.2. Comparison of neural activity during atypical versus typical emotional experiences. From Wilson-Mendenhall, Barrett, and Barsalou (2013b).

nals with the sensory and social context constructed during scenario immersion (to inform valence judgments). Illustrated in Figure 4.2B, activity was observed in the anterior insula and anterior cingulate, hubs in the salience network (Seeley et al., 2007).

Consistent with other recent work in social neuroscience, this study suggests that it is critical to study dimensions of socioemotional experiences, such as typicality and ambiguity (Jenkins & Mitchell, 2010), in addition to types of social cognition (e.g., emotions, beliefs, preferences). Emotions are traditionally discussed as distinct from other forms of cognition. As discussed in this chapter, though, another view is that conceptualization processes operate similarly during emotional and other forms of experience (e.g., Lindquist & Barrett, 2008a; Wilson-Mendenhall et al., 2011). The importance of typicality, as a property of categories, is clear in cognitive science research: It is one of the most important predictors of performance on categorization

tasks (category learning, verification, etc.). As demonstrated in this study, typicality also predicts patterns of brain activity, suggesting that it deserves further study in the domain of emotions.

Conceptualizing and Experiencing Compassion

In recent work, we also explored variations in valence among instances of the emotion category *compassion* (Condon & Barrett, in press). Compassion is usually categorized as a positive emotion, but it may feel unpleasant in some instances. In one study, laboratory inductions of compassion that featured images depicting poverty and vulnerable infants simultaneously increased reports of compassion and distress (Simon-Thomas et al., 2012). Yet previous research has demonstrated that people categorize compassion as being similar to other pleasant feelings, such as love and warmth (Shaver, Schwartz, Kirson, & O'Connor, 1987). These divergent findings suggest that experiences of compassion may differ from the prototypical representation of compassion obtained from semantic comparisons of emotion states. We predicted and found that the category *compassion* includes pleasant and unpleasant instances of experience, but prototypical conceptualizations of compassion are pleasant.

To examine prototypical conceptualizations of compassion, we asked people to rate the similarity of the feeling *compassionate* to a number of other emotion-related adjectives (e.g., *sad, distressed, happy, sad, grateful*) following *neutral* and *compassion* emotion inductions. We also asked the same people to rate their own internal state along a variety of typical positive (e.g., *excited, happy, grateful*) and typical negative (e.g., *angry, afraid, sad*) emotion categories. Both sets of judgments followed laboratory-based *compassion* or *neutral* inductions that included audio clips of people describing events from their lives. Neutral stories focused on themes related to encounters with famous people and events related to work. Compassion stories focused on themes related to others' suffering through disease and loss.

Multidimensional scaling analyses of the similarity judgments rendered two-dimensional maps of the emotion concepts in relation to each other, which yields a prototypical conceptualization of the emotion concepts. Consistent with prior work, these similarity ratings were best depicted using a two-dimensional solution, in which one dimension represented arousal (e.g., alert/excited at one end and quiet/tired at the other) and the other valence (e.g., sad/afraid at one end and happy/grateful at the other). Across all conditions, compassion was located in the low arousal, pleasant quadrant on the circumplex, suggesting that people typically conceptualize compassion as pleasant even after exposure to other-suffering stimuli (cf., Shaver et al., 1987). The pattern of results for self-reported feeling states proved more variable, however.

Following the compassion induction, participants reported feeling increased compassion along with a number of unpleasant states. Furthermore, ratings of compassion correlated with typical unpleasant states (i.e., *sadness, sorrow, sympathy, upset*) but not with typical pleasant states (i.e., *happy, excited, proud, awed*) following the compassion induction. The opposite pattern emerged following the neutral induction: Participants' moderate feelings of compassion correlated with pleasant states (i.e., *happy, excited, awed, proud*), but not unpleasant states (i.e., *sadness, sorrow, sympathy, upset*). These results replicated across two studies implementing within- and between-subjects designs.

These data demonstrated that feeling states within a single emotion category (i.e., compassion) vary in experience. The prototypical cognitive representation of an emotion (e.g., compassion as pleasant) can be different from what people experience (e.g., compassion as unpleasant). Just as the typical conceptualization of fear is unpleasant, people can experience pleasant instances of it (Wilson-Mendenhall et al., 2013a). Together, these data support theoretical views that predict heterogeneity within an emotion category (cf. Barrett, 2009b).

What is a Positive Emotion?: Prospects for Positive Emotion Theory and Research

Emotion categories are goal-directed categories that develop to guide action (see Barrett, 2006b). The most typical members of a goal-directed category are those that maximally achieve the goal of that the category is organized around, not necessarily those that are most frequently encountered (see the earlier discussion on ideals; see also Barsalou, 1991, 2003). Of course, goals can change across situations and context, suggesting that typicality is a dynamic phenomenon (Barsalou, 1985, 2005, 2008). The most typical instances of an emotion category represent the ideal form of the category—that is, whatever is ideal for meeting the goal that the category is organized around—not those that most commonly appear as instances of the category. One goal that surrounds the category anger, for example, is *to remove an obstacle in the environment*. Thus, a highly arousing and unpleasant experience of anger is ideal in the extent to which it achieves the goal of removing the obstacle. Goals that surround the superordinate category *positive emotion* might include *to feel pleasant, to achieve a desirable outcome*, or *to seize an opportunity*. In turn, the instances of positive emotion that maximally achieve a goal such as *to seize an opportunity* will be most typical. Thus, the answer to the question "What is a positive emotion?" or "What counts as a positive emotion?" is a matter of a person's goals.[6] In general, understanding a person's goal(s) will allow a researcher to make predictions about which states that person will find typical or ideal for an emotion category.

A situated conceptualization approach also emphasizes individual differences in people's experience of atypical emotions. We predict that individual differences will be found to the extent that people construct emotional categories around different goals. We predict that a number of individual differences and forms of cultural experience (including experiences with different religions, different regions of a country, different socioeconomic status; see Cohen, 2009) will result in systematic differences in goals surrounding different emotion categories and will therefore result in varying tendencies to experience atypical emotions. Recent work capitalized on the different goals endorsed by individuals across cultures and demonstrated that different situations are perceived as more frequent to the extent that they elicit the condoned emotion (Boiger, Mesquita, Uchida, & Barrett, 2013). Americans, for example, condone experiences of anger that facilitate the goal to maintain dignity and feel good about one-self. Those in Japanese culture, however, condone experiences of shame, which facilitates the goal of harmony. In this study, U.S. and Japanese students rated the frequency of various situation they encountered in their daily lives. Across cultures, a situation was perceived as more frequent to the extent that the situation elicited stronger condoned emotions (anger in the United States, shame in Japan) and as less frequent to extent that the situation elicited stronger condemned emotions (shame in the United States, anger in Japan). This pattern of results occurred despite the fact that pilot data demonstrated the two cultures did not differ in the amount to which they actually experienced the particular situations. These data demonstrate that cultural goals are particularly relevant to the extent to which a person and a culture experiences particular emotions. In this view, individual differences, as they relate to differences in

endorsed goals, will likely explain a person's tendency to experience atypical emotions.

We also predict that individual differences in emotion differentiation will influence the experience of atypical and typical emotions. Substantial individual differences exist in the degree to which individuals label their affective experiences with discrete and specific emotion categories—a phenomenon called "emotion granularity." Individuals with high granularity report on their affective states using terms such as *afraid, angry,* and *sad* to refer to different emotional states, whereas individuals with low granularity report on their affective states using the same terms to refer to a global, unspecified state (Barrett, 2004; Barrett, Gross, Christensen, & Benvenuto, 2001; Demiralp et al., 2012; Feldman, 1995; Lindquist & Barrett, 2008b). High emotion granularity is an adaptive skill because discrete emotion labels provide precise information about appropriate behavior in varying emotional situations (Barrett et al., 2001; Condon, Wilson-Mendenhall, & Barrett, 2014). While emotion granularity has typically been assessed by examining a person's use of labels to distinguish between emotion categories, it is likely that individuals vary in their ability to distinguish among instances of an emotion within a single category. For example, the ability to distinguish between the fear of snakes and the fear of public speaking may represent a type of granularity that offers further advantages. Atypical fear experiences might be atypical because they are less threatening (i.e., they are less likely to match the ideal of the category, which is centered around the goal *to escape threat*). The ability to make this distinction and to recognize atypical fear experiences might be adaptive and conducive to well-being. Yet our understanding of how emotion categories develop for different individuals remains limited and awaits further empirical study.

Positive emotions have been distinguished from negative emotions in their ability to broaden thought–action repertoires and build resources (Fredrickson, 1998, 2001). In turn, positive emotions have been examined from a functionalist perspective, with the aim of discovering the different adaptive consequences of awe, compassion, pride, gratitude, and other positive emotions. Each emotion construct represents a unique combination of ingredients and refers to different situated conceptualizations. Across situated conceptualizations, these emotions will have different adaptive outcomes. Heterogeneity within an emotion category means that all emotions will have a variety of adaptive outcomes across contexts. A general adaptive outcome of atypical emotions—because they are produced from situated conceptualizations—is that they guide situated actions. With atypical emotions, actions are tailored to the situation at hand. Thus, pleasant fear may motivate one to take advantage of resources (e.g., in a job interview, or a challenging performance in front of a crowd; see examples in Table 4.1) rather than avoid the threatening situation. These atypical pleasant emotions may act as social glue and bind people together, for example, when sharing a pleasant fear experience of watching a horror film. Pleasant fear may contribute to experiences of *flow* (Csikszentmihalyi, 1990), for example, in an energizing competition. Recent work examined the ability of fear to promote positive aesthetic experiences of art (Eskine, Kacinik, & Prinz, 2012). Following a short fear-inducing video, participants had more positive impressions of artwork than those who watched a happiness-inducing video. Eskine and colleagues (2012) suggested that fear may enhance the appreciation of art through its ability to remove a person from daily life and thereby grab his or her interest and attention. To the extent that fear causes people to focus attention and experience a pleasant moment or *flow* as a result, they may accrue resources, attain goals, and enhance overall well-being as a result. Pleasant sadness (e.g., reflections on a lost loved one) may signify the importance of relationships and motivate relationship-building pursuits with others. The functional outcomes produced by the situated conceptualizations of atypical emotions remain an area ripe for empirical research.

Examining the variation in behavioral adaptations supported by different instances of a single emotion category may expand the scope of affective science. Some fears might feel good and promote beneficial consequences. In a clinical setting, for example, not all "fears" should be treated the same, just as not all "angers" should be avoided. Indeed, the ability to experience anger in some contexts (e.g., in confrontation, nego-

tiation) can be useful and is preferred by some people (Tamir & Ford, 2012]; Tamir, Mitchell, & Gross, 2008). The ability to tailor one's situated conceptualization in a manner appropriate to the situation at hand will prove beneficial for well-being (see also Condon et al., 2014).

We propose that a significant step in the science of emotion will occur when researchers focus on the heterogeneity of emotional life, studying both typical and atypical instances within various discrete emotion categories. Rather than a sole focus on the typical positive and negative emotions (while keeping these phenomena separate), we suggest that it will be more fruitful to examine the various situated conceptualizations that describe the atypical and typical instances within each positive and negative emotion category. A fine-grained analysis of the population of instances within a given category will ultimately yield greater understanding and predictive power of the situations that produce emotional experience and behavior. In particular, an understanding of unpleasant experiences of *gratitude, awe,* and *hope,* and pleasant experiences of *fear, disgust,* and *sadness* will provide a more dynamic account of emotion and well-being.

Notes

1. Scenarios were developed as part of Christine D. Wilson-Mendenhall's dissertation (see Wilson-Mendenhall, Barrett, & Barsalou, 2013b).

2. Positive emotions are called "positive" because (1) they feel pleasant, (2) the events that preceded the emotional feeling are goal-congruent, or (3) the affective state produces desirable consequence (cf. Harmon-Jones, Harmon-Jones, Abramson, & Peterson, 2009). In this chapter, we use the terms "positive" and "negative" to refer to categories that exist in psychology, but the terms "pleasant" and "unpleasant" to refer to instances of specific mental states.

3. From the conventions of emotion research, gratitude, love, pride, and joy are typical instances of the category *positive emotion* and anger, fear, sadness, and disgust are typical instances of the category *negative emotion* (although no empirical data have demonstrated that nonresearchers share this view). An emotion such as *schaden-*

freude, on the other hand, represents a possible atypical instance of the category *positive emotion*. Furthermore, variations in typicality exist within a category, as suggested by our opening examples of atypical fear and atypical happiness.

4. The conceptual act theory of emotion was introduced in 2006 and has been elaborated through a series of theoretical and empirical papers (Barrett, 2006b, 2009a, 2011, 2012, 2013; Barrett & Bliss-Moreau, 2009; Barrett & Kensinger, 2010; Barrett, Mesquita, Ochsner, & Gross, 2007; Barrett, Ochsner, & Gross, 2007; Lindquist & Barrett, 2008a,b; Lindquist, Wager, Kober, Bliss-Moreau, & Barrett, 2012; Wilson-Mendenhall, Barrett, Simmons, & Barsalou, 2011). In this chapter, we present a summarized view.

5. In some cases, the ideal prototype of a category may not exist in nature even though it fits the goal of the category. We revisit this issue later.

6. Our discussion of ideals parallels work on ideal affect by Jeanne Tsai and colleagues (for a review, see Tsai, 2007), who have demonstrated that ideal affect, the affective experiences that a person wants to feel, differs from actual affect, the affective experiences that a person actually feels. Several variables predict differences in ideal affect, including culture, religion, age, and experience with meditation (Koopman-Holm, Sze, Ochs, & Tsai, 2013; Scheibe, English, Tsai, & Carstensen, 2013; Tsai, Knutson, & Fung, 2006; Tsai, Miao, & Seppala, 2007). Westerners, for example, want to feel high-arousal positive affect. Tsai and colleagues emphasize ideal forms of affect along dimensions of valence and arousal, but our emphasis here is that a person's goals also determine the ideal form of a particular emotion category (e.g., fear, gratitude).

References

Andrews-Hanna, J. R., Reidler, J. S., Sepulcre, J., Poulin, R., & Buckner, R. L. (2010). Functional-anatomic fractionation of the brain's default network. *Neuron, 65,* 550–562.

Bar, M. (2007). The proactive brain: Using analogies and associations to generate predictions. *Trends in Cognitive Science, 11,* 280–289.

Barrett, L. F. (2004). Feelings or words?: Understanding the content in self-report ratings of experienced emotion. *Journal of Personality and Social Psychology, 87,* 266–281.

Barrett, L. F. (2006a). Are emotions natural kinds? *Perspectives on Psychological Science, 1,* 28–58.

Barrett, L. F. (2006b). Solving the emotion paradox: Categorization and the experience of emotion. *Personality and Social Psychology Review, 10,* 20–46.

Barrett, L. F. (2006c). Valence as a basic building block of emotional life. *Journal of Research in Personality, 40,* 35–55.

Barrett, L. F. (2009a). The future of psychology: Connecting mind to brain. *Perspectives on Psychological Science, 4,* 326–339.

Barrett, L. F. (2009b). Variety is the spice of life: A psychological constructionist approach to understanding variability in emotion. *Cognition and Emotion, 23,* 1284–1306.

Barrett, L. F. (2011). Was Darwin wrong about emotional expressions? *Current Directions in Psychological Science, 20,* 400–406.

Barrett, L. F. (2012). Emotions are real. *Emotion, 12,* 413–429.

Barrett, L. F. (2013). Psychological construction: The Darwinian approach to the science of emotion. *Emotion Review, 5,* 379–389.

Barrett, L. F., & Bar, M. (2009). See it with feeling: Affective predictions during object perception. *Philosophical Transactions of the Royal Society B, 364,* 1325–1334.

Barrett, L. F., & Bliss-Moreau, E. (2009). Affect as a psychological primitive. *Advances in Experimental Social Psychology, 41,* 167–218.

Barrett, L. F., Gross, J., Christensen, T. C., & Benvenuto, M. (2001). Knowing what you're feeling and knowing what to do about it: Mapping the relation between emotion differentiation and emotion regulation. *Cognition and Emotion, 15,* 713–724.

Barrett, L. F., & Kensinger, E. A. (2010). Context is routinely encoded during emotion perception. *Psychological Science, 21,* 595–599.

Barrett, L. F., Lindquist, K., Bliss-Moreau, E., Duncan, S., Gendron, M., Mize, J., et al. (2007). Of mice and men: Natural kinds of emotion in the mammalian brain? *Perspectives on Psychological Science, 2,* 297–312.

Barrett, L. F., Mesquita, B., & Gendron, M. (2011). Context in emotion perception. *Current Directions in Psychological Science, 20,* 286–290.

Barrett, L. F., Mesquita, B., Ochsner, K. N., & Gross, J. J. (2007). The experience of emotion. *Annual Review of Psychology, 58,* 373–403.

Barrett, L. F., Ochsner, K. N., & Gross, J. J. (2007). On the automaticity of emotion. In J. Bargh (Ed.), *Social psychology and the uncon-*

scious: The automaticity of higher mental processes (pp. 173–217). New York: Psychology Press.

Barrett, L. F., & Satpute, A. (2013). Large-scale brain networks in affective and social neuroscience: Towards an integrative architecture of the human brain. *Current Opinion in Neurobiology, 23,* 1–12.

Barrett, L. F., Wilson-Mendenhall, C. D., & Barsalou, L. W. (2014). A psychological construction account of emotion regulation and dysregulation: The role of situated conceptualizations. In J. J. Gross (Ed.), *Handbook of emotion regulation* (2nd ed., pp. 447–465). New York: Guilford Press.

Barsalou, L. W. (1985). Ideals, central tendency, and frequency of instantiation as determinants of graded structure in categories. *Journal of Experimental Psychology: Learning, Memory, and Cognition, 11,* 629–654.

Barsalou, L. W. (1991). Deriving categories to achieve goals. In G. H. Bower (Ed.), *The psychology of learning and motivation: Advances in research and theory* (Vol. 27, pp.1–64). New York: Academic Press.

Barsalou, L. W. (1999). Perceptual symbol systems. *Behavioral and Brain Sciences, 22,* 577–660.

Barsalou, L. W. (2003). Situated simulation in the human conceptual system. *Language and Cognitive Processes, 18,* 513–562.

Barsalou, L. W. (2005). Situated conceptualization. In H. Cohen & C. Lefebvre (Eds.), *Handbook of categorization in cognitive science* (pp. 619–650). New York: Elsevier.

Barsalou, L. W. (2008). Situating concepts. In P. Robbins & M. Aydede (Eds.), *Cambridge handbook of situated cognition* (pp. 236–263). New York: Cambridge University Press.

Barsalou, L. W., & Ross, B. H. (1986). The roles of automatic and strategic processing in sensitivity to superordinate and property frequency. *Journal of Experimental Psychology: Learning, Memory, and Cognition, 12,* 116–134.

Boiger, M., Mesquita, B., Uchida, Y., & Barrett, L. F. (2013). Condoned or condemned: The situational affordance of anger and shame in the US and Japan. *Personality and Social Psychology Bulletin, 39,* 540–553.

Buck, R. (1999). The biological affects: A typology. *Psychological Review, 106,* 301–336.

Buckner, R. L., Andrews-Hanna, J. R., & Schacter, D. L. (2008). The brain's default network: anatomy, function, and relevance to disease. *Annals of the New York Academy of Science, 1124,* 1-38.

Buckner, R. L., & Carroll, D. C. (2007). Self-projection and the brain. *Trends in Cognitive Sciences, 11*(2), 49–57.

Cacioppo, J. T., Berntson, G. G., Larsen, J. T., Poehlmann, K. M., & Ito, T. A. (2000). The psychophysiology of emotion. In M. Lewis & J. M. Haviland-Jones (Eds.), *Handbook of emotions* (2nd ed., pp. 173–191). New York: Guilford Press.

Cacioppo, J. T., Gardner, W. L., & Berntson, G. G. (1997). Beyond bipolar conceptualizations and measures: The case of attitudes and evaluative space. *Personality and Social Psychological Review, 1,* 3–25.

Cacioppo, J. T., Gardner, W. L., & Berntson, G. G. (1999). The affect system has parallel and integrative processing components: Form follows function. *Journal of Personality and Social Psychology, 76,* 839–855.

Charles, S. T. (2005). Viewing injustice: Greater emotional heterogeneity with age. *Psychology and Aging, 20,* 159–164.

Clore, G. L., & Ortony, A. (2008). Appraisal theories: How cognition shapes affect into emotion. In M. Lewis, J. M. Haviland-Jones, & L. F. Barrett (Eds.), *Handbook of emotions* (3rd ed., pp. 628–642). New York: Guilford Press.

Cohen, A. B. (2009). Many forms of culture. *American Psychologist, 64,* 194–204.

Condon, P., & Barrett, L. F. (in press). Conceptualizing and experiencing compassion. *Emotion.*

Condon, P., Wilson-Mendenhall, C. D., & Barrett, L. F. (2014). The psychological construction of positive emotion as a window onto well-being. In J. Gruber & J. Moskowitz (Eds.), *Positive emotion: Integrating the light sides and dark sides* (pp. 11–33). New York: Oxford University Press.

Csikszentmihalyi, M. (1990). *Flow.* New York: Harper & Row.

Davis, M. (1992). The role of the amygdala in fear and anxiety. *Annual Review of Neuroscience, 15,* 353–375.

Demiralp, E., Thompson, R. J., Mata, J., Jaeggi, S. M., Buschkuehl, M., Barrett, L. F., et al. (2012). Feeling blue or turquoise?: Emotional differentiation in major depressive disorder. *Psychological Science, 23,* 1410–1416.

Dreyfus, G. (2002). Is compassion an emotion?: A cross-cultural exploration of mental typologies. In R. J. Davidson & A. Harrington (Eds.), *Visions of compassion: Western scientists and Tibetan Buddhists examine human nature* (pp. 31–45). New York: Oxford University Press.

Dreyfus, G., & Thompson, E. (2007). Asian perspectives: Indian theories of mind. In P. D. Zelazo, M. Moscovitch, & E. Thompson (Eds.), *The Cambridge handbook of consciousness* (pp. 89–114). Cambridge, UK: Cambridge University Press.

Duffy, E. (1934). Emotion: An example of the need for reorientation in psychology. *Psychological Review, 41,* 184–198.

Edelman, G. M., & Tononi, G. (2000). *A universe of consciousness.* New York: Basic Books.

Ekman, P. (1972). Universal and cultural differences in facial expressions of emotion. In J. R. Cole (Ed.), *Nebraska Symposium on Motivation, 1971* (Vol. 19, pp. 207–283). Lincoln: University of Nebraska Press.

Ekman, P., & Cordaro, D. (2011). What is meant by calling emotions basic? *Emotion Review, 3,* 364–370.

Ellsworth, P. C., & Scherer, K. R. (2003). Appraisal processes in emotion. In R. J. Davidson, K. R. Scherer, & H. H. Goldsmith (Eds.), *The handbook of affective science* (pp. 572–595). New York: Oxford University Press.

Eskine, K. J., Kacinik, N. A., & Prinz, J. J. (2012). Stirring images: Fear, not happiness or arousal, makes art more sublime. *Emotion, 12,* 1071–1074.

Fehr, B., & Russell, J. A. (1991). The concept of love viewed from a prototype perspective. *Journal of Personality and Social Psychology, 60,* 425–438.

Fehr, B., & Sprecher, S. (2009). Prototype analysis of the concept of compassionate love. *Personal Relationships, 16,* 343–364.

Feldman, L. A. (1995). Valence focus and arousal focus: Individual differences in the structure of affective experience. *Journal of Personality and Social Psychology, 69,* 153–166.

Fredrickson, B. L. (1998). What good are positive emotions? *Review of General Psychology, 2,* 300–319.

Fredrickson, B. L. (2001). The role of positive emotions in positive psychology: The broaden-and-build theory of positive emotions. *American Psychologist, 56,* 218–226.

Frijda, N. H. (1986). *The emotions.* New York: Cambridge University Press.

Gendron, M., & Barrett, L. F. (2009). Reconstructing the past: A century of ideas about emotion in psychology. *Emotion Review, 1,* 1–24.

Gray, J. A. (2004). *Consciousness.* New York: Oxford University Press.

Harmon-Jones, E., Harmon-Jones, C., Abramson, L. Y., & Peterson, C. K. (2009). PANAS positive activation is associated with anger. *Emotion, 9,* 183–196.

Harrison, B. J., Pujol, J., Lopez-Sola, M., Hernandez-Ribas, R., Deus, J., Ortiz, H., et al. (2008). Consistency and functional specialization in the default mode brain network. *Proceedings of the National Academy of Sciences, 105,* 9781–9786.

Hunt, W. A. (1941). Recent developments in the field of emotion. *Psychological Bulletin, 38,* 249–276.

Izard, C. E. (1971). *The face of emotion.* New York: Appleton-Century-Crofts.

Izard, C. E. (1993). Four systems for emotion activation: Cognitive and noncognitive processes. *Psychological Review, 100,* 68–90.

Jenkins, A. C., & Mitchell, J. P. (2010). Mentalizing under uncertainty: Dissociated neural responses to ambiguous and unambiguous mental state inferences. *Cerebral Cortex, 20,* 404–410.

Kagan, J. (2007). *What is emotion?: History, measures, meanings.* New Haven, CT: Yale University Press.

Kirkland, T., & Cunningham, W. A. (2012). Mapping emotions through time: How affective trajectories inform the language of emotion. *Emotion, 12,* 268–282.

Kober, H., Barrett, L. F., Joseph, J., Bliss-Moreau, E., Lindquist, K. A., & Wager, T. D. (2008). Functional networks and cortical-subcortical interactions in emotion: A meta-analysis of neuroimaging studies. *NeuroImage, 42,* 998–1031.

Koopmann-Holm, B., Sze, J., Ochs, C., & Tsai, J. L. (2013). Buddhist-inspired meditation increases the value of calm. *Emotion, 13,* 497–505.

Lambert, N. M., Graham, S. M., & Fincham, F. D. (2009). A prototype analysis of gratitude: Varieties of gratitude experiences. *Personality and Social Psychology Bulletin, 35,* 1193–1207.

Larsen, J. T., McGraw, A. P., & Cacioppo, J. T. (2001). Can people feel happy and sad at the same time? *Journal of Personality and Social Psychology, 81,* 684–696.

Larsen, J. T., & Stastny, B. J. (2011). It's a bit-tersweet symphony: Simultaneously mixed emotional responses to music with conflicting cues. *Emotion, 11,* 1469–1473.

LeDoux, J. E. (2000). Emotion circuits in the brain. *Annual Review of Neuroscience, 23,* 155–184.

Levenson, R. W. (1994). Human emotion: A functional view. In P. Ekman & R. J. Davidson (Eds.), *The nature of emotion: Fundamental questions* (pp. 123–126). New York: Oxford University Press.

Lindquist, K. A., & Barrett, L. F. (2008a). Con-structing emotion: The experience of fear as a conceptual act. *Psychological Science, 19,* 898–903.

Lindquist, K. A., & Barrett, L. F. (2008b). Emotional complexity. In M. Lewis, J. M. Haviland-Jones, & L. F. Barrett (Eds.), *Handbook of emotions* (3rd ed., pp. 513–530). New York: Guilford Press.

Lindquist, K. A., Wager, T. D., Kober, H., Bliss-Moreau, E., & Barrett, L. F. (2012). The brain basis of emotion: A meta-analytic review. *Behavioral and Brain Sciences, 35,* 121–143.

Lynch, E. B., Coley, J. D., & Medin, D. L. (2000). Tall is typical: Central tendency, ideal dimensions, and graded structure among tree experts and novices. *Memory and Cognition, 28,* 41–50.

Mandler, G. (1975). *Mind and emotion.* New York: Wiley.

Matsumoto, D. (1990). Cultural similarities and differences in display rules. *Motivation and Emotion, 14,* 195–214.

Mauss, I. B., & Robinson, M. D. (2009). Mea-sures of emotion: A review. *Cognition and Emotion, 23,* 209–237.

McDougall, W. (1921). *An introduction to social psychology.* Boston: John W. Luce. (Original work published 1908)

Menon, V., & Uddin, L. Q. (2010). Saliency, switching, attention and control: A network model of insula function. *Brain Structure and Function, 214,* 655–667.

Mitchell, J. P. (2009). Inferences about men-tal states. *Philosophical Transactions of the Royal Society B, 364,* 1309–1316.

Miyamoto, Y., Uchida, Y., & Ellsworth, P. C. (2010). Culture and mixed emotions: Co-occurrence of positive and negative emotions in Japan and the United States. *Emotion, 3,* 404–415.

Murphy, G. L. (2002). *The big book of concepts.* Cambridge, MA: MIT Press.

Niedenthal, P. M. (2008). Emotion concepts. In M. Lewis, J. M. Haviland-Jones, & L. F. Bar-rett (Eds.), *Handbook of emotions* (3rd ed., pp. 587–600). New York: Guilford Press.

Nowlis, V., & Nowlis, H. H. (1956). The descrip-tion and analysis of mood. *Annals of the New York Academy of Sciences, 65,* 345–355.

Ortony, A., & Turner, T. J. (1990). What's basic about basic emotions? *Psychological Review, 97,* 315–331.

Panksepp, J. (1998). *Affective neuroscience: The foundations of human and animal emotions.* New York: Oxford University Press.

Panksepp, J., & Watt, D. (2011). What is basic about basic emotions?: Lasting lessons from affective neuroscience. *Emotion Review, 3,* 387–396.

Rips, L. J. (1975). Inductive judgments about natural categories. *Journal of Verbal Learning and Verbal Behavior, 14,* 665–681.

Rosch, E. (1975). Cognitive representations of semantic categories. *Journal of Experimental Psychology: General, 104,* 192–233.

Rosch, E., & Mervis, C. B. (1975). Family resemblances: Studies in the internal struc-ture of categories. *Cognitive Psychology, 7,* 573–605.

Rosch, E., Simpson, C., & Miller, R. S. (1976). Structural bases of typicality effects. *Journal of Experimental Psychology: Human Percep-tion and Performance, 2,* 491–502.

Roseman, I. J. (2011). Emotional behaviors, emotivational goals, emotion strategies: Mul-tiple levels of organization integrate variable and consistent responses. *Emotion Review, 3,* 434–443.

Russell, J. A. (1991). In defense of a prototype approach to emotion concepts. *Journal of Per-sonality and Social Psychology, 60,* 37–47.

Russell, J. A. (2003). Core affect and the psycho-logical construction of emotion. *Psychological Review, 110,* 145–172.

Russell, J. A., Bachorowski, J., & Fernandez-Dols, J. (2003). Facial and vocal expressions of emotion. *Annual Review of Psychology, 54,* 329–349.

Russell, J. A., & Barrett, L. F. (1999). Core affect, prototypical emotional episodes, and other things called emotion: Dissecting the elephant. *Journal of Personality and Social Psychology, 76,* 805–819.

Russell, J. A., & Carroll, J. M. (1999). On the bipolarity of positive and negative affect. *Psy-chological Bulletin, 125,* 3–30.

Russell, J. A., & Fehr, B. (1994). Fuzzy concepts

in a fuzzy hierarchy: Varieties of anger. *Journal of Personality and Social Psychology, 67,* 186–205.

Scheibe, S., English, T., Tsai, J. L., & Carstensen, L. L. (2013). Striving to feel good: Ideal affect, actual affect, and their correspondence across adulthood. *Psychology and Aging, 28,* 160–171.

Scherer, K. R. (2009). Emotions are emergent processes: They require a dynamic computational architecture. *Philosophical Transactions of the Royal Society B, 364,* 3459–3474.

Scollon, C. N., Diener, E., Oishi, S., & Biswas-Diener, R. (2005). An experience sampling and cross-cultural investigation of the relation between pleasant unpleasant affect. *Cognition and Emotion, 19,* 27–52.

Seeley, W. W., Menon, V., Schatzberg, A. F., Keller, J., Glover, G. H., Kenna, H., et al. (2007). Dissociable intrinsic connectivity networks for salience processing and executive control. *Journal of Neuroscience, 27,* 2349–2356.

Shariff, A. F., & Tracy, J. L. (2011). What are emotion expression for? *Current Directions in Psychological Science, 5,* 772–775.

Shaver, P., Schwartz, J., Kirson, D., & O'Connor, C. (1987). Emotion knowledge: Further explorations of a prototype approach. *Journal of Personality and Social Psychology, 52,* 1061–1086.

Simon-Thomas, E. R., Godzik, J., Castle, E., Antonenko, O., Ponz, A., Kogan, A., et al. (2012). An fMRI study of caring vs. self-focus during induced compassion and pride. *Social Cognitive and Affective Neuroscience, 7,* 635–648.

Smith, C. A., & Ellsworth, P. C. (1985). Patterns of cognitive appraisal in emotion. *Journal of Personality and Social Psychology, 48,* 813–838.

Tamir, M., & Ford, B. Q. (2012). When feeling bad is expected to be good: Emotion regulation and outcome expectancies in social conflicts. *Emotion, 12,* 807–816.

Tamir, M., Mitchell, C., & Gross, J. J. (2008). Hedonic and instrumental motives in anger regulation. *Psychological Science, 19,* 324–328.

Tomkins, S. S. (1962). *Affect, imagery, consciousness: Vol. 1. The positive affects.* New York: Springer.

Tomkins, S. S. (1963). *Affect, imagery, consciousness: Vol. 2. The negative affects.* New York: Springer.

Tsai, J. L. (2007). Ideal affect: Cultural causes and behavioral consequences. *Perspectives on Psychological Science, 2,* 242–259.

Tsai, J. L., Knutson, B., & Fung, H. H. (2006). Cultural variation in affect valuation. *Journal of Personality and Social Psychology, 90,* 288–307.

Tsai, J. L., Miao, F., & Seppala, E. (2007). Good feelings in Christianity and Buddhism: Religious differences in ideal affect. *Personality and Social Psychology Bulletin, 33,* 409–421.

Turner, T. J., & Ortony, A. (1992). Basic emotions: Can conflicting criteria converge? *Psychological Review, 99,* 566–571.

Wilson-Mendenhall, C. D., Barrett, L. F., & Barsalou, L. W. (2013a). Neural evidence that human emotions share core affective properties. *Psychological Science, 24,* 947–956.

Wilson-Mendenhall, C. D., Barrett, L. F., & Barsalou, L. W. (2013b). *Variety in emotional life: Typicality of emotion experiences is associated with neural activity in large-scale brain networks.* Manuscript under review.

Wilson-Mendenhall, C. D., Barrett, L. F., Simmons, W. K, & Barsalou, L. W. (2011). Grounding emotion in situated conceptualization. *Neuropsychologia, 49,* 1105–1127.

Wilson-Mendenhall, C. D., Simmons, W. K., Martin, A., & Barsalou, L. W. (2013). Contextual processing of abstract concepts reveals neural representations of non-linguistic semantic content. *Journal of Cognitive Neuroscience, 25,* 920–935.

Wittgenstein, L. (1953). *Philosophical investigations.* Malden, MA: Blackwell.

Yik, M. S. M., Russell, J. A., & Barrett, L. F. (1999). Structure of self-reported current affect: Integration and beyond. *Journal of Personality and Social Psychology, 77,* 600–619.

CHAPTER 5

Personality and Positive Emotion

Kimberly M. Livingstone
Sanjay Srivastava

Are some people happier, prouder, or more content than others, and if so, why? How do a person's goals and the ways they pursue them affect their emotional lives? How are people's emotional lives affected by the ways they select, interpret, and respond to situations and manage their emotions? To answer such questions, personality psychology has increasingly focused on understanding the critical role that emotions play in people's lives. Much like other areas of psychology, in recent years, there has been a particular uptick of interest in understanding positive emotions.

Personality psychology is concerned with the organization of attributes and processes that characterize the whole person. Researchers working within this diverse and vibrant field take a variety of approaches that vary in their emphases, methods, and assumptions. Our goal in this chapter is to review selectively and highlight some of the approaches that have investigated positive emotions and personality. We have organized this chapter around three major approaches to studying emotion from a personality perspective. First, we examine individual differences in the tendency to experience and express positive emotions by examining links between personality traits and positive emotion.

Second, we examine how motivational processes produce and affect positive emotional experiences. Third, we focus on regulatory and coping processes by which people generate, modulate, and alter positive emotions.

Trait Approaches

Although the term "trait" does not have a single, universal definition in personality psychology, trait approaches generally focus on identifying characteristic patterns of behavior, thought, or feeling that are stable over substantial time intervals and that differ between individuals. Within the domain of individual differences in experience and behavior, there are several ways to use trait approaches to understand positive emotions. First, we can examine how positive emotions fit into a larger model of personality structure. In this chapter, we focus on the role of positive emotions within the Big Five model of personality traits. Second, because emotions have experiential, cognitive, and behavioral components, it is also possible to examine positive emotions themselves from a trait perspective. Researchers using this approach examine individual differences in the tendency to experience positive emotional states, as well as in cognitive and behavioral aspects of emotional processes.

How Are Positive Emotions Related to the Big Five Personality Traits?

Over the last 30 years or so, many researchers have consolidated their efforts around a unifying structural model of traits, the Big Five (also known as the five-factor model). The Big Five first emerged from analyses of the trait words represented in the English lexicon; factor analyses of ratings of these traits revealed five replicable factors. Later work has replicated this structure in a number of other languages, and although questions remain about its universality across different cultures, it has proven to be a useful framework for many research purposes (Saucier & Srivastava, in press). The Big Five organizes personality traits into five broad domains: Extraversion, Neuroticism, Agreeableness, Conscientiousness, and Openness. Rather than providing a complete model of personality traits, these five domains represent one level of a hierarchy, with finer-grained distinctions possible within each of these domains, and perhaps higher-order groupings possible among them (Digman, 1997; John, Hampson, & Goldberg, 1991).

Extraversion, Neuroticism, and Emotion

Of the Big Five trait domains, Extraversion and Neuroticism have been most closely linked to individual differences in emotional experience and behavior. Extraversion (vs. introversion) is a continuum of individual differences defined by adjectives such as *talkative, assertive, active, energetic*, and *outgoing* at the high end, and *quiet, reserved, shy*, and *silent* at the low end (John & Srivastava, 1999). Although these adjectives do not explicitly refer to emotions, Extraversion has been consistently associated with measures of positive affect, as well as with the frequency of positive affective states in daily life (Costa & McCrae, 1980; Lucas & Fujita, 2000; Watson & Clark, 1997).

Neuroticism (vs. emotional stability) is a continuum of individual differences defined by the tendency to feel anxious, nervous, sad, and tense at the high end and calm, even-tempered, and emotionally stable at the low end (John & Srivastava, 1999).

Neuroticism has consistently been linked to the experience of negative affect (Costa & McCrae, 1980; Lucas & Fujita, 2000; Watson & Clark, 1997). At a descriptive level, there is fairly robust evidence showing that highly extraverted people tend to experience more positive affect than less extraverted people, and highly neurotic people tend to experience more negative affect than less neurotic people (see also DeNeve & Cooper, 1998). Research has supported the hypothesis that extraversion (but not neuroticism) is a significant predictor of positive mood susceptibility, whereas neuroticism (but not extraversion) is a significant predictor of negative mood susceptibility (e.g., Costa & McCrae, 1980; Larsen & Ketelaar, 1991).

In addition to broadly measured positive affect, extraversion is related to measures of a variety of discrete positive emotions. In one study, extraversion was related to self-reports of all seven positive emotions that were measured: joy, contentment, pride, love, compassion, amusement, and awe (Shiota, Keltner, & John, 2006), supporting the relationship between extraversion and positive emotions in general. Relationships between neuroticism and positive affect and emotion have been less robust, although neuroticism has been linked to the experience of less self-reported joy, contentment, pride, and love (Shiota et al., 2006).

Temperamental Explanations. Several theories offer explanations for the mechanisms linking extraversion and neuroticism to emotional experience. Temperamental accounts point to biologically based individual differences in positive and negative reactivity and in self-regulation that emerge early in development (Evans & Rothbart, 2007). Research using parent reports, behavioral observation, and laboratory assessment has identified extraversion/surgency and negative affectivity as dimensions of individual differences early in life (Rothbart, 2007; Rothbart, Ahadi, & Evans, 2000). Research in adults has shown that these dimensions of temperament are related to extraversion and neuroticism, respectively (Rothbart et al., 2000).

More specifically, other theorists have proposed that extraversion and neuroticism reflect individual differences in biologically based systems of response to reward and punishment. J. A. Gray (1970) proposed two systems: a behavioral activation system (BAS) that is sensitive to signals of reward, motivates approach behavior, and is characterized by positive emotion; and a behavioral inhibition system (BIS) that is sensitive to signals of punishment, motivates avoidance behavior, and is characterized by negative emotion. Eysenck conceptually linked BAS with Extraversion and BIS with Neuroticism (Eysenck & Eysenck, 1985). A later factor analysis linked together the traits of reward sensitivity, BAS, Extraversion, and positive affect on the one hand, and the traits of punishment sensitivity, BIS, Neuroticism, and negative affect on the other. The authors found that the first factor predicted daily positive affect, and the latter predicted daily negative affect (Zelinski & Larsen, 1999).

Transactional Explanations. Whereas temperamental accounts propose a biologically based direct link between traits and emotion, transactional accounts propose that extraverts engage differently with the social world than do introverts; that is, extraverts differ from introverts in their proactive or reactive person–environment transactions. Proactive transactions occur when people consciously or unconsciously select their situations or modify the situations in which they find themselves. For example, the sociability of extraverts offers one explanation for their greater positive emotion: Social relationships are a frequent and important source of positive emotions (e.g., Clark & Watson, 1988; Diener & Seligman, 2002), and it is possible that extraverts experience more positive emotion because they engage in more social activity (the *social participation hypothesis*; Srivastava, Angelo, & Vallereux, 2008). Reactive transactions occur when different people experience the same situation in different ways. For example, it is possible that extraverts derive greater enjoyment from socializing with others, leaving them with greater net positive affect than introverts (the *social reactivity hypothesis*; Srivastava et al., 2008). Independent, replicated empirical tests have supported the social participation hypothesis but not the social reactivity hypothesis. Specifically, people at the high and low ends of the extraversion continuum respond with similar degrees of positive

emotion to social situations, but extraverts spend more time with others (Lucas, Le, & Dyrenforth, 2008; Srivastava et al., 2008). Even after social participation is statistically controlled for, however, a majority of the association between extraversion and positive affect remains unexplained, suggesting that social participation is only part of the story.

Motivational Explanations. Recent research suggests that extraversion is related to which emotional states people want to have and value. Although people have a general preference for positive over negative affect (Kämpfe & Mitte, 2009; Västfjäll, Gärling, & Kleiner, 2001), individuals also differ in the value they place on various emotional states. Consistent with the transactional approach, part of why extraverts experience greater positive emotions may be because they *want to* and actively seek out opportunities to experience positive emotions. For example, when participants rate typical affective experience and desired affective experience, those who score higher on extraversion report desiring greater pleasant affect than do more introverted people, a pattern that matches what they report feeling on average (Augustine, Hemenover, Larsen, & Shulman, 2010; Kämpfe & Mitte, 2009; Rusting & Larsen, 1995). In a longitudinal study over the course of a semester, extraversion was related to greater desire for both low- and high-activation positive affect (Augustine et al., 2010). In another study, extraverts preferred to experience happiness in effortful situations (e.g., taking a test), compared to introverts (Tamir, 2009a).

The *type* of positive emotion a person wants to feel also varies across people. "Ideal affect" refers to the types of emotions that individuals would like to experience in general. For example, some people value high-arousal positive emotions such as enthusiasm and excitement, whereas other people might value low-arousal positive affect, such as calm and relaxation. Ideal affect varies across cultures, as well as within cultures as a function of individual differences, including Extraversion (Tsai, Knutson, & Fung, 2006).

In addition to desiring and valuing positive affect, extraverts are also more likely to try to create, maintain, and increase their experience of positive emotion using a variety of emotion regulation strategies (Livingstone & Srivastava, 2012). In particular, they are more likely to spend time with friends and seek out positive people in order to satisfy their goal of experiencing positive emotions, and more likely to savor the positive experiences when they do arise (Livingstone & Srivastava, 2012; see also Bryant, 2003). These conscious actions may explain why higher extraversion has been linked with a smaller discrepancy between desired and actual affect (e.g., Kämpfe & Mitte, 2009). We return to this research in more detail later in this chapter, when we discuss positive emotion regulation.

Other Big Five Traits and Positive Emotions

Although most research on positive emotions and the Big Five has focused on Extraversion, the other three traits of Agreeableness, Conscientiousness, and Openness to Experience are also related to positive emotion, if more indirectly. Agreeableness is defined by characteristics such as *trustworthy, cooperative, modest*, and *altruistic* (John & Srivastava, 1999). Like Extraversion, it is related to interpersonal style, but it focuses on the intimacy of social connection and on maintaining warm, close relationships (DeNeve & Cooper, 1998; Tobin, Graziano, Vanman, & Tassinary, 2000). In a meta-analysis of the relationship between personality traits and well-being, the correlation between agreeableness-related traits and the experience of positive emotion was not significantly different than the correlation between extraversion-related traits and positive emotion (DeNeve & Cooper, 1998). Agreeableness also distinguishes very happy people from moderately happy people (Diener & Seligman, 2002).

Agreeableness has been linked with positive emotions related to interpersonal relationships, such as intimacy and cooperation: Those who score higher on agreeableness report experiencing more love and compassion, and their peers rate them as experiencing more love, supporting the link between agreeableness and positive interpersonal emotions (Shiota et al., 2006; see also Mitte & Kämpfe, 2008). Tobin and colleagues (2000) found that people who scored higher on agreeableness reported devoting more effort to regulating their emotions, which is consistent with their greater sensitivity to the feelings of others.

Conscientiousness is defined by characteristics such as *organized, thorough, reliable*, and *persevering*, and represents a tendency to engage in self-regulation and to strive toward goals (John & Srivastava, 1999). Although one meta-analysis found that goal- and control-related traits did not predict greater positive affect in general (DeNeve & Cooper, 1998), some research supports an indirect link between Conscientiousness and positive emotion (McCrae & Costa, 1991). Goal pursuit has been linked to the experience of positive emotion—particularly progress toward goals and an increase in the perceived rate of progress toward those goals (Carver & Scheier, 1990; Carver, Sutton, & Scheier, 2000). Indeed, some research has shown that people who score higher in conscientiousness report feeling greater agency-focused emotions, specifically joy, contentment, and pride (Shiota et al., 2006), although other research has found that conscientiousness is related to slightly lower joy (Mitte & Kämpfe, 2008).

Openness to Experience is defined by characteristics such as *original, curious*, and *imaginative*, and involves preferences for novelty and aesthetic stimulation (John & Srivastava, 1999). It has been linked to self-ratings of joy, love, compassion, amusement, and awe, as well as to peer ratings of awe (Shiota et al., 2006). In other research, those scoring higher on Openness reported more interest, and slightly more contentment and love, compared to those scoring lower on Openness (Mitte & Kämpfe, 2008). Like Conscientiousness, it is likely that relationships between Openness and general positive affect are indirect (McCrae & Costa, 1991), via new and interesting experiences.

In summary, Extraversion has been linked broadly overall positive emotion, whereas Agreeableness, Conscientiousness, and Openness to Experience have been linked with discrete positive emotions that are more directly relevant to their domains. Though a relatively large amount of research links Extraversion to positive emotion, much more research is needed to explore the mechanisms linking specific positive emotions to the remaining Big Five traits. In addition, future research should investigate how subdomains of the Big Five factors, as well as possible higher-order traits, are related both to positive emotions in general and to specific positive emotions such as contentment, love, interest, and awe.

The Trait Approach to Positive Emotions

A second way to investigate positive emotions from a trait perspective involves identifying and examining characteristic patterns of feeling, thought, and behavior that are linked to positive emotions. Because emotions have experiential, cognitive, and behavioral components, individual differences in these components can be examined from a trait perspective. Researchers using this approach have investigated individual differences in the tendencies to feel general positive affect and specific positive emotions, in appraisal patterns that give rise to positive emotions, and in expressive behavior associated with the experience of positive emotions.

Subjective Experience

When positive emotion is measured as a state of subjective experience, it is possible to identify reliable individual differences in a tendency to experience happiness and other positive emotions. For example, in a 3-week daily diary study, the amount of variance in positive emotion between people was similar to the amount of variance within people (Nezlek & Kuppens, 2008). Studies that have taken a more short-term approach to measuring positive emotion over time have also found significant between-person variability (e.g., Srivastava et al., 2008). Thus, although almost every person experiences fluctuations in his or her own levels of happiness from moment to moment or day to day, there are reliable individual differences in average or typical levels of happiness.

Global measures of positive emotion also have trait-like properties, supporting the idea that some people are generally happier than others. The heritability of trait subjective well-being has been estimated to be around 50% (Lykken & Tellegen, 1996), and the heritability of trait positive affect has been estimated at around 30–40%, with the remaining variance largely reflect-

ing nonshared environment (Eid, Riemann, Angleitner, & Borkenau, 2003; Tellegen et al., 1988). These percentages are similar to heritability estimates for Big Five personality traits. Longitudinal studies of rank-order stability suggest that individual differences in positive affect are reasonably stable in adulthood. For example, in a sample of young adults in their 20s, positive affect had retest correlations of around .4 over a 6- to 7-year interval (Watson & Walker, 1996). By comparison, in a sample of older adults (ages 70–103), the 4-year stability of positive affect was about .7 (Kunzmann, Little, & Smith, 2000). This increase in stability with age is consistent with a broader finding in the personality change literature that rank-order stability of traits increases with age (Roberts & DelVecchio, 2000). Thus, there is substantial consistency over the course of the lifespan in terms of the experience of positive emotion.

Theorists have proposed individual differences in the "set point" of happiness: People differ in how happy they are in general, and life events cause only temporary fluctuations away from a person's baseline (Headey & Wearing, 1989). Research has shown that the set point model is probably overly simplistic: Major life events such as changes in employment and marital status produce relatively large changes in happiness in the short term, after which people partially (but not fully) return toward their preevent levels of happiness (Diener, Lucas, & Scollon, 2006; Lucas, 2007). Thus, similar to contemporary views of Big Five personality traits, happiness seems to have a substantial but not complete core of stability, with room for life experiences and other factors to produce meaningful changes.

Beyond happiness or general positive affect, researchers have begun to examine specific positive emotions from a trait perspective as well. For example, research by Tracy and Robins (2007) has shown that individual differences in pride come in two varieties. Authentic pride, grounded in prosocial achievements, is positively associated with adjustment and with traits such as extraversion and agreeableness. In contrast, hubristic pride, grounded in self-aggrandizement, is associated with traits such as narcissism and shame-proneness.

Cognition and Appraisal

From a cognitive perspective, individual differences in emotional experience can arise from differences in the tendency to appraise events in certain ways, for example, "agency thinking," or the tendency to believe that goals can be obtained (Tong, Fredrickson, Chang, & Lim, 2010). Differences in appraisals are likely to stem from a combination of affective traits, such as extraversion (the tendency to appraise events as potentially rewarding or positive) and neuroticism (the tendency to appraise events as potentially threatening or negative) on the one hand, and cognitive traits such as optimism (the tendency to expect positive outcomes), locus of control (the tendency to attribute events to oneself or external sources), and self-efficacy (belief in one's coping ability; Ellsworth & Scherer, 2003).

Happy people also have patterns of cognition that reinforce their experience of positive affect (Abbe, Tkach, & Lyubomirsky, 2003; Lyubomirsky, 2001): They remember past events more positively, and react more positively to hypothetical scenarios and standardized situations than less-happy people (Lyubomirsky & Tucker, 1998). Thus, even when the events that the experiences are controlled, happy people seem to perceive, interpret, and remember events that they encountered more positively than unhappy people.

Behavior and Expression

Research also shows that people vary in their tendencies to express positive emotions, and that these differences have implications for the experience of positive emotion and well-being in general. Using self-report data, Gross and John (1997) found that trait-level positive expressivity was related to experienced positive affect, ego resilience, and lower depressive symptoms, whereas masking—hiding inner experience, or experiencing a discrepancy between inner experience and outer display—was associated with greater levels of experienced negative affect and depression.

Expanding on this idea, Mauss, Shallcross, and colleagues (2011) suggest that accurately expressing positive emotions is crucial to social connection and enhances well-being. Dissociation between participants' self-reported online ratings of positive affect and independent coders' ratings of positive expression was associated with greater depressive symptoms and lower life satisfaction, measured 6 months later. This relationship emerged even when researchers controlled for actual and experienced and expressed positive emotion, suggesting that the discrepancy, rather than raw levels, contributes to well-being. Furthermore, this relationship was mediated by lower social connectedness (lower perceived social support and greater loneliness) experienced by those with greater experience–behavior dissociation (Mauss, Shallcross, et al., 2011).

In summary, personality psychologists have examined individual differences in positive emotion both by use of existing trait frameworks (e.g., the Big Five) and investigation of patterns of feeling, thought, and behavior in positive affect and discrete positive emotions. Although traits are a key concept within personality psychology, the scope of personality psychology goes beyond broad, stable dispositions to include within-person processes that are more sensitive to context than are traits (McAdams, 2010). Next, we examine two areas of personality research that have explored individual differences in such contextualized processes: motivation and the self-regulation of emotions.

Motivational Approaches

The motivational perspective within personality psychology emphasizes individual differences in what people want and need, and processes by which they go about trying to achieve those aims. Whereas trait approaches characterize broad patterns of feeling, cognition, and behavior, motivational approaches often focus on contextualized processes that may change over time or across situations. The two approaches are often complementary. For example, at the level of broad traits, we can say that extraverted people typically desire to feel positive emotions; from a motivational approach, we might study how a person's BAS influences behavior in situations that offer opportunities for rewards, and from an integrated perspective, we might examine how BAS functioning covaries with individual differences in extraversion.

Although there is no central theory of motivation that is comparable to the Big Five in the trait approach, many motivational approaches share some common characteristics. First, most models propose that discrepancies between one's current state and a particular end state motivate *approach* behaviors toward desired end states and *avoidance* behaviors away from undesired end states (Carver & Scheier, 1990; Carver & White, 1994; Elliot, 1999; Higgins, 1996; Markus & Nurius, 1986). Second, many personality models of motivation are hierarchical, with abstract, long-term concerns and values influencing time- and context-dependent goals that influence concrete behaviors (Elliot & Church, 1997; Emmons, 1986; Ryan & Deci, 2000).

Positive Emotions as Motivation

One important distinction within motivation literature is between approach and avoidance. Whereas negative emotions are typically associated with the motivation to avoid undesirable outcomes, positive emotions are generally associated with the motivation to approach desired outcomes (e.g., Elliot & Thrash, 2002). Approach motivation is thought to arise from the BAS, which is sensitive to cues of reward and motivates appetitive behavior (J. A. Gray, 1990). At the individual difference level, people vary in three facets of BAS activity: fun seeking, a desire for excitement and the tendency to seek out potentially fun situations; drive, a willingness to persevere to attain a desired outcome; and reward responsiveness, a tendency to experience strong positive affective reactions to rewarding events (Carver & White, 1994). All three BAS facets correlate moderately with Extraversion, positive affect, and with each other (Carver & White, 1994).

Individual differences in BAS activity have indirect implications for a person's typical experience of positive affect, via a person's dynamic interaction with the situation (Carver & White, 1994; Gable, Reis, & Elliot, 2000). Rather than implying high-baseline positive emotion, high BAS activity is associated with greater *sensitivity* to reward in the environment. In a laboratory study, trait extraversion predicted a person's starting happiness, whereas trait measures of drive and reward responsiveness predicted greater sensitivity to cues of reward (Carver & White, 1994). Other research suggests that higher BAS activity is associated with greater *exposure* to positive events: In a series of diary studies (Gable et al., 2000), participants who scored higher on BAS not only experienced more daily positive affect (Studies 2 and 3) but also experienced more daily positive events, which mediated the relationship between BAS and positive affect (Study 3). Focusing on the appetitive nature of the BAS, the authors suggested that the BAS might motivate people to seek out possibly rewarding experiences rather than influence their reactions to positive events. Research has also shown that BAS is associated with greater sensitivity to conditioned incentives, even when the stimulus might have been unpleasant prior to conditioning (Berkman, Lieberman, & Gable, 2009). This has important implications for understanding goal pursuit because many goals require doing an unpleasant task to achieve a desired outcome.

Several specific positive emotions also motivate approach-related behaviors. For example, although the emotion of pride is often thought of an outcome of a successfully achieved goal (e.g., Pekrun, Elliot, & Maier, 2006), there is some indication that pride may also serve to motivate further perseverance in goal-directed behavior (Williams & DeSteno, 2008). Recent research on individual differences in specific emotions has highlighted their role in motivational processes.

A second important distinction in motivational processes involves the difference between intrinsic and extrinsic motivation. Intrinsically motivated activities are pursued because they are enjoyable or interesting, whereas extrinsically motivated activities are pursued in order to attain a desired outcome such as a reward or long-term goal, but are not intrinsically enjoyable (Ryan & Deci, 2000). According to self-determination theory, activities that satisfy the fundamental human needs of autonomy, competence, and relatedness are intrinsically rewarding and produce positive emotion throughout engagement. In contrast, activities that are extrinsically motivated produce positive emotions only when the end goal is attained; the process itself, though it may be important, is not in itself enjoyable (Ryan & Deci, 2000).

One positive experience associated with intrinsic motivation is "flow," which occurs when a person is engaged in an intrinsically interesting activity that provides a good balance between the task's challenge and the person's skill (Csikszentmihalyi, 1990). In a state of flow, the person becomes absorbed in the task and loses awareness of the self and of the passage of time. Flow is associated with momentary feelings of interest, challenge, and competence, and is theorized to be associated with greater long-term positive affect. People who are prone to experience flow are described as "autotelic" (e.g., Nakamura & Csikszentmihalyi, 2002). Autotelic individuals tend to experience greater psychological well-being in a number of domains (see Asakawa, 2010), but the relationship between the autotelic personality and the experience of specific positive emotions has yet to be investigated.

Related to flow are the positive emotions of interest (Izard, 1977) and curiosity (Kashdan, Rose, & Fincham, 2004). Interest, which occurs in novel or complex situations, motivates a desire to explore the environment and gather information, which may serve to promote personal growth, creativity, and intelligence (Fredrickson, 1998; Izard, 1977). Similarly, curiosity, a pleasurable emotional state that motivates approach behavior in the presence of novelty and challenge, includes two facets: exploration (the tendency to seek out novel and complex information) and absorption (the tendency to become fully engaged in intrinsically interesting experiences), an experience closely related to flow (Kashdan et al., 2004). Trait differences in curiosity have been linked both to greater subjective experience of positive affect, positive expectations for the future, and overall well-being, and to greater commitment, effort, and progress in goal pursuit (Kashdan et al., 2004).

Positive Emotion as Feedback

In addition to serving as motivation, emotion provides feedback about goal-related behav-

ior and our status in achieving or avoiding certain end states (Carver & Scheier, 1990; Higgins, 1987). One common view is that emotions arise from evaluations regarding the distance between one's current state and the goal. For example, Higgins (1987, 1996) proposed that people have internal representations of the person that they are (actual self), as well as the people they want to be in the future (ideal selves) and the people that society and others expect them to be (ought selves). In this model, positive emotions derive from perceived congruence between one's perceived self on the one hand, and ought and ideal selves on the other. That is, the closer one's perceived self is to one's desired self, the more happiness, contentment, and pride one should feel.

Carver and Scheier (1990) proposed an alternative model in which emotions arise not from evaluations about the distance between one's current state and one's goal, but from evaluations regarding the rate of progress made toward or away from such a goal. Specifically, positive emotions serve to signal sufficient progress: Elation or excitement occurs when a person perceives that he or she is reducing the distance between the current state and a desired goal at a rate faster than necessary, and relief, serenity, or contentment occur when the person perceives that he or she is increasing the distance between the current state and an aversive goal at a rate faster than necessary (Carver, 2003; Carver et al., 2000). In this case, positive emotion may serve to signal that a person can ease up on efforts related to that particular goal and focus attention elsewhere (Carver, 2003). Others have suggested that positive emotions such as pride may further motivate perseverance in future endeavors (Williams & DeSteno, 2008).

The Content and Organization of Goals

Whether motivating approach behavior or indicating sufficient progress toward an outcome, emotions arise in response to events that are relevant to a person's well-being and goals (Frijda, 1988). In other words, people vary in terms of which emotions are likely to arise in a given situation because they differ in terms of what matters to them: in the values they consider important (Schwartz, 1992), the personal strivings they are typically trying to achieve (Emmons, 1986), and in the types of goals they are trying to pursue (Dweck & Leggett, 1988; Elliot & Thrash, 2002).

Goal *content* theories suggest that the type of goal or motive itself influences the experience of emotion. According to self-determination theory, people who pursue (Kasser & Ryan, 1993) and attain (Sheldon & Kasser, 1998) intrinsically motivated goals, such as developing fulfilling social relationships and personal growth, experience greater positive emotion and well-being than those who pursue extrinsically motivated goals, such as obtaining wealth or social status. People also differ in their tendencies to adopt approach or avoidance goals. In one model, emotions arise from cognitive constructions of what people might become—either desired or feared possible selves—that vary among people and have implications for emotional experience (Markus & Nurius, 1986). Similarly, ideal and ought selves can be either promotion-focused (i.e., approach) or prevention-focused (i.e., avoidance) (Higgins, 1996). Elliot and Thrash (2002) linked approach goals to extraversion, positive temperament, and BAS, and avoidance goals to neuroticism, negative temperament, and BIS.

Self-efficacy also matters in determining which type of goal a person will adopt: When people perceive their competence within a domain to be high, they are more likely to form approach-oriented mastery goals (e.g., to learn as much as possible) or approach-oriented performance goals (e.g., to get a good grade) that orient them toward positive outcomes and emotions, whereas when people perceive their competence to be low, they are more likely to form avoidance-oriented performance goals (e.g., to avoid getting a bad grade) that orient them toward negative outcomes and emotions (Elliot & Church, 1997). Having a mastery goal is associated with the experience of greater positive affect in the face of a challenge, as well as with the experience of enjoyment, hope, and pride (Pekrun, Elliot, & Maier, 2006). In contrast, having a performance goal is only associated with pride, and only when the goal is approach- (e.g., "pass this exam"), rather than avoidance-oriented (e.g., "don't fail"; Pekrun et al., 2006).

Goal *organization* theories suggest that emotions are influenced by whether short-term goals and behaviors are consistent within a person's system of higher-order motives and values (Elliot & Thrash, 2002; Kasser & Ryan, 1993). As previously noted, many theories propose a hierarchical structure of motivation within a person, and hypothesize that motivation is easier and more successful when the hierarchy is aligned. According to this perspective, people experience positive emotions and well-being when their goals are in line with their values, and when their actions support those goals. Indeed, positive emotions are more likely to arise when one's behavior is consistent with deeply held values (Sheldon & Kasser, 1995). For example, Cantor (1991) found that in a sample of college women, participants reported more positive emotions when they were engaged in situations that were relevant to important life tasks—that is, when behavior and values aligned.

In summary, positive emotions play important roles in the patterns of motivation that drive a person's behavior. As motivators of approach behavior, individual differences in positive emotions have implications for people's tendencies to seek out and obtain rewards. As feedback for successful goal progress or achievement, positive emotions reinforce successful behavior and maintain motivation. In addition, individual differences in the content and organization of goals, as well as differences in progress toward and achievement of goals, influence people's experience of positive emotion.

Emotions are dynamic processes and play multiple roles in personality systems. Specifically, emotions can be both regulating, in that they drive and motivate behavior, and regulated, in that people can interact with those emotions in a way that influences how they unfold (Cole, Martin, & Dennis, 2004). Motivational accounts of positive emotion illustrate emotions as regulating. Next, we turn to emotions as regulated, where people proactively or reactively change how they feel.

Coping and Emotion Regulation Approaches

Over the course of development, people learn to understand and manage their emotions, and to increase their emotional competence—a process that involves learning over time (Buck, 1994). Personality psychologists who investigate these issues examine individual differences in the ways that people react to and cope with stressful situations, and the ways they regulate their positive and negative emotions—both reactively and proactively.

Positive Emotions in Negative Emotion Regulation and Coping

Emotion regulation refers to the processes by which a person attempts to change the emotions he or she feels, and how and when they are expressed (Gross, 1998). Most research has focused on strategies people use to decrease their feelings of negative emotions; some of these strategies have implications for the experience of positive emotion as well. For example, in correlational studies, trait-level use of *cognitive reappraisal*—changing the way you think in order to change your emotions—as a regulation strategy is associated with greater trait-level positive emotion, as well as less trait-level negative emotion (Gross & John, 2003). This may be in part because people who rely on reappraisal can transform negative experiences into neutral or positive ones. In contrast, trait use of *expressive suppression*, an emotion regulation strategy in which a person hides his or her display of emotion from others, has been associated with greater experience of negative emotion and less experience of positive emotion (Gross & John, 2003), though this is not necessarily the case for all cultures (Butler, Lee, & Gross, 2007).

People can also use mood repair strategies that draw upon positive emotions to get out of a negative mood: Relaxation-focused strategies (e.g., meditating, lying in the sun) can help people come out of a negative mood by drawing upon emotions such as contentment; pleasure-focused strategies (e.g., fantasize about pleasant things, comfort eating) can draw upon enjoyment and physical pleasure; and mastery-focused strategies (e.g., plan things to do, tidy up) can draw upon feelings of competence and pride (Parkinson & Totterdell, 1999). According to the absorption hypothesis of mood repair, these strategies help repair negative moods by redirecting working memory resources from negative thoughts and feelings to thoughts and activities that are not compatible with negative mood (e.g., enjoyment; Erber, 1996). Thus, people can draw upon positive emotions in order to down-regulate negative emotions, and those who rely on strategies that do so are likely to experience more positive emotion.

In comparison to emotion regulation, *coping* refers to the thoughts and behaviors that people use to deal with situations that they appraise as stressful. Whereas emotion and mood regulation are typically responses to temporary states, coping includes attempts to manage one's emotions in the context of both short- and long-term stressors, such as a chronic illness (Gross, 1998). Coping can refer to an action taken in response to a stressful situation, or to an action taken in response to one's emotions within the situation (Folkman & Lazarus, 1980).

Despite definitional focus on negative situations and experiences, studies of coping in daily life reveal that positive emotions occur frequently even within stressful situations (e.g., Folkman & Moskowitz, 2000). Positive emotions can provide temporary relief from constant negative affect during a stressful experience, provide cognitive and physical energy to cope with the problem at hand, and preserve social relationships during the stressful experience (Folkman & Lazarus, 1980). Certain coping strategies utilize positive emotions in coping with stressful events. For example, positive reappraisal involves cognitively framing a situation in a positive way (Folkman & Moskowitz, 2000; see also Gross, 1998), and problem-focused coping can increase a sense of control over the situation, and therefore feelings of competence and mastery. Individual differences in the use of positive emotions during stressful encounters should have implications for efficacy of the coping process itself and for long-term well-being. Both strategies have been associated with greater positive emotion, even in times of intense distress, such as caring for someone with AIDS (Folkman & Moskowitz, 2000).

Additional research demonstrates that positive emotions play a role in *resilience*—the ability to adapt to and cope with negative situations and to recover quickly from such experiences. In one study, participants who scored higher on trait resilience appraised a stressful task as less threatening and experienced a shorter period of cardio-vascular arousal, an effect mediated by the experience of greater positive emotion during the task (Tugade & Fredrickson, 2004). Even when the appraisal of threat was experimentally manipulated, people who scored higher on trait resilience experienced greater positive emotion during the stressor, which mediated cardiovascular recovery. In another study, people who scored higher on trait resilience before the September 11, 2001, terrorist attacks experienced greater positive emotions in combination with nega-tive emotions, which in turn predicted psy-chological growth in the form of subjective well-being, tranquility, and optimism, in the wake of the attacks (Fredrickson, Tugade, Waugh, & Larkin, 2003). Thus, it appears that in times of stress, resilient individuals utilize positive emotions that contribute to quicker physical and psychological recovery.

Up-Regulation of Positive Emotions

More recently, researchers have focused their attention on the up-regulation of posi-tive emotions—the ways that people create, maintain, or enhance experiences of posi-tive emotion for their own sake. Research suggests that people view the regulation of positive emotions as distinct from the reg-ulation of negative emotions: People have separable beliefs about their abilities to cope with negative emotions and to up-regulate their positive emotions (Bryant, 1989). Bry-ant (2003) distinguishes among three forms of positive emotion up-regulation: savoring the present moment, reminiscing about the past, and anticipating positive experiences in the future. Self-reported individual differ-ences in each of these processes are associ-ated with the greater experience of positive emotion (Bryant, 2003).

Larsen and Prizmic (2004) include *savor-ing*—ruminating on the present—in their list of strategies people can use to up-regulate their positive emotions, along with helping others and using humor. Tkach and Lyubomirsky (2006) investigated the ways college students increase happiness (broadly defined) by asking them what they typically do to increase their happiness. A factor anal-ysis revealed eight general strategies: social

affiliation, partying and clubbing, mental control, instrumental goal pursuit, passive leisure, active leisure, religion, and direct attempts. Some of these strategies (e.g., social affiliation, active leisure) were asso-ciated greater trait-level happiness, whereas others were unrelated to (e.g., passive lei-sure) or negatively associated with (e.g., mental control of negative thoughts) trait-level happiness.

In a series of studies, we systematically investigated the ways in which people up-regulate their positive emotions in everyday life, by consulting the research literature on coping, emotion regulation, and well-being, as well as participant-nominated strategies (Livingstone & Srivastava, 2012). In a pre-liminary study, we asked a sample of young adults to list the activities in which they engage when they want to create, maintain, or increase positive emotions. Supplement-ing this list with strategies suggested by the literature, we factor-analyzed 75 different activities and found three general strategy domains. In a second study, we examined self-reported individual differences in use of the three strategy domains and their relationships to trait positive emotion and well-being. In a third study, we examined the relationship between emotion regulation and positive emotion at a state level, using the day reconstruction method (Kahneman, Krueger, Schkade, Schwarz, & Stone, 2004).

Engagement strategies focus on interact-ing in a positive way with others and with the present moment, through savoring and social interaction. *Betterment* strategies focus on self-improvement goals and spiri-tual fulfillment. *Indulgence* strategies focus on the pursuit of momentary pleasure and include seeking immediate reward (by eat-ing, shopping, or relaxing) and escapism (fantasizing). We examined correlations between these three strategy domains and positive emotion, both at the trait and state levels. Engagement strategies had a robust relationship with a variety of positive emo-tions at both trait and state levels. Better-ment strategies were related to greater trait positive emotion, but lower state positive emotion, indicating a tradeoff between lower temporary pleasure but higher long-term satisfaction. Indulgence strategies were related to greater state positive emotion, but lower trait positive emotion, indicating a tradeoff between momentary pleasure and long-term dissatisfaction.

Different positive emotion regulation strategies have implications for specific positive emotions. Presented below are correlations between the three strategy domains and specific emotions measured using either several items (composite measures) or a single item. Table 5.1 presents zero-order and partial correlations (controlling for the other two strategies) between strategy domains and specific positive emotions.

Engagement strategies were related to all specific positive emotions (with the exception of inspiration), even when we controlled for use of the other strategies. Betterment strategies, in contrast, were particularly related to agency-focused positive emotions such as interest, pride, and inspiration, as well as to future-oriented emotions such as hope and optimism. Indulgence strategies were unrelated to positive emotions, but when

we controlled for use of the other strategies, indulgence was related to lower levels of joy, happiness, contentment, and optimism. Thus, not all strategies for regulating positive emotions are equal in their relationships with the experience of positive emotion (see also Tkach & Lyubomirsky, 2006).

On the other hand, up-regulating emotions may not always be appropriate or functional. In some circumstances, overvaluing happiness was associated with lower well-being (Mauss, Tamir, Anderson, & Savino, 2011). Specifically, for those with low life stress, individual differences in strongly valuing happiness (e.g., "I am concerned with my happiness even when I am happy") predicted lower well-being. When valuing happiness was experimentally manipulated, those who valued happiness experienced lower hedonic tone during a positive situation, but not a negative one. This suggests that placing too much emphasis on positive emotions can be counterproductive.

TABLE 5.1. Zero-Order and Partial Correlations between Trait-Level Positive Emotion Regulation Strategy Domains and Specific Positive Emotions

	Engagement		Betterment		Indulgence	
	r	pr	r	pr	r	pr
Composite measures						
Amusement	.30	.30	.07	−.12	.13	.01
Hope	.50	.46	.24	−.01	.12	−.12
Interest	.37	.26	.29	.15	.10	−.07
Joy	.51	.50	.21	−.07	.09	**−.17**
Love	.38	.36	.12	−.09	.14	−.02
Pride	.43	.31	.34	.18	.13	−.10
Single items						
Inspired	.30	.13	**.41**	.34	.09	−.10
Optimistic	.52	.52	.22	−.05	.07	**−.18**
Happy	.47	.49	.16	−.09	.06	−.19
Content	.42	.40	.22	.03	.02	−.20
Excited	.42	.40	.11	−.14	.18	.00
Enthusiastic	.40	.38	.15	−.07	.15	−.04
Pleased	.38	.28	.23	.04	.18	.04
Love	.35	.37	.08	−.11	.07	−.10
Affection	.29	.23	.12	−.04	.18	.07

*Note. N = 270. Correlations greater than r = .20 are in **bold**.*

Down-Regulation of Positive Emotions

Regulating positive emotions can also involve down-regulation, or dampening them (Gross, 1998). Down-regulation of positive emotions has received relatively less attention from researchers, but a few investigations have suggested that it is an important (if sometimes overlooked) domain of emotion regulation. Parrott (1993) suggested several motives for down-regulating a good mood, including social (e.g., to be considerate of others), nonsocial (e.g., to avoid distraction and improve concentration), and idiosyncratic (e.g., to prevent bad fortune) motives. Specifically, these motives for dampening positive emotions served to influence cognition and motivation in the service of some goal. Thus, the flexible down-regulation of positive emotions (and up-regulation of negative emotions) may serve to enhance psychological and social well-being.

In a similar vein, Tamir (2009b) proposed an instrumental theory of emotion regulation, in which people might (consciously or unconsciously) decrease positive emotions or increase negative ones if they expect the emotions to help them attain long-term goals. For example, in one study, people preferred to be in a neutral mood when meeting a stranger, and therefore dampened both positive and negative emotions (Erber, Wegner, & Therriault, 1996).

On the other hand, habitual and frequent down-regulation of positive emotions has been linked with negative well-being variables. For example, one series of studies found that, across a range of types of events, individuals with low self-esteem were more likely to dampen feelings of positive emotion and to have difficulty savoring positive emotion (Wood, Heimpel, & Michela, 2003).

Conclusion

In this chapter, we have focused on trait, motivational, and self-regulatory approaches to studying positive emotions from a personality perspective. These approaches have provided a better understanding of individual differences in the experience and expression of emotion, and the processes that drive those individual differences. For example, we know that some people are happier, prouder, and more content than others, and we have some insight into why. We know that the goals people hold, and their progress toward them, shape their experiences of positive emotion, and vice versa. We know that people vary in the ways that they select, interpret, and respond to emotional situations, and that the ways in which people manage their emotions (both positive and negative) have implications for how they experience them.

Personality psychology is a diverse and vibrant field, and although we have focused on three major areas of research in this chapter, personality psychologists have taken a variety of other approaches to studying links between the person and positive emotion. For example, the narrative approach to personality examines personality as a life story, in which a person constructs a coherent account of his or her life, including characters, recurring themes, and identity-shaping events (e.g., McAdams, 1995). A person's narrative self-history has possible implications for the experience of positive emotion and well-being, for example, through a sequence of positive transformation after difficulty (Pals, 2006). The very act of writing or telling such a redemptive narrative may promote psychological and somatic health (Pasupathi, McLean, & Weeks, 2009; Pennebaker, 2000).

Another area of personality research we have not covered extensively in this chapter is neuroscience approaches. Researchers working in this area have studied a variety of topics relevant to positive emotions, including how individual differences in positive emotional responses are instantiated in the brain (e.g., Canli et al., 2001), and how individual differences in BAS correspond to neural processing efficiency during a task that requires cognitive control (J. R. Gray et al., 2005). In short, although there has been increasing interest in the links between personality and positive emotion in recent years, there is still much more to learn and substantial opportunity to apply the diverse theories, methods, and emphases within the field of personality psychology.

References

Abbe, A., Tkach, C., & Lyubomirsky, S. (2003). The art of living by dispositionally happy people. *Journal of Happiness Studies, 4,* 385–404.

Asakawa, K. (2010). Flow experience, culture, and well-being: How do autotelic Japanese college students feel, behave, and think in their daily lives. *Journal of Happiness Studies, 11,* 205–223.

Augustine, A. A., Hemenover, S. H., Larsen, R. J., & Shulman, T. E. (2010). Composition and consistency of the desired affective state: The role of personality and motivation. *Motivation and Emotion, 34,* 133–134.

Berkman, E. T., Lieberman, M. D., & Gable, S. L. (2009). BIS, BAS, and response conflict: Testing predictions of the revised reinforcement sensitivity theory. *Personality and Individual Differences, 46,* 586–591.

Bryant, F. B. (1989). A four-factor model of perceived control: Avoiding, coping, obtaining, and savoring. *Journal of Personality, 57,* 773–797.

Bryant, F. B. (2003). Savoring Beliefs Inventory (SBI): A scale for measuring beliefs about savoring. *Journal of Mental Health, 12,* 175–196.

Buck, R. (1994). Nonverbal behavior and the theory of emotion: The facial feedback hypothesis. *Journal of Personality and Social Psychology, 38,* 811–824.

Butler, E. A., Lee, T. L., & Gross, J. J. (2007). Emotion regulation and culture: Are the social consequences of emotion suppression culture-specific? *Emotion, 7,* 30–48.

Canli, T., Zhao, Z., Desmond, J. E., Kang, E., Gross, J. J., & Gabrieli, J. D. E. (2001). An fMRI study of personality influences on brain reactivity to emotional stimuli. *Behavioral Neuroscience, 115,* 33–42.

Cantor, N. (1991). From thought to behavior: "Having" and "doing" in the study of personality and cognition. *American Psychologist, 45,* 735–750.

Carver, C. S. (2003). Pleasure as a sign you can attend to something else: Placing positive feelings within a general model of affect. *Cognition and Emotion, 17,* 241–261.

Carver, C. S., & Scheier, M. (1990). Origins and functions of positive and negative affect: A control-process view. *Psychological Review, 97,* 19–35.

Carver, C. S., Sutton, S. K., & Scheier, M. F. (2000). Action, emotion, and personality: Emerging conceptual integration. *Personality and Social Psychology Bulletin, 26,* 741–751.

Carver, C. S., & White, T. L. (1994). Behavioral inhibition, behavioral activation, and affective responses to impending reward and punishment: The BIS/BAS scales. *Journal of Personality and Social Psychology, 67,* 319–333.

Clark, L. A., & Watson, D. (1988). Mood and the mundane: Relations between daily life events and self-reported mood. *Journal of Personality and Social Psychology, 54,* 296–308.

Cole, P. M., Martin, S. E., & Dennis, T. A. (2004). Emotion regulation as a scientific construct: Methodological challenges and directions for child development research. *Child Development, 75,* 317–333.

Costa, P. T., & McCrae, R. R. (1980). Influence of extraversion and neuroticism on subjective well-being: Happy and unhappy people. *Journal of Personality and Social Psychology, 38,* 668–678.

Csikszentmihalyi, M. (1990). *Flow: The psychology of optimal experience.* New York: Harper & Row.

DeNeve, K. M., & Cooper, H. (1998). The happy personality: A meta-analysis of 137 personality traits and subjective well-being. *Psychological Bulletin, 124,* 197–229.

Diener, E., Lucas, R. E., & Scollon, C. N. (2006). Beyond the hedonic treadmill: Revising the adaptation theory of well-being. *American Psychologist, 61,* 305–314.

Diener, E., & Seligman, M. E. P. (2002). Very happy people. *Psychological Science, 13,* 81–84.

Digman, J. M. (1997). Higher-order factors of the Big Five. *Journal of Personality and Social Psychology, 73,* 1246–1256.

Dweck, C. S., & Leggett, E. L. (1988). A social-cognitive approach to motivation and personality. *Psychological Review, 95,* 256–273.

Eid, M., Riemann, R., Angleitner, A., & Borkenau, P. (2003). Sociability and positive emotionality: Genetic and environmental contributions to the covariation between difference facets of extraversion. *Journal of Personality, 71,* 319–346.

Elliot, A. J. (1999). Approach and avoidance motivation and achievement goals. *Educational Psychologist, 34,* 169–189.

Elliot, A. J., & Church, M. A. (1997). A hierarchical model of approach and avoidance achievement motivation. *Journal of Personality and Social Psychology, 72,* 218–232.

Elliot, A. J., & Thrash, T. M. (2002). Approach–avoidance motivation in personality: Approach and avoidance temperaments and goals. *Journal of Personality and Social Psychology, 82,* 804–818.

Ellsworth, P. C., & Scherer, K. R. (2003). Appraisal processes in emotion. In R. J. Davidson, H. Goldsmith, & K. R. Scherer (Eds.), *Handbook of affective sciences* (pp. 572–595). New York: Oxford University Press.

Emmons, R. A. (1986). Personal strivings: An approach to personality and subjective well-being. *Journal of Personality and Social Psychology, 51,* 1058–1068.

Erber, R. (1996). The self-regulation of moods. In L. L. Martin & A. Tesser (Eds.), *Striving and feeling: Interactions among goals, affect, and self-regulation* (pp. 251–275). Mahwah, NJ: Erlbaum.

Erber, R., Wegner, D. M., & Therriault, N. (1996). On being cool and collected: Mood regulation in anticipation of social interaction. *Journal of Personality and Social Psychology, 70,* 757–766.

Evans, D. E., & Rothbart, M. K. (2007). Developing a model for adult temperament. *Journal of Research in Personality, 41,* 868–888.

Eysenck, H. J., & Eysenck, M. W. (1985). *Personality and individual differences: A natural science approach.* New York: Plenum Press.

Folkman, S., & Lazarus, R. S. (1980). An analysis of coping in a middle-aged community sample. *Journal of Health and Social Behavior, 21,* 219–239.

Folkman, S., & Moskowitz, J. T. (2000). Positive affect and the other side of coping. *American Psychologist, 55,* 647–654.

Fredrickson, B. L. (1998). What good are positive emotions? *Review of General Psychology, 2,* 300–319.

Fredrickson, B. L., Tugade, M. M., Waugh, C. E., & Larkin, G. R. (2003). What good are positive emotions in crises?: A prospective study of resilience and emotions following the terrorist attacks on the United States on September 11th, 2001. *Journal of Personality and Social Psychology, 84,* 365–376.

Frijda, N. H. (1988). The laws of emotion. *American Psychologist, 43,* 349–358.

Gable, S. L., Reis, H. T., & Elliot, A. J. (2000). Behavioral activation and inhibition in everyday life. *Journal of Personality and Social Psychology, 78,* 1135–1149.

Gray, J. A. (1970). The psychophysiological basis of introversion–extraversion. *Behaviour Research and Therapy, 8,* 249–266.

Gray, J. A. (1990). Brain systems that mediate both emotion and cognition. *Cognition and Emotion, 4,* 269–288.

Gray, J. R., Burgess, G. C., Schaefer, A., Yarkoni, T., Larsen, R. J., & Braver, T. (2005). Affective personality differences in neural processing efficiency confirmed using fMRI. *Cognitive, Affective, and Behavioral Neuroscience, 5,* 182–190.

Gross, J. J. (1998). The emerging field of emotion regulation: An integrative review. *Review of General Psychology, 2,* 271–299.

Gross, J. J., & John, O. P. (1997). Revealing feelings: Facets of emotional expressivity in self-reports, peer ratings, and behavior. *Journal of Personality and Social Psychology, 72,* 435–448.

Gross, J. J., & John, O. P. (2003). Individual differences in two emotion regulation processes: Implications for affect, relationships, and well-being. *Journal of Personality and Social Psychology, 85,* 348–362.

Headey, B., & Wearing, A. (1989). Personality, life events, and subjective well-being: Toward a dynamic equilibrium model. *Journal of Personality and Social Psychology, 57,* 731–739.

Higgins, E. T. (1987). Self-discrepancy: A theory relating self and affect. *Psychological Review, 94,* 319–340.

Higgins, E. T. (1996). Ideals, oughts, and regulatory focus: Affect and motivation from distinct pains and pleasures. In P. M. Gollwitzer & J. A. Bargh (Eds.), *The psychology of action: Linking cognition and motivation to behavior* (pp. 91–114). New York: Guilford Press.

Izard, C. E. (1977). *Human emotions.* New York: Plenum Press.

John, O. P., Hampson, S. E., & Goldberg, L. R. (1991). The basic level in personality-trait hierarchies: Studies of trait use and accessibility in different contexts. *Journal of Personality and Social Psychology, 60,* 348–361.

John, O. P., & Srivastava, S. (1999). The Big-Five trait taxonomy: History, measurement, and theoretical perspectives. In L. Pervin & O. P. John (Eds.), *Handbook of personality: Theory and research* (2nd ed., pp. 102–138). New York: Guilford Press.

Kahneman, D., Krueger, A. B., Schkade, D. A., Schwartz, N., & Stone, A. A. (2004). A survey method for characterizing daily life experience: The day reconstruction method. *Science, 306,* 1776–1780.

Kämpfe, N., & Mitte, K. (2009). What you wish is what you get?: The meaning of individual variability in desired affect and affective discrepancy. *Journal of Research in Personality, 43,* 409–418.

Kashdan, T. B., Rose, P., & Fincham, F. D. (2004). Curiosity and exploration: Facilitating positive subjective experiences and personal growth opportunities. *Journal of Personality Assessment, 82,* 291–305.

Kasser, T., & Ryan, R. M. (1993). A dark side of the American Dream: Correlates of financial success as a central life aspiration. *Journal of Personality and Social Psychology, 65,* 410–422.

Kunzmann, U., Little, T. D., & Smith, J. (2000). Is age-related stability of subjective well-being a paradox?: Cross-sectional and longitudinal evidence from the Berlin Aging Study. *Psychology and Aging, 15,* 511–526.

Larsen, R. J., & Ketelaar, T. (1991). Personality and susceptibility to positive and negative emotional states. *Journal of Personality and Social Psychology, 61,* 132–140.

Larsen, R. J., & Prizmic, Z. (2004). Affect regulation. In R. F. Baumeister & K. D. Vohs (Eds.). *Handbook of self-regulation* (pp. 40–61). New York: Guilford Press.

Livingstone, K. M., & Srivastava, S. (2012). Up-regulating positive emotions in everyday life: Strategies, individual differences, and associations with positive emotion and well-being. *Journal of Research in Personality, 46,* 504–516.

Lucas, R. E. (2007). Adaptation and the set-point model of subjective well-being: Does happiness change after major life events? *Current Directions in Psychological Science, 16,* 75–79.

Lucas, R. E., & Fujita, F. (2000). Factors influencing the relation between extraversion and positive affect. *Journal of Personality and Social Psychology, 79,* 1039–1056.

Lucas, R. E., Le, K., & Dyrenforth, P. S. (2008). Explaining the extraversion/positive affect relation: Sociability cannot account for extraverts' greater happiness. *Journal of Personality, 76,* 385–414.

Lykken, D., & Tellegen, A. (1996). Happiness is a stochastic phenomenon. *Psychological Science, 7,* 186–189.

Lyubomirsky, S. (2001). Why are some people happier than others?: The role of cognitive and motivational processes in well-being. *American Psychologist, 56,* 239–249.

Lyubomirsky, S., & Tucker, K. L. (1998). Implications of individual differences in subjective happiness for perceiving, interpreting, and thinking about life events. *Motivation and Emotion, 22,* 155–186.

Markus, H., & Nurius, P. (1986). Possible selves. *American Psychologist, 41,* 954–969.

Mauss, I. B., Shallcross, A. J., Troy, A. S., John, O. P., Ferrer, E., Wilhelm, F. H., et al. (2011). Don't hide your happiness!: Positive emotion dissociation, social connectedness, and psychological functioning. *Journal of Personality and Social Psychology, 100,* 738–748.

Mauss, I. B., Tamir, M., Anderson, L., & Savino, N. S. (2011). Can seeking happiness make people unhappy?: Paradoxical effects of valuing happiness. *Emotion, 11,* 807–815.

McAdams, D. P. (1995). What do we know when we know a person? *Journal of Personality, 63,* 365–396.

McAdams, D. P. (2010). Personality development: Continuity and change over the life course. *Annual Review of Psychology, 61,* 517–542.

McCrae, R. R., & Costa, P. R. (1991). Adding *liebe und arbeit:* The full five-factor model and well-being. *Personality and Psychology Bulletin, 17,* 227–232.

Mitte, K., & Kämpfe, N. (2008). Personality and the four faces of positive affect: A multitrait-multimethod analysis using self- and peer-report. *Journal of Research in Personality, 42,* 1370–1375.

Nakamura, J., & Csikszentmihalyi, M. (2002). The concept of flow. In C. R. Snyder & S. J. Lopez (Eds.), *The handbook of positive psychology* (pp. 89–105). New York: Oxford University Press.

Nezlek, J. B., & Kuppens, P. (2008). Regulating positive and negative emotions in daily life. *Journal of Personality, 76,* 561–579.

Pals, J. L. (2006). Narrative identity processing of difficult life experiences: Pathways of personality development and positive self-transformation in adulthood. *Journal of Personality, 74,* 1079–1110.

Parkinson, B., & Totterdell, P. (1999). Classifying affect-regulation strategies. *Cognition and Emotion, 13,* 277–303.

Parrott, W. G. (1993). Beyond hedonism: Motives for inhibiting good moods and for maintaining bad moods. In D. M. Wegner & J. W. Pennebaker (Eds.), *Handbook of mental control* (pp. 278–305). Englewood Cliffs, NJ: Prentice-Hall.

Pasupathi, M., McLean, K. C., & Weeks, T. (2009). To tell or not to tell: Disclosure and the narrative self. *Journal of Personality, 77,* 89–124.

Pekrun, R., Elliot, A. J., & Maier, M. A. (2006). Achievement goals and discrete achievement emotions: A theoretical model and prospective test. *Journal of Educational Psychology, 98,* 583–597.

Pennebaker, J. W. (2000). Telling stories: The health benefits of narrative. *Literature and Medicine, 19,* 3–18.

Roberts, B. W., & DelVecchio, W. F. (2000). The rank-order consistency of personality traits from childhood to old age: A quantitative review of longitudinal studies. *Psychological Bulletin, 126,* 3–25.

Rothbart, M. K. (2007). Temperament, development, and personality. *Current Directions in Psychological Science, 103,* 55–66.

Rothbart, M. K., Ahadi, S. A., & Evans, D. E. (2000). Temperament and personality: Origins and outcomes. *Journal of Personality and Social Psychology, 78,* 122–135.

Rusting, C. L., & Larsen, R. J. (1995). Moods as sources of stimulation: Relationships between personality and desired mood states. *Personality and Individual Differences, 3,* 321–329.

Ryan, R. M., & Deci, E. L. (2000). Intrinsic and extrinsic motivations: Classic definitions and new directions. *Contemporary Educational Psychology, 25,* 54–67.

Saucier, G., & Srivastava, S. (in press). What are the most important dimensions of personality?: A review and critique of studies of descriptors in diverse languages. In M. Mikulincer & P. R. Shaver (Series Eds.) and M. L. Cooper & R. J. Larsen (Vol. Eds.), *Handbook of social and personality psychology: Vol. 3. Personality processes and individual differences.* Washington, DC: American Psychological Association.

Schwartz, S. H. (1992). Universals in the content and structure of values: Theoretical advances and empirical tests in 20 countries. *Advances in Experimental Social Psychology, 25,* 1–65.

Sheldon, K. M., & Kasser, T. (1995). Coherence and congruence: Two aspects of personality integration. *Journal of Personality and Social Psychology, 68,* 531–543.

Sheldon, K. M., & Kasser, T. (1998). Pursuing personal goals: Skills enable progress, but not all progress is beneficial. *Personality and Social Psychology Bulletin, 24,* 1319–1331.

Shiota, M. N., Keltner, D., & John, O. P. (2006). Positive emotions dispositions differentially associated with Big Five personality and attachment style. *Journal of Positive Psychology, 1,* 61–71.

Srivastava, S., Angelo, K. M., & Vallereux, S. R. (2008). Extraversion and positive affect: A day reconstruction study of person–environment transactions. *Journal of Research in Personality, 42,* 1613–1618.

Tamir, M. (2009a). Differential preferences for happiness: Extraversion and trait-consistent emotion regulation. *Journal of Personality, 77,* 448–470.

Tamir, M. (2009b). What do people want to feel and why?: Pleasure and utility in emotion regulation. *Current Directions in Psychological Science, 18,* 101–105.

Tellegen, A., Lykken, D. T., Bouchard, T. J., Wilcox, K. J., Segal, N. L., & Rich, S. (1988). Personality similarity in twins reared apart and together. *Journal of Personality and Social Psychology, 54,* 1031–1039.

Tkach, C., & Lyubomirsky, S. (2006). How do people pursue happiness?: Relating personality, happiness-increasing strategies, and well-being. *Journal of Happiness Studies, 7,* 183–225.

Tobin, R. M., Graziano, W. G., Vanman, E. J., & Tassinary, L. G. (2000). Personality, emotional experience, and efforts to control emotions. *Journal of Personality and Social Psychology, 79,* 656–669.

Tong, E. M. W., Fredrickson, B. L., Chang, W., & Lim, Z. X. (2010). Re-examining hope: The roles of agency thinking and pathways thinking. *Cognition and Emotion, 24,* 1207–1215.

Tracy, J. L., & Robins, R. W. (2007). The psychological structure of pride: A tale of two facets. *Journal of Personality and Social Psychology, 92,* 506–525.

Tsai, J. L., Knutson, B., & Fung, H. H. (2006). Cultural variation in affect valuation. *Journal of Personality and Social Psychology, 90,* 288–307.

Tugade, M. M., & Fredrickson, B. L. (2004). Resilient individuals use positive emotions to bounce back from negative emotional experiences. *Journal of Personality and Social Psychology, 86,* 320–333.

Västfjäll, D., Gärling, T., & Kleiner, M. (2001). Does it make you happy feeling this way?:

A core affect account of preferences for current mood. *Journal of Happiness Studies, 2,* 337–354.

Watson, D., & Clark, L. A. (1997). Extraversion and its positive emotional core. In R. Hogan, J. A. Johnson, & S. R. Briggs (Eds.), *Handbook of personality* (pp. 767–793). San Diego, CA: Academic Press.

Watson, D., & Walker, L. M. (1996). The long-term stability and predictive validity of trait measures of affect. *Journal of Personality and Social Psychology, 70,* 567–577.

Williams, L. A., & DeSteno, D. (2008). Pride and perseverance: The motivational role of pride. *Journal of Personality and Social Psychology, 94,* 1007–1017.

Wood, J. V., Heimpel, S. A., & Michela, J. L. (2003). Savoring versus dampening: Self-esteem differences in regulating positive affect. *Journal of Personality and Social Psychology, 85,* 566–580.

Zelinski, J. M., & Larsen, R. J. (1999). The distribution of basic emotions in everyday life: A state and trait perspective from experience sampling data. *Journal of Research in Personality, 34,* 178–197.

PART II

The Biology
of Positive Emotion

CHAPTER 6

Approach Motivation and Its Relationship to Positive and Negative Emotions

Eddie Harmon-Jones
Tom F. Price
Philip A. Gable
Carly K. Peterson

Approach motivation is often considered to be closely related to positive affect (Watson, 2000). Indeed, some theories consider approach motivation to involve only positive affect, and avoidance motivation to involve only negative affect (Lang & Bradley, 2013; Watson, 2000). In this chapter, we review theory and research on the relationship between approach motivation and affective states and traits. We start by reviewing theory and research on asymmetrical frontal cortical activity and its relationship with affective valence (positive vs. negative) and motivational direction (approach vs. avoidance). Within this body of research, much work has examined anger because it is an emotion that may assist in disentangling approach motivation from affective valence. That is, anger is often associated with approach motivation even though it is experienced as a negative affective state. After reviewing work on asymmetrical frontal cortical activity and affective valence/motivational direction, we review research suggesting positive affective states that vary in approach motivational intensity differ in their relationships with asymmetrical frontal cortical activity and other psychophysiological responses. Then, we review another line of research, inspired by the former research, which suggests that positive affective states varying in approach motivational intensity differentially influence some cognitive processes. We conclude that despite differing in affective valence, high-approach positive affects share some similarities with approach-oriented anger.

Our Definitions

We begin by presenting definitions of concepts we have used in our program of research given the diversity of definitions used in emotions research (Izard, 2010). Emotions are multifaceted processes comprised of more basic components such as feelings of pleasure or pain, outward displays (e.g., facial expressions, body postures), motivational changes, and changes in physiology (Lang, 1995). Moreover, these components are not perfectly correlated with each other (Lang, 1995).

Motivational direction (approach or avoidance) is an important component of emotion. We conceptualize approach motivation as the urge to move toward something, whereas avoidance motivation is the urge to move away (E. Harmon-Jones, C. Harmon-Jones, & Price, 2013). As noted earlier, theories often posit that approach motivation is associated with positive affect, whereas avoidance motivation is associated with negative affect. In this chapter, we review research suggesting that approach motivation can also be associated with the negative affective experience of anger (Carver & E. Harmon-Jones, 2009). Motivational direction, therefore, can be independent of affective valence.

Arousal is often posited to be a proxy for motivational intensity, where increased positive or negative arousal indicates increased approach or avoidance activation, respectively (Bradley & Lang, 2007). While an increase in motivational intensity might be associated with an increase in arousal, an increase in arousal might not necessarily indicate an increase in motivational intensity. Humor and amusement, for example, are arousing positive states (Fredrickson & Branigan, 2005; Gable & E. Harmon-Jones, 2008a), but they are often low in approach motivation. Similarly, caffeine and physical exercise might increase arousal but not the motivation to approach or avoid something (Gable & E. Harmon-Jones, 2013a).

Affective valence can be defined in at least one of three ways; that is, emotions or affective states can be positive or negative (1) because of the conditions that evoked the emotion; (2) because of an emotion's adaptive consequences; (3) or because of the emotion's subjective feel (Lazarus, 1991). Most appraisal theorists regard the first definition—the appraised situation—as the primary definition for affective valence (Lazarus, 1991), and according to this definition, positive emotions occur in positively appraised (goal-congruent or desirable) situations, whereas negative emotions occur in negatively appraised (goal-incongruent or undesirable) situations. According to this definition, anger is a negative emotion because it is evoked in situations that are evaluated as negative or goal-incongruent.

The second definition of affective valence is difficult to use, in our opinion, because functional accounts of emotion (see Shiota, Chapter 3, this volume) would regard all emotions as having positive adaptive fitness consequences. Thus, all emotions would be positive. Even if functional accounts are not acceptable, this definition is problematic because of the difficulty of defining consequences: Are they consequences for the self, another person, society, the species, or what? Are they short-term or long-term consequences?

The third definition—the subjective evaluation of the feeling state—has been subjected to scientific scrutiny recently and is the one that we prefer when defining an emotion as negative or positive. Research has revealed that individuals have distinct attitudes toward different emotions such as joy, anger, fear, disgust, and sadness (E. Harmon-Jones, C. Harmon-Jones, Amodio, & Gable, 2011). Across all participants, joy is evaluated more positively than anger, fear, disgust, and sadness, and these latter emotions are generally evaluated as negative (rarely do individuals evaluate these latter emotions as positive; E. Harmon-Jones, 2004). These results are consistent with the intuition that joy is positive and the other emotions are negative.

However, individuals differ in how positively they regard joy and how negatively they regard anger, fear, disgust, and sadness. Moreover, these individual differences in attitudes toward specific emotions predict interest in viewing different types of stimuli associated with these emotions (E. Harmon-Jones, C. Harmon-Jones, Amodio, et al., 2011, Study 2). In addition, these attitudes toward emotions correlate with trait emotions, but the direction of these correlations depends on whether the emotion being examined is approach- or withdrawal-oriented (E. Harmon-Jones, C. Harmon-Jones, Amodio, et al., 2011, Study 3). That is, individuals with high trait levels of approach-oriented emotions (e.g., joy, anger) like these emotional states more, whereas individuals with high trait levels of withdrawal-oriented emotions (e.g., disgust, fear) dislike these emotional states more. In addition, more positive attitudes toward approach-oriented emotions caused greater experienced approach-oriented emotions, whereas more positive attitudes toward withdrawal-oriented emotions caused less experienced withdrawal-oriented emotions when they were evoked in the laboratory (E. Harmon-Jones, C. Harmon-Jones, Amodio, et al., 2011, Study 4).

Asymmetrical Frontal Cortical Activity, Affective Valence, and Motivational Direction

The left and right frontal cortices are involved in different emotive processes. This was originally observed in World War I soldiers who experienced changes in positive affect (approach motivation) or negative affect (withdrawal motivation) after damage to the right or left anterior cortex, respectively (Goldstein, 1939). Later research supported these findings using the Wada test, which involves injecting sodium amytal (barbiturate) into the left or right carotid artery within the neck. Injections into the left interior artery, suppressing left-hemispheric brain activation, caused depressive symptoms. Injections into the right interior artery, suppressing right-hemispheric brain activation, caused euphoria (Terzian & Cecotto, 1959). These results suggested that the right and left hemispheres of the brain exert inhibitory effects on one another, such that when the right (left) hemisphere is inhibited with sodium amytal, the left (right) hemisphere becomes disinhibited and produces euphoria (depression).

Positive and Negative Affect

Additional research revealed that individuals with lesions to the left frontal region were more likely to show depressive symptoms (Gainotti, 1972; Robinson & Price, 1982), whereas those with lesions to the right frontal region were more likely to show manic symptoms (Gainotti, 1972; Robinson & Price, 1982). Nonhuman animals show similar effects. That is, asymmetries associated with appetitive and avoidant behaviors have been found in animals ranging from apes and reptiles to pigeons, amphibians, spiders, and dogs (Quaranta, Siniscalchi, & Vallortigara, 2007; see review by Vallortigara & Rogers, 2005).

Other research supported these findings using electroencephalographic (EEG) methodologies and measuring cortical activity

with EEG alpha power, which is inversely associated with regional brain activity (Cook, O'Hara, Uijtdehaage, Mandelkern, & Leuchter 1998). In this research, asymmetrical frontal cortical activation is measured in homologous areas in the left and right frontal regions. Difference scores are used in this research; their use is consistent with the aforementioned amytal and lesion studies that suggest a reciprocal relationship between the left and right frontal regions.

EEG research has revealed that greater left than right frontal cortical activity at resting baseline is associated with more trait approach motivation (Amodio, Master, Yee, & Taylor, 2008; E. Harmon-Jones & Allen, 1997), more trait positive activation and less trait negative activation (Tomarken, Davidson, Wheeler, & Doss, 1992), more promotion (vs. prevention) focus (Amodio, Shah, Sigelman, Brazy, & E. Harmon-Jones, 2004), and less depression (Thibodeau, Jorgensen, & Kim, 2006). Low relative left frontal activity predicts the onset of depression (Nusslock et al., 2011). Moreover, greater relative left frontal activity predicts the conversion from less severe forms of bipolar disorder to more severe forms (bipolar I; Nusslock et al., 2012), a psychological disorder that has been associated with overactive approach motivation sensitivity (Urošević, Abramson, Harmon-Jones, & Alloy, 2008). Similarly, individuals with bipolar disorder respond with greater relative left frontal activity to challenging tasks that promise rewards (E. Harmon-Jones et al., 2008).

Greater relative left frontal activity at baseline has also been found to predict reduced sensitivity to negative outcomes, as measured by error-related negativities in response to behavioral errors committed on speeded reaction time tasks (Nash, Inzlicht, & McGregor, 2012). In addition, greater relative right frontal activity at baseline has been found to predict more empathic reactions to others in need of help (Tullett, E. Harmon-Jones, & Inzlicht, 2012). It is important to note, however, that although resting baseline frontal asymmetry is often regarded as a trait measure, research using multiple recording sessions has found that roughly half of the variance in baseline recordings is due to state influences and half is due to trait influences (Hagemann,

Naumann, Thayer, & Bartussek, 2002). In line with this, situational variables such as time of day, time of year (Peterson & E. Harmon-Jones, 2009), and attractiveness of the opposite sex experimenter (Wacker, Mueller, Pizzagalli, Hennig, & Stemmler, 2013) influence asymmetrical frontal cortical activity and its relationship with other variables such as behavioral activation sensitivity (BAS).

Situational manipulations of emotive states also influence asymmetrical frontal cortical activity. That is, relative left frontal activity was increased by manipulations of positive affective states using stimuli such as directed facial expressions (Coan, Allen, & E. Harmon-Jones, 2001), humorous film clips (Davidson, Ekman, Saron, Senulis, & Friesen, 1990), film clips of an actress generating a happy facial expression (Davidson & Fox, 1982), and pleasant words (Cunningham, Espinet, DeYoung, & Zelazo, 2005). Newborn infants (2–3 days old) evidenced greater relative left-sided activation in frontal regions in response to sucrose as compared with water (Fox & Davidson, 1986). Relative right frontal activity was increased by manipulations of negative affective states using stimuli such as directed facial expressions to evoke disgust and fear (Coan et al., 2001), film clips to evoke disgust (Jones & Fox, 1992), and unpleasant words (Cunningham et al., 2005).

Manipulations of relative left frontal activity also influence affective variables, providing even more evidence of a causal relationship between these variables. For instance, experiments using biofeedback (Allen, E. Harmon-Jones, & Cavender, 2001) and unilateral hand contractions (E. Harmon-Jones, 2006) have found that manipulated increases in relative left frontal activity influence positive affective responses to appetitive stimuli. Moreover, a manipulated increase in relative left frontal activity (using repetitive transcranial magnetic stimulation; see below) is an effective treatment for depression (Schutter, 2009).

Some past research on asymmetrical frontal cortical activity and emotion has failed to produce predicted results (see reviews by Murphy, Nimmo-Smith, & Lawrence, 2003; Pizzagalli, Shackman, & Davidson, 2003). Studies using affective pictures are particularly noteworthy for their failures to produce predicted results (Hagemann, Naumann, Becker, Maier, & Bartussek, 1998). Pictures may not evoke sufficient emotional intensity to engage asymmetrical frontal cortical activations for *all* individuals. Also, the intermixing of multiple types of affective stimuli may weaken motivational effects (Gable & E. Harmon-Jones, 2009). One way to address these issues is to examine whether individual differences in emotion-related variables would predict asymmetrical frontal cortical activity in response to pictures. Studies have revealed that individuals with stronger emotive tendencies (e.g., longer time since they have eaten, more liking for dessert) toward positive stimuli (e.g., pictures of desserts) showed greater relative left frontal activation to those stimuli but not to neutral stimuli (Gable & E. Harmon-Jones, 2008b; E. Harmon-Jones & Gable, 2009). In these studies, the affective pictures alone did not cause significant changes in asymmetrical frontal cortical activity.

These studies led to the suggestion that relative left frontal cortical activity was associated with approach motivation and positive affective valence, whereas greater relative right frontal cortical activity was associated with withdrawal motivation and negative affect (Davidson, 1998). Another interpretation is that motivational direction was confounded with affective valence in past studies. That is, studies had typically examined positive emotions high in approach motivation and negative emotions high in avoidance motivation. Thus, research was needed to address this confound. An emotion that might assist in deconfounding motivational direction and affective valence is anger because it is considered to be negative in valence but approach-oriented.

Anger and Asymmetrical Frontal Cortical Activity

Anger and Approach Motivation

The idea that anger is negatively valenced is well accepted, but the idea that it is associated with approach motivation is less well established. Several theorists have posited that anger evokes behavioral tendencies of approach (e.g., Darwin, 1872; Plutchik, 1980). Of course, emotions such as anger are complex phenomena that may evoke approach or withdrawal tendencies depending on the situation. However, as we review below, most evidence suggests that the dominant behavioral tendency associated with anger is approach (Carver & E. Harmon-Jones, 2009).

In the animal behavior literature, offensive or irritable aggression is distinguished from defensive aggression (e.g., Moyer, 1976). Offensive aggression is posited to be associated with anger, attack, and no attempts to escape, whereas defensive aggression is posited to be associated with fear, attempts to escape, and attack only if escape is impossible (Blanchard & Blanchard, 1984; Lagerspetz, 1969). In support of this relationship between offensive aggression and approach motivation, Lagerspetz (1969) found that under certain conditions mice would cross an electrified grid to attack another mouse.

Another way anger is linked with approach motivation is in terms of the triggering stimulus. Anger often results from goal blockage, when organisms are obstructed from obtaining expected, desired outcomes (Carver & E. Harmon-Jones, 2009). Consistent with these ideas, Lewis, Alessandri, and Sullivan (1990; Lewis, Sullivan, Ramsey, & Alessandri, 1992) taught infants to pull a string to receive a reward. They found that infants who displayed anger when the reward was withdrawn demonstrated the highest levels of joy, interest, and required arm pull when the learning portion of the task was reinstated. Thus, subsequent to frustrating events, anger may maintain and increase task engagement and approach motivation.

In response to anger-arousing situations, self-reported state anger increases, as does positive activation (PA) (E. Harmon-Jones, C. Harmon-Jones, Abramson, & Peterson, 2009), as measured by the Positive and Negative Affect Schedule (PANAS; which includes words such as *strong, determined,* and *active* [Watson, 2000]). Moreover, anger correlates directly with PA. Studies within this article by E. Harmon-Jones and colleagues (2009) revealed that these effects are not due to anger being evaluated as positive, but are instead due to both anger and PA being associated with approach motivation. Consequently, we suggest that the PA of the PANAS means "pounce affect"; thus, PA can occur in positively or negatively valenced affective situations.

Trait anger relates to high levels of assertiveness and competitiveness (Buss & Perry, 1992) and optimistic expectations (whereas fear is associated with pessimistic expectations; Lerner & Keltner, 2001). Happiness is also associated with optimism, making anger and happiness more similar to each other in their relationship with optimism than are fear and anger.

Other individual-differences studies support the hypothesis that trait anger is related to trait approach motivation, or more specifically, trait behavioral activation sensitivity (BAS). Carver and White (1994) designed a scale to measure BAS, as well as behavioral inhibition sensitivity (BIS) or punishment sensitivity. Sample items from the BIS scale include "I worry about making mistakes" and "I have very few fears compared to my friends" (reverse scored). Sample items from the BAS include "It would excite me to win a contest," "I go out of my way to get things I want," and "I crave excitement and new sensations." Studies have revealed that trait BAS is positively related to trait anger (E. Harmon-Jones, 2003).

Other research has found that trait levels of BAS relate to self-reported anger responses to laboratory manipulations of anger. Carver (2004) found that trait BAS predicts state anger in response to situational anger manipulations. Putman, Hermans, and van Honk (2004) found that trait BAS predicts attentional vigilance to angry faces, suggesting that individuals with stronger approach motivational sensitivities selectively attend to angry faces, as in a dominance confrontation. And E. Harmon-Jones and Peterson (2008) found that individuals high in BAS who were primed with approach motivation showed the most aggressive inclinations after being insulted.

Trait Anger and Asymmetrical Frontal Cortical Activity

To test the relation of anger with asymmetrical frontal cortical activity, researchers examined trait anger and resting, baseline EEG activity. Trait anger was found to be associated with greater relative left frontal cortical activity (E. Harmon-Jones, 2004; E. Harmon-Jones & Allen, 1998), even among young male psychiatric patients (ages 5–17) with a history of impulsive aggression (Rybak, Crayton, Young, Herba, & Konopka, 2006) and imprisoned violent offenders (Keune et al., 2012). In addition, greater relative left frontal cortical activity in response to anger-evoking stimuli is predicted by trait anger (E. Harmon-Jones, 2007), trait hypomania (E. Harmon-Jones et al., 2002), and trait approach motivation (Gable & Poole, in press).

State Anger Influences Asymmetrical Frontal Cortical Activity

Experiments that have manipulated anger have revealed that anger causes greater relative left frontal activity (E. Harmon-Jones & Sigelman, 2001; E. Harmon-Jones, Vaugh-Scott, Mohr, Sigelman, & C. Harmon-Jones, 2004; Jensen-Campbell, Knack, Waldrip, & Campbell, 2007). In these experiments, anger was evoked using insulting interpersonal feedback (E. Harmon-Jones & Sigelman, 2001), social ostracism (E. Harmon-Jones, Peterson, & Harris, 2009; Peterson, Gravens, & E. Harmon-Jones, 2011), and physical stressors such as annoying high-pressure air blasts delivered to the throat (Verona, Sadeh, & Curtin, 2009). Subsequent experiments revealed that when individuals were angry and expected to act on their anger (a manipulation of approach motivation), they showed greater relative left frontal activity. These results suggest that the approach motivation that often accompanies anger is the critical variable underlying the relative left frontal activity increase during anger (E. Harmon-Jones, Lueck, Fearn, & C. Harmon-Jones, 2006; E. Harmon-Jones, Sigelman, Bohlig, & C. Harmon-Jones, 2003). Also, when individuals are in a supine body position and insulted, which undermines approach motivation (see below), they do not respond with an increase in relative left frontal activity (E. Harmon-Jones & Peterson, 2009).

Manipulating Asymmetrical Frontal Cortical Activity Influences Anger

In order to establish a stronger causal link between relative left frontal activity and anger, researchers have used noninvasive brain stimulation techniques such as repetitive transcranial magnetic stimulation (rTMS) and transcranial direct current stimulation (tDCS). For example, d'Alfonso, van Honk, Hermans, Postma, and de Haan (2000) used slow rTMS to inhibit the left or right prefrontal cortex. Slow rTMS reduces cortical excitability, so that rTMS applied to the right prefrontal cortex decreases its activation and causes the left prefrontal cortex to become more active, while rTMS applied to the left prefrontal cortex causes activation of the right prefrontal cortex. They found that rTMS applied to the right prefrontal cortex caused selective attention toward angry faces, whereas applied to the left prefrontal cortex caused selective attention away from angry faces. Thus, an increase in left prefrontal activity led participants to approach angry faces attentionally, as in an aggressive confrontation. In contrast, an increase in right prefrontal activity led participants to avoid angry faces attentionally, as in a fear-based avoidance. The interpretation of these results is supported by research demonstrating that attention toward angry faces is associated with high levels of anger, BAS, and testosterone, and that attention away from angry faces is associated with high levels of social anxiety and cortisol (see review by van Honk & Schutter, 2007). These results have been conceptually replicated using rTMS by van Honk and Schutter (2006) and by Peterson, Shackman, and E. Harmon-Jones (2008) using hand contractions and a behavioral measure of aggression.

tDCS uses two electrodes: The anodal electrode increases cortical excitability, whereas the cathodal one decreases it (Nitsche & Paulus, 2000). When placed over the left and right frontal regions, tDCS is perfect for examining the influence of asymmetrical cortical activity on psychobehavioral processes. One tDCS study revealed that increasing relative left frontal cortical activity promotes aggressive responses in individuals who are angry (Hortensius, Schutter, & E. Harmon-Jones, 2012). In another study, increasing relative right frontal cortical activity led to more rumination after an anger provocation that could not be acted upon (Kelley, Hortensius, & E. Harmon-Jones, 2013). This latter study is consistent with other research suggesting that when angry expressions are blocked, relatively greater right frontal activation may occur, and the anger may be mixed with anxiety

(Zinner, Brodish, Devine, & E. Harmon-Jones, 2008).

In summary, the idea that anger is associated with approach motivational tendencies is supported by behavioral and neurophysiological evidence. However, some instances of anger, such as anger mixed with anxiety, may be associated with withdrawal motivational tendencies (Zinner et al., 2008), which may associated with rumination (Kelley et al., 2013). Also, anger may not be the only negative emotion associated with approach motivation. During guilt, individuals may evidence more approach motivation as they attempt to make reparations for the action that caused their guilt. In one study testing this idea, individuals evidenced greater relative right frontal activity when first exposed to information that made them feel guilt, but they later showed greater relative left frontal activity when provided an opportunity to make amends for their guilt (Amodio, Devine, & E. Harmon-Jones, 2007).

Positive Affects Varying in Approach and Asymmetrical Frontal Cortical Activity

In past research relating positive affect with greater relative left frontal activity, it was unknown how well the examined positive affect related to approach motivation. That is, if positive affect and approach motivation are separable and perhaps independent constructs, then positive affect may vary in approach motivation. If asymmetrical frontal cortical activity indeed reflects the intensity of motivational direction, then positive affects that vary in motivational intensity should also vary in degree of relative left frontal cortical activity.

Only a few studies have examined whether positive affective states that vary in approach motivational intensity influence asymmetrical frontal cortical activity. In one experiment, participants described steps needed to obtain a desired goal (positive action-oriented), a normal day (neutral), or a past event that made them feel good without personal action (positive, non-action-oriented; E. Harmon-Jones, C. Harmon-Jones, Fearn, Sigelman, & Johnson, 2008; Experiment 2). Results indicated that self-reported positivity (*enthusiastic, interested, happy, proud,* and *feel good about myself*) was greater in the action- and non-action-oriented posi-

tive conditions than in the neutral condition. More importantly, participants in the positive action-oriented condition had greater relative left frontal cortical activity than did participants in the other two conditions. Thus, high-approach, compared to low-approach positive affective states causes greater relative left frontal cortical activity.

Other research provided converging evidence using different manipulations of high- and low-approach positive affect. For example, E. Harmon-Jones, Gable, and Price (2011) had participants adopt high-approach leaning-forward or low-approach reclining-backward postures (e.g., Price & E. Harmon-Jones, 2010). While in one of these two postures, participants viewed appetitive (dessert) and neutral (rock) pictures. Thus, there were four conditions in this experiment: high-approach appetitive (leaning toward desserts), high-approach neutral (leaning toward rocks), low-approach appetitive (reclining from desserts), and low-approach neutral (reclining from rocks). Results indicated that posture moderated the effects of picture type. Those in the high-approach, forward-leaning posture showed greater relative left frontal activity in response to appetitive dessert as compared to neutral rock pictures. Those in the low-approach reclining posture, however, did not show this picture type difference in asymmetrical frontal cortical activity. Thus, these motivational postures promoted relative left frontal cortical activity in response to appetitive but not neutral pictures.

Based on work suggesting that determination is a positive emotion associated with higher approach motivation than is satisfaction (C. Harmon-Jones, Schmeichel, Mennitt, & E. Harmon-Jones, 2011), it is was predicted that determination would cause greater relative left frontal activity than satisfaction, even though both emotions are positive in valence. In this experiment, participants were asked to express determination, satisfaction, or neutrality on their faces while EEG was recorded (Price, Hortensius, & E. Harmon-Jones, 2013). After making the expression of the emotion for 1 minute, participants worked on a puzzle task that included some insolvable puzzles, so that task persistence could be assessed. Results indicated that the determination facial expression caused greater relative left frontal activity, and this cortical activity was correlated with more behavioral persistence on the task.

Other Psychophysiological Responses Influenced by Positive Affects Varying in Approach

So far this chapter has focused on asymmetrical frontal cortical activity and its relationship with approach motivation. Other psychophysiological, neural, chemical, and hormonal responses are involved in approach motivation as well. However, given space limitations, we now turn to a brief review of some of those responses, focusing on psychophysiological ones.

Event-Related Potentials

The late positive potential (LPP) of the event-related potential (ERP) is one such example (for review, see Hajcak, Weinberg, MacNamara, & Foti, 2012). The LPP is a positive deflection in the ERP occurring 300 ms following stimulus onset and lasting for several 100 ms at central parietal regions of the scalp. It is thought to reflect motivated attention. Functional magnetic resonance imaging (fMRI) and EEG studies have revealed multiple neural generators of the LPP, such as the occipitotemporal cortex, parietal cortex, and the amygdala (Sabatinelli, Lang, Keil, & Bradley, 2007). Research has also indicated that LPPs are larger to motivationally significant positive (e.g., erotica) and negative (e.g., mutilations) stimuli than to less motivationally significant positive (e.g., sports scenes), negative (e.g., scenes of loss), and neutral stimuli (Hajcak et al., 2012).

Based on this prior research, Price, Dieckman, and E. Harmon-Jones (2012) predicted that high compared to low approach motivation should cause greater motivated attention (e.g., larger LPPs) in response to positive stimuli. The motivational manipulation was not predicted to influence LPP response to less motivationally significant neutral stimuli. In this experiment, participants adopted high-approach forward-leaning or low-approach reclining postures while viewing erotic scenes with men and women, or neutral scenes with two individuals. Participants were initially prescreened to

ensure that they were not offended by erotica. Self-reported emotions to pictures confirmed that erotic images were rated more positively than neutral images. LPP results at central-parietal regions of the scalp, furthermore, were in line with predictions: Leaning compared to reclining caused larger LPPs in response to erotica, whereas posture did not influence LPPs to neutral stimuli. Similar effects emerged for even earlier ERP components (e.g., 100 ms after stimulus onset), suggesting that the motivational manipulation influenced early attentional processes toward positive stimuli as well, and are consistent with other research examining ERPs related to positive affects high in approach motivation (Gable & Harmon-Jones, 2013b). These results suggest that manipulating motivational intensity influences how individuals attend to positive stimuli.

Startle Reflex

Some reflexive responses are also influenced by motivational factors, for example, the startle eyeblink reflex (Lang, 1995). The startle reflex causes the orbicularis oculi muscle to contract around the eye, protecting it from sudden aversive events. Startle responses are often induced by loud (100 dB), unexpected bursts of white noise with instantaneous rise time (100-ms duration). Experiments have demonstrated that the affective content of pictures modulates startle eyeblink responses. In particular, larger blinks occur while viewing negative rather than neutral pictures. Smaller blinks occur while viewing positive rather than neutral pictures (Lang, 1995). These effects are often interpreted with the response-matching hypothesis, which states that the startle response is a defensive reaction that is sensitive to affective cues. Negative pictures or aversive cues add to the avoidant motivation of the startling sound, causing larger startle blinks. Positive pictures or appetitive cues clash with the avoidant motivation of the startling sound; these inconsistent motivational states cause smaller startle blinks. Animal research has indicated that nuclei within the amygdala are critical for the affective modulation of the startle response (Lang, 1995).

Consistent with the motivational interpretation of the response-matching hypothesis, manipulations of high- and low-approach motivation influence startle responses to positive pictures. For example, forward leaning compared to reclining body position causes smaller startle responses in participants viewing erotic but not neutral stimuli (Price et al., 2012). These results suggest that higher approach motivation elicits a greater appetitive response (e.g., smaller startle blink) to positive but not neutral images.

In addition, trait levels of approach motivation have been linked to startle responses to positive pictures. Amodio and E. Harmon-Jones (2011), for example, measured participants' trait levels of enjoyment and surprise. Results indicated that higher levels of these traits correlated with greater blink inhibition in response to positive pictures. In addition, higher levels of trait anger also correlated with greater blink inhibition in response to positive pictures. These results suggest that trait anger, though typically negative in valence, is associated with an approach-oriented response to appetitive stimuli at a basic, reflexive level.

Together, this work suggests that positive affects vary in approach motivational intensity, as revealed by asymmetrical frontal cortical activity, the LPP, and the startle eyeblink response. Given this, we have also examined whether positive affects varying in approach motivational intensity have different cognitive consequences; that is, do positive affective states that are low rather than high in approach motivation produce different cognitive outcomes?

Cognitive Scope, Positive Affect, and Approach Motivation

One cognitive variable that relates to affect is "cognitive scope," or how broadly or narrowly one attends to or categorizes information. Past research has suggested that positive affective states broaden cognitive scope and negative affective states narrow it (Easterbrook, 1959; Fredrickson, 2001). This research measured cognitive scope in a number of ways, such as local–global attention (Fredrickson & Branigan, 2005), cognitive categorization (Isen & Daubman, 1984), and unusualness of associations (Isen, Johnson, Mertz, & Robinson, 1985).

This work, however, may have only examined positive affective states low in motivational intensity, such as amusement, and negative affective states high in motivational intensity, such as fear (E. Harmon-Jones & Gable, 2008). In the past research on positive affect and cognitive scope, positive affect was created with gifts (Isen & Daubman, 1984), recall of past positive events (Gasper & Clore, 2002), or clips of humorous or satisfying events (Fredrickson & Branigan, 2005). We suggest that these manipulations created positive affective states that were low in approach motivation.

Positive affects that are high in approach motivation may instead narrow cognitive scope, which might be functional in goal pursuit and acquisition. That is, during appetitive states, positive affect may facilitate a focus on specific goals that assists in eliminating potentially distracting peripheral details. As such, the organism may be more likely to obtain the desired goal. In contrast, positive affects with lower approach motivation often occur after goals have been acquired, and during this period, cognitive scope becomes broadened, so that the organism can find new opportunities to pursue later.

High- versus Low-Approach Positive Affect Influences Attentional Scope

In the first experiment testing the effects of low- versus high-approach positive affect on attentional scope (Gable & E. Harmon-Jones, 2008a; Experiment 1), low-approach positive affect was created with a film clip of funny cats, and high-approach positive affect with a film clip of desirable desserts. Self-report manipulation checks indicated that positive affect was evoked without any negative affect. In support of the hypothesis, the dessert film (causing high-approach positive affect) compared to the funny cats film (causing low-approach positive affect) caused less broadening of attention on the Kimchi and Palmer (1982) task (see Figure 6.1 for a description of the task).

This initial experiment, however, lacked a neutral condition. Therefore, it could not examine whether high-approach positive affect narrowed attention relative to a neutral condition. Further experiments clarified this point; dessert pictures presented

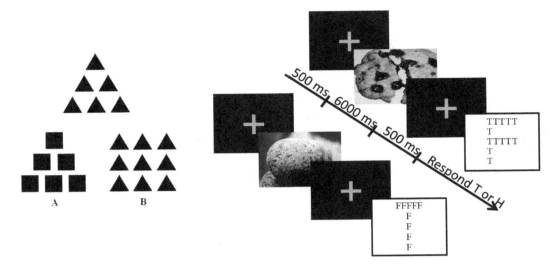

FIGURE 6.1. Kimchi and Palmer task stimuli (left) and Navon letter task trial order (right).

before Navon (1977; see Figure 6.1) letters caused more narrowing of attention than neutral rock pictures presented before letter targets (Gable & E. Harmon-Jones, 2008a; Experiment 2). Converging evidence also indicated that these effects were associated with trait levels of approach motivation. For example, individuals who scored higher in trait approach motivation showed even more narrowing of attention following appetitive pictures (Gable & E. Harmon-Jones, 2008a; Experiment 3). Leading individuals to believe they would get to eat desserts following picture viewing (a manipulation further increasing approach motivation) caused even more narrowing of attention (Gable & E. Harmon-Jones, 2008a; Experiment 4). Alcohol-related pictures, furthermore, caused narrowed attention for individuals motivated to consume alcohol (Hicks, Friedman, Gable, & Davis, 2012). These positive affect manipulations increase self-reported positive affect (e.g., excited, enthusiastic) but not negative affect.

Monetary Manipulations of High-versus Low-Approach Positive Affect

This hypothesis has also been tested with different manipulations of high- versus low-approach positive affect. One experiment used a monetary incentive delay paradigm that creates low-approach (postgoal) com-

pared to high-approach (pregoal) positive affective states (Knutson & Wimmer, 2007). Pre- and postgoal cues are presented in this reaction time task. Pregoal cues indicate the possibility of gaining money on an upcoming trial, whereas postgoal cues indicate whether a reward was obtained after a trial. Targets in this task are neutral words presented centrally or peripherally after pre- and postgoal cues. Gable and E. Harmon-Jones (2010a) found that participants displayed superior memory for centrally displayed words after pregoal compared with postgoal positive affect cues. Memory for peripherally presented words, however, was superior after postgoal rather than pregoal positive affect cues. A second experiment replicated these findings with pictures of dessert compared to neutral rock pictures; dessert pictures caused better memory for centrally compared to peripherally presented words. Peripherally presented words, however, were better remembered after neutral rather than appetitive dessert pictures. In addition, pregoal compared to postgoal monetary incentive cues caused narrowed attention measured with Navon's (1977) task (Gable & E. Harmon-Jones, 2011a).

Collectively, these results suggest that high-approach-motivated positive affect narrows attention and memory. Low-approach-motivated positive affect, on the other hand, broadens attention and memory.

Cognitive Categorization

Previous research has indicated that positive and negative affect differentially influence how individuals categorize related information. Positive compared to negative affect was found to broaden categorization. This past research, however, manipulated positive affect potentially lower in approach motivation, by giving participants a free gift or having them watch an amusing film (Isen & Daubman, 1984). Price and E. Harmon-Jones (2010) tested if high- compared to low-approach positive affect influences cognitive categorization. High-approach positive affect was manipulated by having participants lean forward in a chair and smile, similar to how someone might lean toward delicious food. Low-approach positive affect, however, was manipulated by having participants recline backwards in the chair while smiling, similar to how someone might recline after consuming a satisfying meal. A moderate-approach, upright smiling condition was also included in these experiments. In each posture, participants completed a cognitive categorization task adapted from Isen and Daubman (1984). In this task, participants were presented with typical (e.g., car) and atypical (e.g., camel) examples of a category (e.g., vehicle) and asked to rate how much they believed each example belonged to the category. Results indicated that participants in the high-approach positive posture rated atypical examples as belonging less to the category (narrowed categorization) compared to participants in the moderate- and low-approach positive postures.

Psychophysiological Responses Underlying the Effect of Approach Motivation on Attentional Narrowing

Finally, we have examined the association between relative left frontal cortical activity and broadening and narrowing of attention. In one experiment (E. Harmon-Jones & Gable, 2009), participants' frontal cortical activity (assessed with EEG alpha power) was measured in response to dessert and neutral picture primes, and attentional scope was measured following each prime using the Navon (1977) letters task. Results indicated that greater relative left frontal cortical activity in response to dessert but not neutral rock pictures predicted attentional narrowing immediately following the dessert picture primes (E. Harmon-Jones & Gable, 2009).

We have also examined the association between LPPs and narrowing–broadening of attention associated with high- and low-approach positive affect. In the Gable and E. Harmon-Jones (2010b) experiment, participants responded to Navon (1977) letters after appetitive dessert and neutral rock picture primes while EEG was recorded. Results indicated that LPPs were larger in response to dessert pictures than to rock pictures. This effect occurred at medial central and parietal regions but also occurred asymmetrically over the frontal cortex. That is, dessert pictures elicited larger LPPs over the left than over the right frontal cortex. Furthermore, LPPs in response to dessert pictures predicted attentional narrowing after viewing dessert pictures.

Manipulation of Attentional Scope and Reactions to Appetitive Stimuli

Given the effect of approach-motivated positive affect on the narrowing of attentional scope and the generally close connection between attention and emotion, we next tested whether a manipulated local attentional scope would cause greater approach motivational processing than a global attentional scope (Gable & E. Harmon-Jones, 2011b). That is, focusing narrowly on an appetitive object may increase desire for the object, whereas attending more broadly to an appetitive object may decrease desire for the object. To test these ideas, we measured ERPs to appetitive and neutral pictures, and focused on the N1 component, one of the earliest ERP components influenced by motivational intensity (Hajcak et al., 2012).

Attentional scope was manipulated prior to each affective or neutral picture by having participants indicate what letter was displayed at the local or global level. Compared to a global attentional scope, a local attentional scope caused a larger N1 in response to appetitive pictures but not neutral pictures. These results suggest that the relationship between narrowed attentional scope and approach-motivated positive affect is bidirectional.

Conclusions

In this chapter, we have reviewed evidence associating approach motivation with greater relative left frontal cortical activity, as well as other psychophysiological responses (LPP, startle magnitude), and with reduced breadth of cognitive scope affecting attention, memory, and categorization processes. We also have reviewed evidence suggesting that approach motivation is not invariably related to positive affect. The research on anger, a negatively valenced affect, provides much evidence suggesting that some instances of approach are subjectively negative. A task for future research will be to uncover other violations of the approach-is-positive mantra. We also have reviewed evidence suggesting that positive affects vary in approach motivational intensity, and that this variation has important implications for understanding not only psychophysiological processes underlying affects but also the influence of affects on cognitive processes. We hope this consideration of motivational direction and intensity as separate from affective valence will continue to generate new research that yields a better understanding of emotion, motivation, cognition, and psychophysiology.

References

Allen, J. J. B., Harmon-Jones, E., & Cavender, J. (2001). Manipulation of frontal EEG asymmetry through biofeedback alters self-reported emotional responses and facial EMG. *Psychophysiology, 38,* 685–693.

Amodio, D. M., Devine, P. G., & Harmon-Jones, E. (2007). A dynamic model of guilt: Implications for motivation and self-regulation in the context of prejudice. *Psychological Science, 18,* 524–530.

Amodio, D. M., & Harmon-Jones, E. (2011). Trait emotions and startle eyeblink responses to affective pictures: On the unique relationship of trait anger. *Emotion, 11,* 47–51.

Amodio, D. M., Master, S. L., Yee, C. M., & Taylor, S. E. (2008). Neurocognitive components of the behavioral inhibition and activation systems: Implications for theories of self-regulation. *Psychophysiology, 45,* 11–19.

Amodio, D. M., Shah, J. Y., Sigelman, J. D., Brazy, P. C., & Harmon-Jones, E. (2004). Implicit regulatory focus associated with rest-ing frontal cortical asymmetry. *Journal of Experimental Social Psychology, 40,* 225–232.

Blanchard, D. C., & Blanchard, R. J. (1984). Affect and aggression: An animal model applied to human behavior. *Advances in the Study of Aggression, 1,* 1–62.

Bradley, M. M., & Lang, P. J. (2007). Emotion and motivation. In J. T. Cacioppo, L. G. Tassinary, & G. Berntson (Eds.), *Handbook of psychophysiology* (3rd ed., pp. 581–607). New York: Cambridge University Press.

Buss, A. H., & Perry, M. (1992). The aggression questionnaire. *Journal of Personality and Social Psychology, 63,* 452–459.

Carver, C. S. (2004). Negative affects deriving from the behavioral approach system. *Emotion, 4,* 3–22.

Carver, C. S., & Harmon-Jones, E. (2009). Anger is an approach-related affect: Evidence and implications. *Psychological Bulletin, 135,* 183–204.

Carver, C. S., & White, T. L. (1994). Behavioral inhibition, behavioral activation, and affective responses to impending reward and punishment: The BIS/BAS scales. *Journal of Personality and Social Psychology, 67,* 319–333.

Coan, J. A., Allen, J. J. B., & Harmon-Jones, E. (2001). Voluntary facial expression and hemispheric asymmetry over the frontal cortex. *Psychophysiology, 38,* 912–925.

Cook, I. A., O'Hara, R., Uijtdehaage, S. H. J., Mandelkern, M., & Leuchter, A. F. (1998). Assessing the accuracy of topographic EEG mapping for determining local brain function. *Electroencephalography and Clinical Neurophysiology, 107,* 408–414.

Cunningham, W. A., Espinet, S. D., DeYoung, C. G., & Zelazo, P. D. (2005). Attitudes to the right- and left: Frontal ERP asymmetries associated with stimulus valence and processing goals. *NeuroImage, 28,* 827–834.

Darwin, C. (1872). *The expression of emotions in man and animals.* New York: Philosophical Library.

d'Alfonso, A. A. L., van Honk, J., Hermans, E., Postma, A., & de Haan, E. H. F. (2000). Laterality effects in selective attention to threat after repetitive transcranial magnetic stimulation at the prefrontal cortex in female subjects. *Neuroscience Letters, 280,* 195–198.

Davidson, R. J. (1998). Anterior electrophysiological asymmetries, emotion, and depression: Conceptual and methodological conundrums. *Psychophysiology, 35,* 607–614.

Davidson, R. J., Ekman, P., Saron, C. D., Senulis, J. A., & Friesen, W. V. (1990). Approach–withdrawal and cerebral asymmetry: Emotional expression and brain physiology I. *Journal of Personality and Social Psychology, 58*, 330–341.

Davidson, R. J., & Fox, N. A. (1982). Asymmetrical brain activity discriminates between positive and negative affective stimuli in human infants. *Science, 218*, 1235–1237.

Easterbrook, J. A. (1959). The effect of emotion on cue utilization and the organization of behavior. *Psychological Review, 66*, 183–201.

Fox, N. A., & Davidson, R. J. (1986). Taste-elicited changes in facial signs of emotion and the asymmetry of brain electrical activity in human newborns. *Neuropsychologia, 24*, 417–422.

Fredrickson, B. L. (2001). The role of positive emotions in positive psychology: The broaden-and-build theory of positive emotions. *American Psychologist, 56*, 218–226.

Fredrickson, B. L., & Branigan, C. (2005). Positive emotions broaden the scope of attention and thought–action repertoires *Cognition and Emotion, 19*(3), 313–332.

Gable, P. A., & Harmon-Jones, E. (2008a). Approach-motivated positive affect reduces breadth of attention. *Psychological Science, 19*, 476–482.

Gable, P. A., & Harmon-Jones, E. (2008b). Relative left frontal activation to appetitive stimuli: Considering the role of individual differences. *Psychophysiology, 45*, 275–278.

Gable, P. A., & Harmon-Jones, E. (2009). Postauricular reflex responses to pictures varying in valence and arousal. *Psychophysiology, 46*, 487–490.

Gable, P. A., & Harmon-Jones, E. (2010a). The effect of low vs. high approach-motivated positive affect on memory for peripherally vs. centrally presented information. *Emotion, 10*, 599–603.

Gable, P. A., & Harmon-Jones, E. (2010b). Late positive potential to appetitive stimuli and local attentional bias. *Emotion, 10*, 441–446.

Gable, P. A., & Harmon-Jones, E. (2011a). Attentional consequences of pre-goal and post-goal positive affects. *Emotion, 11*, 1358–1367.

Gable, P. A., & Harmon-Jones, E. (2011b). Attentional states influence early neural responses associated with motivational processes: Local vs. global attentional scope and N1 amplitude to appetitive stimuli. *Biological Psychology, 87*, 303–305.

Gable, P. A., & Harmon-Jones, E. (2013a). Does arousal per se account for the influence of

appetitive stimuli on attentional scope and the late positive potential? *Psychophysiology, 50*, 344–350.

Gable, P. A., & Harmon-Jones, E. (2013b). Trait behavioral approach sensitivity (BAS) relates to early (< 150 ms) electrocortical responses to appetitive stimuli. *Social Cognitive Affective Neuroscience, 8*, 795–798.

Gable, P. A., & Poole, B. D. (in press). Influence of trait behavioral inhibition and behavioral approach motivation systems on the LPP and frontal asymmetry to anger pictures. *Social Cognitive Affective Neuroscience.*

Gainotti, G. (1972). Emotional behavior and hemispheric side of the lesion. *Cortex, 8*, 41–55.

Gasper, K., & Clore, G. L. (2002). Attending to the big picture: Mood and global versus local processing of visual information. *Psychological Science, 13*, 34–40.

Goldstein, K. (1939). *The organism: An holistic approach to biology, derived from pathological data in man.* New York: American Book.

Hagemann, D., Naumann, E., Becker, G., Maier, S., & Bartussek, D. (1998). Frontal brain asymmetry and affective style: A conceptual replication. *Psychophysiology, 35*, 372–388.

Hagemann, D., Naumann, E., Thayer, J. F., & Bartussek, D. (2002). Does resting EEG asymmetry reflect a trait?: An application of latent state–trait theory. *Journal of Personality and Social Psychology, 82*, 619–641.

Hajcak, G., Weinberg, A., MacNamara, A., & Foti, D. (2012). ERPs and the study of emotion. In S. J. Luck & E. S. Kappenman (Eds.), *Oxford handbook of ERP components* (pp. 441–474). New York: Oxford University Press.

Harmon-Jones, C., Schmeichel, B. J., Mennitt, E., & Harmon-Jones, E. (2011). The expression of determination: Similarities between anger and approach-related positive affect. *Journal of Personality and Social Psychology, 100*, 172–181.

Harmon-Jones, E. (2003). Anger and the behavioural approach system. *Personality and Individual Differences, 35*, 995–1005.

Harmon-Jones, E. (2004). On the relationship of anterior brain activity and anger: Examining the role of attitude toward anger. *Cognition and Emotion, 18*, 337–361.

Harmon-Jones, E. (2006). Unilateral right-hand contractions cause contralateral alpha power suppression and approach motivational affective experience. *Psychophysiology, 43*, 598–603.

Harmon-Jones, E. (2007). Trait anger predicts relative left frontal cortical activation to anger-inducing stimuli. *International Journal of Psychophysiology, 66,* 154–160.

Harmon-Jones, E., Abramson, L. Y., Nusslock, R., Sigelman, J. D., Urošević, S., Turonie, L., et al. (2008). Effect of bipolar disorder on left frontal cortical responses to goals differing in valence and task difficulty. *Biological Psychiatry, 63,* 693–698.

Harmon-Jones, E., Abramson, L. Y., Sigelman, J., Bohlig, A., Hogan, M. E., & Harmon-Jones, C. (2002). Proneness to hypomania/mania or depression and asymmetrical frontal cortical responses to an anger-evoking event. *Journal of Personality and Social Psychology, 82,* 610–618.

Harmon-Jones, E., & Allen, J. J. B. (1997). Behavioral activation sensitivity and resting frontal EEG asymmetry: Covariation of putative indicators related to risk for mood disorders. *Journal of Abnormal Psychology, 106,* 159–163.

Harmon-Jones, E., & Allen, J. J. B. (1998). Anger and prefrontal brain activity: EEG asymmetry consistent with approach motivation despite negative affective valence. *Journal of Personality and Social Psychology, 74,* 1310–1316.

Harmon-Jones, E., & Gable, P. A. (2008). Incorporating motivational intensity and direction into the study of emotions: Implications for brain mechanisms of emotion and cognition–emotion interactions. *Netherlands Journal of Psychology, 64,* 132–142.

Harmon-Jones, E., & Gable, P. A. (2009). Neural activity underlying the effect of approach-motivated positive affect on narrowed attention. *Psychological Science, 20,* 406–409.

Harmon-Jones, E., Gable, P. A., & Price, T. F. (2011). Leaning embodies desire: Evidence that leaning forward increases relative left frontal cortical activation to appetitive stimuli. *Biological Psychology, 87,* 311–313.

Harmon-Jones, E., Harmon-Jones, C., Abramson, L. Y., & Peterson, C. K. (2009). PANAS positive activation is associated with anger. *Emotion, 9,* 183–196.

Harmon-Jones, E., Harmon-Jones, C., Amodio, D. M., & Gable, P. A. (2011). Attitudes toward emotions. *Journal of Personality and Social Psychology, 101,* 1332–1350.

Harmon-Jones, E., Harmon-Jones, C., Fearn, M., Sigelman, J. D., & Johnson, P. (2008). Action orientation, relative left frontal corti- cal activation, and spreading of alternatives: A test of the action-based model of dissonance. *Journal of Personality and Social Psychology, 94,* 1–15.

Harmon-Jones, E., Harmon-Jones, C., & Price, T. F. (2013). What is approach motivation? *Emotion Review, 5*(3), 291–295.

Harmon-Jones, E., Lueck, L., Fearn, M., & Harmon-Jones, C. (2006). The effect of personal relevance and approach-related action expectation on relative left frontal cortical activity. *Psychological Science, 17,* 434–440.

Harmon-Jones, E., & Peterson, C. K. (2008). Effect of trait and state approach motivation on aggressive inclinations. *Journal of Research in Personality, 42,* 1381–1385.

Harmon-Jones, E., & Peterson, C. K. (2009). Supine body position reduces neural response to anger evocation. *Psychological Science, 20,* 1209–1210.

Harmon-Jones, E., Peterson, C. K., & Harris, C. R. (2009). Jealousy: Novel methods and neural correlates. *Emotion, 9,* 113–117.

Harmon-Jones, E., & Sigelman, J. (2001). State anger and prefrontal brain activity: Evidence that insult-related relative left prefrontal activation is associated with experienced anger and aggression. *Journal of Personality and Social Psychology, 80,* 797–803.

Harmon-Jones, E., Sigelman, J. D., Bohlig, A., & Harmon-Jones, C. (2003). Anger, coping, and frontal cortical activity: The effect of coping potential on anger-induced left frontal activity. *Cognition and Emotion, 17,* 1–24.

Harmon-Jones, E., Vaughn-Scott, K., Mohr, S., Sigelman, J., & Harmon-Jones, C. (2004). The effect of manipulated sympathy and anger on left and right frontal cortical activity. *Emotion, 4,* 95–101.

Hicks, J. A., Friedman, R. S., Gable, P. A., & Davis, W. E. (2012). Interactive effects of approach motivational intensity and alcohol cues on the scope of perceptual attention. *Addiction, 107,* 1074–1080.

Hortensius, R., Schutter, D. J. L. G., & Harmon-Jones, E. (2012). When anger leads to aggression: Induction of relative left frontal cortical activity with transcranial direct current stimulation increases the anger–aggression relationship. *Social Cognitive and Affective Neuroscience, 7,* 342–347.

Isen, A. M., & Daubman, K. A. (1984). The influence of affect on categorization. *Journal of Personality and Social Psychology, 47,* 1206–1217.

Isen, A. M., Johnson, M. M., Mertz, E., & Robinson, G. F. (1985). The influence of positive affect on the unusualness of word associations. *Journal of Personality and Social Psychology, 48,* 1413–1426.

Izard, C. E. (2011). The many meanings/aspects of emotion: Definitions, functions, activation, and regulation. *Emotion Review, 2,* 363–370.

Jensen-Campbell, L. A., Knack, J. M., Waldrip, A. M., & Campbell, S. D. (2007). Do Big Five personality traits associated with self-control influence the regulation of anger and aggression? *Journal of Research in Personality, 41,* 403–424.

Jones, N. A., & Fox, N. A. (1992). Electroencephalogram asymmetry during emotionally evocative films and its relation to positive and negative affectivity. *Brain and Cognition, 20,* 280–299.

Kelley, N. J., Hortensius, R., & Harmon-Jones, E. (2013). When anger leads to rumination: Induction of relative right frontal cortical activity with transcranial direct current stimulation increases anger-related rumination. *Psychological Science, 24*(4), 475–481.

Keune, P. M., van der Heiden, L., Várkuti, B., Konicar, L., Veit, R., & Birbaumer, N. (2012). Prefrontal brain asymmetry and aggression in imprisoned violent offenders. *Neuroscience Letters, 515,* 191–195.

Kimchi, R., & Palmer, S. E. (1982). Form and texture in hierarchically constructed patterns. *Journal of Experimental Psychology: Human Perception and Performance, 8,* 521–535.

Knutson, B., & Wimmer, G. E. (2007). Reward: Neural circuitry for social valuation. In E. Harmon-Jones & P. Winkielman (Eds.), *Social neuroscience: Integrating biological and psychological explanations of social behavior* (pp. 157–175). New York: Guilford Press.

Lagerspetz, K. M. J. (1969). Aggression and aggressiveness in laboratory mice. In S. Garattini & E. B. Sigg (Eds.), *Aggressive behavior* (pp. 77–85). New York: Wiley.

Lang, P. J. (1995). The emotion probe. *American Psychologist, 50,* 372–385.

Lang, P. J., & Bradley, M. M. (2013). Appetitive and defensive motivation: Goal-directed or goal-determined? *Emotion Review, 5*(3), 230–234.

Lazarus, R. S. (1991). *Emotion and adaptation.* New York: Oxford University Press.

Lerner, J. S., & Keltner, D. (2001). Fear, anger, and risk. *Journal of Personality and Social Psychology, 81,* 146–159.

Lewis, M., Alessandri, S. M., & Sullivan, M. W. (1990). Violation of expectancy, loss of control, and anger expressions in young infants. *Developmental Psychology, 26,* 745–751.

Lewis, M., Sullivan, M. W., Ramsey, D. S., & Alessandri, S. M. (1992). Individual differences in anger and sad expressions during extinction: Antecedents and consequences. *Infant Behavior and Development, 15,* 443–452.

Moyer, K. E. (1976). *The psychobiology of aggression.* New York: Harper & Row.

Murphy, F. C., Nimmo-Smith, I., & Lawrence, A. D. (2003). Functional neuroanatomy of emotion: A meta-analysis. *Cognitive, Affective, and Behavioral Neuroscience, 3,* 207–233.

Nash, K., Inzlicht, M., & McGregor, I. (2012). Approach-related left prefrontal EEG asymmetry predicts muted error-related negativity. *Biological Psychology, 91,* 96–102.

Navon, D. (1977). Forest before trees: The precedence of global features in visual perception. *Cognitive Psychology, 9,* 353–383.

Nitsche, M. A., & Paulus, W. (2000). Excitability changes induced in the human motor cortex by weak transcranial direct current stimulation. *Journal of Physiology, 527,* 633–639.

Nusslock, R., Harmon-Jones, E., Alloy, L. B., Urošević, S., Goldstein, K., Abramson, L. Y. (2012). Elevated left mid-frontal cortical activity prospectively predicts conversion to bipolar I disorder. *Journal of Abnormal Psychology, 121*(3), 592–601.

Nusslock, R., Shackman, A. J., Harmon-Jones, E., Alloy, L. B., Coan, J. A., & Abramson, L. Y. (2011). Cognitive vulnerability and frontal brain asymmetry: Common predictors of first prospective depressive episode. *Journal of Abnormal Psychology, 120,* 497–503.

Peterson, C. K., Gravens, L., & Harmon-Jones, E. (2011). Asymmetric frontal cortical activity and negative affective responses to ostracism. *Social Cognitive and Affective Neuroscience, 6,* 277–285.

Peterson, C. K., & Harmon-Jones, E. (2009). Circadian and seasonal variability of resting frontal EEG asymmetry. *Biological Psychology, 80,* 315–320.

Peterson, C. K., Shackman, A. J., & Harmon-Jones, E. (2008). The role of asymmetrical frontal cortical activity in aggression. *Psychophysiology, 45,* 86–92.

Pizzagalli, D., Shackman, A. J., & Davidson, R. J. (2003). The functional neuroimaging of human emotion: Asymmetric contributions of cortical and subcortical circuitry. In K. Hugdahl & R. J. Davidson (Eds.), *The asymmetrical brain* (pp. 511–532). Cambridge, MA: MIT Press.

Plutchik, R. (1980). *Emotion: A psychoevolutionary synthesis.* New York: Harper & Row.

Price, T. F., Dieckman, L., & Harmon-Jones, E. (2012). Embodying approach motivation: Body posture influences startle eyeblink and event-related potential responses to appetitive stimuli. *Biological Psychology, 90,* 211–217.

Price, T. F., & Harmon-Jones, E. (2010). The effect of embodied emotive states on cognitive categorization. *Emotion, 10,* 934–938.

Price, T. F., Hortensius, R., & Harmon-Jones, E. (2013). Neural and behavioral associations of manipulated determination facial expressions. *Biological Psychology, 94*(1), 221–227.

Putman, P., Hermans, E., & van Honk, J. (2004). Emotional Stroop performance for masked angry faces: It's BAS, not BIS. *Emotion, 4,* 305–311.

Quaranta, A., Siniscalchi, M., & Vallortigara, G. (2007). Asymmetric tail-wagging responses by dogs to different emotive stimuli. *Current Biology, 17,* R199–R201.

Robinson, R. G., & Price, T. R. (1982). Poststroke depressive disorders: A follow-up study of 103 patients. *Stroke, 13,* 635–641.

Rybak, M., Crayton, J. W., Young, I. J., Herba, E., & Konopka, L. M. (2006). Frontal alpha power asymmetry in aggressive children and adolescents with mood and disruptive behavior disorders. *Clinical EEG and Neuroscience, 37,* 16–24.

Sabatinelli, D., Lang, P. J., Keil, A., & Bradley, M. M. (2007). Emotional perception: Correlation of functional MRI and event-related potentials. *Cerebral Cortex, 17,* 1085–1091.

Schutter, D. J. L. G. (2009). Antidepressant efficacy of high-frequency transcranial magnetic stimulation over the left dorsolateral prefrontal cortex in double-blind sham-controlled designs: A meta-analysis. *Psychological Medicine, 39,* 65–75.

Terzian, H., & Cecotto, C. (1959). Determination and study of hemispheric dominance by means of intracarotid sodium amytal injection in man: II. Electroencephalographic effects. *Bolletino della Societa Italiana Sperimentale, 35,* 1626–1630.

Thibodeau, R., Jorgensen, R. S., & Kim, S. (2006). Depression, anxiety, and resting frontal EEG asymmetry: A meta-analytic review. *Journal of Abnormal Psychology, 115,* 715–729.

Tomarken, A., Davidson, R. J., Wheeler, R. E., & Doss, R. C. (1992). Individual differences in anterior brain asymmetry and fundamental dimensions of emotion. *Journal of Personality and Social Psychology, 62,* 676–687.

Tullett, A. M., Harmon-Jones, E., & Inzlicht, M. (2012). Right-frontal cortical asymmetry predicts empathic reactions: Support for a link between withdrawal motivation and empathy. *Psychophysiology, 49*(8), 1145–1153.

Urošević, S., Abramson, L. Y., Harmon-Jones, E., & Alloy, L. B. (2008). Dysregulation of the behavioral approach system (BAS) in bipolar spectrum disorders: Review of theory and evidence. *Clinical Psychology Review, 28,* 1188–1205.

Vallortigara, G., & Rogers, L. J. (2005). Survival with an asymmetrical brain: Advantages and disadvantages of cerebral lateralization. *Behavioral and Brain Sciences, 28,* 575–633.

van Honk, J., & Schutter, D. J. (2006). From affective valence to motivational direction: The frontal asymmetry of emotion revised. *Psychological Science, 17,* 963–965.

van Honk, J., & Schutter, D. J. L. G. (2007). Vigilant and avoidant responses to angry facial expressions: Dominance and submission motives. In E. Harmon-Jones & P. Winkielman (Eds.), *Social neuroscience: Integrating biological and psychological explanations of social behavior* (pp. 197–223). New York: Guilford Press.

Verona, E., Sadeh, N., & Curtin, J. J. (2009). Stress-induced asymmetric frontal brain activity and aggression risk. *Journal of Abnormal Psychology, 118,* 131–145.

Wacker, J., Mueller, E. M., Pizzagalli, D. A., Hennig, J., & Stemmler, G. (2013). Dopamine D2 receptor blockade reverses the association between trait approach motivation and frontal asymmetry in an approach-motivation context. *Psychological Science, 24*(4), 489–497.

Watson, D. (2000). *Mood and temperament.* New York: Guilford Press.

Zinner, L., Brodish, A., Devine, P. G., & Harmon-Jones, E. (2008). Anger and asymmetrical frontal cortical activity: Evidence for an anger–withdrawal relationship. *Cognition and Emotion, 22,* 1081–1093.

CHAPTER 7

Animal Neuroscience of Positive Emotion

Jeffrey S. Burgdorf
Jaak Panksepp
Joseph R. Moskal

In this chapter we review key issues and core findings in animal research on the neuroscience of positive emotion. The rapid development of neuroimaging technology in recent decades has enabled a burgeoning field of human affective neuroscience. However, animal neuroscience remains an important tool for studying the neural substrates of emotion, with far greater ability experimentally to manipulate brain activity and observe the effects on behavior than is generally possible with humans.

The main aims of animal positive emotional neuroscience research are (1) to identify animal behaviors that are putative homologues to human emotional experiences; (2) to elucidate the neural and molecular mechanisms of these behaviors, and, most importantly (3) to translate these observations to therapeutics for the treatment of psychiatric disorders. This chapter is structured accordingly. We begin by addressing the problem of measuring positive emotion in animals, summarizing our own extensive program of research on 50-Hz ultrasonic vocalizations in rats as an example of a solution to this problem. Next we discuss the mesolimbic dopaminergic SEEKING system, and the robust evidence linking activation in this system to appetitive behavior. Third, we consider other neural systems whose activation might be involved in specific states often considered, in the human literature, to be positive emotions (i.e., the sensory pleasure, PLAY, LUST, and CARE systems). We conclude by discussing future directions in positive emotion neuroscience with animals, with a particular emphasis on molecular mechanisms, as well as implications of animal research on the neural substrates of positive emotion for treating human pathologies involving emotion.

Measuring Positive Emotion in Animal Behavior

In order to investigate the neural substrates of some putative psychological state, researchers must have a reliable and valid way to measure the occurrence of that state—in this case, positive emotion. In humans, "positive emotions" can be defined as positively valenced feeling states that are associated with the propensity toward approach and/or consummatory behavior. The primary function of positive emotions is to elicit and maintain appetitive and consummatory behavior, as well as to produce positive reinforcement. This definition suggests the existence of two main classes of positive emotion: appetitive positive emotional states associated with approach behavior (e.g., enthusiasm, joy), and sensory pleasure associated with consummatory behavior. In humans, such states are elicited primarily by rewarding social interaction, food, and exercise, and are decreased by negative affective stimuli (Csikszentmihalyi & Hunter, 2003; Kahneman & Krueger, 2006; Stone et al., 2006). In empirical research with human subjects, positive emotion is measured primarily through the self-report of subjective feelings, and sometimes behaviorally through facial–vocal displays such as Duchenne smiling (Ekman, Davidson, & Friesen, 1990).

In laboratory animal experiments, where we can rely only on observed behaviors with no possibility of semantic report of subjective states, we must identify facial or vocal displays that reliably predict changes in approach behavior. In order to establish that an animal display reflects a positive affective state, several criteria must be met. First, the same categories of appetitive stimuli that increase positive emotion in humans (i.e., desired social interaction, food, and exercise) should also increase the animal's facial–vocal display, and aversive stimuli should decrease it. Second, what is known about the neurobiological mechanisms of the facial–vocal displays in animals should be consistent with the neurobiological mechanisms of human positive affective states.

Finally, from a more strictly neuroscientific perspective, the "gold standard" is that the display should be observed during certain central nervous system states in animals, as provoked by local brain stimulation, whether chemical or electrical (Ikemoto, 2010; Panksepp, 1998), already known to serve as rewards in various learning tasks. This approach has been well documented ever since the work of Olds and Milner (1954), as well as validated psychologically with human brain stimulation studies (Heath, 1972).

Importantly, neither the frequency of a given display nor the fact that it is associated with reinforcement, broadly speaking, is sufficient to indicate the presence of positive affect (by those who acknowledge such intrapsychic processes in animals). In humans, there is not a clear positive relationship between the frequency at which a behavior is performed and the level of positive affect associated with that behavior. For example, among Americans, watching television is only weakly hedonic, but it is engaged in more frequently than more hedonic activities such as prosocial behavior and exercise. In addition, working, cleaning, and commuting are high-frequency behaviors that are nonhedonic (unless one is recruiting the positive side of the SEEKING system, an ethological, primary-process concept, which is still mistakenly called the "brain reward system" because of cultural traditions in the field; Panksepp & Moskal, 2008).

With respect to reinforcement, many conceptual difficulties in the field arise from the general failure of scientists to acknowledge a central nervous emotional system that can generate states that are rewarding and punishing in diverse ways (Panksepp, 1998). Operant responding alone is not a sufficient (i.e., a conceptually clear) index of a positive emotional state. Rates of operant responding (i.e., bar pressing) can be increased both by positive affective stimuli (positive reinforcement) and the avoidance of aversive stimuli (negative reinforcement). In traditional behavioral terminology, only positive reinforcements are specific to positive affective states, whereas negative reinforcements (i.e., withdrawal of punishing stimuli) are not—at least not as clearly. Negative reinforcements probably operate by reducing negative affective states, and surely such reductions have their own affective consequences, namely, feelings such as "relief" and "relaxation" from tense states of mind. Such effects are even evident in studies of rat behavior. For instance, rats undergoing simple pain-induced fear conditioning show a remarkable response when they are provided with safety signals indicating that no shocks will be forthcoming for a while. As soon as such safety signals come on, animals relax, and emit a measureable "sigh of relief"—a double inspiration similar to the one humans exhibit when they experience relief after a period of active stress (Soltysik & Jelen, 2005). Although this "negative reinforcement" state is still an affective state, at least in humans, of considerable importance for feelings of composure, it is not the same as having directly increased a positive emotional state.

In summary, there are three criteria for identifying an animal display as a marker of positive affect: (1) elicitation by desired social interaction, food, and/or exercise; (2) evidence for shared neurobiological mechanisms of the display across humans and nonhuman animals; and (3) observation during certain central nervous system states and other behaviors previously associated with positive reinforcements/rewards. To date, only two such animal behaviors meet all of these criteria. The first, emission of 50-kHz ultrasonic vocalizations (USVs) by rats, is discussed in detail below. The other is hedonic taste reactivity, reviewed by Berridge (2003), although in this latter case the rewardingness of the underlying circuits have not been directly evaluated in the "taste plume" areas of the basal forebrain, to the extent that they have been for rats' 50-kHz USVs (Burgdorf, Wood, Kroes, Moskal, & Panksepp, 2007).

50-kHz USVs in Rats

In our own, long-standing program of research, we have sought to develop a vocal output measure of animals' positive affective states, analogous to the way that screaming expresses states of pain induced by nociceptive simuli. In research involving laboratory rodents, emotional vocalizations in the ultrasonic range have been proposed as potential nonsemantic "self-report" measures indicating that animals are in positive affective space (Knutson, Burgdorf, & Panksepp, 2002; Panksepp, Knutson, & Burgdorf, 2002), especially one with a social-affective tone.

The use of USVs as an index of affect in rats is not limited to positive affect. Adult rat 22-kHz USVs and infant rat distress calls (35–40 kHz) may reflect a negative emotional state analogous to human anxiety and/or depressive states (e.g., aversive facial expressions such as crying, and behavioral inhibition; Knutson et al., 2002). Despite significant sonographic differences between the adult and infant vocalizations, they share similar characteristics in aversive and dan-

gerous situations. In humans, these affective states are often elicited by social loss and anticipation of perceived threats (Knutson et al., 2002). In infant rat pups, 35- to 40-kHz USVs are best elicited by separating the pup from the mother, which in typical testing leads to a rapid reduction in core temperature (possibly indicating a general distress call rather than a discrete social separation–distress call; Panksepp, Newman, & Insel, 1992). In adult rats 22-kHz USVs are best elected by social defeat and the presence of a predator (Blanchard & Blanchard, 1989; Brunelli & Hofer, 2007; Panksepp, Burgdorf, Beinfeld, Kroes, & Moskal, 2007). Emission of 22-kHz USVs is strongly related to avoidance behavior and freezing during social defeat testing (Panksepp et al., 2007). Environments paired with drugs causing aversive states also elicit 22-kHz USVs. Rates of emitted calls are positively correlated with drug-induced conditioned place avoidance (Burgdorf, Knutson, Panksepp, & Shippenberg, 2001). Anxiolytic benzodiazepines and antidepressants reduce rates of 22-kHz calls and 35- to 40-kHz USVs (Carden & Hofer, 1990; Covington & Miczek, 2003).

Using social defeat as a method to elicit negative emotional states associated with 22-kHz USVs, we conducted a transcriptomic analysis of gene expression in the periaqueductal gray (PAG), one of the regions found to be critical for the generation of negative affect and 22-kHz USVs in rats (Kroes, Burgdorf, Otto, Panksepp, & Moskal, 2007). These studies revealed that messenger RNA (mRNA) expression of genes associated with acetylcholine metabolism and receptor function was altered in the PAG following social defeat. This finding is consistent with the previously reported role of tegmental cholinergic system in the generation of 22-kHz USVs (Brudzynski, 2001). Studies in humans have demonstrated that depressed patients have altered cholinergic transmission (Wang, Liang, Burgdorf, Wess, & Yeomans, 2008), and scopolamine has been shown to be a potent a rapid antidepressant (Furey & Drevets, 2006).

In contrast, 50-kHz USVs have been shown to reflect a positive affective state in rats, especially the frequency-modulated varieties of those calls. The less complex, "flat" variety may be a social-exploration/

contact signaling mechanism that is less indicative of positive affect. Rewarding social interactions (i.e., mating and rough-and-tumble play in juveniles), anticipation of food, and action of euphorigenic drugs of abuse increased number of emitted 50-kHz USVs (Burgdorf, Knutson, & Panksepp, 2000; Budgdorf, Knutson, Panksepp, & Ikemoto, 2001; Burgdorf et al., 2007, 2008; Panksepp & Burgdorf, 2000), whereas aversive stimuli such as social defeat, frustrative nonrewarding situations, sickness-inducing doses of lithium chloride, and foot shock all decreased the number of 50-kHz USVs (Burgdorf et al., 2000, 2008; Burgdorf, Knutson, et al., 2001). The rewarding (i.e., positively reinforcing) value of stimuli eliciting positive affective states was positively correlated with rates of 50-kHz USVs elicited by positive social, drug, and electrical brain stimulation rewards (Burgdorf et al., 2007, 2008).

Mu-opiate and dopamine agonists, as well as electrical brain stimulation of the mesolimbic dopamine system, also increased rates of 50-kHz USVs in rats (Burgdorf et al., 2000, 2007). Thus, the desire for intravenous injections of cocaine can be monitored not only by conditioned lever presses but also simply by measuring 50-KHz USVs, which were not formally conditioned in those operant tasks (Browning et al., 2011, and other studies cited therein).

Alternative nonhedonic interpretations of 50-kHz USVs (e.g., non-positively valenced arousal, non-positively valenced seeking behavior, or nonaffective social contacts) are not supported by the available experimental data (see Table 7.1 for details). Furthermore, this measure has already proved useful in studies of drug addiction, characterizing resilient and nonresilient rats in studies of the neuroanatomical regions that are impacted most by stressors that promote depression (Kanarik et al., 2011; Mällo, Matrov, Koiv, & Harro, 2009). Indeed, tickling, a way to evoke 50-kHz USVs quickly in rats (Burgdorf & Panksepp, 2006; Panksepp & Burgdorf, 2000), has positive effects on hippocampal neurogensis, which is widely considered a marker of antidepressant effects (Wöhr et al., 2009). We note that the tickling procedure can be used as a formal assay of this type of affect in rat studies, providing opportunities for new drug discovery and affective-state monitoring in animal models (Burgdorf, Panksepp, & Moskal, 2011).

TABLE 7.1. Nonaffective Hypotheses of 50-kHz USV Significance, with Rebuttals

Alternate hypothesis	Rebuttal
50-kHz USVs are an artifact of locomotor activity-induced thoratic compressions (Blumberg, 1992).	Only 10% of 50-kHz USVs were coincident with thoratic compressions and could be dissociated from locomotion (Panksepp & Burgdorf, 2003).
50-kHz USVs are a nonaffective contact call (Schwarting et al., 2007).	"Flat" 50-kHz calls appear to be a contact call, occurring at highest rates during nonpositive affect social interactions. Frequency-modulated 50-kHz calls appeared to be selective for social positive affect (Burgdorf et al., 2008).
50-kHz calls are evident during aggression (Berridge, 2003).	50-kHz calls occur primarily before onset of aggression, and the vast majority of calls associated with aggression were of the nonaffective, "flat" variety (Burgdorf et al., 2008; Panksepp & Burgdorf, 2003)
50-kHz calls reflect a nonpositive affective "wanting" state (Schwarting et al., 2007).	50-kHz USVs increased in the anticipation of delivered reward (Knutson et al., 2001). However, during extinction bursts or "frustrative nonreward," rates of 50-kHz calls decreased, and rates of aversive 22-kHz calls increased (Burgdorf et al., 2000).
Ultrasonic calls reflect a state of high arousal that is not specific to positive affective states (Bell, 1974).	Highly arousing aversive stimuli, such as predatory odor, foot shock, and bright light, decrease rates of 50-kHz calls, whereas rewarding stimuli increase rates of 50-kHz calls (Knutson et al., 2002)

Selective Breeding for Differential Rates of 50-kHz and 22-kHz USVs

In order to elucidate further the molecular mechanisms involved in the regulation of positive and negative emotional states, rats were selectively bred for differential rates of hedonic 50-kHz USVs (Burgdorf et al., 2008). Animals selectively bred for low rates of 50-kHz USVs (Low Line) had a concomitant increase in 22-kHz USVs and showed elevated levels of anxiety in the open field, in the social contact test, and in infant distress vocalization tests compared to randomly bred animals (Burgdorf et al., 2008). Conversely, animals selectively bred for high rates of 50-kHz USVs (High Line) had a concomitant decrease in the 22-kHz USVs, showed lower levels of anxiety in the open field test, decreased rates of aggression, and increased sensitivity to sucrose reward compared to randomly breed animals (Burgdorf et al., 2009).

These animals have been selectively bred for 18 generations to date and have displayed stable differences in USVs from adolescence through adulthood (3 months). Regrettably, because of inbreeding reproductive problems, the lines have recently been lost. Studies of the molecular mechanisms associated with the USV patterns of the High Line and Low Line animals to date are consistent with depressant-resilient and depressant-prone phenotypes as discussed earlier. For example, High Line animals exhibited higher levels of the mu-opiate acting met-enkephalin-like immunoreactivity in the hypothalamus and other related limbic structures (Burgdorf et al., 2008). Injections of the mu-opiate agonist DAMGO into the ventral tegmental area (a region included in the hypothalamus dissection) increased rates of 50-kHz USVs and was rewarding to the animals (Burgdorf et al., 2007). Low Line animals exhibited higher levels of cholecystokinin (CCK)-like immunoreactivity in the posterior neocortex. CCK content in the posterior cortex was elevated by social defeat, and was correlated with 22-kHz USVs rate of the defeated animal (Panksepp, Burgdorf, Beinfeld, Kroes, & Moskal, 2007).

Although in this chapter we emphasize the utility of 50-kHz USVs as markers of positive affect in animal neuroscience studies, they have proved useful in other lines of research as well. For example, genes specific to positive affective states can be uncovered by examining transcripts that are upregulated by hedonic play but not aversive social defeat (Burgdorf, Kroes, Beinfeld, Panksepp, & Moskal, 2010). We have developed an in-house fabricated focused microarray platform that can detect families of genes that are specifically upregulated following hedonic rough-and-tumble play when coupled with appropriate bioinformatics tools. These mRNA changes are corroborated by quantitative reverse transcription polymerase chain reaction (qrtPCR) and quantitative protein assays (radioimmunoassay, enzyme-linked immunosorbent assay [ELISA], western blots).

These studies identified both the insulin-like growth factor 1 (IGF1) and the N-methyl-D-aspartate (NMDA) NR2B receptor subunit as being specifically upregulated by hedonic rough-and-tumble play. Gain and loss of function studies with IGF1 and NR2B demonstrate that they play a functional role in positive affective states (Burgdorf et al., 2010). Intracerebroventricular (icv) injections of IGF1 increase hedonic USVs in an IGF1 receptor (IGFIR)-dependent manner, whereas icv injections of an IGFIR-specific siRNA decrease rates of hedonic USVs. Peripheral injections of the NMDA receptor (NMDAR) NR2B–preferring glycine site partial agonist, GLYX-13, increase rates of hedonic USVs, whereas the NR2B receptor antagonist, ifenprodil, decreases rates of hedonic USVs. Microinjections of GLYX-13 into the medial prefrontal cortex (but not dorsal control sites) increases rates of hedonic USVs.

Studies of this kind can have important applications in the treatment of human psychiatric disorders. For example, modulation of glutamatergic transmission has become a major target in the development of antidepressants for biogenic-amine antidepressant-resistant patients (Hashimoto, 2009; Machado-Vieira, Salvadore, DiazGranados, & Zarate, 2009; Skolnick, Popik, & Trullas, 2009). NMDAR is now a validated target for depression, and GLYX-13 is in Phase II clinical development for the treatment of depression (Burgdorf et al., 2011). Recent human clinical studies with known NMDAR antagonists CP-101,606 and ketamine have found significant reductions in depression scores in patients with treatment-resistant depression. Ketamine was also shown to produce a robust antidepressant effect in patients with treatment-resistant bipolar disorder (Zarate et al., 2006). Although these drugs produced clinically unacceptable dissociative side effects, the efficacy in these studies was significant (greater than 50% response rate in resistant subjects, fast onset of action, and long duration of effect up to 7 or more days following a single dose), and confirmed NMDAR as a novel target of high interest in the treatment of depression.

The Neuroanatomy of Positive Emotion

As noted earlier, positive emotions are thought to serve the important function of promoting appetitive and consummatory behavior in the presence of rewards. This definition suggests the existence of two main classes of positive emotion: appetitive positive emotional states associated with approach behavior (e.g., enthusiasm, joy), and sensory pleasure associated with consummatory behavior. In this section we summarize evidence from both animal and human research regarding the neuroanatomical systems linked to the two types of positive affect.

SEEKING and the Mesolimbic Dopamine System

In both animal and human research, the neuroanatomical underpinnings of positive emotional states have been associated primarily with the ascending mesolimbic dopamine system that includes the ventral tegmental area, nucleus accumbens, and medial prefrontal and orbital frontal cortices (Burgdorf & Panksepp, 2006). Experimental activation of this system (i.e., electrical or chemical stimulation) has been found to sustain self-stimulation reward in animals. Human studies have primarily relied on correlational brain imaging (i.e., fMRI or positron emission tomography), along with abundant studies of addictive drugs, as well as occasional studies of electrical brain stimulation reward in humans.

Human brain imaging studies involving recall of positive affective memories (Dama-sio et al., 2000), listening to positive music (Blood & Zatorre, 2001), male orgasm (Holstege et al., 2003), and positive anticipation of monetary reward (Knutson, Adams, Fong, & Hommer, 2001), have all shown activation in components of this system. In pharmacological studies, the euphoric effects of intravenous amphetamine have been shown to be directly related to dopamine activity in the nucleus accumbens (Drevets et al., 2001; Oswald et al., 2005). Direct electrical brain stimulation of the accumbens has been found to elicit Duchenne smiles and laughter, as well as self-reports of positive affect (Okun et al., 2004). Patients given the opportunity to self-administer electrical stimulation to the nucleus accumbens (sometimes called the nucleus accumbens septi, as a ventral extension of the lateral septum), or to an area at or near the ventral tegmental area, repeatedly self-administer this stimulation and report that it elicits a positive affective state (Heath, 1963, 1972). The evidence for the role of dopamine in positive affect is reviewed in Table 7.2.

It is important to note that this type of emotional positive affect is distinctly different from the pleasure of sensory affect. The feeling is one of eager anticipation, enthusiasm, and euphoria rather than discrete sensory pleasures such as those evoked by food, massage or orgasm. The names we chose to help reflect the concurrent behavioral and psychological functions of this system were EXPECTANCY and SEEKING (Panksepp, 1981, 1982, 1998). The constructs of EXPECTANCY and SEEKING are quite similar to the concept of "wanting," which is thought to mediate "incentive salience" (Robinson & Berridge, 2001). However, there is a substantial difference between incentive salience, which is fundamentally a sensory–perceptual process, and SEEKING, which certainly is linked strongly to the pleasure–displeasure gradient of experience (since each emotional system performs sensory–perceptual gating functions) but is also an integrated motor–action process that conveys an emotional feeling tone (i.e., this positive emotional action systems allows organisms to pursue enthusiastically *all* of the resources needed for survival; Panksepp & Moskal, 2008). SEEKING is tightly linked to the primary-process instinctual-action

TABLE 7.2. Evidence that Dopamine Modulates an Appetitive Type of Positive Affective (PA) State

Finding	Key cite(s)
Psychostimulant-induced PA associated with dopamine activity in the ventral striatum	Drevets et al. (2001); Martinez et al. (2003); Volkow & Swanson (2003)
Psychostimulant-induced PA attenuated by dopamine receptor antagonists	Jönsson et al. (1971); Newton et al. (2001); Romach et al. (1999)
People with 9/9 dopamine transporter polymorphisms show diminished subjective and physiological effects of amphetamine (including euphoric effects)	Lott et al. (2005)
Personality trait of extraversion (highly correlated with PA) associated with dopamine functioning	Depue & Collins (1999)
Dysphoric effects of dopamine receptor antagonists associated with striatal dopamine binding	Voruganti et al. (2001)
Drugs of abuse (but not aversive stimuli) increase dopamine levels in accumbens shell region of rat brain	Di Chiara (2002); Di Chiara & Imperato (1988)
50-kHz ultrasonic vocalizations, a rat model of PA, modulated by dopamine	Knutson et al. (2002)

aspects of an organism and to the sensory inputs that the system harvests. Thus, we are focusing primarily on the evolved primary processes of the affective–emotional mind. "Wanting" lies at the secondary process-learning level, and many other cognitive processes such as "reward prediction error" involve related, higher tertiary process levels (see Panksepp, 2011a, for a full discussion of evolutionary levels of control within the brain).

Sensory Pleasure and the Orbitofrontal Cortex

Whereas the anticipation of reward has been linked to activation of the ascending meso-limbic dopamine system, the experience of sensory pleasure or enjoyment has been linked to activation a brain region known as the orbitofrontal cortex. Activation of the orbitofrontal (i.e., behind and above the eyes) cortex has been observed in fMRI of positive emotional states related to taste-induced positive affect (Kringelbach, O'Doherty, Rolls, & Andrews, 2003), olfaction-induced positive affect (Rolls, Kringelbach, & De Araujo, 2003), and somatosensory-induced positive affect (Rolls, O'Doherty, et al., 2003). Positive affective states induced by

music (Blood & Zatorre, 2001), as well those observed in mothers viewing pictures of their newborn babies (Nitschke et al., 2004), have also been linked to increased orbitofrontal activity. In nonhuman primates, a subset of orbitofrontal cortex neurons are activated specifically by taste stimuli that are palatable to the monkey (Thorpe, Rolls, & Maddison, 1983).

Lesion studies show definitively that the right frontal cortex is especially important in the neurobiology of positive affect, consistent with the long-standing thesis of lateralized positive versus negative affect in humans. Patients with right frontal lesions are more likely to present with symptoms of mania, whereas patients with left frontal lesions are more likely to present with depression (Robinson, Boston, Starkstein, & Price, 1988; Robinson, Kubos, Starr, Rao, & Price, 1984; Sackeim et al., 1982). Additional evidence for the laterality of PA comes from EEG studies, with generalized PA states associated with increased left cortical power in the alpha frequency compared to the right hemisphere, and generalized negative affective states associated with decreased left cortical activation (e.g., Davidson, 2004; Tomarken, Davidson, Wheeler, & Kinney, 1992).

The Molecular Underpinnings of Positive Affective States

The molecular mechanisms involved in the regulation of positive affective states are not as clearly understood as the neuroanatomical substrates. The best-understood mechanisms include brain dopamine mechanisms supporting appetitive motivations (as in the SEEKING system discussed earlier) and endogenous brain opioid mechanisms mediating various sensory pleasures and bodily satisfactions, including social rewards (Panksepp, 1981). Specifically, endogenous opiates acting on mu-type receptors (endomorphins, met-enkephalin, and beta-endorphin) and dopamine have been the most extensively examined (see Burgdorf & Panksepp, 2006, for an extensive review). Mu-type opiate and dopamine levels in the mesolimbic positive affect circuit have been positively correlated with the euphoric effects of exercise and amphetamine, respectively (Boecker et al., 2008; Drevets et al., 2001), and intravenous administration of mu-opiate and dopamine agonists produces positive affective states in humans (Drevets et al., 2001; Zacny et al., 1994). Mu-type opiate antagonists have been shown to blunt the positive affective state elicited by exercise and alcohol (Davidson, Palfai, Bird, & Swift, 1999; Janal, Colt, Clark, & Glusman, 1984). Similarly, dopamine antagonists decrease positive affective states associated with psychostimulants (Jönsson, Anggård, & Gunne, 1971; Newton, Ling, Kalechstein, Uslaner, & Tervo, 2001; Romach et al., 1999) and produce a state of dysphoria (Voruganti et al., 2001). The endogenous cannabinoids may also be involved in the regulation of positive affective states, as they appear to modulate many emotional processes, including the intensity of sensory pleasure, as well as social enjoyment associated with physical play (Moreira & Lutz, 2008; Trezza, Baarendse, & Vanderschuren, 2010).

Aversive stimuli also increase mu-opiate and dopamine levels in the nucleus accumbens (Marinelli, Quirion, & Gainoulakis, 2004; Tidey & Miczek, 1996). This suggests that the mu-opiate and dopamine systems are not completely specific to subjectively positive-valence emotions. However, these effects are completely consistent with a SEEKING interpretation of the ascending mesolimbic "brain reward" system, as that circuitry also operates when animals are seeking safety (i.e., actively pursuing so-called "negative reinforcement" states).

In order to develop a more comprehensive affective neuroscience strategy for identification of new hedonic pathways, we need to consider the criteria that would allow us to study relevant underlying molecular processes that instigate and regulate affective states in animal models. To establish a causal link between a particular molecular mechanism and positive affect, the following conditions must be fulfilled:

1. Concentrations of key molecules associated with the mechanism under investigation must be significantly altered in critical brain regions following positive affective stimuli.
2. These molecular changes will change in the opposite direction, or not change significantly at all, following presentation of negative affective stimuli.
3. Direct injection of the target molecules or agonists will produce a positive affective state.
4. Pharmacological agonism–antagonism of the key molecules will increase–decrease positive affective states.

Thus far, no molecular mechanism has been characterized as meeting all four of these criteria.

The PLAY, LUST, and CARE Systems

The cases for SEEKING and sensory pleasure/enjoyment as exemplars of positive emotion are especially strong given both the subjective experience associated with these states in human research and the association between neural substrates and functional, reward-oriented behavior in studies of both humans and animals. However, there is also some evidence for additional neurobehavioral systems that appear, at least in humans, to involve pleasurable emotional feelings. Although a detailed review of these systems is beyond the scope of this chapter (see Panksepp, 1998, for such a review), we briefly discuss three such systems here.

The Rough-and-Tumble PLAY System

Young animals crave rough-and-tumble, socially engaged, physical play. When made hungry for play, rats will pounce on each other, engendering bouts of chasing and wrestling, all accompanied by joyful 50-kHz chirps signaling an intense social joy. Wherever in the brain one can evoke these chirps with electrical stimulation, animals will eagerly self-stimulate the circuitry, suggesting that one motivation for play is the dopamine-energized SEEKING system (Burgdorf et al., 2007). If humans tickle rats, these vocalizations become very intense, but when any negative affect is induced, these vocalizations cease. A key function of the social PLAY system is to help young animals to acquire the social knowledge and to refine subtle social interactions that they will need to thrive. Thus, PLAY maybe one of the major emotional forces that promotes the epigenetic construction of higher social brain functions, perhaps even including mirror neurons.

The LUST Systems

Sexual urges are mediated by specific brain circuits and chemistries that are overlapping, but also quite distinct, for males and females. These circuits and the associated feelings are aroused by male and female sex hormones, which regulate a variety of neuropeptides. Brain oxytocin transmission, facilitated by estrogen, promotes sexual readiness in females, whereas male assertiveness ("pushiness"?) is regulated by vasopressin, a neuropeptide that is invigorated by testosterone. These brain chemistries help create gender-specific sexual tendencies. Although distinct male and female sexual proclivities are constructed into LUST networks early in life, they are brought to full bloom by the hormonal tides of puberty. Because brain and bodily sex characteristics are independently organized, in all mammals, genetically male animals may exhibit female sexual urges, and genetic females can exhibit male-typical urges.

Certain ancestral chemistries of sexuality, for instance, oxytocin, have been redeployed for crafting maternal CARE—nurturance and social bonding—suggesting evolutionary continuities between female sexual rewards and maternal satisfaction.

The CARE Maternal Nurturance System

Brain evolution has provided safeguards to ensure that parents take care of offspring, with mammalian mothers generally being more devoted than fathers. The massive hormonal changes at the end of pregnancy (declining progesterone and increasing estrogen, prolactin, and oxytocin) set the stage for activation of maternal urges a few days before the young are born. These hormonal and neurochemical tides facilitate maternal moods and promote social bonding with offspring. Similar neurochemicals, especially oxytocin and endogenous opioids, promote infant bonding to the mother. These changes are foundational for a fundamental love: mother–infant bonding.

Conclusion

Affective neuroscience approaches provide coherent methodologies to decipher neural mechanisms for the generation of appetitive and sensory positive emotion states. In addition, by studying diverse primary process forms of positive, prosocial emotional states (e.g., the LUST, CARE, and PLAY networks in rats; Panksepp, 2011a), the neuroanatomical basis and molecular mechanisms of various types of positive affect can be understood. Although animal neuroscience presents distinct challenges for the study of emotion (i.e., the issue of operationalizing "positive affect" in the absence of language), it also presents opportunities that go beyond what can currently be examined with human participants. We are confident that behavioral indices such as 50-kHz USVs express positive emotional states because all of the brain sites concentrated in SEEKING circuits that generate these sounds also sustain self-stimulation behavior (Burgdorf et al., 2007), a critical criterion for positive affect processes of the brain.

The implications of these developments for psychiatric medicine are increasingly evident. For instance, depressive disorders can be ameliorated by promoting various positive emotions, whether psychobehaviorally or pharmacologically. The discovery that 50-kHz USVs reflect a positive affective state in rats allows this measure to be used effectively to monitor hedonic states in animal models of addictions (Panksepp et al., 2002), and in various models of disorders characterized by imbalanced mood states, especially depression. Our working hypothesis is that these vocalizations directly reflect bursting of ventral tegmental dopamine neurons within the mesolimbic reward-SEEKING dopamine circuits. Our prediction is that 50-kHz "chirps" are emitted in close relationship to the bursting of dopamine cells, a neurophysiological condition that promotes active dopamine release.

These findings have direct implications for new therapeutics in biological psychiatry, as well as psychotherapeutic approaches to achieve affective homeostasis. For example, as discussed earlier, the use of affective neuroscience approaches led to the discovery that the NR2B NMDA receptor subunit plays a functional role in hedonic USVs. In an important application of this basic finding, GLYX-13 (a NMDAR glycine site functional partial agonist) is in a Phase II clinical development program for the treatment of depression. Clearly, the next generation of science on neuropsychiatric disorders needs to integrate the growing knowledge about affective brain circuits more fully and explicitly into new experimental approaches to treatment, and conversations are sorely needed on how we can better use limited research resources to promote new medicinal discoveries.

Acknowledgments

This work was supported by the Ralph and Marian Falk Medical Research Trust, Chicago, Illinois (to Joseph R. Moskal), the Hope for Depression Research Foundation (to Jaak Panksepp and Joseph R. Moskal), and National Institute of Mental Health Grant No. 1-R01-MH094835 (to Jeffrey S. Burgdorf).

References

Bell, R. W. (1974). Ultrasounds in small rodents: Arousal-produced and arousal-producing. *Developmental Psychobiology, 7*(1), 39–42.

Berridge, K. C. (2003). Pleasures of the brain. *Brain and Cognition, 52*(1), 106–128.

Blanchard, R. J., & Blanchard, D. C. (1989). Antipredator defensive behaviors in a visible burrow system. *Journal of Comparative Psychology, 103*(1), 70–82.

Blood, A. J., & Zatorre, R. J. (2001). Intensely pleasurable responses to music correlate with activity in brain regions implicated in reward and emotion. *Proceedings of the National Academy of Sciences, 98*(20), 11818–11823.

Blumberg, M. S. (1992). Rodent ultrasonic short calls: Locomotion, biomechanics, and communication. *Journal of Comparative Psychology, 106*(4), 360–365.

Boecker, H., Sprenger, T., Spilker, M. E., Henriksen, G., Koppenhoefer, M., Wagner, K. J., et al. (2008). The runner's high: Opioidergic mechanisms in the human brain. *Cerebral Cortex, 18*(11), 2523–2531.

Browning, J. R., Browning, D. A., Maxwell, A. O., Dong, Y., Jansen, H. T., Panksepp, J., et al. (2011). Positive affective vocalizations during cocaine and sucrose self-administration: A model for spontaneous drug desire in rats. *Neuropharmacology, 61*(1), 268–275.

Brudzynski, S. M. (2001). Pharmacological and behavioral characteristics of 22 kHz alarm calls in rats. *Neuroscience and Biobehavioral Reviews, 25*(7), 611–617.

Brunelli, S. A., & Hofer, M. A. (2007). Selective breeding for infant rat separation-induced ultrasonic vocalizations: Developmental precursors of passive and active coping styles. *Behavioural Brain Research, 182*(2), 193–207.

Burgdorf, J., Knutson, B., & Panksepp, J. (2000). Anticipation of rewarding electrical brain stimulation evokes ultrasonic vocalization in rats. *Behavioral Neuroscience, 114*(2), 320–327.

Burgdorf, J., Knutson, B., Panksepp, J., & Ikemoto, S. (2001). Nucleus accumbens amphetamine microinjections unconditionally elicit 50-kHz ultrasonic vocalizations in rats. *Behavioral Neuroscience, 115*(4), 940–944.

Burgdorf, J., Knutson, B., Panksepp, J., & Shippenberg, T. S. (2001). Evaluation of rat ultrasonic vocalizations as predictors of the conditioned aversive effects of drugs. *Psychopharmacology, 155*, 35–42.

Burgdorf, J., Kroes, R. A., Beinfeld, M. C., Panksepp, J., & Moskal, J. R. (2010). Uncovering the molecular basis of positive affect using rough-and-tumble play in rats: A role for insulin-like growth factor I. *Neuroscience, 168*(3), 769–777.

Burgdorf, J., Kroes, R. A., Moskal, J. R., Pfaus, J. G., Brudzynski, S. M., & Panksepp, J. (2008). Ultrasonic vocalizations of rats (*Rattus norvegicus*) during mating, play, and aggression: Behavioral concomitants, relationship to reward, and self-administration of playback. *Journal of Comparative Psychology, 122*(4), 357–367.

Burgdorf, J., & Panksepp, J. (2006). The neurobiology of positive emotions. *Neuroscience and Biobehavioral Reviews, 30*(2), 173–187.

Burgdorf, J., Panksepp, J., Brudzynski, S. M., Beinfeld, M. C., Cromwell, H. C., Kroes, R. A., et al. (2009). The effects of selective breeding for differential rates of 50-kHz ultrasonic vocalizations on emotional behavior in rats. *Developmental Psychobiology, 51*(1), 34–46.

Burgdorf, J., Panksepp, J., & Moskal, J. R. (2011). Frequency-modulated 50 kHz ultrasonic vocalizations: A tool for uncovering the molecular substrates of positive affect. *Neuroscience and Biobehavioral Reviews, 35*(9), 1831–1836.

Burgdorf, J., Wood, P. L., Kroes, R. A., Moskal, J. R., & Panksepp, J. (2007). Neurobiology of 50-kHz ultrasonic vocalizations in rats: Electrode mapping, lesion, and pharmacology studies. *Behavioural Brain Research, 182*(2), 274–283.

Carden, S. E., & Hofer, M. A. (1990). Independence of benzodiazepine and opiate action in the suppression of isolation distress in rat pups. *Behavioral Neuroscience, 104*(1), 160–166.

Covington, H. E., & Miczek, K. A. (2003). Vocalizations during withdrawal from opiates and cocaine: Possible expressions of affective distress. *European Journal of Pharmacology, 467*(1), 1–13.

Csikszentmihalyi, M., & Hunter, J. (2003). Happiness in everyday life: The uses of experience sampling. *Journal of Happiness Studies, 4*(2), 185–199.

Damasio, A. R., Grabowski, T. J., Bechara, A., Damasio, H., Ponto, L. L., Parvizi, J., et al. (2000). Subcortical and cortical brain activity during the feeling of self-generated emotions. *Nature Neuroscience, 3*, 1049–1056.

Davidson, D., Palfai, T., Bird, C., & Swift, R. (1999). Effects of naltrexone on alcohol self-administration in heavy drinkers. *Alcoholism: Clinical and Experimental Research, 23*(2), 195–203.

Davidson, R. J. (2004). What does the prefrontal cortex "do" in affect: Perspectives on frontal EEG asymmetry research. *Biological Psychology, 67*(1), 219–234.

Depue, R. A., & Collins, P. F. (1999). Neurobiology of the structure of personality: Dopamine, facilitation of incentive motivation, and extraversion. *Behavioral and Brain Sciences, 22*(3), 491–517.

Di Chiara, G. (2002). Nucleus accumbens shell and core dopamine: Differential role in behavior and addiction. *Behavioural Brain Research, 137*(1–2), 75–114.

Di Chiara, G., & Imperato, A. (1988). Drugs abused by humans preferentially increase synaptic dopamine concentrations in the mesolimbic system of freely moving rats. *Proceedings of the National Academy of Sciences, 85*(14), 5274–5278.

Drevets, W. C., Gautier, C., Price, J. C., Kupfer, D. J., Kinahan, P. E., Grace, A. A., et al. (2001). Amphetamine-induced dopamine release in human ventral striatum correlates with euphoria. *Biological Psychiatry, 49*(2), 81–96.

Ekman, P., Davidson, R. J., & Friesen, W. V. (1990). The Duchenne smile: Emotional expression and brain physiology: II. *Journal of Personality and Social Psychology, 58*(2), 342–353.

Furey, M. L., & Drevets, W. C. (2006). Antidepressant efficacy of the antimuscarinic drug scopolamine: A randomized, placebo-controlled clinical trial. *Archives of General Psychiatry, 63*(10), 1121–1129.

Hashimoto, K. (2009). Emerging role of glutamate in the pathophysiology of major depressive disorder. *Brain Research Reviews, 61*(2), 105–123.

Heath, R. G. (1963). Electrical self-stimulation of the brain in man. *American Journal of Psychiatry, 120*(6), 571–577.

Heath, R. G. (1972). Pleasure and brain activity in man: Deep and surface electroencephalograms during orgasm. *Journal of Nervous and Mental Disease, 154*(1), 3–18.

Holstege, G., Georgiadis, J. R., Paans, A. M., Meiners, L. C., van der Graaf, F. H., & Reinders, A. S. (2003). Brain activation during human male ejaculation. *Journal of Neuroscience, 23*(27), 9185–9193.

Ikemoto, S. (2010). Brain reward circuitry beyond the mesolimbic dopamine system: A neurobiological theory. *Neuroscience and Biobehavioral Reviews, 35*(2), 129–150.

Janal, M. N., Colt, E. W., Clark, W. C., & Glusman, M. (1984). Pain sensitivity, mood and plasma endocrine levels in man following long-distance running: Effects of naloxone. *Pain, 19*(1), 13–25.

Jönsson, L. E., Anggård, E., & Gunne, L. M. (1971). Blockade of intravenous amphetamine euphoria in man. *Clinical Pharmacology and Therapeutics, 12*(6), 889–896.

Kahneman, D., & Krueger, A. B. (2006). Developments in the measurement of subjective well-being. *Journal of Economic Perspectives, 20*(1), 3–24.

Kanarik, M., Alttoa, A., Matrov, D., Kõiv, K., Sharp, T., Panksepp, J., et al. (2011). Brain responses to chronic social defeat stress: Effects on regional oxidative metabolism as a function of a hedonic trait, and gene expression in susceptible and resilient rats. *European Neuropsychopharmacology, 21*(1), 92–107.

Knutson, B., Adams, C. M., Fong, G. W., & Hommer, D. (2001). Anticipation of increasing monetary reward selectively recruits nucleus accumbens. *Journal of Neuroscience, 21*(16), 1–5.

Knutson, B., Burgdorf, J., & Panksepp, J. (2002). Ultrasonic vocalizations as indices of affective states in rats. *Psychological Bulletin, 128*(6), 961–977.

Kringelbach, M. L., O'Doherty, J., Rolls, E. T., & Andrews, C. (2003). Activation of the human orbitofrontal cortex to a liquid food stimulus is correlated with its subjective pleasantness. *Cerebral Cortex, 13*(10), 1064–1071.

Kroes, R. A., Burgdorf, J., Otto, N. J., Panksepp, J., & Moskal, J. R. (2007). Social defeat, a paradigm of depression in rats that elicits 22-kHz vocalizations, preferentially activates the cholinergic signaling pathway in the periaqueductal gray. *Behavioural Brain Research, 182*(2), 290–300.

Lott, D. C., Kim, S. J., Cook, E. H., & de Wit, H. (2004). Dopamine transporter gene associated with diminished subjective response to amphetamine. *Neuropsychopharmacology, 30*(3), 602–609.

Machado-Vieira, R., Salvadore, G., DiazGranados, N., & Zarate, C. A., Jr. (2009). Ketamine and the next generation of antidepressants with a rapid onset of action. *Pharmacology and Therapeutics, 123*(2), 143–150.

Mällo, T., Matrov, D., Koiv, K., & Harro, J. (2009). Effect of chronic stress on behavior and cerebral oxidative metabolism in rats with high or low positive affect. *Neuroscience, 164*(3), 963–974.

Marinelli, P. W., Quirion, R., & Gianoulakis, C. (2004). An *in vivo* profile of β-endorphin release in the arcuate nucleus and nucleus accumbens following exposure to stress or alcohol. *Neuroscience, 127*(3), 777–784.

Martinez, D., Slifstein, M., Broft, A., Mawlawi, O., Hwang, D. R., Huang, Y., et al. (2003). Imaging human mesolimbic dopamine transmission with positron emission tomography: Part II. Amphetamine-induced dopamine release in the functional subdivisions of the striatum. *Journal of Cerebral Blood Flow and Metabolism, 23*(3), 285–300.

Moreira, F. A., & Lutz, B. (2008). The endocannabinoid system: Emotion, learning and addiction. *Addiction Biology, 13*(2), 196–212.

Newton, T. F., Ling, W., Kalechstein, A. D., Uslaner, J., & Tervo, K. (2001). Risperidone pre-treatment reduces the euphoric effects of experimentally administered cocaine. *Psychiatry Research, 102*(3), 227-233.

Nitschke, J. B., Nelson, E. E., Rusch, B. D., Fox, A. S., Oakes, T. R., & Davidson, R. J. (2004). Orbitofrontal cortex tracks positive mood in mothers viewing pictures of their newborn infants. *NeuroImage, 21*(2), 583–592.

Olds, J., & Milner, P. (1954). Positive reinforcement produced by electrical stimulation of septal area and other regions of rat brain. *Journal of Comparative and Physiological Psychology, 47*(6), 419–427.

Okun, M. S., Bowers, D., Springer, U., Shapira, N. A., Malone, D., Rezai, A. R., et al. (2004). What's in a "smile?": Intra-operative observations of contralateral smiles induced by deep brain stimulation. *Neurocase, 10*(4), 271–279.

Oswald, L. M., Wong, D. F., McCaul, M., Zhou, Y., Kuwabara, H., Choi, L., et al. (2005). Relationships among ventral striatal dopamine release, cortisol secretion, and subjective responses to amphetamine. *Neuropsychopharmacology, 30*(4), 821–832.

Panksepp, J. (1981). Hypothalamic integration of behavior: Rewards, punishments, and related psychobiological process. *Handbook of the Hypothalamus, 3*(Pt. A), 289–487.

Panksepp, J. (1982). Toward a general psychobiological theory of emotions. *Behavioral and Brain Sciences, 5*(03), 407–422.

Panksepp, J. (1998). *Affective neuroscience: The foundations of human and animal emotions.* New York: Oxford University Press.

Panksepp, J. (2011a). The basic emotional circuits of mammalian brains: Do animals have affective lives? *Neuroscience and Biobehavioral Reviews, 35,* 1791–1804.

Panksepp, J. (2011b). Cross-species affective neuroscience decoding of the primal affective experiences of humans and related animals. *PloS ONE, 6*(9), e21236.

Panksepp, J., & Burgdorf, J. (2000). 50-kHz chirping (laughter?) in response to conditioned and unconditioned tickle-induced reward in rats: effects of social housing and genetic variables. *Behavioural Brain Research, 115*(1), 25–38.

Panksepp, J., & Burgdorf, J. (2003). "Laughing" rats and the evolutionary antecedents of human joy?. *Physiology and Behavior, 79*(3), 533–547.

Panksepp, J., Burgdorf, J., Beinfeld, M. C., Kroes, R. A., & Moskal, J. R. (2004). Regional brain cholecystokinin changes as a function of friendly and aggressive social interactions in rats. *Brain Research, 1025*(1), 75–84.

Panksepp, J., Burgdorf, J., Beinfeld, M. C., Kroes, R. A., & Moskal, J. R. (2007). Brain regional neuropeptide changes resulting from social defeat. *Behavioral Neuroscience, 121*(6), 1364–1371.

Panksepp, J., Knutson, B., & Burgdorf, J. (2002). The role of brain emotional systems in addictions: A neuro-evolutionary perspective and new "self-report" animal model. *Addiction, 97*(4), 459–469.

Panksepp, J., & Moskal, J. (2008). Dopamine and SEEKING: Subcortical "reward" systems and appetitive urges. In A. J. Elliot (Ed.), *Handbook of approach and avoidance motivation* (pp. 67–87). Mahwah, NJ: Erlbaum.

Panksepp, J., Newman, J. D., & Insel, T. R. (1992). Critical conceptual issues in the analysis of separation distress systems of the brain. In K. T. Strongman (Ed.), *International review of studies on emotion* (Vol. 2, pp. 51–72). New York: Wiley.

Robinson, T. E., & Berridge, K. C. (2001). Incentive-sensitization and addiction. *Addiction, 96*(1), 103–114.

Robinson, R. G., Boston, J. D., Starkstein, S. E., & Price, T. R. (1988). Comparison of mania and depression after brain injury: Causal factors. *American Journal of Psychiatry, 145*(2), 172–178.

Robinson, R. G., Kubos, K. L., Starr, L. B., Rao, K., & Price, T. R. (1984). Mood disorders in stroke patients: Importance of location of lesion. *Brain, 107*(1), 81–93.

Rolls, E. T., Kringelbach, M. L., & De Araujo, I. E. (2003). Different representations of pleasant and unpleasant odours in the human brain. *European Journal of Neuroscience, 18*(3), 695–703.

Rolls, E. T., O'Doherty, J., Kringelbach, M. L.,

Francis, S., Bowtell, R., & McGlone, F. (2003). Representations of pleasant and painful touch in the human orbitofrontal and cingulate cortices. *Cerebral Cortex, 13*(3), 308–317.

Romach, M. K., Glue, P., Kampman, K., Kaplan, H. L., Somer, G. R., Poole, S., et al.(1999). Attenuation of the euphoric effects of cocaine by the dopamine D1/D5 antagonist ecopipam (SCH 39166). *Archives of General Psychiatry, 56*(12), 1107–1108.

Sackeim, H. A., Greenberg, M. S., Weiman, A. L., Gur, R. C., Hungerbuhler, J. P., & Geschwind, N. (1982). Hemispheric asymmetry in the expression of positive and negative emotions: Neurologic evidence. *Archives of Neurology, 39*(4), 210–218.

Schwarting, R. K., Jegan, N., & Wöhr, M. (2007). Situational factors, conditions and individual variables which can determine ultrasonic vocalizations in male adult Wistar rats. *Behavioural Brain Research, 182*(2), 208–222.

Skolnick, P., Popik, P., & Trullas, R. (2009). Glutamate-based antidepressants: 20 years on. *Trends in Pharmacological Sciences, 30*(11), 563–569.

Soltysik, S., & Jelen, P. (2005). In rats, sighs correlate with relief. *Physiology and Behavior, 85*(5), 598–602.

Stone, A. A., Schwartz, J. E., Schkade, D., Schwarz, N., Krueger, A., & Kahneman, D. (2006). A population approach to the study of emotion: Diurnal rhythms of a working day examined with the Day Reconstruction Method. *Emotion, 6*(1), 139–149.

Thorpe, S. J., Rolls, E. T., & Maddison, S. (1983). The orbitofrontal cortex: Neuronal activity in the behaving monkey. *Experimental Brain Research, 49*(1), 93–115.

Tidey, J. W., & Miczek, K. A. (1996). Social defeat stress selectively alters mesocorticolimbic dopamine release: An in vivo microdialysis study. *Brain Research, 721*(1), 140–149.

Tomarken, A. J., Davidson, R. J., Wheeler, R. E., & Kinney, L. (1992). Psychometric properties of resting anterior EEG asymmetry: Temporal stability and internal consistency. *Psychophysiology, 29*(5), 576–592.

Trezza, V., Baarendse, P. J., & Vanderschuren, L. J. (2010). The pleasures of play: Pharmacological insights into social reward mechanisms. *Trends in Pharmacological Sciences, 31*(10), 463–469.

Volkow, N. D., & Swanson, J. M. (2003). Variables that affect the clinical use and abuse of methylphenidate in the treatment of ADHD.

American Journal of Psychiatry, 160(11), 1909–1918.

Voruganti, L., Slomka, P., Zabel, P., Costa, G., So, A., Mattar, A., et al. (2001). Subjective effects of AMPT-induced dopamine depletion in schizophrenia-correlation between dysphoric responses and striatal D2 binding ratios on SPECT imaging. *Neuropsychopharmacology, 25*(5), 642–650.

Wang, H., Liang, S., Burgdorf, J., Wess, J., & Yeomans, J. (2008). Ultrasonic vocalizations induced by sex and amphetamine in M2, M4, M5 muscarinic and D2 dopamine receptor knockout mice. *PLoS ONE, 3*(4), e1893.

Wöhr, M., Kehl, M., Borta, A., Schänzer, A., Schwarting, R. K., & Höglinger, G. U. (2009). New insights into the relationship of neurogenesis and affect: tickling induces hippocampal cell proliferation in rats emitting appetitive 50-kHz ultrasonic vocalizations. *Neuroscience, 163*(4), 1024–1030.

Zacny, J. P., Lichtor, J. L., Thapar, P., Coalson, D. W., Flemming, D., & Thompson, W. K. (1994). Comparing the subjective, psychomotor and physiological effects of intravenous butorphanol and morphine in healthy volunteers. *Journal of Pharmacology and Experimental Therapeutics, 270*(2), 579–588.

Zarate, C. A., Jr., Singh, J. B., Carlson. P. J., Brutsche, N. E., Ameli, R., Luckenbaugh, D. A., et al. (2006). A randomized trial of an N-methyl-D-aspartate antagonist in treatment-resistant major depression. *Archives of General Psychiatry, 63*(8), 856–864.

CHAPTER 8

Autonomic Nervous System Aspects of Positive Emotions

Sylvia D. Kreibig

A pounding heart, changes in breathing, and sweaty palms are prototypical examples of the physiological changes occurring in fear. Might similar, possibly less vigorous, changes also appear in pride, amusement, and other positive emotions? Although physiological changes are often described as a defining characteristic of emotion, alongside changes in subjective experience and facial and vocal expression (Scherer, 2001), they have been less well studied in positive than in negative emotions.

In this chapter, I illustrate how an affective psychophysiology approach (Kreibig, Schaefer, & Brosch, 2010) can be applied to the study of autonomic changes in positive emotions. The core idea of affective psychophysiology involves a twofold approach: (1) psychological theories are used to predict and explain how emotions influence autonomic nervous system (ANS) functioning, and (2) analysis of autonomic response patterns is used to generate integrative psychological models of emotion. As will be seen, this approach can identify both commonalities and differences among positive emotions. Based on this approach, I outline several models of ANS responding in positive emotions that suggest one emotion merges into another as a situation evolves.

Table 8.1 serves as a road map throughout this chapter. As it illustrates, I focus on positive emotions in action and interpersonal contexts. Within action contexts, I address the families of agentic and epistemological emotions; within interpersonal contexts, I address the families of affiliative and other-oriented emotions. This is not to claim that these are the only positive emotions. There are many other positive emotions that could be subjected to similar analysis. These four broad emotion families were selected as reflecting the major contexts in which individuals interact with their environment. To structure and integrate core findings regarding ANS effects of positive emotions, I frequently return to Table 8.1. Before delving into this discussion, however, I first introduce some general principles relating to the structure and measurement of the ANS.

Structure and Measurement of the ANS

The ANS controls many of the involuntary physiological changes associated with emotion. It consists of a system of nerves that regulates organ functioning throughout the human body, including the viscera, vasculature, glands, and other tissues, excepting

TABLE 8.1. Core Findings of Autonomic Nervous System Effects of Positive Emotions

| | Positive emotions in action contexts | | | | | | Positive emotions in interpersonal contexts | | | |
| | Agentic emotions | | | Epistemological emotions | | | Affiliative emotions | | Other-oriented emotions | |
	Joy	Flow	Pride	Surprise	Interest	Amusement	Love, anticipatory	Love, consummatory	Compassion	Gratitude
Response measure										
HR	+	+	+	−	+	=	+	−	−	
PEP	−	=	−	=	−	+				
SV										
CO			+		+	−				
PTT	−				+					
SBP	+	−	+	+	+	=	−			−
DBP	+	+	+	+	+	+	−			−
TPR			+		+	+				
FPA				−		−				
FT				−	+	+				
SCL	+	+	+		+	−			+	
SCR	+		+	+		−	+			
nsSCRR				+						
RSA/HF-HRV		−	+	=	−	+		+		+
LF-HRV	+				+					+
Response systems										
Sympathetic nervous system										
Cardiac	+	=	+	=	+	−	+/=?	−	−/=?	
Vascular	+	+	+	+	+/−	+		−		−
Electrodermal	+	+	+	+	+	−	+		+	
Parasympathetic nervous system										
Cardiac RM		−	+	=	−	+	−	+	+/=?	+
Cardiac BRM	+				+					+

Note. +, increased activation; −, decreased activation; =, unchanged activation; ?, unclear implications; blank fields signify absence of empirical findings; RM, respiration-mediated; BRM, baroreflex-mediated; for other abbreviations, see Table 8.2.

striated muscle fibers (Jänig, 2003; Langley, 1921). The ANS comprises several subsystems, including the sympathetic (SNS) and parasympathetic (PNS) nervous systems. These two systems differ in their anatomical structure, neurotransmitters used for synaptic communication, and innervation targets. Central innervation targets of the SNS include the heart, vasculature, erector pili muscles, pupils, lungs, sweat and salivary glands, and the adrenal medulla. Central innervation targets of the PNS include the heart's pacemaker cells and atria, smooth muscles and glands of the airways, intraocular smooth muscles, and exocrine glands of the head.

Autonomic regulation of target tissues is normally fast, occurring within a time range of less than a second. Autonomic regulation is also highly differentiated. Both SNS and PNS subsume several different, functionally distinct subsystems, which innervate different types of target tissues. Little or no cross talk between these various subsystems (Jänig & Häbler, 2000) results in a highly differentiated organization that brings about a large repertoire of distinct autonomic responses (Folkow, 2000; Jänig, 2003). This constitutes the basis for differentiated autonomic responses in emotion.

Various measures allow inferences about the state of ANS functioning. These can be organized into five primary groups (see Table 8.2). A first group relates to the heart's sympathetic activation level. Although heart rate is commonly used in this context, it is a relatively unspecific measure. The heart is dually innervated by the SNS and PNS, and both systems can evoke heart rate changes. Increases in heart rate can mean increased sympathetic influence, decreased parasympathetic influence, or both. A more specific measure of sympathetic effects on the heart is obtained through quantification of pre-ejection period (PEP), the time interval from the beginning of electrical stimulation of the ventricles to the opening of the aortic valve (i.e., electrical systole), relating to myocardial contractility.

A second group of measures addresses effects of the SNS on the vasculature, which can lead to vasodilation and vasoconstriction. Measures of arterial functioning, such as diastolic blood pressure, total peripheral

TABLE 8.2. Overview of Indicator Functions of Primary Autonomic Response Measures According to Autonomic Branch, Effector Organ, Receptor Type, and Response Direction

Autonomic branch	Effector organ	Receptor type	Response measure	Abbreviation	Response direction
SNS	Heart	Beta-adrenergic	Heart rate[†]	HR	+
			Pre-ejection period	PEP	−
			Stroke volume	SV	+
			Cardiac output	CO	+
			Pulse transit time	PTT	−
			Systolic blood pressure	SBP	+
	Vasculature	Alpha-adrenergic	Diastolic blood pressure	DBP	+
			Total peripheral resistance	TPR	+
			Finger pulse amplitude	FPA	−
			Finger temperature (surface)	FT	−
	Eccrine sweat glands/ electrodermal	Cholinergic	Skin conductance level	SCL	+
			Skin conductance response amplitude	SCR	+
			Skin conductance response rate	nsSCRR	+
PNS	Heart/ respiration-mediated	Cholinergic	Heart rate[†]	HR	−
			Root mean squared successive differences	RMSSD	+
			Peak–valley respiratory sinus arrhythmia	p-v RSA	+
			High-frequency heart rate variability	HF-HRV	+
	Heart/ baroreflex-mediated	Alpha- and beta-adrenergic	Low-frequency heart rate variability	LF-HRV	+

Note. SNS, sympathetic nervous system; PNS, parasympathetic nervous system; †, unspecific index due to dual control through SNS and PNS; +, increase with increasing autonomic influence; −, decrease with increasing autonomic influence.

resistance, pulse amplitude, and peripheral surface temperature, allow assessment of peripheral sympathetic effects and gauge their impact on central cardiac processes.

A third group of measures assesses sympathetic effects on the electrodermal system, including skin conductance level, response rate, and amplitude. Although measures of the electrodermal system are a reliable index of sympathetic activity, it is of note that this system is solely controlled by the SNS and, in contrast to other sympathetic effector organs, its influence is mediated by cholinergic rather than adrenergic transmitters (Schütz et al., 2008; Shields, MacDowell, Fairchild, & Campbell, 1987). Hence, inferences of sympathetic functioning obtained from the electrodermal system may not apply to other organ systems.

A fourth group of measures allows assessment of parasympathetic vagal influences on the heart, specifically respiration-mediated vagal effects, which impact the high-frequency component of heart rate variability. During inspiration, vagal activity is attenuated and heart rate accelerates, whereas during expiration, vagal activity is reinstated and heart rate slows. This phenomenon is referred to as respiratory sinus arrhythmia (RSA) and can be quantified through various variability measures of heart rate.

A fifth group of measures relates to baroreflex-mediated cardiac vagal effects (Goldstein, Bentho, Park, & Sharabi, 2011), which impact the low-frequency component of heart rate variability. Spectral analysis of heart rate variability allows quantification of this component. The baroreflex describes the mechanism through which increases in blood pressure lead to reflexive decreases in heart rate, cardiac output, and total peripheral resistance, illustrating the complex interaction between vascular and cardiac processes.

Given the possibility of complex interactions, as well as nonuniform ANS functioning at different organ sites, multiple measures of end organ activity are necessary to infer ANS functioning. Hence, these five primary groups of cardiovascular and electrodermal response measures and their autonomic index function, as summarized in Table 8.2, constitute the focus of the present chapter.

Positive Emotions in Action Contexts

In this section I address positive emotions that occur in action contexts, including two types of emotion families. The first family, that of positive agentic emotions, occurs in achievement contexts (Depue & Collins, 1999): We strive to reach an achievement goal by performing certain actions that are expected to produce the desired outcome. Occurrence of positive agentic emotions informs us that execution and progress of actions proceeds as planned (Carver & Scheier, 1998). That is, expectations of the outcomes of our actions are confirmed or even overconfirmed, our actions are successful, and we are reaching ambitious goals. One may say that positive agentic emotions arise when we navigate in "a world as we know it."

Epistemological emotions (Keltner & Shiota, 2003) comprise a second family of emotions that occur in action contexts. Positive epistemological emotions arise when we are confronted with a (benign) world "as we *don't* know it," that is, when the world operates in ways that are incongruous with our knowledge or expectations, such as deviation from generally accepted social norms or standards. In positive epistemological emotions, these deviations are appraised both as comprehensible and as not impacting the individual negatively (Silvia, 2005). Accordingly, positive epistemological emotions motivate thinking, exploring, and learning in order to foster growth of knowledge.

Positive Agentic Emotions: Joy, Flow, and Pride

Goal-directed behavior involves planned action geared toward reaching a goal—a cognitive representation of a future object that an individual is committed to approach or avoid (Elliot & Fryer, 2008). Although it may seem linear, goal striving, particularly in achievement contexts, is an intricately recursive process: setting a goal, undertaking action to come closer to the goal, evaluating whether one's action has had the desired effect and whether the goal has already been achieved, and looping back into action (Carver & Scheier, 1998; Miller, Galanter, & Pribram, 1960). More often than not, achieving one goal opens up new aspirations. The end of one achievement striving merges fluently into the start of a new one. While different stages throughout the goal-striving process give rise to different feeling qualia, the physiological response elicited by each stage shares a common denominator—the mobilization of resources, as will be seen below. Possibly because of the recursiveness of the goal-striving process, the agentic emotion family illustrates common physiological factors among positive emotions.

That goal-directed behavior is not always affectively laden is both theoretically (Heckhausen & Gollwitzer, 1987) and empirically supported (Gendolla, 1999; Gendolla & Richter, 2005). Nonetheless, when an obstacle has to be overcome, progress is fast, or an activity goes superbly smoothly, the pleasure of exerting a skill or performing at the limit of one's ability can occur during goal striving (Frijda, 2007). Three types of success events in the goal-striving process can be distinguished and are associated with different positive emotions. While we are engaged in a task, small events signal stepwise successes—turning over another page, fitting in another piece of a puzzle, looking back downhill at a divide. Such intermittent success events can arise from both external and internal evaluations of one's task performance, signaling that "things are going well." Intermittent external success events during task performance elicit joy, based on the appraisal that progress toward a goal is achieved at a rate higher than one's standard (Carver & Scheier, 1998). Self-generated success events during task performance (e.g., feel-right experiences; Kruglanski, 2006) arise when an activity goes superbly smoothly. Improved performance and pleasant feelings result. Enjoyment or flow is the emotion experienced in the context of effortless, yet highly focused, task performance (Csikszentmihalyi, 1990).

When these successive successes come to a climactic completion—reading the final page of a book, finishing the 500-piece puzzle, reaching the mountaintop—there may be an extended sense of goal attainment. Pride is experienced from goal attainment appraised as being caused by stable aspects of the self, including ability (Weiner, 1985, 2000). Although sustained success events involve a sense of closure, from a broader perspective they have a penultimate charac-

ter. The next book, the 1,000-piece puzzle, and the next higher mountain are already in sight. Completion of one goal striving opens up more advanced goals.

Joy and the Pursuit of Achievement Goals

Joy is commonly defined as "the emotion evoked by well-being, success, or good fortune or by the prospect of possessing what one desires" (Merriam-Webster Online, 2012a). It involves a desirable event that contributes to the realization of an individual's goals (Ortony, Clore, & Collins, 1988) and the appraisal that an event's implications are relevant and highly conducive to the attainment of those goals (Scherer, 2001). Thus, joy arises on the way to goals rather than at their attainment (Carver & Scheier, 1998). More specifically, progress toward a goal at a rate higher than one's standard is said to elicit joy (Carver & Scheier, 1998). Joy has been characterized as an energizing emotion that reinforces the process of goal pursuit.

Motivational theories of resource mobilization or effort investment allow prediction of the physiological effects of emotion during goal pursuit. Resource mobilization (i.e., the effort invested in goal striving) corresponds to task difficulty when a task has clearly defined and known performance standards (Brehm & Self, 1989). The importance of success sets an upper limit, beyond which all effort is withdrawn (e.g., if success is viewed as impossible or requiring more effort than warranted by its importance). When a task calls for a subject's "best performance," effort corresponds directly to the importance of success (Richter & Gendolla, 2009). Given that success feedback promotes optimistic appraisals of one's ability to master the challenge successfully, and of the attractiveness and likelihood of success, joy is expected to lead to increased effort investment under conditions of subsequently increasing difficulty level or "do your best" instructions. In contrast, failure feedback incites more pessimistic appraisals, such that disappointment will lead to decreased effort investment under such conditions (cf. mood influences; Gendolla, 2000).

Physiologically, resource mobilization relates to sympathetic beta-adrenergic cardiovascular activation (Wright, 1996), most directly quantified through measures of PEP and systolic blood pressure. Diastolic blood pressure and heart rate show less consistent results, as these measures are multiply determined. Other research has also related electrodermal activity to resource mobilization (Gendolla & Richter, 2005; Pecchinenda & Smith, 1996).

Intermittent success events signal successive progress toward a goal. Such events elicit phasic (i.e., short-lived) event-related physiological responses of increased heart rate, shortened pulse transit time, and increased electrodermal activity (Ravaja, Saari, Salminen, Laarni, & Kallinen, 2006; Ravaja, Turpeinen, Saari, Puttonen, & Keltikangas-Järvinen, 2008; van Reekum et al., 2004). This response pattern reflects increased effort mobilization. Success feedback also enhances task-related effort expenditure; tonic or sustained physiological changes during subsequent task performance include shortened PEP and increased heart rate, and systolic and diastolic blood pressure (Tomaka & Palacios-Esquivel, 1997). This contrasts with the physiological responses elicited by intermittent failure events, which elicit phasic physiological responses of depressed cardiac reactivity (e.g., heart rate and pulse transit time) and stronger increases in electrodermal activity. Failure feedback after a successful start also leads to withdrawal of mobilized resources during subsequent task performance: Tonic physiological activation indicates a return to baseline of the initially decreased PEP and increased systolic and diastolic blood pressure, and a lowering of the initially increased heart rate (Tomaka & Palacios-Esquivel, 1997; see also Annis, Wright, & Williams, 2001). Taken together, and as summarized in Table 8.1, autonomic responses during joy consist of increased beta-adrenergic cardiovascular and electrodermal sympathetic activation.

Flow and Optimal Performance

Flow is a subjective state of optimal experience during performance of a nontrivial task, whose difficulty is on par with the skill level of the subject (Csikszentmihalyi, 1990). Flow is positively associated with quality of performance and may function as a reward signal that promotes repeated engagement in a task. de Manzano, Theorell, Harmat, and Ullén (2010) suggested that the focused

yet effortless attention characteristic of flow results from an interaction between a high degree of selective attention (high mental effort) and positive affect.

Physiologically, then, flow may be expressed in a superposition of response patterns characteristic of these two processes: As discussed in the previous section, effort mobilization leads to increased sympathetic activation, reflected in both sympathetic beta-adrenergic cardiovascular (Richter, Friedrich, & Gendolla, 2008; Richter & Gendolla, 2009) and electrodermal effects (Gendolla & Richter, 2005; Pecchinenda & Smith, 1996). Positive affect is often associated with increased heart rate variability (McCraty, Atkinson, Tiller, Rein, & Watkins, 1995). Although the high-frequency component of heart rate variability (i.e., RSA) has been the main focus of research, there may also be grounds for associating the low-frequency component (i.e., baroreflex-mediated vagal modulation) (Goldstein et al., 2011) with positive affect. A shift from respiration-mediated to baroreflex-mediated vagal drive has been interpreted as a decrease in entropic tendencies in the cardiovascular system (Wu et al., 2009). The resulting decrease in homeostatic demand on the body is believed to facilitate positive affect. Taken together, such a response pattern would signify sympathetic and parasympathetic coactivation, providing precise control of response direction and magnitude, as well as fine-tuning of target organ function (Berntson, Cacioppo, & Quigley, 1991).

Flow experiences have been experimentally elicited in the context of gaming (Nacke & Lindley, 2009), Web browsing (Mauri, Cipresso, Balgera, Villamira, & Riva, 2011), piano playing (de Manzano et al., 2010), and performing a low-load attentional task after a pride-eliciting social interaction (Fourie et al., 2011). In line with predictions of increased sympathetic activation, flow has been associated with increased skin conductance level (Fourie et al., 2011; Mauri et al., 2011; Nacke & Lindley, 2009) and increased diastolic blood pressure (de Manzano et al., 2010), but decreased systolic blood pressure and unchanged PEP. Supporting predictions of parasympathetic coactivation, increased heart rate, and decreased high-frequency and increased low-frequency heart rate variability suggest a shift from respiration- to baroreflex-mediated vagal drive (de Manzano et al., 2010; Fourie et al., 2011). Taken together, peripheral sympathetic activation of the vasculature and sweat glands and cardiac vagal control increase, while central cardiac sympathetic beta-adrenergic drive remains unchanged or decreases (see Table 8.1). Fourie and colleagues (2011, p. 898) suggested that "this transient non-cardiac [SNS] arousal . . . can be viewed as 'being in the zone,' i.e., [SNS]-aroused but not stressed, relaxed yet focused—a pleasurable feeling that should encourage future [flow]-eliciting behaviors." Peripheral sympathetic and baroreflex-mediated parasympathetic coactivation hence appears to be a plausible hypothesis for the affective state of flow during task performance (cf. Table 8.1).

Pride in Attaining Achievement Goals

Pride arises in response to personal achievements (C. A. Smith & Ellsworth, 1985). Specifically, pride is elicited when a highly valued accomplishment is attained, and the success is interpreted as caused by oneself (Frijda, Kuipers, & ter Schure, 1989; Lazarus, 1991). Thus, pride involves appraisals of high goal relevance, goal congruence, and self-agency. Pride gives rise to exuberant action tendencies—approach, expansiveness, a strong desire to pay attention, an urge to share the achievement with others, and envisioning greater achievements in the future (Frijda et al., 1989; Lazarus, 1991; Lewis, 1993; C. A. Smith & Ellsworth, 1985). Continued engagement in similar or more challenging tasks and taking leadership roles often follow (Williams & DeSteno, 2008, 2009).

The self-reinforcing effect of pride fuels achievement motivation (Fredrickson, 2004; Lewis, 1993) and forms the stepping-stone for future achievement strivings (cf. penultimate character). Physiologically, such behavioral activation is associated with the cardiac response system (Fowles, 1980; Kreibig, 2012). Specifically, to support attentional engagement with the valued object or positive performance feedback, an orienting response is expected, involving decreased heart rate and increased skin conductance level (cf. section on "Positive Epistemological Emotions"). To support continued engagement with the environment for "broadening and building" (e.g., continued task engagement, communication with others; Fredrickson, 2001), increased autonomic regulation, which comprises sympathetic activation for energy mobilization (Bandler, Keay, Floyd, & Price, 2000; Recordati, 2003) and parasympathetic coactivation, as found under conditions of optimal autonomic functioning (Berntson et al., 1991), is predicted. In contrast, a disengagement response, involving resignation and attentional withdrawal, is expected to lead to decreased autonomic regulation (sympathetic–parasympathetic co-inhibition) under conditions of goal nonattainment.

A relatively pure probe of the psychophysiological response of pride can be obtained from laboratory paradigms that disentangle goal attainment from goal pursuit. This can be achieved by creating task conditions that do not allow monitoring of one's performance during goal pursuit. Presentation of positive performance feedback, then, constitutes goal attainment as the pride-eliciting event. Based on this paradigm, studies have found sympathetic–parasympathetic coactivation, including shortened PEP and increased cardiac output, increased RSA, increased blood pressure, and increased nonspecific skin conductance response rate for pride (Kreibig, Gendolla, & Scherer, 2010, 2012). Variable effects on heart rate (i.e., either increases or decreases) are caused by the unspecific expression of sympathetic–parasympathetic coactivation on heart rate. This response pattern reflects the predicted components of the physiological response of pride, including responding to the reward, increased attentional engagement, and effort investment in a task. In contrast, disappointment leads to lower RSA, lengthened PEP, decreased blood pressure, and decreased electrodermal activity (Kreibig et al., 2012). This disengagement response is related to feelings of resignation and disengagement from the task.

Taken together, a physiologically activating response accompanies the elicitation of pride in response to goal attainment, whereas a physiologically deactivating response accompanies the elicitation of disappointment in response to goal nonattainment. As summarized in Table 8.1, pride has effects on cardiovascular variables related to alpha- and beta-adrenergic sympathetic activation in combination with cardiac parasympathetic coactivation.

Summary

By looking at different types of success events, it becomes evident that autonomic responding in positive agentic emotions elicited in achievement contexts is positively effort mobilizing, whether the success is a brief external event during task performance, the experience of great ease during task performance, or an extended sense of success upon penultimate goal attainment. While sympathetic activation is a common denominator of positive agentic emotions, the experience of optimal functioning in flow and pride adds a component of parasympathetic coactivation not observed in joy (see Table 8.1).

Applications

The first evidence for generalization of this response pattern beyond the laboratory comes from a pioneering study in which heart rate reactivity was investigated in relation to students' emotional experience in the classroom while working on math problems (Ahmed, van der Werf, & Minnaert, 2010). Consistent with the response found in the laboratory, nonverbal expressions of pride were reliably associated with heart rate increases.

The autonomic response pattern evoked by agentic emotions may become maladaptive when pride is made contingent upon meeting excessively high performance standards, as in Type A behavior (Friedman & Rosenman, 1959; Price, 1982), or when pride becomes hubristic, as in narcissism (Campbell, Foster, & Burnell, 2004; Tracy & Robins, 2004). Higher cardiovascular reactivity, including greater heart rate and systolic and diastolic blood pressure, has been noted for Type A behavior during and after task performance in various achievement contexts (Harbin, 1989). Similarly, high narcissism leads to greater PEP decreases in task contexts, suggesting greater cardiovascular reactivity and heightened effort (Kelsey et al., 2000). In the long term, the heightened cardiovascular reactivity found in Type A behavior and narcissism may be associated with greater risk for coronary atherosclerosis and heart disease.

Positive Epistemological Emotions: Surprise, Interest, and Amusement

When a benign world acts in mildly unexpected ways, currently activated expectations or knowledge structures are disconfirmed. Successfully integrating an incongruous stimulus event into alternative knowledge structures satisfies the goal of meaning making. Surprise, interest, and amusement are the positive epistemological emotions that arise under these conditions. In what follows, I focus on humor comprehension, as it exemplifies all three emotions in sequential occurrence and illustrates their close interrelationship.

The epistemological emotion family serves as an illustration of superposition of physiological response patterns, which likely results from the close temporal succession of these emotions. Humor comprehension involves a two-stage process (cf. incongruity resolution theory; Suls, 1972): the detection of incongruity, followed by its resolution. Three emotions occur during this process. An incongruous stimulus event first generates surprise, signaling deviation from the expected. Surprise functions to interrupt ongoing action and orient the individual to a potentially significant event. In order to resolve the incongruity and transform nonsense into humorous sense, a frame shift is necessary (i.e., conceptual reinterpretation; Coulson, 1997). This engagement with the incongruous stimulus is experienced as interest when the event is appraised as novel and complex, but comprehensible (Silvia, 2005). Successfully achieving integration into an alternative frame resolves the incongruity and leads to amusement—or terms often used interchangeably with it, such as *mirth, happiness,* and *exhilaration.* Amusement is associated with a state of pleasurable, relaxed excitation (Ruch, 1993) and playful, nonserious interaction with the environment. Each of the emotions leads to specific effects on the ANS. The following sections outline theoretically derived predictions and empirical observations of autonomic response patterns associated with each emotion, stressing their sequential and super-posed expression as the emotion transitions from surprise over interest to amusement.

Surprise and the Detection of Incongruity

Surprise, a hedonically neutral, short-lived emotion triggered by events that disconfirm expectations (Ellsworth & Smith, 1988), is elicited by a single appraisal, that of unexpectedness (Roseman, Antoniou, & Jose, 1996; Scherer, 1984). Effects of surprise are believed to appear quickly, with latency of only a few hundred milliseconds (Delplanque et al., 2009; Grandjean & Scherer, 2008; Horstmann, 2006; Niepel, 2001), but also to subside quickly because subsequent appraisals differentiate the emotion almost immediately (Scherer, 1987). Surprise alerts and stimulates (Izard, 1991). It interrupts ongoing cognitive and motor processes, and refocuses attention to the discrepant event; if warranted, it may lead to effortful, conscious, and deliberate analysis of the event (Horstmann, 2006; Meyer, Reisenzein, & Schützwohl, 1997). Surprise arouses epistemic motivation and impels investigatory and exploratory behavior. In this way, surprise functions to monitor a person's schemas or belief system, and to update them when facing unexpected conditions (Reisenzein, 2000). Thus, surprise serves the goal of predicting environmental events (Scherer, 1987).

Surprise has been associated with the orienting response (Reisenzein, Meyer, & Schützwohl, 1996), which constitutes "a complex of automatic, pre-attentive changes in brain activity and peripheral reflex responses to unexpected, novel changes in the environment" (Stekelenburg & van Boxtel, 2002, p. 707). It involves a "tuning of the receptor" (e.g., eye and head movements); inhibition of gross body movements (including respiration); and autonomic changes, including heart rate deceleration (bradycardia), peripheral vasoconstriction, and increased electrodermal activity (Niepel, 2001; Siddle, 1991; Sokolov, 1990). Coactivation of vagal and sympathetic branches characterizes the cardiac component of the orienting response (Sokolov & Cacioppo, 1997). The combination of these effects facilitates the uptake, transmission, and analysis of environmental information. The transient effects of the generalized orienting response subserve involuntary orienting to an unexpected nonsignal stimulus that primarily elicits surprise.

Empirical support for an orienting response as characterizing early-onset autonomic changes during humor processing comes from studies of humorous stimuli of short to intermediate duration. For example, 10-second presentations of incongruous pictures (e.g., a young woman with shaving cream on her face and an electric razor in her hand) lead to decreased heart rate, mildly increased skin conductance response amplitude, and no effects on respiration (Klorman, Weissberg, & Wiesenfeld, 1977; Klorman, Wiesenfeld, & Austin, 1975). Humorous film clips of 20 seconds to 3 minutes also elicit decreased heart rate, increased skin conductance response amplitude and response rate, and increased respiratory rate (Britton, Taylor, Berridge, Mikels, & Liberzon, 2006; Demaree, Schmeichel, Robinson, & Everhart, 2004; Herring, Burleson, Roberts, & Devine, 2011; Kreibig, Samson, & Gross, 2013; Shiota, Neufeld, Yeung, Moser, & Perea, 2011). Results also indicate peripheral vasoconstriction (e.g., decreased finger temperature, decreased finger pulse amplitude; Giuliani, McRae, & Gross, 2008; Gross & Levenson, 1997). Decreased PEP and RSA may indicate reciprocal sympathetic activation (Kreibig, Samson, et al., 2013), although other studies indicate no change on these measures (Demaree et al., 2004; Herring et al., 2011; Shiota et al., 2011). Taken together, autonomic changes, as summarized in Table 8.1, reflect the predicted peripheral vasoconstriction and electrodermal activation but do not clearly indicate the expected sympathetic–parasympathetic coactivation at the heart.

Interest in and Engagement with an Incongruous Stimulus

Interest arises from two central appraisals—evaluating an event as new, unexpected, complex, and unfamiliar (a high novelty–complexity appraisal) and as comprehensible (a high coping-potential appraisal; Silvia, 2005). Clearly, surprise and interest are closely related: Appraising an event as new predicts surprise; adding in comprehensibility transforms the emotion into interest (Silvia, 2005). Because the appraisal structure of interest is still fairly simple, interest, too, transforms into other emotions as the appraisal process continues to unfold (Ellsworth & Smith, 1988; Silvia, 2005).

The outcome of the novelty–complexity appraisal creates a subjective feeling of uncertainty; the event is perceived as demanding or deserving attention, leading to high attentional activity; and the disrupted or dysfluent processing gives rise to the experience that the event is hard to process (Ellsworth & Smith, 1988; Silvia, 2005). *Coping potential* broadly refers to estimates of resources, power, abilities, and control for dealing with an event. In the context of knowledge, the appraisal of coping potential evaluates whether one can achieve the goal of understanding (Silvia, 2005). Evaluating a poorly understood event as understandable implies that the event deserves high effort (Ellsworth & Smith, 1988). Within a couple of seconds, interest leads to intense and persistent motivational engagement in the processing of information (Reeve & Nix, 1997). Thus, interest both holds attention to the eliciting event and mobilizes sustained effort, supporting the urge to explore and seek out new information and experiences (Ellsworth & Smith, 1988).

Physiologically, interest has autonomically activating effects, supporting orientation, attention direction, concentration, behavioral activation, and approach-oriented action (Libby, Lacey, & Lacey, 1973; Silvia, 2008). Sustained attention and effort investment are key components of autonomic change in interest. The voluntary and sustained attention to a signal stimulus (Stekelenburg & van Boxtel, 2002), characteristic of interest, is associated with a local orienting response. However, rather than the transient effects of the generalized orienting response for surprise, effects of the local orienting response during interest are persistent. In particular, unexpected, novel, and complex stimuli sustain the inhibitory response pattern, with deeper and sustained heart rate deceleration, peripheral vasoconstriction, and skin conductance responses than for surprise (Libby et al., 1973; Turpin, Schaefer, & Boucsein, 1999).

In addition to the orienting response, effects of increased effort (i.e., resource mobi-

lization for engagement with the event) are predicted for interest. As detailed in the section "Positive Agentic Emotions," resource mobilization is subserved by predominantly sympathetic beta-adrenergic activation (Wright, 1996) and is expressed in decreased PEP, increased heart rate, increased cardiac output, and increased electrodermal activity. Thus, whereas attentional aspects of interest lead to sympathetic–parasympathetic coactivation in the orienting response, as characteristic for novel or challenging environments (Sokolov & Cacioppo, 1997), effort mobilizing aspects of interest lead to (beta-adrenergic) sympathetic activation. These mixed autonomic influences are expected to lead to variable expression of, particularly dually controlled, response measures, such as the heart rate response.

Studies that experimentally manipulated interest in game and task contexts found evidence for cardiovascular activation, as indicated by increased heart rate, decreased PEP and increased cardiac output, increased systolic and diastolic blood pressure, and increased total peripheral resistance (Kreibig et al., 2010; Muth, Koch, Stern, & Thayer, 1999; Waldstein, Bachen, & Manuck, 1997; van Reekum et al., 2004). These response variables point to increased alpha- and beta-adrenergic sympathetic cardiovascular activation. Skin conductance level was also increased, additionally indicating activation of the electrodermal system. Faster rise of finger temperature and longer pulse transit time suggest peripheral vasodilation. Furthermore, increased low-frequency and decreased high-frequency heart rate variability indicate vagal withdrawal. Taken together, this pattern of broad sympathetic activation, peripheral vasodilation, and decreased respiration but increased baroreflex-mediated cardiac vagal activation (see Table 8.1) supports the hypothesis of attentional and effort-related processes contributing to the physiological response underlying interest.

Amusement and the Resolution of Incongruity

Amusement involves the enjoyment of play, humor, and entertainment. Its elicitation is based on a sequence of appraisals: the appraisal of unexpectedness identifies an incongruity; the appraisal of coping potential evaluates it as comprehensible; and an appraisal of alternative meaning of diminished value can resolve the incongruity, which the appraisal of motive consistency evaluates as not impinging on one's goals (Suls, 1972; Wyer & Collins, 1992). As these appraisals suggest, amusement is closely tied to surprise and interest (Ludden, Hekkert, & Schifferstein, 2006). Adding in appraisals of motive consistency and diminished value transforms these emotions into amusement. In support of this sequence hypothesis, emotional response components of amusement occur with a greater latency than those of surprise or interest (Cunningham & Derks, 2005; Derks, Staley, & Haselton, 1998; Keltner, 1995). Amusement leads to readiness to approach, to attend, and to be exuberant, as expressed in free activation, such as participating in physical or intellectual play (Frijda et al., 1989). By practicing new physical and cognitive skills, amusement broadens an individual's thought–action repertoire (Fredrickson, 2000).

The physiological amusement response is predicted to include components of attentional orienting toward the incongruous event, resource mobilization for engaging with the incongruous event, adoption of an alternative processing mode for comprehending it, and enjoyment upon successfully resolving the incongruity. Given that amusement is experienced upon completing incongruity resolution, beta-adrenergic sympathetic effects of mental effort should be less evident, possibly giving way to cardiac vagal control, whereas attention-related vasoconstriction may persist. These predictions are consistent with assuming a process of emotional conflict adaptation upon engrossment with the humorous material. Repetitive incongruity resolution is believed to facilitate processes of conflict regulation, situated in the anterior cingulate cortex that inhibits amygdala activation (Etkin, Prater, Hoeft, Menon, & Schatzberg, 2010). Activation of the anterior cingulate cortex has been previously related to increased blood pressure reactivity and parasympathetic activity (Critchley, Corfield, Chandler, Mathias, & Dolan, 2000; Matthews, Paulus, Simmons, Nelson, & Dimsdale, 2004), whereas deactivation of the amygdala relates to decreased electrodermal activity (Boucsein, 1992;

Critchley, 2002). Patterned SNS activation, comprising vascular activation and cardiac and electrodermal deactivation, and cardiac vagal activation are therefore predicted for the state of pleasurable, relaxed excitation associated with amusement. Effects of amusement are predicted to dominate autonomic responding, once incongruity resolution has become the predominant mode of information processing.

Effects of amusement are believed to predominate upon longer presentation of humorous material. Time course analyses by Hubert and de Jong-Meyer (1990, 1991) suggest a shift in autonomic activation between 1 and 3 minutes of continuous humor processing. This change may be obscured if exclusively analyzing condition averages. Rather than the early inhibitory orienting response, a state more consistent with pleasurable, relaxed excitation (Ruch, 1993) arises. First, continued peripheral vasoconstriction, as expressed in increased diastolic blood pressure and total peripheral resistance, and decreased finger temperature and finger pulse amplitude (Averill, 1969; Harrison et al., 2000), likely reflects sustained attention. Second, decreased beta-adrenergic (increased PEP, unchanged systolic blood pressure, and decreased cardiac output; Averill, 1969; Harrison et al., 2000) and cholinergic activation to a level below resting state (decreased skin conductance level and response rate; Averill, 1969; Hubert & de Jong-Meyer, 1990, 1991), may be taken to indicate decreased cognitive effort and increased relaxation. Third, an increase in cardiac vagal influence may occur (Carruthers & Taggart, 1973). Finally, accompanying heart rate is at base level (Averill, 1969; Hubert & de Jong-Meyer, 1990; Harrison et al., 2000) or decreased (Carruthers & Taggart, 1973; Hubert & de Jong-Meyer, 1991). In summary, empirical findings support the hypothesis of peripheral vasoconstriction, decreased beta-adrenergic and cholinergic sympathetic activation, and increased cardiac vagal influence during amusement (see Table 8.1).

As a side note, laughter can occur during episodes of amusement, involving diaphragmatic convulsions that disrupt the regular breathing pattern (see Owren & Amoss, Chapter 9, this volume). This poses the question of whether apparent autonomic effects of amusement are merely due to the pronounced autonomic effects of laughter. A number of findings suggest that autonomic effects of amusement and laughter are reasonably distinguishable. Findings document different brain areas for the generation of amusement and laughter (Arroyo et al., 1993; Iwasa et al., 2002). The inhibitory response of amusement noted earlier is incompatible with stimulatory autonomic effects of laughter, for example, marked increases in heart rate and blood pressure (Buchowski et al., 2007; Fry, 1992; Fry & Savin, 1988), substantial decreases in lung volume, increased inspiratory pause time, and decreased inspiratory time (Boiten, 1998; Filippelli et al., 2001). Correlations suggest that changes in autonomic variables are related to subjective feelings of amusement rather than to the amount of laughter (Averill, 1969; Hubert & de Jong-Meyer, 1990). Brief and sporadic occurrences of laughter cannot account for the consistent autonomic changes observed during amusement episodes (Averill, 1969; Filippelli et al., 2001). Thus, it seems unlikely that autonomic effects of laughter underlie the changes observed during episodes of amusement.

Summary

This discussion of autonomic responding during humor processing highlights the multiplicity of emotional processes in this context. The sequential elicitation of emotions leads to distinguishable autonomic effects: a generalized orienting response for surprise; a localized orienting response and effort mobilization for interest; and pleasurable, relaxed excitation, including components of attention, decreased effort, and enjoyable engrossment, for amusement (cf. Table 8.1). Superposition of the autonomic response patterns was suggested for their integrated occurrence in humor processing more generally.

Applications

Beyond mere entertainment, humor processing and its autonomic signature have far-reaching implications: Experiencing amusement subsequent to a negative emotion brings about faster heart rate recovery (Fredrickson & Levenson, 1998; Fredrick-

son, Mancuso, Branigan, & Tugade, 2000) and larger increases in high-frequency heart rate variability (Llera & Newman, 2010). Beneficial effects of dispositional amusement have been observed at the endocrine level (Lai et al., 2010) but have yet to be explored systematically with respect to ANS functioning.

Because amusement arises in response to an individual's understanding of the external world (Keltner, Gruenfeld, & Anderson, 2003), it has proved useful to study individual differences in autonomic reactivity to amusement inductions in the context of psychopathologies and their prognosis. For example, amusement reactivity may serve as an index of the behavioral approach system, which gives rise to a variety of positive emotions. Depression is one disorder in which positive emotional reactivity is impaired (Allen, Trinder, & Brennan, 1999; Sloan, Strauss, Quirk, & Sajatovic, 1997). Interestingly, greater heart rate reactivity in response to an amusement film has been found to predict subsequent recovery from depression (Rottenberg, Kasch, Gross, & Gotlib, 2002), possibly indicating less impairment of the behavioral approach system. The study of autonomic responses during amusement may also help to elucidate mechanisms that underlie impairments in the expression of amusement, as found in cases of pathological laughter and crying in amyotrophic lateral sclerosis (Olney et al., 2011).

Positive Emotions in Interpersonal Contexts

In this section, I address positive emotions in interpersonal contexts, where two emotion families can be distinguished. The first family, positive affiliative emotions, occurs in close personal relationships involving kinship or romance. Positive affiliative emotions elicit and reinforce the goal of close proximity with loved ones who signal affection, care, and safety. The arousal of positive affiliative emotions may act as incentive to establish and maintain intimate bonds (Depue & Morrone-Strupinsky, 2005). Other-oriented emotions constitute a second emotion family that occurs in interpersonal contexts. Positive other-oriented emotions arise when we enter altruistic exchange relationships with individuals who are not necessarily affiliated with us. They build on the appraisal that one can ameliorate another's situation, or that another has ameliorated one's own situation (Lazarus, 2006). They signal feeling good about helping or being helped. Their arousal may promote group cohesion beyond close personal relationships.

Positive Affiliative Emotions: Anticipatory and Consummatory Aspects of Love

Love involves feelings of strong affection and personal attachment (Merriam-Webster Online, 2012b). It is experienced in "important, pleasant situations in which things are going as desired, and in which the focus is on another person" (Ellsworth & Smith, 1988, p. 329). Because love has different implications depending on the degree of physical proximity, the affiliative emotion family serves as an illustration of physiological response pattern differentiation within one emotion construct: Love motivates approach when distant from the loved one, whereas it motivates expression of affection when physically close. Partitioning love into these goal-striving and goal-attainment phases creates a structure similar to the distinction between anticipatory and consummatory stages of reward striving in classical theories of metabolic demand (Di Chiara & North, 1992). The anticipatory stage involves energy expenditure—release of fat stores, sympathetic arousal, and activation of motor behavior. The consummatory stage, in contrast, involves energy restoration—building up of organs and tissues through protein synthesis and muscle growth, activation of the PNS, and rest and sedation (Di Chiara & North, 1992). These response patterns are, for example, evident under conditions of anticipatory food collection and consummatory food ingestion. I suggest that anticipatory and consummatory aspects of love can similarly be distinguished.

The Anticipatory Aspect of Love: Distal Cues of Loved Ones

An anticipatory phase of love is evoked when perceiving distal cues of a loved one, such as facial features and smiles, friendly vocalizations and gestures, and bodily features (Depue & Collins, 1999). Feelings of desire, wanting, excitement, and elation arise. Perceiving the other person is deeply valued (i.e., goal relevant and goal congruent) and increasing physical closeness is both highly desirable and feasible (high ability and high effort). This constellation elicits appraisals of enthusiasm, energy, potency, and self-efficacy. The anticipatory aspect of love is associated with highly activated preparation, effort expenditure, and appetitive approach. Thus, the anticipatory aspect of love functions to achieve increased physical closeness.

Physiologically, desire for closeness is predicted to lead to metabolic and behavioral mobilization through SNS activation. This supports forward locomotion as a means of bringing individuals into close proximity (Depue & Collins, 1999; Di Chiara & North, 1992; Porges, 1998). Increased SNS activation is expressed in measures such as increased heart rate, cardiac contractility, and electrodermal activity. Support for the prediction of a sympathetically activated response in the anticipatory phase of love can be derived from a sequence of studies that probed autonomic responding to pictures of the faces of loved ones, including the romantic partner, parents, siblings, second-degree relatives, and friends. Whereas the perception of famous, unknown, baby, and neutral faces leads to heart rate deceleration (suggesting an orienting response; compare the section "Positive Epistemological Emotions"), the perception of loved faces leads to heart rate acceleration, and the perception of one's romantic partner leads to particularly pronounced skin conductance responses (Guerra et al., 2011; Vico, Guerra, Robles, Vila, & Anllo-Vento, 2010). Similarly, whereas seeing or hearing an unfamiliar infant elicits heart rate deceleration and smaller skin conductance responses in mothers, their own infants elicit heart rate acceleration and larger skin conductance responses (Wiesenfeld & Klorman, 1978; Wiesenfeld, Malatesta, & DeLoach, 1981; Wiesenfeld, Malatesta, Whitman, Granrose, & Uili, 1985). Appetitive approach may also be induced by stimuli perceived as "cute," signaling youth, helplessness, and the need for care (cf. "baby schema"; Lorenz, 1971). Slides of baby animals also lead to increased heart and respiration rates and decreased RSA, as do slides of attachment figures (e.g., Papa Smurf, Big Bird; Shiota et al., 2011).

Cardiac acceleration in response to perceiving loved ones may serve to support the motor behavior involved in increasing proximity between oneself and the loved one. Taken together, as summarized in Table 8.1, the autonomic response underlying the anticipatory aspect of love is suggested to involve increased SNS and decreased PNS activation.

The Consummatory Aspect of Love: Physical Proximity with Loved Ones

When close proximity to a loved one has been achieved, the anticipatory response gives way to a consummatory response. Feelings of pleasure, gratification, and liking arise (Depue & Collins, 1999). The individual feels safe and secure. Appraisals of high goal relevance and goal congruence and low effort characterize the situation. The consummatory aspect of love leads to expression of affection toward the loved one, for example, courtship, gentle stroking and grooming, mating, and certain maternal patterns such as breastfeeding (Depue & Collins, 1999). These conditions are conducive to relaxation and pair-bonding.

The autonomic state subserving the consummatory aspect of love is generally thought to be one of physiological quiescence, characterized by increased release of oxytocin and predominance of PNS activity. The vagus nerve of the PNS and its source nuclei in particular have been hypothesized to form a "social engagement system" (Beauchaine, 2001; Porges, 1995, 2001). Central to the consummatory aspect of love, this system supports attachment and caregiving behaviors, such as facial and vocal displays, looking and listening activities, and motor behaviors (e.g., tactile contact). Activation of the vagus nerve can be inferred from measures of RSA. This physiologically quieting response is predicted to be expressed both in benign conditions, when exchanging expressions of affection, and in overruling the physiological stress response under emotionally challenging conditions (Depue & Morrone-Strupinsky, 2005; Taylor et al., 2000).

Animal models show that administration of oxytocin decreases blood pressure (Petersson, Alster, Lundeberg, & Uvnas-Moberg, 1996), and oxytocin release can be provoked by regular ventral stroking in animals. In humans, this translates into various forms of physical touch. For example, 10 minutes of warm contact with a loved one, such as one's partner, leads to decreased systolic blood pressure (Grewen, Girdler, Amico, & Light, 2005). Similarly, frequent hugs and high perceived partner support are associated with lower resting-state blood pressure and lower heart rate (Grewen et al., 2005; Light, Grewen, & Amico, 2005). Sexually active, cohabiting couples show lower diastolic blood pressure and greater heart rate variability than do noncohabiting couples (Brody, Veit, & Rau, 2000), and self-reported marital quality is positively associated with resting high-frequency heart rate variability (T. W. Smith et al., 2011).

Consistent with the stress-buffering effects of oxytocin under emotionally challenging conditions, Schneiderman, Zilberstein-Kra, Leckman, and Feldman (2011) demonstrated that new lovers (i.e., individuals who had begun a romantic relationship 2 to 16 weeks prior to the experiment) lacked the decrease in heart rate variability that singles demonstrated in response to emotionally negative film clips. Likewise, mothers who nursed their babies evidenced lower systolic blood pressure reactivity in response to a speech stressor than did mothers who bottle-fed their babies (Light et al., 2000). As summarized in Table 8.1, the hypothesized increased release of oxytocin associated with the consummatory component of love leads to autonomic effects of increased parasympathetic activation and a dampening of the sympathetic stress response under both benign and challenging conditions.

Summary

More than for any other emotion, eliciting affiliative emotions in the laboratory underscores the importance of a dimension of personal relevance, such as perceiving or being with one's spouse, parent, or child, or other idiosyncratic love stimuli. Two contrasting autonomic response patterns appear to underlie the affiliative emotions, as summarized in Table 8.1. Findings on visual or auditory perception of cues of loved ones suggest increased sympathetic and decreased cardiac vagal influences as characteristic of the anticipatory component of love. Findings on close interactions with loved ones or being in a close relationship document decreased sympathetic reactivity and increased cardiac vagal influences as characteristic of the consummatory aspect of love.

Applications

Investigation of autonomic response patterns in love may contribute to a better understanding of disorders characterized by aberrant social interactions and attachment relationships, such as autism, schizophrenia, conduct disorder, and depression (Lee, Macbeth, Pagani, & Young, 2009). For example, children with autism, unlike typically developing controls, do not show greater skin conductance responses when responding to their mothers' faces compared to a plain paper cup (Hirstein, Iversen, & Ramachandran, 2001). Children with autism also show higher heart rate and higher blood pressure than do normally developing children during social interactions with either a parent or familiar teacher (Kootz & Cohen, 1981). These findings may indicate impairment of the anticipatory and consummatory aspects of love. Porges (2004) has suggested diminished functioning of the vagus nerve in autism. Still, specific emotional impairments related to love await systematic study in this and other disorders.

Positive, Other-Oriented Emotions: Compassion and Gratitude

Giving and receiving are fundamental themes in interpersonal exchange. Altruistic behavior arises in response to the needs and sufferings of others, as well as the reciprocation of favors received. Compassion and gratitude are the emotions elicited in this context. Compassion is experienced in response to another person's suffering, whereas gratitude is experienced by the target of altruistic acts (Eisenberg & Fabes, 1990; Lazarus & Lazarus, 1994). These are considered other-directed and empathic emotions because both direct attention outward, to other individuals. Both emotions require an understanding of the other person's mental state—inferring the other person's needs and sufferings in compassion, and the other person's positive intentions in gratitude. This process of theory of mind builds on an exteroceptive mode of outward attention and attunement with another's thoughts, knowledge, beliefs, emotions, and desires. This final section revisits physiological concepts of the orienting response and attachment system in interpersonal helping contexts that support the other-directedness of compassion and gratitude. These two emotions serve as examples for the recurrence of key physiological response patterns across emotion families.

Compassion in the Face of Another's Suffering

Compassion is the emotion evoked by the suffering of others. It includes feelings of sympathy, attachment, and tenderness. Concern for the other's welfare lies at the core of compassion (Goetz, Keltner, & Simon-Thomas, 2010). It is elicited by appraisals of undeserved suffering, that is, judgments of whether the target's suffering is self-inflicted (responsibility and controllability), as well as benefits and costs of aiding the other involving evaluations of how important the other is to one's well-being (self- and goal-relevance) and one's resources and abilities in relation to the costs and threats of providing help (coping potential; Goetz et al., 2010). Compassion promotes attention to the needs of others, orients the individual to social approach, and motivates caretaking behavior to enhance others' welfare (e.g., comforting, helping, or otherwise alleviating suffering; Oveis, Horberg, & Keltner, 2010). Thus, compassion facilitates cooperation and protection of vulnerable others.

Compassion is distinct from personal distress, which is an alternative response to another's suffering. Personal distress is aroused given a sense of helplessness and inability to alleviate the other's suffering (Mikulincer & Shaver, 2005). It brings about an attentional shift from the other's needs to one's own distress, focusing on self-protective concerns and motivating escape from the source of distress. The distinction between compassion and personal distress was addressed in early, pioneering research by Eisenberg and colleagues. Eisenberg and colleagues (1989) reasoned that compassion should be associated with interest in the other, focusing one's attention outward, and taking in information concerning the other. Notably, neural circuits subserving theory of mind (i.e., inferring another person's state of mind) and reorienting overlap (Corbetta, Patel, & Shulman, 2008).

Physiologically, the orienting response (cf. the section "Positive Epistemological Emotions") leads to decreased heart rate (Lacey, Kagan, Lacey, & Moss, 1963). In contrast, a personal distress response to another's suffering, entailing self-oriented, aversive emotional reactions such as apprehension, anxiety, or discomfort, will lead to processing of information relevant to one's own situation. Such cognitive elaboration and active coping should be expressed physiologically in increased heart rate (Lacey et al., 1963), which is part of defensive responding. Thus, personal distress reactions should be more arousing than compassionate reactions, both subjectively, as in the experience of restlessness, excitation, and agitation, and physiologically, as indexed by electrodermal activity. Personal distress would therefore be expected to entail higher skin conductance than would compassion.

A series of studies offers convergent findings in support of this reasoning. Film clips that induced either compassion or personal distress were found to elicit differential heart rate responses: heart rate deceleration during compassion and heart rate acceleration during personal distress (Eisenberg, Fabes, et al., 1988; Eisenberg, Schaller, et al., 1988). A person's idiosyncratic response—that is, compassion or personal distress—to another person's suffering also influences the direction of autonomic response: Heart rate decreased more strongly given stronger helping intentions (i.e., commitment of more volunteer hours); heart rate and skin conductance increased more strongly given verbal or facial expression of distress (Eisenberg et al., 1989; Eisenberg, Fabes, Schaller, Carlo, & Miller, 1991). In summary, these studies suggest heart rate deceleration and decreased skin conductance responses as autonomic markers of compassion (see Table 8.1).

Gratitude and the Receipt of Benefit

Gratitude arises in the context of a dyadic relationship in which a donor has given a benefit to a recipient (Emmons & Crumpler, 2000; Lazarus, 1991). It is marked by strong feelings of appreciation and thankfulness (Fredrickson, 2004). At its core, gratitude involves benefit and praiseworthiness appraisals (Wood, 2008). These comprise the perception that a valuable outcome for oneself has been brought about by the intentional, effortful, and voluntary actions of another (Tesser, Gatewood, & Driver, 1968; Weiner, 1985) who expressed thoughtfulness, making one feel cared for, understood, and valued (Algoe, Haidt, & Gable, 2008). Prerequisites for these appraisals are insight into the perspective and desires of the benefactor (Fredrickson, Cohn, Coffey, Pek, & Finkel, 2008) and acceptance of dependence on the benefactor (cf. attachment; Emmons & Crumpler, 2000).

Gratitude is a moderately activating emotion (Reisenzein, 1994). It functions as a "detection-and-response system to help find, remind, and bind ourselves to attentive others" (Algoe et al., 2008, p. 429). It alerts individuals to the value of receiving a benefit from a benefactor, focuses attention on others, especially the need and deservingness of the original benefactor, and motivates moving toward others to reciprocate the kindness and form relationships with attentive others (Algoe et al., 2008; McCullough, Kilpatrick, Emmons, & Larson, 2001).

Predictions generally center on activation of the attachment system in gratitude. As detailed in the section "Positive Affiliative Emotions," the attachment system is hypothesized to be associated with activation of the PNS. This system leads to higher heart rate variability while feeling safe and decreased heart rate variability while feeling unsafe (Porges, 2007). Thus, receiving compassionate care, support, and kindness is believed to have a calming and soothing effect on the grateful individual whose distress has been alleviated (Bowlby, 1969).

Gratitude inductions, such as sincerely focusing on feelings of appreciation experienced toward others (McCraty et al., 1995; Rash, Matsuba, & Prkachin, 2011) or engaging in prayers of gratefulness (Stanley, 2009), have been found to increase low-frequency heart rate variability. Increased low-frequency heart rate variability reflects increased baroreceptor-afferent activity (Goldstein et al., 2011), causing increased parasympathetic and decreased sympathetic efferent outflow, as expressed in increased heart rate variability and decreased vaso-constriction. This shift in sympathovagal balance may underlie the previously noted positive health effects of gratitude (Emmons & McCullough, 2003).

Consistent with the notion of gratitude as requiring the beneficiary to accept indebted-ness (i.e., entering into a recipient relation-ship), attachment style has been found to moderate the emotional response to receiv-ing compassion. When invoking the image of feeling cared for, change in heart rate variability was positively related to secure attachment and social safeness, whereas it was negatively related to anxious attach-ment and self-criticism (Rockliff, Gilbert, McEwen, Lightman, & Glover, 2008). Further research points to an interaction between ability to direct compassion at oth-ers and ability to receive and benefit from others' compassion: When provided with social support during a social stress task, individuals who scored high in trait compas-sion responded with lower blood pressure reactivity (a measure of sympathetic acti-vation) and increased high-frequency heart rate variability (an indicator of parasym-pathetic function), whereas their low-trait-compassion counterparts showed a classical stress response (Cosley, McCoy, Saslow, & Epel, 2010). This suggests that having com-passion *for* others may increase one's ability to accept compassion *from* others, leading to a more adaptive physiological response in stressful conditions. Taken together, empiri-cal findings suggest that increased vagal activity, both respiration- and baroreflex-mediated, and decreased sympathetic activ-ity at the heart and vasculature underlie the autonomic response of gratitude, as summa-rized in Table 8.1.

Summary

Taken together, the positive other-oriented emotions are associated with an autonomic response pattern that orients the individual outwardly, toward the feelings, struggles, and benevolent acts of others. The orienting response constitutes the physiological basis of compassion, directing attention toward misfortunes of others that one may be able to ameliorate. Thus, compassion was reli-ably indicated by heart rate deceleration and reduced skin conductance. The physiologi-cally soothing effects of experiencing and expressing gratitude, supported by increased PNS and decreased SNS activation, give individuals the capacity to reciprocate and bond with the attentive other when receiving compassionate deeds (cf. Table 8.1).

Applications

Heart rate deceleration and decreased skin conductance reactivity are also sensitive indicators of impaired levels of compassion; adolescents with disruptive behavior disor-der, specifically those with highly callous traits, show smaller heart rate deceleration in response to others' suffering (De Wied, van Boxtel, Matthys, & Meeus, 2012; De Wied, van Boxtel, Posthumus, Goudena, & Matthys, 2009). By contrast, individu-als with Williams syndrome have a strong interest in social interactions that manifests in increased attention to human faces, high compassion toward people in distress, and approach behavior. Correspondingly, in response to viewing dynamic negative emo-tional faces, stronger heart rate decelera-tion reflecting increased interest in the other person and decreased skin conductance response amplitude reflecting low personal distress have both been found in this popu-lation (Skwerer et al., 2009).

Autonomic differentiation between com-passion and gratitude can also be demon-strated using their respective autonomic markers. Interventions in the context of an interpersonal offense with either a focus on compassion or benefit finding (culti-vating gratitude) indicate decreased heart rate reactivity for compassion-focused reappraisal, and increased high-frequency heart rate variability for benefit-focused reappraisal (vanOyen Witvliet, Knoll, Hin-man, & DeYoung, 2010). Parasympathetic engagement may be a common physiologi-cal pathway through which compassion- and benefit-finding strategies lead to the generally observed health benefits of these emotions (Bower, Moskowitz, & Epel, 2009).

Conclusion and Future Directions

This chapter has applied an affective psychophysiology approach to the study of physiological changes in positive emotions, resulting in three key outcomes: First, inspection of autonomic response patterns, summarized in Table 8.1, suggests four major categories of positive emotions, each of which show a fairly coherent profile. Second, within each category, rather than a single ANS profile, a sequence of ANS profiles reflects the evolution of emotion over the course of the eliciting situation. Third, the ANS is a complex system with multifaceted activation states. A sound understanding of its functional activation states necessitates study of response profiles across multiple organ systems. The attempt to map ANS activation onto a single dimension of arousal, for example, by using heart rate, conflates a number of distinct autonomic mechanisms.

Table 8.1, summarizing core findings of ANS effects of positive emotions, served as a road map throughout this chapter. It may serve as a similar road map for future research. Its numerous blank entries highlight areas in which research has been lacking so far. Given the strong need for replication of the autonomic response patterns summarized herein, I hope that Table 8.1 will motivate additional research in areas where preliminary empirical results exist.

To conclude, I offer one central future direction, which I believe emerges from this chapter as a key question. Throughout the discussion of ANS aspects of positive emotions, key concepts of physiological responses surfaced: the orienting response (as contrasted to a defensive response); sympathetic (beta-adrenergic) activation for energy mobilization; sympathetic–parasympathetic coactivation under conditions of optimal functioning; and parasympathetic activation given activation of the attachment system. It is important to investigate whether the conceptualization of emotion-specific autonomic response patterns can be maintained, or whether it needs to give way to a conceptualization of a smaller set of basic, underlying physiological responses (cf. Folkow, 2000). This chapter clearly demonstrates that autonomic responses differ between and within positive emotion families. Only systematic future research can answer the question of the degree of autonomic specificity among positive emotions.

Acknowledgments

I thank Guido H. E. Gendolla and Andrea C. Samson for helpful comments on earlier versions of this chapter. Writing of this chapter was supported by the Swiss National Science Foundation (Grant Nos. PBGEP1-125914 and PA00P1-139593).

References

Ahmed, W., van der Werf, G., & Minnaert, A. (2010). Emotional experiences of students in the classroom: A multimethod qualitative study. *European Psychologist, 15*, 142–151.

Algoe, S. B., Haidt, J., & Gable, S. L. (2008). Beyond reciprocity: Gratitude and relationships in everyday life. *Emotion, 8*, 425–429.

Allen, N. B., Trinder, J., & Brennan, C. (1999). Affective startle modulation in clinical depression: Preliminary findings. *Biological Psychiatry, 46*, 542–550.

Annis, S., Wright, R. A., & Williams, B. J. (2001). Interactional influence of ability perception and task demand on cardiovascular response: Appetitive effects at three levels of challenge. *Journal of Applied Behavioral Research, 6*, 82–107.

Arroyo, S., Lesser, R. P., Gordon, B., Uematsu, S., Hart, J., Schwerdt, P., et al. (1993). Mirth, laughter and gelastic seizures. *Brain, 116*, 757–780.

Averill, J. R. (1969). Autonomic response patterns during sadness and mirth. *Psychophysiology, 5*, 399–414.

Bandler, R., Keay, K. A., Floyd, N., & Price, J. (2000). Central circuits mediating patterned autonomic activity during active vs. passive emotional coping. *Brain Research Bulletin, 53* (1), 95–104.

Beauchaine, T. (2001). Vagal tone, development, and Gray's motivational theory: Toward an integrated model of autonomic nervous system functioning in psychopathology. *Development and Psychopathology, 13*, 183–214.

Berntson, G. G., Cacioppo, J. T., & Quigley, K. S. (1991). Autonomic determinism: The modes of autonomic control, the doctrine of autonomic space, and the laws of autonomic constraint. *Psychological Review, 98*, 459–487.

Boiten, F. A. (1998). The effects of emotional behaviour on components of the respiratory cycle. *Biological Psychology, 48,* 29–51.

Boucsein, W. (1992). *Electrodermal activity.* New York: Plenum Press.

Bower, J. E., Moskowitz, J. T., & Epel, E. (2009). Is benefit finding good for your health?: Pathways linking positive life changes after stress and physical health outcomes. *Current Directions in Psychological Science, 18,* 337–341.

Bowlby, J. (1969). *Attachment and loss: Attachment* (Vol. 3). New York: Basic Books.

Brehm, J. W., & Self, E. A. (1989). The intensity of motivation. *Annual Review of Psychology, 40,* 109–131.

Britton, J. C., Taylor, S. F., Berridge, K. C., Mikels, J. A., & Liberzon, I. (2006). Differential subjective and psychophysiological responses to socially and nonsocially generated emotional stimuli. *Emotion, 6,* 150–155.

Brody, S., Veit, R., & Rau, H. (2000). A preliminary report relating frequency of vaginal intercourse to heart rate variability, valsalva ratio, blood pressure, and cohabitation status. *Biological Psychology, 52,* 251–257.

Buchowski, M. S., Majchrzak, K. M., Blomquist, K., Chen, K. Y., Byrne, D. W., & Bachorowski, J.-A. (2007). Energy expenditure of genuine laughter. *International Journal of Obesity, 31,* 131–137.

Campbell, K., Foster, J. D., & Burnell, A. B. (2004). Running from shame or reveling in pride?: Narcissism and the regulation of self-conscious emotions. *Psychological Inquiry, 15,* 150–153.

Carruthers, M., & Taggart, P. (1973). Vagotonicity of violence: Biochemical and cardiac responses to violent films and television programmes. *British Medical Journal, 3,* 384–389.

Carver, C. S., & Scheier, M. F. (1998). *On the self-regulation of behavior.* Cambridge, UK: Cambridge University Press.

Corbetta, M., Patel, G., & Shulman, G. L. (2008). The reorienting system of the human brain: From environment to theory of mind. *Neuron, 58,* 306–324.

Cosley, B. J., McCoy, S. K., Saslow, L. R., & Epel, E. S. (2010). Is compassion for others stress buffering?: Consequences of compassion and social support for physiological reactivity to stress. *Journal of Experimental Social Psychology, 46,* 816–823.

Coulson, S. (1997). *Semantic leaps: Frame-shifting and conceptual blending in meaning construction.* Cambridge, UK: Cambridge University Press.

Critchley, H. D. (2002). Electrodermal responses: What happens in the brain. *The Neuroscientist, 8,* 132–142.

Critchley, H. D., Corfield, D. R., Chandler, M. P., Mathias, C. J., & Dolan, R. J. (2000). Cerebral correlates of autonomic cardiovascular arousal: A functional neuroimaging investigation in humans. *Journal of Physiology, 523,* 259–270.

Csikszentmihalyi, M. (1990). *Flow: The psychology of optimal experience.* New York: Harper & Row.

Cunningham, W. A., & Derks, P. (2005). Humor appreciation and latency of comprehension. *Humor, 18,* 389–403.

Delplanque, S., Grandjean, D., Chrea, C., Coppin, G., Aymard, L., Cayeux, I., et al. (2009). Sequential unfolding of novelty and pleasantness appraisals of odors: Evidence from facial electromyography and autonomic reactions. *Emotion, 9,* 316–328.

de Manzano, O., Theorell, T., Harmat, L., & Ullén, F. (2010). The psychophysiology of flow during piano playing. *Emotion, 10,* 301–311.

Demaree, H. A., Schmeichel, B., Robinson, J., & Everhart, D. E. (2004). Behavioural, affective, and physiological effects of negative and positive emotional exaggeration. *Cognition and Emotion, 18,* 1079–1097.

Depue, R. A., & Collins, P. F. (1999). Neurobiology of the structure of personality: Dopamine, facilitation of incentive motivation, and extraversion. *Behavioral and Brain Sciences, 22,* 491–569.

Depue, R. A., & Morrone-Strupinsky, J. V. (2005). A neurobehavioral model of affiliative bonding: Implications for conceptualizing a human trait of affiliation. *Behavioral and Brain Sciences, 28,* 313–395.

Derks, P., Staley, R. E., & Haselton, M. G.. (1998). "Sense" of humor: Perception, intelligence, or expertise? In W. Ruch (Ed.), *The sense of humor: Explorations of a personality characteristic* (pp. 143–158). Berlin: de Gruyter.

De Wied, M., van Boxtel, A., Matthys, W., & Meeus, W. (2012). Verbal, facial and autonomic responses to empathy-eliciting film clips by disruptive male adolescents with high versus low callous-unemotional traits. *Journal of Abnormal Child Psychology, 40,* 211–223.

De Wied, M., van Boxtel, A., Posthumus, J. A., Goudena, P. P., & Matthys, W. (2009). Facial

EMG and heart rate responses to emotion-inducing film clips in boys with disruptive behavior disorders. *Psychophysiology, 46,* 996–1004.

Di Chiara, G., & North, R. A. (1992). Neurobiology of opiate abuse. *Trends in Pharmacological Sciences, 13,* 185–193.

Eisenberg, N., & Fabes, R. A. (1990). Empathy: Conceptualization, measurement, and relation to prosocial behavior. *Motivation and Emotion, 14,* 131–149.

Eisenberg, N., Fabes, R. A., Bustamante, D., Mathy, R. M., Miller, P. A., & Lindholm, E. (1988). Differentiation of vicariously induced emotional reactions in children. *Developmental Psychology, 24,* 237–246.

Eisenberg, N., Fabes, R. A., Miller, P. A., Fultz, J., Shell, R., Mathy, R. M., et al. (1989). Relation of sympathy and personal distress to prosocial behavior: A multimethod study. *Journal of Personality and Social Psychology, 57,* 55–66.

Eisenberg, N., Fabes, R. A., Schaller, M., Carlo, G., & Miller, P. A. (1991). The relations of parental characteristics and practices to children's vicarious emotional responding. *Child Development, 62,* 1393–1408.

Eisenberg, N., Schaller, M., Fabes, R. A., Bustamante, D., Mathy, R. M., Shell, R., et al. (1988). Differentiation of personal distress and sympathy in children and adults. *Developmental Psychology, 24,* 766–775.

Elliot, A. J., & Fryer, J. W. (2008). The goal construct in psychology. In J. Y. Shah & W. L. Gardner (Eds.), *Handbook of motivation science* (pp. 235–250). New York: Guilford Press.

Ellsworth, P. C., & Smith, C. A. (1988). Shades of joy: Patterns of appraisal differentiating pleasant emotions. *Cognition and Emotion, 2* (4), 301–331.

Emmons, R. A., & Crumpler, C. A. (2000). Gratitude as a human strength: Appraising the evidence. *Journal of Social and Clinical Psychology, 19,* 56–69.

Emmons, R. A., & McCullough, M. E. (2003). Counting blessings versus burdens: An experimental investigation of gratitude and subjective well-being in daily life. *Journal of Personality and Social Psychology, 84,* 377–389.

Etkin, A., Prater, K. E., Hoeft, F., Menon, V., & Schatzberg, A. F. (2010). Failure of anterior cingulate activation and connectivity with the amygdala during implicit regulation of emotional processing in generalized anxiety disorder. *American Journal of Psychiatry, 167,* 545–554.

Filippelli, M., Pellegrino, R., Iandelli, I., Misuri, G., Rodarte, J. R., Duranti, R., et al. (2001). Respiratory dynamics during laughter. *Journal of Applied Physiology, 90,* 1441–1446.

Folkow, B. (2000). Perspectives on the integrative functions of the "sympatho-adrenomedullary system." *Autonomic Neuroscience: Basic and Clinical, 83,* 101–115.

Fourie, M. M., Rauch, H. G. L., Morgan, B. E., Rellis, G. F. R., Jordaan, E. R., & Thomas, K. G. F. (2011). Guilt and pride are heartfelt, but not equally so. *Psychophysiology, 48,* 888–899.

Fowles, D. C. (1980). The three arousal model: Implications of Gray's two-factor learning theory for heart rate, electrodermal activity, and psychopathy. *Psychophysiology, 17*(2), 87–104.

Fredrickson, B. L. (2000). Cultivating positive emotions to optimize health and well-being. *Prevention and Treatment, 3,* 1–25.

Fredrickson, B. L. (2001). The role of positive emotions in positive psychology: The broaden-and-build theory of positive emotions. *American Psychologist, 56,* 218–226.

Fredrickson, B. L. (2004). Gratitude, like other positive emotions, broadens and builds. In R. A. Emmons & M. E. McCullough (Eds.), *The psychology of gratitude* (pp. 145–166). New York: Oxford University Press.

Fredrickson, B. L., Cohn, M. A., Coffey, K. A., Pek, J., & Finkel, S. M. (2008). Open hearts build lives: Positive emotions, induced through loving-kindness meditation, build consequential personal resources. *Journal of Personality and Social Psychology, 95,* 1045–1062.

Fredrickson, B. L., & Levenson, R. W. (1998). Positive emotions speed recovery from the cardiovascular sequelae of negative emotions. *Cognition and Emotion, 12,* 191–220.

Fredrickson, B. L., Mancuso, R. A., Branigan, C., & Tugade, M. M. (2000). The undoing effect of positive emotions. *Motivation and Emotion, 24,* 237–258.

Friedman, M., & Rosenman, R. H. (1959). Association of specific overt behavior pattern with blood and cardiovascular findings. *Journal of the American Medical Association, 169,* 1286–1296.

Frijda, N. H. (2007). *The laws of emotion.* Mahwah, NJ: Erlbaum.

Frijda, N. H., Kuipers, P., & ter Schure, E. (1989). Relations among emotion, appraisal, and emotional action readiness. *Journal of Personality and Social Psychology, 57*(2), 212–228.

Fry, W. F. (1992). The physiologic effects of humor, mirth, and laughter. *Journal of the American Medical Association, 267*, 1857–1858.

Fry, W. F., & Savin, W. M. (1988). Mirthful laughter and blood pressure. *Humor, 1*, 49–62.

Gendolla, G. H. E. (1999). Self-relevance of performance, task difficulty, and task engagement assessed as cardiovascular response. *Motivation and Emotion, 23*, 45–66.

Gendolla, G. H. E. (2000). On the impact of mood on behavior: An integrative theory and a review. *Review of General Psychology, 4*, 378–408.

Gendolla, G. H. E., & Richter, M. (2005). Ego-involvement and mental effort: Cardiovascular, electrodermal, and performance effects. *Psychophysiology, 42*, 595–603.

Giuliani, N. R., McRae, K., & Gross, J. J. (2008). The up- and down-regulation of amusement: Experiential, behavioral, and autonomic consequences. *Emotion, 8*(5), 714–719.

Goetz, J. L., Keltner, D., & Simon-Thomas, E. (2010). Compassion: An evolutionary analysis and empirical review. *Psychological Bulletin, 136*, 351–374.

Goldstein, D. S., Bentho, O., Park, M.-Y., & Sharabi, Y. (2011). Low-frequency power of heart rate variability is not a measure of cardiac sympathetic tone but may be a measure of modulation of cardiac autonomic outflows by baroreflexes. *Experimental Physiology, 96*, 1255–1261.

Grandjean, D., & Scherer, K. R. (2008). Unpacking the cognitive architecture of emotion processes. *Emotion, 8*(3), 341–351.

Grewen, K. M., Girdler, S. S., Amico, J. A., & Light, K. C. (2005). Effects of partner support on resting oxytocin, cortisol, norepinephrine, and blood pressure before and after warm partner contact. *Psychosomatic Medicine, 67*, 531–538.

Gross, J. J., & Levenson, R. W. (1997). Hiding feelings: The acute effects of inhibiting negative and positive emotion. *Journal of Abnormal Psychology, 106*, 95–103.

Guerra, P., Campagnoli, R. R., Vico, C., Volchan, E., Anllo-Vento, L., & Vila, J. (2011). Filial versus romantic love: Contributions from peripheral and central electrophysiology. *Biological Psychology, 88*, 196–203.

Harbin, T. J. (1989). The relationship between the Type A behavior pattern and physiological reactivity: A quantitative review. *Psychophysiology, 26*, 110–119.

Harrison, L., Carroll, D., Burns, V., Corkill, A., Harrison, C., Ring, C., et al. (2000). Cardiovascular and secretory immunoglobulin A reactions to humorous, exciting, and didactic film presentations. *Biological Psychology, 52*, 113–126.

Heckhausen, H., & Gollwitzer, P. M. (1987). Thought contents and cognitive functioning in motivational versus volitional states of mind. *Motivation and Emotion, 11*, 101–120.

Herring, D. R., Burleson, M. H., Roberts, N. A., & Devine, M. J. (2011). Coherent with laughter: Subjective experience, behavior, and physiological responses during amusement and joy. *International Journal of Psychophysiology, 79*, 211–218.

Hirstein, W., Iversen, P., & Ramachandran, V. S. (2001). Autonomic responses of autistic children to people and objects. *Proceedings of the Royal Society of London B: Biological Sciences, 268*, 1883–1888.

Horstmann, G. (2006). Latency and duration of the action interruption in surprise. *Cognition and Emotion, 20*(2), 242–273.

Hubert, W., & de Jong-Meyer, R. (1990). Psychophysiological response patterns to positive and negative film stimuli. *Biological Psychology, 31*, 73–93.

Hubert, W., & de Jong-Meyer, R. (1991). Autonomic, neuroendocrine, and subjective responses to emotion-inducing film stimuli. *International Journal of Psychophysiology, 11*, 131–140.

Iwasa, H., Shibata, T., Mine, S., Koseki, K., Yasuda, K., Kasagi, Y., et al. (2002). Different patterns of dipole source localization in gelastic seizure with or without a sense of mirth. *Neuroscience Research, 43*, 23–29.

Izard, C. E. (1991). *The psychology of emotions.* New York: Plenum Press.

Jänig, W. (2003). The autonomic nervous system and its coordination by the brain. In R. J. Davidson, K. R. Scherer, & H. H. Goldsmith (Eds.), *Handbook of affective sciences* (pp. 135–186). New York: Oxford University Press.

Jänig, W., & Häbler, H.-J. (2000). Specificity in the organization of the autonomic nervous system: A basis for precise neural regulation of homeostatic and protective body functions. *Progress in Brain Research, 122*, 351–367.

Kelsey, R. M., Blascovich, J., Leitten, C. L.,

Schneider, T. R., Tomaka, J., & Wiens, S. (2000). Cardiovascular reactivity and adaptation to recurrent psychological stress: The moderating effects of evaluative observation. *Psychophysiology, 37,* 748–756.

Keltner, D. (1995). Signs of appeasement: Evidence for the distinct displays of embarrassment, amusement, and shame. *Journal of Personality and Social Psychology, 68,* 441–454.

Keltner, D., Gruenfeld, D. H., & Anderson, C. (2003). Power, approach, and inhibition. *Psychological Review, 110,* 265–284.

Keltner, D., & Shiota, M. N. (2003). New displays and new emotions: A commentary on Rozin and Cohen (2003). *Emotion, 3,* 86–91.

Klorman, R., Weissberg, R. P., & Wiesenfeld, A. R. (1977). Individual differences in fear and autonomic reactions to affective stimulation. *Psychophysiology, 14,* 45–51.

Klorman, R., Wiesenfeld, A. R., & Austin, M. L. (1975). Autonomic responses to affective visual stimuli. *Psychophysiology, 12,* 553–560.

Kootz, J. P., & Cohen, D. J. (1981). Modulation of sensory intake in autistic children. *Journal of the American Academy of Child Psychiatry, 20,* 692–701.

Kreibig, S. D. (2012). Emotion, motivation, and cardiovascular response. In R. A. Wright & G. H. E. Gendolla (Eds.), *How motivation affects cardiovascular response: Mechanisms and applications* (pp. 93–117). Washington, DC: American Psychological Association.

Kreibig, S. D., Gendolla, G. H. E., & Scherer, K. R. (2010). Psychophysiological effects of emotional responding to goal attainment. *Biological Psychology, 84,* 474–487.

Kreibig, S. D., Gendolla, G. H. E., & Scherer, K. R. (2012). Goal relevance and goal conduciveness appraisals lead to differential autonomic reactivity in emotional responding to performance feedback. *Biological Psychology, 91,* 365–375.

Kreibig, S. D., Samson, A. C., & Gross, J. J. (2013), The psychophysiology of mixed emotional states. *Psychophysiology, 50,* 799–811.

Kreibig, S. D., Schaefer, G., & Brosch, T. (2010). Psychophysiological response patterning in emotion: Implications for affective computing. In K. R. Scherer, T. Baenziger, & E. Roesch (Eds.), *Blueprint for affective computing: A sourcebook* (pp. 105–130). Oxford, UK: Oxford University Press.

Kruglanski, A. W. (2006). The nature of fit and the origins of "feeling right": A goal-systemic perspective. *Journal of Marketing Research, 43,* 11–14.

Lacey, J. I., Kagan, J., Lacey, B. C., & Moss, H. A. (1963). The visceral level: Situational determinants and behavioral correlates of autonomic response patterns. In P. Knapp (Ed.), *Expressions of the emotions in man* (pp. 161–196). New York: International University Press.

Lai, J. C. L., Chong, A. M. L., Siu, O. T., Evans, P., Chan, C. L. W., & Ho, R. T. H. (2010). Humor attenuates the cortisol awakening response in healthy older men. *Biological Psychology, 84*(2), 375–380.

Langley, J. N. (1921). *The autonomic nervous system* (Pt. 1). Cambridge, UK: Heffer.

Lazarus, R. S. (1991). Progress on a cognitive-motivational-relational theory of emotion. *American Psychologist, 46*(8), 819–834.

Lazarus, R. S. (2006). Emotions and interpersonal relationships: Toward a person-centered conceptualization of emotions and coping. *Journal of Personality, 74,* 9–46.

Lazarus, R. S., & Lazarus, B. N. (1994). *Passion and reason: Making sense of our emotions.* New York: Oxford University Press.

Lee, H. J., Macbeth, A. H., Pagani, J. H., & Young, W. S., III. (2009). Oxytocin: The great facilitator of life. *Progress in Neurobiology, 88,* 127–151.

Lewis, M. (1993). Self-conscious emotions: Embarrassment, pride, shame, and guilt. In M. Lewis & J. M. Haviland-Jones (Eds.), *Handbook of emotions* (pp. 563–573). New York: Guilford Press.

Libby, W. L., Lacey, B. C., & Lacey, J. I. (1973). Pupillary and cardiac activity during visual attention. *Psychophysiology, 10,* 270–294.

Light, K. C., Grewen, K. M., & Amico, J. A. (2005). More frequent partner hugs and higher oxytocin levels are linked to lower blood pressure and heart rate in premenopausal women. *Biological Psychology, 69,* 5–21.

Light, K. C., Smith, T. E., Johns, J. M., Brownley, K. A., Hofheimer, J. A., & Amico, J. A. (2000). Oxytocin responsivity in mothers of infants: A preliminary study of relationships with blood pressure during laboratory stress and normal ambulatory activity. *Health Psychology, 19,* 560–567.

Llera, S. J., & Newman, M. G. (2010). Effects of worry on physiological and subjective reactivity to emotional stimuli in generalized anxiety disorder and nonanxious control participants. *Emotion, 10,* 640–650.

Lorenz, K. (1971). Part and parcel in animal and

human societies. In *Studies in animal and human behavior* (Vol. 2, pp. 115–195). Cambridge, MA: Harvard University Press.

Ludden, G. D. S., Hekkert, P., & Schifferstein, H. N. (2006, September). Surprise and emotion. In P. Desmet, M. Karlsson, & J. van Erp (Eds.), *Proceedings of 5th International Conference on Design and Emotion*. Goteborg, Sweden. Available at *http://studiolab.io.tudelft.nl/manila/gems/ludden/DE2006luddensurprise.pdf*.

Matthews, S. C., Paulus, M. P., Simmons, A. N., Nelson, R. A., & Dimsdale, J. E. (2004). Functional subdivisions within anterior cingulate cortex and their relationship to autonomic nervous system function. *NeuroImage, 22*, 1151–1156.

Mauri, M., Cipresso, P., Balgera, A., Villamira, M., & Riva, G. (2011). Why is Facebook so successful?: Psychophysiological measures describe a core flow state while using Facebook. *Cyberpsychology, 14*, 723–731.

McCraty, R., Atkinson, M., Tiller, W., Rein, G., & Watkins, A. D. (1995). The effects of emotions on short-term power spectrum analysis of heart rate variability. *American Journal of Cardiology, 76*, 1089–1093.

McCullough, M. E., Kilpatrick, S. D., Emmons, R. A., & Larson, D. B. (2001). Is gratitude a moral affect? *Psychological Bulletin, 127*, 249–266.

Merriam-Webster Online. (2012a). Joy. In *Merriam-Webster's online dictionary*. Retrieved from *www.merriam-webster.com/dictionary/joy*.

Merriam-Webster Online. (2012b). Love. In *Merriam-Webster's online dictionary*. Retrieved from *www.merriam-webster.com/dictionary/love*.

Meyer, W.-U., Reisenzein, R., & Schützwohl, A. (1997). Toward a process analysis of emotions: The case of surprise. *Motivation and Emotion, 21*, 251–274.

Mikulincer, M., & Shaver, P. R. (2005). Attachment theory and emotions in close relationships: Exploring the attachment-related dynamics of emotional reactions to relational events. *Personal Relationships, 12*, 149–168.

Miller, G. A., Galanter, E., & Pribram, K. H. (1960). *Plans and the structure of behavior*. New York: Holt, Rinehart & Winston.

Muth, E. R., Koch, K. L., Stern, R. M., & Thayer, J. F. (1999). Effect of autonomic nervous system manipulations on gastric myoelectrical activity and emotional responses in healthy human subjects. *Psychosomatic Medicine, 61*(3), 297–303.

Nacke, L. E., & Lindley, C. A. (2009). Affective ludology, flow and immersion in a first-person shooter: Measurement of player experience. *Journal of the Canadian Game Studies Association, 3*, 1–21.

Niepel, M. (2001). Independent manipulation of stimulus change and unexpectedness dissociates indices of the orienting response. *Psychophysiology, 38*(1), 84–91.

Olney, N. T., Goodkind, M. S., Lomen-Hoerth, C., Whalen, P. K., Williamson, C. A., Holley, D. E., et al. (2011). Behaviour, physiology and experience of pathological laughing and crying in amyotrophic lateral sclerosis. *Brain, 12*, 3455–3466.

Ortony, A., Clore, G. L., & Collins, A. (1988). *The cognitive structure of emotions*. Cambridge, UK: Cambridge University Press.

Oveis, C., Horberg, E. J., & Keltner, D. (2010). Compassion, pride, and social intuitions of self-other similarity. *Journal of Personality and Social Psychology, 98*, 618–630.

Pecchinenda, A., & Smith, C. A. (1996). The affective significance of skin conductance activity during a difficult problem-solving task. *Cognition and Emotion, 10*, 481–503.

Petersson, M., Alster, P., Lundeberg, T., & Uvnas-Moberg, K. (1996). Oxytocin causes a long-term decrease in BP in female and male rats. *Physiology and Behavior, 60*, 1311–1315.

Porges, S. W. (1995). Orienting in a defensive world: Mammalian modifications of our evolutionary heritage: A polyvagal theory. *Psychophysiology, 32*, 301–318.

Porges, S. W. (1998). Love: An emergent property of the mammalian autonomic nervous system. *Psychoneuroendocrinology, 23*, 837–861.

Porges, S. W. (2001). The polyvagal theory: Phylogenetic substrates of a social nervous system. *International Journal of Psychophysiology, 42*, 123–146.

Porges, S. W. (2004). The vagus: A mediator of behavioral and physiological features associated with autism. In M. L. Bauman (Ed.), *Neurobiology of autism* (pp. 65–79). Baltimore: Johns Hopkins University Press.

Porges, S. W. (2007). The polyvagal perspective. *Biological Psychology, 74*, 116–143.

Price, V. A. (1982). What is Type A?: A cognitive social learning model. *Journal of Occupational Behavior, 3*, 109–129.

Rash, J. A., Matsuba, M. K., & Prkachin, K. M. (2011). Gratitude and well-being: Who benefits the most from a gratitude intervention? *Applied Psychology: Health and Well-Being, 3*, 350–369.

Ravaja, N., Saari, T., Salminen, M., Laarni, J., & Kallinen, K. (2006). Phasic emotional reactions to video game events: A psychophysiological investigation. *Media Psychology, 8*(4), 343–367.

Ravaja, N., Turpeinen, M., Saari, T., Puttonen, S., & Keltikangas-Järvinen, L. (2008). The psychophysiology of James Bond: Phasic emotional responses to violent video game events. *Emotion, 8*(1), 114–120.

Recordati, G. (2003). A thermodynamic model of the sympathetic and parasympathetic nervous systems. *Autonomic Neuroscience: Basic and Clinical, 103*, 1–12.

Reeve, J., & Nix, G. (1997). Expressing intrinsic motivation through acts of exploration and facial displays of interest. *Motivation and Emotion, 21*, 237–250.

Reisenzein, R. (1994). Pleasure-arousal theory and the intensity of emotions. *Journal of Personality and Social Psychology, 67*, 525–539.

Reisenzein, R. (2000). Exploring the strength of association between the components of emotion syndromes: The case of surprise. *Cognition and Emotion, 14*, 1–38.

Reisenzein, R., Meyer, W.-U., & Schützwohl, A. (1996). Reactions to surprising events: A paradigm for emotion research. In N. Frijda (Ed.), *Proceedings of the 9th Conference of the International Society for Research on Emotions* (pp. 292–296). Toronto: International Society for Research on Emotions.

Richter, M., Friedrich, A., & Gendolla, G. H. E. (2008). Task difficulty effects on cardiac activity. *Psychophysiology, 45*, 869–875.

Richter, M., & Gendolla, G. H. E. (2009). The heart contracts to reward: Monetary incentives and preejection period. *Psychophysiology, 46*, 451–457.

Rockliff, H., Gilbert, P., McEwen, K., Lightman, S., & Glover, D. (2008). A pilot exploration of heart rate variability and salivary cortisol responses to compassion-focused imagery. *Clinical Neuropsychiatry, 5*, 132–139.

Roseman, I. J., Antoniou, A. A., & Jose, P. E. (1996). Appraisal determinants of emotions: Constructing a more accurate and comprehensive theory. *Cognition and Emotion, 10*, 241–277.

Rottenberg, J., Kasch, K. L., Gross, J. J., & Gotlib, I. H. (2002). Sadness and amusement reactivity differentially predict concurrent and prospective functioning in major depressive disorder. *Emotion, 2*, 135–146.

Ruch, W. (1993). Exhilaration and humor. In M. Lewis & J. M. Haviland (Eds.), *Handbook of emotions* (pp. 605–616). New York: Guilford Press.

Scherer, K. R. (1984). Emotion as a multi-component process: A model and some cross-cultural data. In P. Shaver (Ed.), *Emotions, relationships, and health* (Vol. 5, p. 37–63). Beverly Hills, CA: Sage.

Scherer, K. R. (1987). Toward a dynamic theory of emotion: The component process model of affective states. *Geneva Studies in Emotion and Communication, 1*, 1–98.

Scherer, K. R. (2001). Appraisal considered as a process of multi-level sequential checking. In K. R. Scherer, A. Schorr, & T. Johnstone (Eds.), *Appraisal processes in emotion: Theory, methods, research* (pp. 92–120). New York/Oxford: Oxford University Press.

Schneiderman, I., Zilberstein-Kra, Y., Leckman, J. F., & Feldman, R. (2011). Love alters autonomic reactivity to emotions. *Emotion, 11*, 1314–1321.

Schütz, B., von Engelhardt, J., Gördes, M., Schäfer, M. K.-H., Eiden, L. E., Monyer, H., et al. (2008). Sweat gland innervation is pioneered by sympathetic neurons expressing a cholinergic/noradrenergic co-phenotype in the mouse. *Neuroscience, 156*, 310–318.

Shields, S. A., MacDowell, K. A., Fairchild, S. B., & Campbell, M. L. (1987). Is mediation of sweating cholinergic, adrenergic, or both?: A comment on the literature. *Psychophysiology, 24*, 312–319.

Shiota, M. N., Neufeld, S. L., Yeung, W. H., Moser, S. E., & Perea, E. F. (2011). Feeling good: Autonomic nervous system responding in five positive emotions. *Emotion, 11*, 1368–1378.

Siddle, D. A. T. (1991). Orienting, habituation, and resource allocation: An associative analysis. *Psychophysiology, 28*, 245–259.

Silvia, P. J. (2005). What is interesting?: Exploring the appraisal structure of interest. *Emotion, 5*, 89–102.

Silvia, P. J. (2008). Interest—the curious emotion. *Current Directions in Psychological Science, 17*, 57–60.

Skwerer, D. P., Borum, L., Verbalis, A., Schofield, C., Crawford, N., Ciciolla, L., et al. (2009). Autonomic responses to dynamic displays of facial expressions in adolescents and adults with Williams syndrome. *Social Cognitive and Affective Neuroscience, 4,* 93–100.

Sloan, D. M., Strauss, M. E., Quirk, S. Q., & Sajatovic, M. (1997). Subjective and expressive emotional responses in depression. *Journal of Affective Disorders, 46,* 135–141.

Smith, C. A., & Ellsworth, P. C. (1985). Patterns of cognitive appraisal in emotion. *Journal of Personality and Social Psychology, 48,* 813–838.

Smith, T. W., Cribbet, M. R., Nealey-Moore, J. B., Uchino, B. N., Williams, P. G., MacKenzie, J., et al. (2011). Matters of the variable heart: Respiratory sinus arrhythmia response to marital interaction and associations with marital quality. *Journal of Personality and Social Psychology, 100,* 103–119.

Sokolov, E. N. (1990). The orienting response, and future directions of its development. *Pavlovian Journal of Biological Science, 25,* 142–150.

Sokolov, E. N., & Cacioppo, J. T. (1997). Orienting and defense reflexes: Vector coding the cardiac response. In P. J. Lang, R. F. Simon, & T. Balaban (Eds.), *Attention and orienting: Sensory and motivational processes* (pp. 1–22). Mahwah, NJ: Erlbaum.

Stanley, R. (2009). Types of prayer, heart rate variability, and innate healing. *Zygon: Journal of Religion and Science, 44,* 825–846.

Stekelenburg, J. J., & van Boxtel, A. (2002). Pericranial muscular, respiratory, and heart rate components of the orienting response. *Psychophysiology, 39,* 707–722.

Suls, J. M. (1972). A two-stage model for the appreciation of jokes and cartoons: An information-processing analysis. In J. H. Goldstein & P. E. McGhee (Eds.), *The psychology of humor: Theoretical perspectives and empirical issues* (pp. 81–100). New York: Academic Press.

Taylor, S. E., Klein, L. C., Lewis, B. P., Gruenwald, T. L., Gurung, R. A., & Updegraff, J. A. (2000). Biobehavioral responses to stress in females: Tend-and-befriend, not fight-or-flight. *Psychological Review, 107*(3), 411–429.

Tesser, A., Gatewood, R., & Driver, M. (1968). Some determinants of gratitude. *Journal of Personality and Social Psychology, 9,* 233–236.

Tomaka, J., & Palacios-Esquivel, R. L. (1997). Motivational systems and stress-related cardiovascular reactivity. *Motivation and Emotion, 21*(4), 275–296.

Tracy, J. L., & Robins, R. W. (2004). Putting the self into self-conscious emotions: A theoretical model. *Psychological Inquiry, 15*(2), 103–125.

Turpin, G., Schaefer, F., & Boucsein, W. (1999). Effects of stimulus intensity, risetime, and duration on autonomic and behavioral responding: Implications for the differentiation of orienting, startle, and defense responses. *Psychophysiology, 36,* 453–463.

vanOyen Witvliet, C., Knoll, R. W., Hinman, N. G., & DeYoung, P. A. (2010). Compassion-focused reappraisal, benefit-focused reappraisal, and rumination after an interpersonal offense: Emotion-regulation implications for subjective emotion, linguistic responses, and physiology. *Journal of Positive Psychology, 5,* 226–242.

van Reekum, C. M., Johnstone, T., Banse, R., Etter, A., Wehrle, T., & Scherer, K. R. (2004). Psychophysiological responses to appraisal dimensions in a computer game. *Cognition and Emotion, 18,* 663–688.

Vico, C., Guerra, P., Robles, H., Vila, J., & Anllo-Vento, L. (2010). Affective processing of loved faces: Contributions from peripheral and central electrophysiology. *Neuropsychologia, 48,* 2894–2902.

Waldstein, S. R., Bachen, E. A., & Manuck, S. B. (1997). Active coping and cardiovascular reactivity: A multiplicity of influences. *Psychosomatic Medicine, 59*(6), 620–625.

Weiner, B. (1985). An attributional theory of achievement motivation and emotion. *Psychological Review, 92,* 548–573.

Weiner, B. (2000). Intrapersonal and interpersonal theories of motivation from an attributional perspective. *Educational Psychological Review, 12,* 1–14.

Wiesenfeld, A. R., & Klorman, R. (1978). The mother's psychophysiological reactions to contrasting affective expressions by her own and an unfamiliar infant. *Developmental Psychology, 14,* 294–304.

Wiesenfeld, A. R., Malatesta, C. Z., & DeLoach, L. L. (1981). Differential parental response to familiar and unfamiliar infant distress signals. *Infant Behavior and Development, 4,* 281–295.

Wiesenfeld, A. R., Malatesta, C. Z., Whitman, P. B., Granrose, C., & Uili, R. (1985). Psychophysiological response of breast- and bottle-feeding mothers to their infants' signals. *Psychophysiology, 22,* 79–86.

Williams, L. A., & DeSteno, D. (2008). Pride and

perseverance: The motivational role of pride. *Journal of Personality and Social Psychology, 94*(6), 1007–1017.

Williams, L. A., & DeSteno, D. (2009). Pride: Adaptive social emotion or seventh sin? *Psychological Science, 20,* 284–288.

Wood, K. C. (2008). *On ambivalence: A facial electromyographic investigation of mixed emotions.* Unpublished master's thesis, Texas Tech University.

Wright, R. A. (1996). Brehm's theory of motivation as a model of effort and cardiovascular response. In P. M. Gollwitzer & J. A. Bargh (Eds.), *The psychology of action: Linking cognition and motivation to behavior* (pp. 424–453). New York: Guilford Press.

Wu, G.-Q., Arzeno, N. M., Shen, L.-L., Tang, D.-K., Zheng, D.-A., Zhao, N.-Q., et al. (2009). Chaotic signatures of heart rate variability and its power spectrum in health, aging and heart failure. *PLoS ONE, 4,* e4323.

Wyer, R. S., Jr., & Collins, J. E., II. (1992). A theory of humor elicitation. *Psychological Review, 99,* 663–688.

CHAPTER 9

Spontaneous Human Laughter

Michael J. Owren
R. Toby Amoss

Laughter is ubiquitous in human social behavior, best known for its association with humor and mirth (O'Connell & Kowal, 2008). But this vocalization is much more than just an adjunct to merriment. In fact, it arguably has no inherent connection to humor at all (e.g., Attardo, 2011; Chafe, 2007; Poyatos, 1993; Provine, 1993; Vettin & Todt, 2004). Instead, laughter occurs across a variety of circumstances and resists easy characterization—even as a necessarily positive event. To better understand laughter as a basic human behavior, in this chapter we examine a range of acoustical, biological, and functional aspects of this vocalization. This review reveals laughter to be a complex phenomenon that is difficult to explain within a single, unified framework. The final section of the chapter, therefore, attempts to do just that, with emotion induction and social bonding given key roles. The focus throughout is on *spontaneous* laughter, referring to unbidden, emotion-triggered sound production that happens as much to the vocalizer as being originated by the vocalizer. These sounds can be contrasted with deliberate, *volitional* versions, which are learned simulations of spontaneous forms. Although distinguishing the two

can be difficult in practice, it is important at least to separate them conceptually. While the ultimate goal is to understand both phenomena, we suggest that the most fruitful approach is to tackle spontaneous laughter first.

Laughter Acoustics

While almost instantly familiar to any human listener (e.g., Bachorowski, Smoski, & Owren, 2001), laughter is difficult to define objectively. One challenge is the surprising diversity of sounds that occur. All are readily recognizable, yet the variety involved is routinely ignored in the prevalent conception of laughter as a simple "ha-ha-ha." For instance, while the perfectly ordinary-sounding laugh shown in Figure 9.1a begins with vowel-like sounds, it then turns into a series of vocal clicks and noise bursts. Thus, understanding spontaneous laughter as a general phenomenon requires starting from an accurate and thorough acoustical description of the sounds involved.

Two rather different approaches have been taken in this regard, creating divergence in associated terminology. On the one

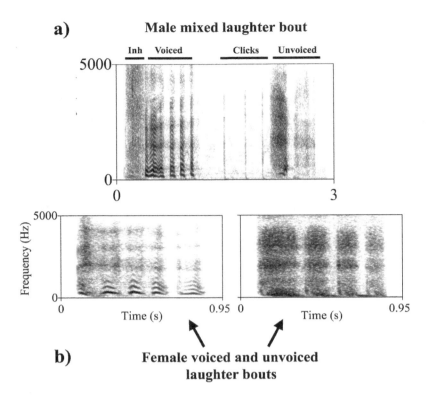

FIGURE 9.1. Spectrograms of adult male (a) and adult female (b) laughter (22,050-Hz sampling rate and 0.03-second Gaussian analysis window). The male laughter bout begins with a sharp inhalation, and is followed by four voiced bursts, three glottal clicks, and four unvoiced bursts. The female laughter bouts illustrate that more uniform structure is also common, and can differ within and across individual vocalizers. This laughter consists of five voiced and four unvoiced bursts, respectively.

hand, scholars perceiving parallels to speech often apply phonetic constructs, labeling laughter sounds as consonant–vowel *syllables* organized in language-like *phrases* (e.g., Edmonson, 1987; Trouvain, 2003). On the other hand, researchers with a more comparative orientation see close ties between laughter and nonhuman vocalizations, with some referring to its individual sounds as *calls* (Bachorowski et al., 2001; Bryant & Aktipis, 2013). Our discussion here draws from both approaches, while aiming to use more generic terminology (e.g., Chafe, 2007). Individual laughter components are therefore labeled as *bursts* of vocal energy (Luschei, Ramig, Finnegan, Baker, & Smith, 2006; Mowrer, LaPointe, & Case, 1987; Titze, Finnegan, Laukkanen, Fuja, & Hoffman, 2008), which in turn are grouped in *bouts*.

Characterizing Laughter Sounds

Edmonson (1987) provided the first systematic, phonetically based analysis of laughter, transcribing recordings from a variety of vocalizers by ear (also see Chafe, 2007; Poyatos, 1993; Trouvain, 2003; Urbain & Dutoit, 2011). One important distinction he pointed out was between vowel-like, *voiced* (*phonated*) bursts produced by vibrating the *vocal folds* (*vocal cords*), and *unvoiced* (*aspirated*) versions consisting of turbulent, noisy airflow occurring without vocal fold involvement (see Figure 9.1). The former involves two basic maneuvers, namely, producing a stream of pressurized air from the lungs while repeatedly bringing the vocal folds together (*adduction*) to produce short bursts of vibration (Bryant & Aktipis, 2013; Luschei et al., 2006). The latter requires only airflow, with the folds held apart (*abducted*) without vibrating. However, vocal fold involvement can also take the form of individual, metallic-sounding pulses (*glottal clicks*; see Figure 9.1) and bursts of rough, irregular voicing.

Edmonson (1987) detected a number of different vowel sounds in his laughter sample, discussed further below. Fewer consonant sounds were discernible, mainly reflecting the degree of adduction at sound onset, whether the mouth was open, closed, or in between, and whether airflow was oral, nasal, or both. The most important distinction was that voiced bursts either began abruptly or were preceded by unvoiced, *h*-like aspiration. Edmonson also found that laughter mainly occurred with outward (*egressive*) airflow, but was sometimes

inward (*ingressive*) as well (also see Chafe, 2007; Urbain & Dutoit, 2011).

Bachorowski and colleagues (2001) conducted the first, large-scale acoustic study of laughter, adopting a *source-filter* analysis strategy. As illustrated in Figure 9.2, this approach views vocalization as a linear combination of an energy source and filtering effects created by the pharyngeal, oral, and nasal cavities that this energy then passes through (reviewed by Stevens, 2000). In most voiced laughter, for example, the energy source is regular vocal fold vibration. The vocal pitch perceived in this kind of sound is largely determined by the phonation rate involved, known as the "fundamental frequency" (F_0; see Figure 9.2). Bachorowski and colleagues found F_0 in voiced laughter to be roughly twice that of conversational

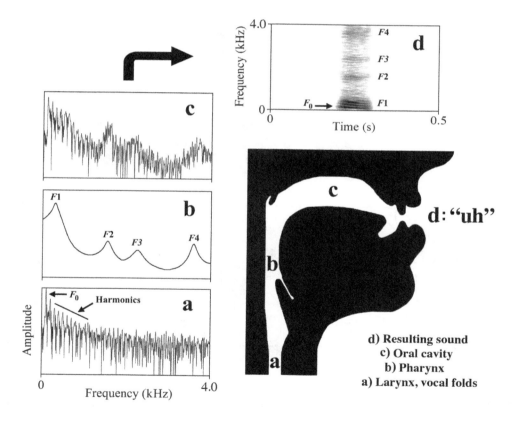

FIGURE 9.2. Schematic view of a human male vocal tract, illustrating source-filter vocal production. (a) and (b) show the frequency spectrum of the laryngeal source energy and the supralaryngeal filter, respectively. (c) presents the frequency characteristics that result when source and filter combine, and (d) shows a spectrogram of the original "uh" sound (also known as "schwa," or /ə/). F_0 refers to the fundamental frequency of vocal-fold vibration, and $F1$–$F4$ designate the first through fourth formants.

speech for both males and females, while often going much higher.

Filtering effects are created by resonances of the cavities above the larynx ("formants"), which strengthen energy in some frequency regions while weakening it in others. As illustrated in Figure 9.2, energy in a voiced source is greatest for F_0, dropping monotonically across higher harmonic components. In contrast, the sound emerging from a vocalizer's mouth exhibits a distinct pattern of frequency peaks and troughs. This patterning is due to the formants, whose detailed effects mirror the sizes and shapes of a given vocalizer's *supralaryngeal* cavities. Formant patterning simultaneously contributes both to the quality of an individual's voice and to creating different vowel sounds.

Spontaneous Laughter Lacks Differentiated Vowel Quality

Like speech, voiced laughter has traditionally been considered to exhibit distinct vowel qualities, including "hah-hah," "he-he," "hoo-hoo," and even "hoe-hoe-hoe"

(e.g., Provine & Yong, 1991). Edmonson's (1987) transcriptions included not only these sounds but also a variety of other vowels. However, as illustrated in Figure 9.3a, differentiated vowels require "articulation"—repositioning of tongue, lips, and jaw so as to change the relationship between the two lowest formants ($F1$ and $F2$). In speech, the overall *vowel space* of a given talker or a particular language can be mapped based on $F1$–$F2$ values, illustrated in Figure 9.3b.

But laughter looks quite different from speech when mapped in this space (Bachorowski et al., 2001; Makagon, Funayama, & Owren, 2008). Rather than falling into the "ee" (/i/), "ah"(/a/), and "oo" (/u/) regions, spontaneous laughter clusters around a central, grunt-like, "uh" known phonetically as *schwa* (/ə/). This sound, produced with the tongue in a relaxed, "neutral" position, is not considered a true vowel.

Some formant variation does occur in laughter, but largely due to the degree of jaw lowering and concomitant mouth opening involved (Makagon et al., 2008). Physically,

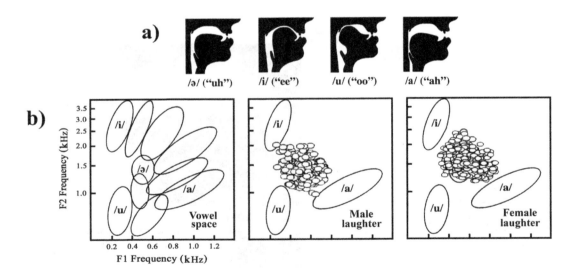

FIGURE 9.3. (a) Tongue positions associated with vowel production, shown in schematic side views of a male vocal tract. (b) The left panel shows American English vowels mapped in $F1$–$F2$ space, with each ellipse illustrating the range of variation occurring when men, women, and children produce a given vowel (redrawn from Peterson & Barney, 1952). The two right panels show $F1$ and $F2$ values from individual male and female voiced laughter bursts, illustrating that these sounds are not articulated vowels, instead clustering around the center of vowel space (redrawn from Bachorowski et al., 2001).

at least, laughter sounds show few clear instances of the /i/, /a/, and /u/ qualities so often attributed to them perceptually (also see Tanaka & Campbell, 2011).

Variability and Individual Distinctiveness

Although laughter has often been described as "stereotyped" or "ritualized" (e.g., Gervais & Wilson, 2005; Grammer & Eibl-Eibesfeldt, 1990; Provine, 2000; Provine & Yong, 1991), acoustically oriented researchers consistently report just the opposite (e.g., Chafe, 2007; Rothgänger, Hauser, Cappellini, & Guidotti, 1998; Vettin & Todt, 2004). In fact, Bachorowski and colleagues (2001) found that variability is virtually a hallmark of spontaneous laughter. In a sample of 97 different laughers, for example, these researchers found that laughter bouts included from as few as one to as many as 30 individual bursts. Furthermore, while voicing is often considered the norm in spontaneous laughter, only about one-third of the 1,024 bouts examined were consistently voiced—the remainder were either unvoiced or mixed. Similarly, while some laughter was produced with an open mouth, at other times, the mouth was closed or changed through the course of the bout. Burst spacing within bouts was also variable, as were F_0 and amplitude patterns. Features of individual bursts varied as well, including duration, source-energy type, F_0, and amplitude.

The argument for stereotyped acoustics might still be salvageable given that overall outcomes could vary as a result of individual laughers each producing somewhat different sounds. That possibility has not been entirely ruled out, although all vocalizers do appear to produce multiple laugh variants (e.g., Bachorowski et al., 2001; Edmonson, 1987). Strong identity indicators are probably present, however, as the regular phonation found in most voiced bursts is a rich source of cues to vocalizer characteristics (known as "indexical cues"; Bachorowski & Owren, 1999). In addition, bout-level temporal, pitch, and amplitude patterning may also be different across individuals (Fry & Rader, 1977). Burst- and bout-level characteristics could thus conceivably combine to create one or more unique, "favored" laughs in every vocalizer's repertoire (Askenasy, 1987; Chafe, 2007; Edmonson, 1987).

Summary: Laughter Acoustics Are Simple but Variable

Examined individually, laughter sounds are relatively straightforward. In basic terms, laughter is made up of separable bursts of air passing through vocal folds that may be adducted or abducted at onset, with the airflow creating vibration or only turbulence, respectively. The resulting acoustic energy then passes through the supralaryngeal vocal tract either orally, nasally, or both. While it is tempting to describe laughter bursts phonetically, taking that approach may encourage important misconceptions—for instance, that laughter sounds are more stereotyped and distinctly articulated than is actually the case. Variability is a prominent feature of laughter at both burst and bout levels, within and across vocalizers. Still, indexical cuing created through phonation and potentially idiosyncratic bout-level patterning makes it probable that spontaneous laughter presents important vocalizer-identity cues.

The Biology of Laughter

This section reviews several kinds of evidence that spontaneous laughter is deeply rooted in primate biology, including data from great apes, laughter ontogeny, and neural circuitry. One emerging theme is that laughter is a relatively primitive and imprecise vocalization—consistent with finding that the individual sounds involved are acoustically simple, yet variable. A second, important point is that spontaneous human laughter is nonetheless critically different from that of its nonhuman counterparts. In the final section of the chapter, those differences are mined for clues to the evolution of laughter.

Laughter in Nonhuman Primates

Primatologists have long argued that human emotional expressions are traceable to our species' primate past, including expressions in both the facial and vocal domains (e.g., Andrew, 1963; van Hooff, 1972). It has been suggested that human laughter derives from calls originally present in a shared, nonhuman ancestor. The best evidence comes from extant great apes—chimpanzees, bonobos, gorillas, and orangutans—all of which have been reported to laugh under certain conditions. Davila-Ross, Owren, and Zimmermann (2009) tested this claim by comparing tickle-induced vocalizations from ape and human youngsters. In great apes, the sounds consistently showed irregular, noisy phonation, and could be either egressive or ingressive. There was notable variation among the various apes as well, however, allowing the investigators to trace possible patterns of "descent" based on the vocalizations of all five species. Results were consistent with the same derivation pattern already known from genetic analyses: Human laughter was most similar to chimpanzee and bonobo vocalizations, more distant from gorilla sounds, and most distant from orangutan versions.

Davila-Ross and colleagues (2009) concluded that tickle-induced vocalizations in great apes and humans probably all have a common evolutionary origin—sounds found in a last common ancestor that lived 10 to 16 million years ago. However, differences between ape and human versions were telling as well. Most importantly, human laughter showed a much higher proportion of egressive airflow and regular voicing than any of the ape vocalizations. The latter occur only in circumstances of play and being tickled (see Davila-Ross, Allcock, Thomas, & Bard, 2011). Taken together, the evidence indicates that while the sounds can legitimately be considered laughter in each case, evolution produced significant changes in both the form and usage of human versions compared to those of the other species.

Ontogeny

The biological basis of spontaneous laughter is even more strongly evident from studies of vocal ontogeny. For example, these sounds emerge early in human development, typically by about 4 months of age (reviewed by Rothbart, 1973; see also Sauter, McDonald, Gangi, & Messinger, Chapter 10, this volume). Such early emergence suggests that direct experience with laughter is not necessary for production, confirmed in the finding that deaf and deaf–blind infants also laugh (e.g., Eibl-Eibesfeldt, 1989). In one study, Scheiner, Hammerschmidt, Jürgens, and Zwirner (2004) examined vocal production in seven hearing-impaired children over the first year of life. They reported that laughter, as well as a variety of other emotion-triggered sounds, appeared on the same timeline shown by typically developing, age-matched comparison infants. Moreover, spontaneous laughter persists into adulthood in deaf individuals; Makagon and colleagues (2008) found that laugh sounds produced by congenitally, bilaterally, and profoundly deaf university students were acoustically comparable to those of their hearing peers.

However, human infants also quickly begin to gain volitional control over vocal production. That control is demonstrated not only by the gradual emergence of deliberate speech, but also by infants learning to simulate emotion-triggered vocalizations. By toddler age, for example, many are using such sounds instrumentally as attention-getting devices, and are coordinating vocalization with gestures and other skeletal motor actions (Bell & Ainsworth, 1982; Gustafson & Green, 1991; Lester & Boukydis, 1992). The upshot is that these vocalizations begin as spontaneous, emotion-triggered events, but human infants are soon able to use them with a level of deliberateness and flexibility that far outstrips what any nonhuman primate can do.

Neural Underpinnings

Studies of the neural pathways underlying vocal production provide further compelling evidence about laughter biology. A comparative perspective is important here as well, with vocalization in nonhuman mammals critically mediated by ancient, emotion-related brainstem circuits (reviewed by Jürgens, 2009). Over the years, many researchers have argued that this same system also controls emotion-triggered vocalizations such as spontaneous laughter and crying in humans. Reviewing the available evidence, for example, Wild, Rodden, Grodd, and Ruch (2003) concluded that activity in a variety of subcortical structures can be important, including amygdala, thalamus, hypo- and subthalamic areas, and dorsal/tegmental brainstem. Vocal output is then ultimately coordinated in the midbrain and hindbrain pons region. While the cerebral cortex can also directly affect spontaneous laughter, its role is mainly inhibitory. In contrast, volitional vocal production in humans has been traced to a newer, specifically cortically based pathway—one not found in nonhuman primates (see Owren, Amoss, & Rendall, 2011). This system bypasses the older structures via direct connections between cortical motor areas and brainstem vocal centers. Volitional laughter is thus believed to originate in frontal cortical areas, with associated neural signals reaching the brainstem via motor cortex.

Critical evidence about both pathways derives from the phenomenon of *pathological laughter*, in which brain damage can result in normal-sounding but socially inappropriate vocal production occurring in a virtual emotional vacuum (Parvizi, Coburn, Shillcutt, Coffey, Lauterbach, & Mendez, 2009). This insidious syndrome has been recognized since the 19th century and can occur secondarily to damage in diverse brain areas when injury gives rise to "autonomous" signaling that ultimately reaches brainstem vocal mechanisms via the emotion-related laughter pathway. When those activations occur close to the brainstem, resulting neural activity can be inaccessible to higher-level control centers. Afflicted individuals thus find themselves producing repeated bouts of empty laughter that they are helpless to inhibit, no matter how hard they try.

Summary: Human Laughter Is Ancient, Yet Unique

Taken together, results from nonhuman primates, vocal ontogeny, and neuroanatomy all point to spontaneous laughter having ancient evolutionary origins. However, evidence from great apes also indicates that laughter underwent important modification, specifically among human ancestors. Changes included the sounds becoming consistently egressive, showing more regular voicing, and being triggered by a wider range of emotions and circumstances. A variety of findings also underscore that spontaneous and volitional laughter are ultimately separable, even if frequently intertwined in everyday life. Spontaneous laughter is organized at the brainstem level and is triggered through the same, emotion-related pathway that controls nonhuman primate

vocalization. At some point, however, direct neural connections evolved between cortex and brainstem vocal circuitry, creating the pathway that mediates volitional sound production in modern humans. Its emergence must have not only allowed human ancestors to begin to simulate laughter and other emotion-related vocalizations but also laid the foundation for eventual speech production.

The Function of Laughter

Historically, more has probably been written about laughter's function than about any other aspect of this behavior. Little has been done to integrate the many ideas described, however, with some suggestions being well reasoned and plausible, and others less so. The review presented here is selective both by necessity and by choice, focusing on ideas that help move the discussion forward. Hypotheses are grouped into four overlapping categories: benefits to vocalizer health, social-status signaling, communicating vocalizer state, and facilitating social bonding. Discussion in each case is brief but designed to create a conceptual foundation for further consideration of the ideas in later sections.

Health

A connection between laughter and health has been suggested since biblical times, with many scholars citing energy release and stress reduction as primary effects (e.g., Askenasy, 1987). The idea of laughter as a curative agent gained its greatest momentum with Cousins's (1979) description of overcoming a debilitating rheumatoid disease through self-prescribed immersion in humor and laughter. Unfortunately, the wave of studies he triggered has not proved conclusive. Reviewing this work, Mora-Ripoll (2010) argued that many studies testing the therapeutic value of laughter have been scientifically unsound, for example, by not using randomized treatment assignment, or by omitting necessary control conditions. Even the stronger work has typically failed to distinguish the impact of laughing per se from other effects, such as mood improvement, positive emotion, and affirmative social interactions resulting from the experimental manipulations (also see R. A. Martin, 2004).

Setting these difficulties aside, the evidence for health benefits of laughter is still equivocal at best (reviewed by R. A. Martin, 2001, 2004; Mora-Ripoll, 2010). Studies measuring key endocrine and cellular markers have provided little support for claims that laughing has positive effects on stress responding or immune system function (Mora-Ripoll, 2010). It is true that laughter requires coordinated and forceful muscular contractions in the diaphragm, abdomen, and rib cage (e.g., Luschei et al., 2006), and that humor-induced sounds are associated with increases in heart rate, respiration, and oxygen consumption. But while the resulting energy expenditure can be as much as 20% higher than that at rest (Buchowski et al., 2007), the effort involved still falls well below that of vigorous exercise.

The most telling effects found so far have been that mirthful laughing can elevate an individual's pain threshold and increase long-term pain tolerance (Mora-Ripoll, 2010). As pain can be induced experimentally under well-controlled conditions, studies in this area tend to be the strongest methodologically. While it is not necessarily clear that pain threshold is important to health outcomes, this finding has at least inspired continued optimism that evidence of more direct benefits will eventually be found.

Social Status Signaling

Researchers have suggested that laughter functions to signal relative social status, especially that lower-status individuals use these sounds to "acknowledge" inferior standing vis-à-vis higher-status companions. While difficult to specify precisely, the message involved in such vocalizations has been variously described as appeasing, compliant, submissive, or subservient (e.g., Adams & Kirkevold, 1978; Mehu & Dunbar, 2008; Provine, 2000). For example, among 1,200 instances of laughter occurring in small, mixed-sex groups, Provine (1993) found that females laughed significantly more than males, an outcome interpreted as reflecting frequent male dominance. He also reported that both females and males laughed less in response to female than to male speakers.

Grammer and Eibl-Eibesfeldt (1990) emphasized the role of gender as well, interpreting female laughter as a submission signal (also see Mehu & Dunbar, 2008).

Fry and Rader (1977) linked laughter to social status in a notably different way. They argued that laughter can provide a means of "currying favor" with others, for instance with lower-status persons laughing more effusively at jokes told by higher-status individuals than the converse. To test this idea, Stillman, Baumeister, and DeWall (2007) gave a confederate experimenter control over the distribution of cash rewards and found that even this temporary power asymmetry affected laughter rates. The confederate told both funny and unfunny jokes during individual interviews with participants, eliciting significantly more laughter from those who believed there was cash on the line than from control individuals who had not been offered money. Rather than signaling subservience, Stillman and colleagues argued that laughter was being used to elicit liking—hence, better treatment.

Communicating Vocalizer State

While social status factors are correlated with rates of laughing, a broader—and more common—proposal is that the primary function of laughter is to communicate the vocalizer's emotional state to others. One interpretation is that laughter is a relatively diffuse signal, reflecting feelings of "tension release," "satisfaction," or "safety" (Rothbart, 1973). Two other suggestions along these lines are Ramachandran's (1998) "safety-signal" and Chafe's (2007) "nonseriousness" hypotheses. The former proposes that human laughter evolved to convey a message of "false alarm" after disturbing events prove harmless (also see Hayworth, 1928), with the emotional trigger being tension release or relief. The latter proposes that the critical element is a state of nonseriousness, a feeling that can also accompany positive and nonpositive emotions alike.

Other researchers have argued that spontaneous laughter communicates more specific states, including positive emotions such as friendliness, happiness, joy, mirth, playfulness, and sexual interest (e.g., Gervais & Wilson, 2005; Grammer & Eibl-Eibesfeldt, 1990; Ruch, 1993). Laughter has also been connected to negative emotions, such as contempt, embarrassment, guilt, nervousness, sadness, and self-consciousness, as well as to feelings that clearly are neither positive nor negative, such as attentiveness, self-deprecation, and surprise (Coates, 2007; Glenn 1991/1992; Keltner & Bonanno, 1997; G. N. Martin & Gray, 1996). Finally, laughter has been linked to situations that can be positive for vocalizers but negative for listeners, including derision, taunting, and *schadenfreude* (e.g., Eibl-Eibesfeldt, 1989). The common thread in each case is that laughter is a kind of "language without words" (DePaulo, 1992, p. 203), implying that its sounds "stand for" or "code for" particular emotions. In this view, laughter functions to transmit information from vocalizer to listener, thereby benefiting both parties. If so, the challenge becomes to "decode" that system, specifying how particular states map onto corresponding laughter acoustics.

Social Bonding Effects

Perhaps the most global proposal is that laughter exists to create social bonds (e.g., Glenn, 2010; Grammer & Eibl-Eibesfeldt, 1990; Mehu & Dunbar, 2008; Provine, 2000). The basic idea is that individuals who laugh together form stronger personal bonds than those who do not, although little is usually said to explain either why such bonding was needed in human evolution or what particular mechanisms are involved. Dunbar (1996, 2004) has proposed a "group-size" interpretation that is an exception to this rule, and discusses both issues. On the evolutionary side, his argument is that as group sizes and concomitant social networks grew larger in human ancestors, the primate-like grooming behavior used to maintain friendly interindividual relationships became too inefficient. In his view, spontaneous laughter arose as a more efficient means of promoting positive relationships, one that eliminated the need for direct physical contact and could occur in parallel with other activities.

On the mechanistic side, Dunbar (1996, 2004) proposed that laughter is linked to social bonding via physical exertion and brain opiates. Specifically, he suggested that the effort involved in laughing triggers endorphin release, much as occurs during strenuous exercise. During intense laughter sessions, these opiates are proposed to produce pleasurable feelings that laughers then associate with the other individuals present—thereby strengthening mutually positive feelings among these parties. This argument is consistent with the evidence of a link between laughter and pain tolerance, allowing Dunbar and colleagues (2012) to use pain reactivity as a proxy measure in testing for laughter-related endorphin release. In this study, pain tolerance was measured after participants watched videos in the laboratory, or attended or performed in a theatrical production. In both cases, the researchers found greater tolerance in participants exposed to comedy than in comparison subjects exposed to more serious material.

Owren and Bachorowski (2001) suggested a different scenario, arguing that human ancestors faced circumstances that put a premium on long-term cooperation between genetically unrelated individuals, and that laughter played an important role in making such relationships possible. A key observation was that while biological kin in many species routinely act favorably toward one another, lasting cooperation among nonkin is much less common. For the latter, immediate, short-term benefits of selfish behavior routinely derail the opportunity to obtain greater, long-term rewards through ongoing cooperation with others. A key issue is that such cooperation often entails one individual behaving favorably toward another, thereby incurring a "cost" that may or may not later be "repaid" by the other party. To become feasible for unrelated individuals, cooperative relationships require that each be able to predict how the other will behave in the future. Owren and Bachorowski proposed that because emotion is important in guiding behavior, reliable external manifestations of emotional state can help provide the predictive power needed.

Two elements were involved, namely, that the cooperating parties be positively disposed toward one another, and that each individual show reliable evidence of that favorable disposition. In essence, each party must know that the other individual is consistently in a positive state when the two are together, reflecting an inherently positive regard that is predictive of favorable future treatment. The predictive value involved increases the more frequently and consistently such interactions occur, thereby making it safer for each individual to behave cooperatively with the other. A strong argument can be made that individual great apes do inherently like (and dislike) others, and in fact have the long-term emotional disposition needed for cooperative relationships (Seyfarth & Cheney, 2012). Remarkably, however, extant apes do little to manifest any associated positive states via emotion-triggered facial and vocal expressions. They have no smile or equivalent expression, for example, and their laughter is very limited in scope.

Owren and Bachorowski (2001) therefore argued that spontaneous laughter in human ancestors evolved to become a broadly used manifestation of positive vocalizer state. As in extant apes, laughter was exclusively positive at first, but expanded usage allowed others to rely on the relative prevalence of these sounds as a predictor of another individual's future behavior. As described, the likelihood of mutual, cooperative behavior increased for any two parties if both consistently manifested this reliable cue to positive state when together. If only one, or if neither individual reliably laughed during such interactions, cooperative behavior was significantly less probable. Owren and Bachorowski's proposal actually went a step further, arguing that laughter also acted mechanistically as a vehicle for learned, emotional responses that could amplify the positive feelings on each side. This point is discussed in more detail below, but the essence is that in cases of mutual liking, each individual would routinely be in a positive state when hearing a companion's laughter. Over repeated interactions, each vocalizer's laughter would itself come to evoke and reinforce positive feelings in the other.

Summary: Many Ideas, Little Integration

Spontaneous laughter and health have been perennially linked in popular imagination, but available data show only that laughter increases aerobic metabolism and pain tolerance to some degree. In contrast, evidence that relative social status plays a role in laughter production suggests a communicative function. Because spontaneous laughter occurs across a wide range of social circumstances, there may be many different signals involved, with particular sounds providing cues to a variety of possible vocalizer emotions. The exact messages involved are hard to specify, however, and no one has provided a principled account of how these states map onto laughter acoustics. An overarching theme is that laughter serves a global function of strengthening social bonds, possibly involving mechanisms of differentiated signaling, bonding through opiate release, or association of the vocalizer's laughter with positive emotions in listeners.

"Contagion," More on Social Mediation, and the Mapping Question

It proves easy to enumerate possible functions for spontaneous laughter, especially if one considers each social context in which the sounds occur to represent functionally distinct usage. The greater challenge is to provide a single, functional account of laughter that can also explain associated acoustic and behavioral phenomena. One such framework is presented at the end of the chapter; in this section we first discuss further evidence and theory of interest in understanding laughter.

Laughter Contagion

A much-remarked upon, yet little understood, aspect of spontaneous laughter is its famously "contagious" quality—which means that just hearing these sounds can trigger smiles, laughter, and positive emotion in others. This effect has long been exploited commercially, including through novelty "laugh records" and use of canned laughter to increase enjoyment of comedy shows (see G. N. Martin & Gray, 1996; Provine, 2000). In a related test, Provine (1992) presented a brief segment of canned laughter to a large student audience, then reported that the sounds elicited visible smiling and audible laughter in many of those present. Given its methodology, the experiment could not rule out that the undergraduates were simply amused by the professor's unusual behavior, or that they found the sounds themselves to be odd and funny. However, subsequent laboratory experiments that presented a variety of laughter recordings have confirmed that these sounds can elicit positive responses even when heard in isolation (Bachorowski & Owren, 2001). Follow-up work also showed these positive reactions to be both automatic and reflective of a true emotional response (Owren et al., 2012).

Of course, the concept of laughter "infecting" others cannot be taken literally, as it is metaphorical rather than explanatory (Hempelmann, 2007). To better explain the effect, Provine (1996) argued that laughter is an evolved, "stereotyped action pattern" that activates a similarly specialized "laugh detector" in listeners—which then automatically triggers laughing. Yet, as discussed in the first section, spontaneous laughter is not acoustically stereotyped. In addition, while developmental data indicate that neural circuitry for laughter production is present from a young age, there is no corresponding evidence of a neural laugh detector. Comparative data instead suggest that experience and learning are probably essential in shaping responses to spontaneous laughter sounds (Owren et al., 2011).

Other evidence demonstrates that the presence or absence of voicing in laughter plays a key role in contagion. Specifically, experiments presenting laughter in isolation found that voiced laughter reliably elicited positive emotion, whereas unvoiced versions did not (Bachorowski & Owren, 2001; Owren et al., 2012; also see Grammer & Eibl-Eibesfeldt, 1990). This is a striking outcome, in that listeners readily recognized both forms as normative laughter and that all the sounds had been drawn from the same, mirthful circumstances. Smoski and Bachorowski (2003a, 2003b) confirmed the importance of voicing in naturalistic situations as well by testing dyads engaged in a series of interactive, game-like tasks. The study focused on "antiphonal" laughter, defined as instances in which laugh sounds from one individual were followed by laughter from the other within 1 second. As might be expected, significantly more antiphonal laughter occurred if dyad members were friends rather than strangers—but only if the initial vocalizer's sounds were voiced. Unvoiced versions did not routinely evoke antiphonal laughter, regardless of the social relationship involved.

Social Mediation

Another basic property of laughter is that it occurs at much higher rates in social, as opposed to solitary, circumstances (Bainum, Lounsbury, & Pollio, 1984; Provine & Fischer, 1989). In an early study of the importance of social factors in laughter, Provine (1993) tallied the number of sounds occurring in groups observed in public places. Most observations were of student dyads, and Provine reported that speakers tended to laugh more than their audience, that individuals in subordinate social positions laughed more than those in dominant roles, and that females laughed more than males. However, the sample did not take group composition into account, nor was any distinction made between spontaneous and volitional laughter.

Mehu and Dunbar (2008) tried to account for both elements when later conducting similar observations in bars and food courts. These researchers catalogued both smiling and laughter in relation to group size and estimated participant age, including only laugh sounds accompanied by a spontaneous-seeming smile. Contrary to Provine's finding, males and females were found to laugh at equivalent overall rates, although younger females in particular were found to laugh more when in different-gender social groups. Older females laughed significantly less, but no age effect was found for males. In other words, while female laughter was strongly affected by the presence of males, males were not much influenced by female presence. Similar outcomes occurred in unpublished data from Bachorowski and colleagues' (2001) study of dyads watching humorous video clips (Owren & Bachorowski, 2003)—a situation in which all the laughter produced was assumed to be spontaneous and positive. Those pairs were either same- or different-gender, and either friends or strangers. Males and females were found to produce comparable amounts of laughter here as well, although females laughed most when paired with males. Females also generally laughed more when teamed with friends—but especially with male friends (also see Smoski & Bachorowski, 2003a). Taken together, the evidence indicates that while males and females produce spontaneous laughter at similar overall rates, they "use" these sounds differently. Social status appears to play an important role, with females—especially young females—commonly assumed to have lower social standing than males.

The finding that laughter rates are importantly affected by who else is present has led to a number of proposals concerning vocal function, including status signaling (Adams & Kirkevold, 1978; Grammer & Eibl-Eibesfeldt, 1990), sexual advertisement (Grammer & Eibl-Eibesfeldt, 1990; Mehu & Dunbar, 2008), and elicitation of liking (Stillman et al., 2007). However, drawing firm conclusions will require more detail about the specific relationships represented in these kinds of studies. In laboratory work, participants have typically been classified only as friends or strangers (but see Smoski & Bachorowski, 2003b). Researchers conducting studies in public have been able to report even less about their participants, with any pair of individuals potentially being family, friends, romantic partners, colleagues, or even enemies or virtual strangers.

Mapping from Vocalizer State to Laughter Acoustics

The question of how internal states map onto the acoustic features of spontaneous laughter is arguably the thorniest issue of all in this area of research. As discussed earlier, one possibility is that laughter is always traceable to a single, generalized feeling, such as tension release or nonseriousness. However, the more common interpretation is that many differentiable states can be involved, each associated with one or more distinctive features in resulting sounds. "Valence," which refers to the kind, or quality, of emotion triggering the laughter, is typically assumed to be the critical factor. Vocalizer "arousal" (or "activation level"), which refers to the intensity of that state, is almost certainly critical in shaping laughter acoustics, but it has rarely been discussed or investigated.

The problem in addressing the mapping question is that direct testing requires comparison of spontaneous laughter recorded from vocalizers in two or more different emotional states. When presenting comedic material, one can be reasonably confident that resulting laughter is both emotion-triggered and specifically positive. In nonmirthful circumstances, it becomes much more difficult to know whether laughter is spontaneous or volitional, and what particular emotion was involved in triggering it. New, imaginative methods are therefore sorely needed to obtain the kinds of recordings required. In an alternative approach, some researchers have tested "faked laughter," which is volitional laughs made by actors simulating what might occur in response to various emotions (Szameitat et al., 2009a, 2009b). Interpreting such studies is problematic, however, due to the inherent contradictions and circularity of testing for natural mappings between vocalizer state and laughter acoustics using stimuli that are deliberately designed to portray such relationships. Emerging evidence that faked laughter is discriminable from spontaneous counterparts also provides reason for caution (Bryant & Aktipis, 2013).

Given that recordings of spontaneous laughter from participants in known, nonmirthful states are so hard to come by, the most telling evidence about the mapping question so far may be the marked variability observed in mirthful laughter alone. Unless these sounds are somehow exceptional, finding so much acoustic variation within this one context makes it difficult to argue that unique, well-differentiated laughter can nonetheless be occurring in other situations. The variability observed instead highlights the likely importance of arousal, in line with expecting vocalizer responses to humorous material to vary dramatically within and across individuals—depending on how funny the comedy is to each person from moment to moment. Although not yet investigated for spontaneous laughter, arousal is generally found to affect a variety of aspects of vocal acoustics in both humans and nonhumans—including the amplitude, F_0, F_0 range, rate, duration, and variability of the sounds produced (Zimmermann, Leliveld, & Schehka, 2013). If arousal does affect laughter in important ways, the chances of finding clear, "one-to-one" relationships between internal states and acoustics become even smaller—requiring any valence-specific features then to be preserved in the face of such effects. Conversely, adding arousal to the equation strengthens the argument for a "one-to-many" mapping, as implied in proposals emphasizing single states such as tension-release or nonseriousness. By the same token, mappings might instead be "many-to-many" or "many-to-one," with multiple valenced states being able to "access" brainstem mechanisms generating spontaneous laughter. Arousal would be primary in shaping acoustics in either of these cases, with significant overlap expected across contexts regardless of vocalizer valence.

Summary: Are Contagion and Function Connected?

Contagion is a remarkable and fundamental aspect of spontaneous laughter, but it has not been well explained. It is also interestingly constrained by being limited to laughter with regular phonation, providing a potential clue to the mechanism involved. Contagiousness is also consistent with the social nature of laughter, showing that this vocalization by itself can have an immediate, meaningful impact on listener emotion. Upon further examination, evidence about social mediation of spontaneous laughter reveals that males and females laugh about the same amount but use their sounds differently, depending on who else is present. Whether that usage involves a strategy of acoustics "standing for" specific states is unclear—too little research has addressed potential mappings between emotional valence and laughter sounds, or the impact of arousal.

"Affect Induction" and the Evolution of Laughter

The previous material on spontaneous laughter covers a variety of evidence and ideas, yet has left a number of loose threads and unanswered questions. For example, why does laughter occur in both spontaneous and volitional forms, each involving a distinct neural pathway? How can one account for the particular changes occurring in spontaneous laughter after human ancestors diverged from apes? If the sounds communicate vocalizer emotion via a differentiated coding system, why is mirthful laughter

in and of itself so variable? Furthermore, if laughter communicates in this language-like way, why do these sounds induce positive emotion in listeners, whereas actually saying "That's funny" has no such effect? Finally, why is it that voiced bursts and bouts are contagious, whereas unvoiced sounds in the same circumstances are not? This final section attempts to address each of these questions within an integrated theory of laughter and its evolution. By necessity, discussion moves quickly and lightly over each topic but nonetheless includes specific proposals about mechanism and function of this vocalization.

Laughter and Associative Learning

The foundational assumption in the account is that the basic function of all communication is to influence behavior in others. While signals that "stand for" something are one means to that end, we assume that other mechanisms are also possible. In other words, communication is not synonymous with "language-like code," but may instead take a variety of forms—particularly in the case of signaling that is not language. One such strategy is for signalers to use sounds to induce emotional responses in listeners (e.g., Owren, Rendall, & Bachorowski, 2005)—precisely the effect labeled as "contagion" in voiced laughter. We suggest that this is a relatively simple phenomenon, at least if one can suppose that spontaneous laughter occurs more often overall in circumstances that are positive for the listener than in either neutral or negative situations. If so, the positive responses evoked upon hearing voiced laughter can be explained as associative learning.

The learning process involved likely begins early in life, for instance, during mutually positive, face-to-face interactions between infants and caregivers—circumstances often accompanied by copious laughter on both sides. Emotional synchrony is key, as the associations require that positive emotion and laughter in one party occurs while the listener is also experiencing a positive state. Of course, there are many instances over a lifetime in which one hears laughter when not in a positive state. However, the argument requires only that an overall correlation exist, with the expectation being that children and adults alike should then—all other things being equal—show a net positive response when hearing laughter. Learning effects are expected to be strongest when hearing sounds from close friends and family members, those with whom an individual most frequently shares positive social interactions. A weaker but still positive response is also expected in response to anonymous laughter, including when these sounds are heard in isolation.

Accounting for Contagion

This overall perspective is an *affect-induction* approach, one that can arguably explain multiple aspects of laughter and its evolution. In this view, laughter contagion becomes a simple consequence of listeners repeatedly hearing laughter while simultaneously experiencing positive states themselves. Associative learning effects can furthermore explain why only regularly voiced laughter sounds are contagious, with unvoiced sounds recorded in the same original circumstances having little effect. The difference lies in the former being notably more salient than the latter—including being louder and being much richer in indexical cues. Even when occurring side by side in a laughter stream, voiced bursts are therefore expected to overshadow unvoiced versions in the learning process. Differences in identity-cueing also make voiced laughter a far better vehicle for both vocalizer-specific and generalized associations. This learning-based account can thereby explain Smoski and Bachorowski's (2003a, 2003b) friend-versus-stranger effect for antiphonal laughter, as well as the fact that stranger-dyads tested over repeated sessions showed increasing amounts of antiphonal laughter as they went on to become friends.

Vocalizer States, Laughter Acoustics, and Listener Perception

As noted earlier, the finding that vocalizers produce spontaneous laughter in response to a variety of emotions in and of itself does not imply that the sounds are carefully calibrated and state-specific. Rather, spontaneous laughter may be quite imprecise, operating via ancient, emotion-related brainstem mechanisms. One likely indicator of such imprecision is that in spite of having very different significance for listeners, voiced and unvoiced bursts can occur almost interchangeably—even within the same bout. Although direct evidence is not available, we suspect that relative arousal is a critical factor, with rising activation levels probabilistically pushing vocalizer output from mostly unvoiced to mostly voiced sounds. Laughter acoustics are therefore likely to provide reliable, arousal-related cueing, but affect induction logic actually argues against that possibility for valence. If the consistent function of spontaneous laughter is to induce positive responses in listeners, then vocalizers in nonpositive states should specifically produce laughter that resembles the sounds triggered by positive emotion.

At first blush, this reasoning seems to be both at odds with listeners being able to draw inferences about vocalizer valence and to contradict the common experience of "hearing" emotion in laughter sounds. However, neither need be the case. Noting the extensive variability in naturally occurring laughter, for instance, Grammer (1990; Grammer & Eibl-Eibesfeldt, 1990) suggested that listeners interpret these sounds within the broader frame of concomitant facial expressions, movements, postures, and other aspects of the situation. Under natural circumstances, listeners actually have still more to go on, including lifelong experience with laughter, and often are familiar with the particular vocalizer involved. In fact, perceptual processing in general is strongly context- and experience-bound, as raw sensory input alone always leaves room for ambiguity. Observers are never directly aware of the extensive, interpretative processing they do, however, instead attributing resultant perceptual inferences to the original input itself. For laughter, the question therefore boils down to understanding the extent to which "hearing" the vocalizer's state reflects valence specificity versus the listener's own enriching, perceptual interpretation of the acoustics involved.

Social Mediation

The view that laughter functions by inducing positive emotion in listeners is consistent with Stillman and colleagues' (2007) proposal that participants laughed at a confederate experimenter's jokes because doing so might elicit more favorable treatment. The affect induction approach is similarly applicable to Provine's (2000) generalizations about who does and does not laugh most in an interaction. Using laughter to evoke positive emotion is clearly pertinent in socially challenging circumstances, such as those that make a vocalizer embarrassed or nervous. In such situations, producing voiced laughter can nudge both friends and strangers toward more supportive behavior than they might otherwise have shown. The affect induction perspective therefore does not argue that females laugh with males to convey subservience, appeasement, or even sexual interest. Instead, it suggests that females are using laughter strategically to shape and manage male emotions and associated behavior. Because males famously (mis)interpret female signals in a biased, self-flattering fashion, using laughter to induce small "hits" of positive emotion in a male can be a fruitful management strategy—especially for younger females (Owren & Bachorowski, 2003).

A Scenario for Laughter Evolution

Based on the evidence, laughter does not appear to have evolved to benefit health. It is also difficult to make a compelling case for laughter acoustics "standing for" particular vocalizer states—although better data are desperately needed. Our interpretation is that human laughter evolved as a mechanism of social bonding and cooperative behavior, particularly among unrelated individuals (Owren & Bachorowski, 2001). Furthermore, the central mechanism proposed is that laughter can be used to induce learned emotion. Based on these ideas, the next paragraphs outline how evolution may have produced the key features that laughter has today.

Initially, spontaneous laughter in human ancestors was ape-like—both ingressive and egressive, irregularly voiced, and mainly occurring in youngsters playing or being tickled. Two changes were most important in transforming these sounds into a potent vehicle for emotional learning, namely, increased identity cueing and expanded usage. For the former, we noted earlier that

regular phonation creates stronger indexical cueing than does irregular vibration—specifically including cues to vocalizer identity. Consistently egressive laughter is therefore proposed to reflect selection for increased identity cueing because phonation is more regular with outward than inward airflow (Eklund, 2008). Modification of the vocal-fold tissues themselves is also likely, contributing to the smooth, self-synchronizing action that is a hallmark of the modern human voice (Titze, 1994). For the latter—expanded usage of laughter—our evolutionary argument focuses on cooperative behavior among adults, which takes usage far beyond play and tickling contexts. With affect induction as the central mechanism, a social-bonding function implies that laughter should evolve to occur in essentially every circumstance in which adult vocalizers and listeners both predictably experience positive emotion.

To summarize, the argument so far is that the first adaptive changes were toward egressive, regularly voiced laughter coming to be triggered by positive emotion across a wide range of social circumstances—thereby increasing cooperative behavior and overall reproductive success among individuals producing these sounds. Once established, however, vocalizations that can induce positive emotion in others become useful in their own right. For example, a vocalizer who experiences challenging social circumstances—and concomitant negative emotions—could also benefit from using laughter to "tweak" listener emotion in a positive direction. Mechanistically, that change may have been quite straightforward, requiring only that nonpositive emotional states also gain neural "access" to brainstem laughter-production circuitry. Vocalizers could use this new capability in a variety of situations—most powerfully with friends and family but also to some effect with virtually any listener.

Although useful to individual vocalizers, expanded laughter usage also diluted the overall association between this vocalization and positive states in listeners—thereby decreasing the effectiveness of these sounds in inducing positive listener emotion. Yet laughter continues to elicit positive emotion even today, in spite of an additional evolutionary step that diluted that association even further. As before, the reasoning is that the power of positive, emotion-triggered laughter to influence others created inherent selection pressure for more strategic deployment, in this case, by using volitional, simulated versions. This change created a new kind of power, allowing vocalizers to produce these potentially emotion-inducing sounds literally at will. While potentially evolving in parallel with nonpositive emotions gaining access to spontaneous laughter circuitry, the neural modifications needed were probably more extensive. However, any evolutionary complications on the neural side were likely dwarfed by the complex behavioral implications of the emergence of volitional vocal control—with our evolving ancestors applying their new capabilities not only to laughter sounds but also eventually to every aspect of vocalization found in modern humans.

Summary: Strategic Affect Induction Using Laughter

This final section has briefly presented an affect induction account of spontaneous laughter behavior, centered on associative learning and serving a larger function of social bonding. The approach potentially accounts for a number of aspects of spontaneous laughter, with its emotional learning perspective on contagion serving to explain both the form and usage of these sounds. The fact that only voiced laughter is contagious is traced to a combination of salience and rich indexical cueing—characteristics that make such sounds an excellent vehicle of associative learning. Unvoiced laughter recorded from the same situations has neither property; therefore, it shows little contagion. While arousal effects are seemingly quite evident in laughter, the affect induction view predicts that valence-specific acoustics are either less prominent or basically absent. The affect induction approach also speaks to social status and gender outcomes, based on the premise that voiced laughter can influence listener emotion and behavior, thereby encouraging more favorable treatment of the vocalizer. If so, one expects the sounds to be used specifically by those who can most benefit from influencing listener state in a given situation, including lower-status individuals of both sexes and younger females when males are present. Viewing laughter from

this perspective suggests stepwise evolutionary emergence—first, as an indexically rich, more widely used version of an existing vocalization; second, by then becoming triggered by nonpositive states; and third, by coming under volitional control via a new, cortical pathway.

Conclusions: Promise and Challenge

This chapter has covered much ground, touching on a diverse range of topics and complexities concerning spontaneous laughter. It has also highlighted that achieving a satisfactory understanding of this behavior will mean going much further. In covering so many different aspects of spontaneous laughter, we hope we have demonstrated that it is a complicated phenomenon—one that combines exacting empirical study with an integrative, "big-picture" theoretical perspective. While generally useful in scientific inquiry, this kind of hybrid approach may hold particular promise in studying laughter. Specifically, we suggest that elucidating the origins, neural organization, and emotional underpinnings of this vocal behavior can be singularly helpful, for instance, in uncovering basic principles of emotional expression that are applicable to wide range of facial and vocal signals.

Yet there are serious practical challenges to overcome in studying laughter. One major impediment is the virtual absence of direct evidence about mapping of internal states to vocal acoustics—particularly with respect to possible valence effects. While little is known about the impact of arousal, that question can be more straightforwardly addressed—for example, by using psychophysiological measures to monitor arousal in participants who are laughing in response to humorous material. An entirely different level of imagination and effort will be needed to determine whether and how valence is differentially represented in laughter acoustics. Here, one must not only ensure that the laughter is genuinely emotion-triggered but also determine what that state specifically is.

In fact, the problem of distinguishing between spontaneous and volitionally produced laughter may prove to be the greatest challenge of all—both theoretically and empirically. So far, scientific treatments of laughter have typically glossed over this distinction, likely because of the difficulty of addressing the issue. The challenge must eventually be met, however, including the possibility that everyday laughter may routinely be neither purely spontaneous nor purely volitional. Exploring the full range of possibilities created by having two underlying neural pathways is likely the key to taking on the full range of basic issues in laughter acoustics, biology, function, and usage. To date, the most common approach has been to focus either on humor-induced sounds that are assumed to be spontaneous and positive, or to rely on accompanying smiles as evidence of triggered emotion. Neither of these strategies will be sufficient in the long run. For instance, both fail to address the possibility that even emotion-triggered laughter need not be positive, and that the two underlying neural systems controlling laughter output may be working either separately or together in any given instance.

Despite these and other difficulties, the study of human laughter well warrants the increased scientific attention it is now receiving. As a ubiquitous component of human behavior, laughter is clearly much more than just a safety valve for tense nervous systems. While laughing in and of itself may not produce the health-related benefits often attributed to this behavior, there is no doubt that laughter is one of the most important of all nonverbal human signals. Given its many complexities, laughter almost certainly "wears many different hats" in human social behavior, figuring into virtually every individual interaction and interindividual relationship. Untangling these myriad roles presents a combination of challenge and promise that should keep laughter researchers fruitfully busy for decades to come.

Acknowledgments

We thank Anaïs Stenson and Michelle Shiota for helpful feedback on earlier versions of this chapter.

References

Adams, R. M., & Kirkevold, B. (1978). Looking, smiling, laughing, and moving in restaurants: Sex and age differences. *Environmental Psychology and Nonverbal Behavior, 3,* 117–121.

Andrew, R. J. (1963). The origin and evolution of the calls and facial expressions of the primates. *Behaviour, 20,* 1–107.

Askenasy, J. J. M. (1987). The functions and dysfunctions of laughter. *Journal of General Psychology, 114,* 317–334.

Attardo, S. (2011). Review of Wallace Chafe, "The importance of not being earnest. The feeling behind lauher and humor." *Pragmatics and Cognition, 19,* 375–382.

Bachorowski, J.-A., & Owren, M. J. (1999). Acoustic correlates of talker sex and individual talker identity are present in a short vowel segment produced in running speech. *Journal of the Acoustical Society of America, 106,* 1054–1063.

Bachorowski, J.-A., & Owren, M. J. (2001). Not all laughs are alike: Voiced but not unvoiced laughter elicits positive affect in listeners. *Psychological Science, 12,* 252–257.

Bachorowski, J.-A., Smoski, M. J., & Owren, M. J. (2001). The acoustic features of human laughter. *Journal of the Acoustical Society of America, 110,* 1581–1597.

Bainum, C. K., Lounsbury, K. R., & Pollio, H. R. (1984). The development of smiling and laughter in nursery school children. *Child Development, 55,* 1946–1957.

Bell, S. M., & Ainsworth, M. D. S. (1972). Infant crying and maternal responsiveness. *Child Development, 43,* 1171–1190.

Bryant, G., & Aktipis, C. A. (2013). *The animal nature of spontaneous human laughter.* Manuscript in review

Buchowski, M. S., Majchrzak, K. M., Blomquist, K., Chen, K. Y., Byrne, D. W., & Bachorowski, J.-A. (2007). Energy expenditure of genuine laughter. *International Journal of Obesity, 31,* 131–137.

Chafe, W. L. (2007). *The importance of not being earnest: The feeling behind laughter and humor* (Vol. 3). Amsterdam: Benjamins.

Coates, J. (2007). Talk in a play frame: More on laughter and intimacy. *Journal of Pragmatics, 39,* 29–49.

Cousins, N. (1979). *Anatomy of an illness as perceived by the patient: Reflections on healing and regeneration.* New York: Norton.

Davila-Ross, M., Allcock, B., Thomas, C., & Bard, K. A. (2011). Aping expressions?: Chimpanzees produce distinct laugh types when responding to laughter of others. *Emotion, 11,* 1013–1020.

Davila-Ross, M., Owren, M. J., & Zimmermann, E. (2009). Reconstructing the phylogeny of laughter in great apes and humans. *Current Biology, 19,* 1106–1111.

DePaulo, B. M. (1992). Nonverbal behavior and self-presentation. *Psychological Bulletin, 111,* 203–243.

Dunbar, R. I. M. (1996). *Grooming, gossip, and the evolution of language.* Cambridge, MA: Harvard University Press.

Dunbar, R. I. M. (2004). Language, music, and laughter in evolutionary perspective. In D. K. Oller & U. Griebel (Eds.), *Evolution of communication systems: A comparative approach* (pp. 257–273). Cambridge, MA: MIT Press.

Dunbar, R. I. M., Baron, R., Frangou, A., Pearce, E., van Leeuwin, E. J. C., Stow, J., et al. (2012). Social laughter is correlated with an elevated pain threshold. *Proceedings of the Royal Society of London B, 279,* 1161–1167.

Edmonson, M. S. (1987). Notes on laughter. *Anthropological Linguistics, 29,* 23–34.

Eibl-Eibesfeldt, I. (1989). *Human ethology.* New York: de Gruyter.

Eklund, R. (2008). Pulmonic ingressive phonation: Diachronic and synchronic characteristics, distribution and function in animal and human sound production and in human speech. *Journal of the International Phonetic Association, 38,* 235–324.

Fry, W. F., & Rader, C. (1977). The respiratory components of mirthful laughter. *Journal of Biological Psychology, 19,* 39–50.

Gervais, M., & Wilson, D. S. (2005). The evolution and functions of laughter and humor: A synthetic approach. *Quarterly Review of Biology, 80,* 395–430.

Glenn, P. (2010). Interviewer laughs: Shared laughter and asymmetries in employment interviews. *Journal of Pragmatics, 42,* 1485–1498.

Glenn, P. J. (1991/1992). Current speaker initiation of two-party shared laughter. *Research on Language and Social Interaction, 25,* 139–162.

Grammer, K. (1990). Strangers meet: Laughter and nonverbal signs of interest in opposite-sex encounters. *Journal of Nonverbal Behavior, 14,* 209–236.

Grammer, K., & Eibl-Eibesfeldt, I. (1990). The ritualization of laughter. In W. Koch (Ed.) *Naturlichkeit der Sprache und der Kultur: Acta Colloquii* [The naturalness of language and culture: Conference proceedings]

(pp. 192–214). Bochum, Germany: Brockmeyer.

Gustafson, G. E., & Green, J. A. (1991). Developmental coordination of cry sounds with visual regard, and gestures. *Infant Behavior and Development, 14,* 51–57.

Hayworth, D. (1928). The social origin and function of laughter. *Psychological Review, 35,* 367–384.

Hempelmann, H. F. (2007). The laughter of the 1962 Tanganyika "laughter epidemic." *Humor, 20,* 49–71.

Jürgens, U. (2009). The neural control of vocalization in mammals: A review. *Journal of Voice, 23,* 1–10.

Keltner, D., & Bonanno, G. A. (1997). A study of laughter and dissociation: Distinct correlates of laughter and smiling during bereavement. *Journal of Personality and Social Psychology, 73,* 687–702.

Lester, B. M., & Boukydis, C. F. Z. (1992). Infantile colic: Acoustic cry characteristics, maternal perception of cry and temperament. *Infant Behavior and Development, 15,* 15–26.

Luschei, E. S., Ramig, L. O., Finnegan, E. M., Baker, K. K., & Smith, M. E. (2006). Patterns of laryngeal electromyography and the activity of the respiratory system during spontaneous laughter. *Journal of Neurophysiology, 96,* 442–450.

Makagon, M. M., Funayama, E. S., & Owren, M. J. (2008). An acoustic analysis of laughter from congenitally deaf and normally hearing college students. *Journal of the Acoustical Society of America, 124,* 472–483.

Martin, G. N., & Gray, C. D. (1996). The effects of audience laughter on men's and women's responses to humor. *Journal of Social Psychology, 136,* 221–231.

Martin, R. A. (2001). Humor, laughter, and physical health: Methodological issues and research findings. *Psychological Bulletin, 127,* 504–519.

Martin, R. A. (2004). Sense of humor and physical health: Theoretical issues, recent findings, and future directions. *Humor, 17,* 1–19.

Mehu, M., & Dunbar, R. I. M. (2008). Naturalistic observations of smiling and laughter in human group interactions. *Behaviour, 145,* 1747–1780.

Mora-Ripoll, R. (2010). The therapeutic value of laughter in medicine. *Alternative Therapies in Health and Medicine, 16,* 56–64.

Mowrer, D. E., LaPointe, L. L., & Case, J.

(1987). Analysis of five acoustic correlates of laughter. *Journal of Nonverbal Behavior, 11,* 191–199.

O'Connell, D. C., & Kowal, S. (2008). *Communicating with one another: Toward a psychology of spontaneous spoken discourse.* New York: Springer-Verlag.

Owren, M. J., Amoss, R. T., & Rendall, D. (2011). Two organizing principles of vocal production: Implications for nonhuman and human primates. *American Journal of Primatology, 73,* 530–544.

Owren, M. J., & Bachorowski, J.-A. (2001). The evolution of emotional expression: A "selfishgene" account of smiling and laughter in early hominids and humans. In T. J. Mayne & G. A. Bonanno (Eds.), *Emotion: Current issues and future directions* (pp. 152–191). New York: Guilford Press.

Owren, M. J., & Bachorowski, J.-A. (2003). Reconsidering the evolution of nonlinguistic communication: The case of laughter. *Journal of Nonverbal Behavior, 27,* 183–200.

Owren, M. J., Philipp, M. C., Vanman, E., Trivedi, N., Schulman, A., & Bachorowski, J.-A. (2012). Understanding spontaneous human laughter: The role of voicing in inducing positive emotion. In E. Altenmüller, S. Schmidt, & E. Zimmermann (Eds.), *Evolution of emotional communication: From sounds in nonhuman mammals to speech and music in man* (pp. 176–190). Oxford, UK: Oxford University Press.

Owren, M. J., Rendall, D., & Bachorowski, J.-A. (2005). Conscious and unconscious emotion in nonlinguistic vocal communication. In L. F. Barrett, P. M. Niedenthal, & P. Winkielman (Eds.), *Emotion and consciousness* (pp. 185–204). New York: Guilford Press.

Parvizi, J., Coburn, K. L., Shillcutt, S. D., Coffey, C. E., Lauterbach, E. C., & Mendez, M. F. (2009). Neuroanatomy of pathological laughing and crying: A report of the American Neuropsychiatric Association Committee on Research. *Journal of Neuropsychiatry and Clinical Neuroscience, 21,* 75–87.

Peterson, G. E., & Barney, H. L. (1952). Control methods used in a study of the vowels. *Journal of the Acoustical Society of America, 24,* 175–184.

Poyatos, F. (1993). The many voices of laughter: A new audible–visual paralinguistic approach. *Semiotica, 93,* 61–81.

Provine, R. R. (1992). Contagious laughter: Laughter is a sufficient stimulus for laughs and smiles. *Bulletin of the Psychonomic Society of America, 30,* 1–4.

Provine, R. R. (1993). Laughter punctuates speech: Linguistic, social and gender contexts of laughter. *Ethology, 95,* 291–298.

Provine, R. R. (1996). Laughter. *American Scientist, 84,* 38–45.

Provine, R. R. (2000). *Laughter: A scientific investigation.* New York: Viking.

Provine, R. R., & Fischer, K. R. (1989). Laughing, smiling, and talking: Relation to sleeping and social context in humans. *Ethology, 83,* 295–305.

Provine, R. R., & Yong, Y. L. (1991). Laughter: A stereotyped human vocalization. *Ethology, 89,* 115–124.

Ramachandran, V. S. (1998). The neurology and evolution of humor, laughter, and smiling: The false alarm theory. *Medical Hypotheses, 51,* 351–354.

Rothbart, M. K. (1973). Laughter in young children. *Psychological Bulletin, 80,* 247–256.

Rothgänger, H., Hauser, G., Cappellini, A. C., & Guidotti, A. (1998). Analysis of laughter and speech sounds in Italian and German students. *Naturwissenschaften, 85,* 394–402.

Ruch, W. (1993). Exhilaration and humor. In M. Lewis & J. M. Haviland (Eds.), *The handbook of emotion* (pp. 605–616). New York: Guilford Press.

Scheiner, E., Hammerschmidt, K., Jürgens, U., & Zwirner P. (2004). The influence of hearing impairment on preverbal emotional vocalizations of infants. *Folia Phoniatrica Logopaedica, 56,* 27–40.

Seyfarth, R. M., & Cheney, D. L. (2012). The evolutionary origins of friendship. *Annual Review of Psychology, 53,* 153–177.

Smoski, M. J., & Bachorowski, J.-A. (2003a). Antiphonal laughter between friends and strangers. *Cognition and Emotion, 17,* 327–340.

Smoski, M. J., & Bachorowski, J.-A. (2003b). Antiphonal laughter in developing friendships. *Annals of the New York Academy of Sciences, 1000,* 300–303.

Stevens, K. N. (2000). *Acoustic phonetics.* Cambridge, MA: MIT Press.

Stillman, T. F., Baumeister, R. F., & DeWall, C. N. (2007). What's so funny about not having money?: The effects of power on laughter. *Personality and Social Psychology Bulletin, 33*(11), 1547–1558.

Szameitat, D. P., Alter, K., Szameitat, A. J., Darwin, C. J., Wildgruber, D., Dietrich, S., et al. (2009a). Differentiation of emotions in laughter at the behavioral level. *Emotion, 9,* 397–405.

Szameitat, D. P., Alter, K., Szameitat, A. J., Wildgruber, D., Sterr, A., & Darwin, C. J. (2009b). Acoustic profiles of distinct emotional expressions in laughter. *Journal of the Acoustical Society of America, 126,* 354–366.

Tanaka, H., & Campbell, N. (2011). Acoustic features of four types of laughter in natural conversational speech. In W.-S. Lee & E. Zee (Eds.), *Proceedings of the 17th International Congress of Phonetic Sciences* (pp. 1958–1961). Hong Kong: City University of Hong Kong.

Titze, I. R. (1994). *Principles of voice production.* New York: Prentice Hall.

Titze, I. R., Finnegan, E. M., Laukkanen, A.-M., Fuja, M., & Hoffman, H. (2008). Laryngeal muscle activity in giggle: A damped oscillation model. *Journal of Voice, 22,* 644–648.

Trouvain, J. (2003). Segmenting phonetic units in laughter. In M.-J. Solé, D. Recasens, & J. Romero (Eds.), *Proceedings of 15th International Congress of Phonetic Sciences* (pp. 2983–2996). Barcelona: Casual Productions.

Urbain, J., & Dutoit, T. (2011). A phonetic analysis of natural laughter, for use in automatic laughter processing systems. *Lecture Notes in Computer Science, 6974,* 397–406.

van Hooff, J. A. R. A. M. (1972). A comparative approach to the phylogeny of laughter and smiling. In R. A. Hinde (Ed.), *Non-verbal communication* (pp. 209–241). Cambridge, UK: Cambridge University Press.

Vettin, J., & Todt, D. (2004). Laughter in conversation: Features of occurrence and acoustic structure. *Journal of Nonverbal Behavior, 28,* 93–115.

Wild, B., Rodden, F. A., Grodd, W., & Ruch, W. (2003). Neural correlates of laughter and humour. *Brain, 126,* 2121–2138.

Zimmermann, E., Leliveld, L., & Schehka, S. (2013). Toward the evolutionary roots of affective prosody in speech and music: Universal affect cues in mammalian voices? In E. Altenmüller, S. Schmidt, & E. Zimmermann (Eds.), *Evolution of emotional communication: From sounds in nonhuman mammals to speech and music in man* (pp. 116–132). Oxford, UK: Oxford University Press.

CHAPTER 10

Nonverbal Expressions of Positive Emotions

Disa A. Sauter
Nicole M. McDonald
Devon N. Gangi
Daniel S. Messinger

Positive emotions affect the tone of our voice, the ways in which we move our body, and the expressions on our face. In this chapter, we review research on the production and comprehension of nonverbal signals of positive emotions. We take a lifespan approach, considering research on infants and children, as well as adults. We first review the literature on the production and perception of positive emotions in the voice, the body, and the face, and provide a summary of its conclusions and limitations. We end the chapter with a general discussion and proposals for future research.

The vast majority of studies on emotional communication do not differentiate among positive emotions. The difficulty with this approach has been recognized for some time, with one theorist noting that "a comparison of results from different studies is virtually impossible if it is unclear whether . . . 'happiness' refers to quiet bliss or bubbling elation" (Scherer, 1986, p. 163; see also Ekman, 1992, for a similar point). Nevertheless, most contemporary studies still treat positive emotion as a unitary category. Increasingly, however, researchers are starting to go beyond a single positive emotion to examine a range of diverse positive states and expressions. That work is the focus of this chapter.

Positive Emotions in the Voice

The human voice is a rich instrument with which to communicate positive emotions: We cheer with triumph, sigh with relief, and laugh with amusement. Some of these vocal expressions emerge early in life, whereas others develop later in childhood. In this section, we first review research on nonverbal vocalizations from infancy through adulthood, then discuss studies of emotional speech intonation in children and adults. Research into laughter is discussed in more detail by Owren and Amoss (Chapter 9, this volume).

Nonverbal Vocalizations in Infants

Vocalization is one of the first ways in which infants communicate their affective states: They coo, laugh, and smack their lips with delight. Vocalizations, including laughter,

gurgling, positively toned babbling, and cooing, appear to have an inherent signal value
and are used as indices of positive affect in
observational research on infant temperament (e.g., Goldsmith & Rothbart, 1999;
Hane, Fox, Henderson, & Marshall, 2008).

Laughter emerges when infants are
between 2 and 5 months of age (Nwokah,
Hsu, Dobrowolska, & Fogel, 1994; Washburn, 1929) and appears to index intense
positive emotion and arousal (Sroufe &
Waters, 1976). Initial laughs sound much
like early vowel-like vocalizations, but
mothers appear to recognize and comment
on them (Nwokah & Fogel, 1993). Laughing
becomes more frequent between the second
month and the second year of life (Nwokah
et al., 1994), and during this period physically stimulating games, such as tickling, are
potent elicitors of laughter (see Owren &
Amoss, Chapter 9, this volume). Between 6
and 12 months of age, infants become more
likely to laugh in response to social games,
such as peekaboo, as they simultaneously
become more active in these games (Sroufe
& Waters, 1976). Furthermore, infant and
mother laugh onsets and offsets occur
increasingly close in time between 12 and
24 months, suggesting that laughter reflects
and supports increasing communicative synchrony in the second year (Nwokah et al.,
1994).

In contrast to laughter, many infant
speech-like vocalizations seem to acquire a
positive signal value for the social partner or
observer because of the behavioral context in
which they occur. Nonverbal vocalizations
in infants are typically thought to express
positive emotions when they occur during
smiles. Yale, Messinger, and Cobo-Lewis
(2003) examined how infants at 3 and 6
months coordinate vocalizations with facial
expressions. They found that vocalizations
were typically embedded within smiles: The
infants smiled, vocalized, finished the vocalization, and only then terminated the smile.
This suggests that the vocalizations may
emphasize the affective message provided
by the smile. In support of this hypothesis,
recent research indicates that listeners show
only moderate agreement when distinguishing the affective tenor of infant vocalizations
from listening to the vocalization alone;
however, agreement increases substantially
when observers listen to the vocalization

as they watch the infant (Franklin, Oller,
Ramsdell, & Jhang, 2011).

Nonverbal Vocalizations in Adults

In contrast with the developmental research
in this area, several studies have differentiated among different kinds of nonverbal positive vocalizations in adults. Schröder (2003),
for example, studied listeners' perception
of affect bursts of admiration, elation, and
relief. Affect bursts are "very brief, discrete,
nonverbal expressions of affect in both face
and voice" (Scherer, 1994, p. 170). The
study found substantial variability in recognition across positive emotions. Whereas
affect bursts of admiration and relief were
well recognized, elation expressions seemed
to lack a clear prototype. Schröder's results,
however, showed that some specific positive
emotions can be communicated via vocal
signals.

Extending this research, Sauter and colleagues have examined nonverbal vocalizations of positive emotions that, unlike affect
bursts, do not include facial expressions and
need not be brief. Sauter and Scott (2007)
tested Ekman's (1992) hypothesis that there
are several positive emotions with distinct
nonverbal vocal expressions, by examining enacted vocalizations of achievement/
triumph, amusement, contentment, sensual pleasure, and relief. Among English
and Swedish speakers, each positive emotion vocalization was well recognized, and
listeners consistently rated vocalizations as
expressing the intended emotion. Sauter,
Eisner, Calder, and Scott (2010) examined
the acoustic cues used by listeners to judge
emotions from nonverbal vocalizations.
They found that each set of emotion ratings
was predicted by a unique combination of
acoustic measures. Relief and achievement
ratings were predicted by different subsets
of spectral and pitch cues, whereas amusement, contentment, and pleasure were predicted by different combinations of spectral
and envelope information. This suggests
that listeners employ different acoustic cues
to distinguish different positive emotions.

In a related study, Sauter, Eisner, Ekman,
and Scott (2010) examined the production
and recognition of emotion vocalizations
among English and Himba individuals,
the latter from remote, culturally isolated

Namibian villages. Different positive emotions yielded different patterns of results. Laughter was recognized bidirectionally, with listeners inferring amusement from laughs by their own and the other group. Triumph and sensual pleasure vocalizations were recognized within each group, but not across groups, suggesting that the development of these vocalizations depends on culture-specific input. Both English and Himba individuals produced acoustically similar sighs in response to relief scenarios. Himba listeners, however, did not recognize relief vocalizations from either group, suggesting that sighs are ambiguous signals that can communicate a range of affective states.

In a follow-up study (Sauter, 2010), English and Himba individuals matched laughter to a smiling facial expression. Nonverbal vocalizations of other positive emotions were not cross-culturally associated with the smiling facial expression. However, only one type of smiling was provided, leaving open the possibility that different positive vocalizations might be associated with different smile configurations.

Simon-Thomas, Keltner, Sauter, Sinicropi-Yao, and Abramson (2009) examined vocalizations of 22 different emotions, including 13 positive states. They found that, as in Sauter and colleagues' (Sauter, Eisner, Calder & Scott, 2010; Sauter, Eisner, Ekman, & Scott, 2010; Sauter & Scott, 2007) work, relief and amusement were the two best-recognized positive emotions. More generally, analysis of listeners' errors revealed that incorrect classifications mainly occurred within emotion families (e.g., "self-conscious," "prosocial"), suggesting that vocal signals of functionally similar emotions may overlap acoustically.

The Development of Positive Prosody

In addition to nonverbal expressions, positive emotions can be expressed vocally through speech prosody. Studies in this area have predominantly focused on the perception, rather than the production, of speech prosody. The early development of prosody perception is often investigated via looking time measures in which infants are "asked" to relate a positive speech segment to a smile. Infants can associate facial and vocal expressions of positive emotion in their par-

ents by 3 months of age (Kahana-Kalman & Walker-Andrews, 2001; Montague & Walker-Andrews, 2002), and can associate these expressions in an unfamiliar adult in the context of a peekaboo game by 4 months (Montague & Walker-Andrews, 2001). Between ages 5 and 7 months, infants can associate facial and vocal positive expressions in unfamiliar adults outside the context of familiar games (Walker-Andrews, 1997). In these studies, infants discriminate positive expressions from neutral and negative expressions. Research on the perception of different types of positive emotion is not available until much later in development.

We know of no research on positive emotional prosody production in older children. Recent research, however, has begun to explore children's ability to distinguish among different types of positive speech alongside nonverbal vocalizations, using adult expressions of triumph, amusement, contentment, and relief as stimuli (Sauter, Panattoni, & Happé, 2013). Using forced-choice tasks, Sauter and colleagues (2013) found that children as young as 5 years of age were proficient in interpreting positive emotional cues from vocal signals, although performance for both nonverbal and verbal stimuli improved through 10 years (the oldest age studied). Consistent with evidence from adults, children's accuracy was higher for nonverbal vocalizations than for speech stimuli (Hawk, Van Kleef, Fischer, & van der Schalk, 2009). This is likely because processing speech automatically engages mechanisms involved in decoding speech, even when it is irrelevant to the task at hand. In contrast, nonverbal vocalizations are not language-like, so resources are fully focused on understanding the nonverbal emotional information. Recognition was better than chance for both speech and nonverbal stimuli for all of the positive emotions studied, however, demonstrating that children are able to infer positive emotional states from different vocal cues. Furthermore, the two tasks were sensitive to individual differences, with high correspondence between children's performance across the tasks.

In adults, listeners across several cultures find "happy" speech more difficult to identify than speech expressing other emotions (e.g., Scherer, Banse, & Wallbott, 2001; but see Pell, Monetta, Paulmann, & Kotz, 2009, for a different pattern of results). Could it be that an array of distinct positive emotions would be better recognized than happiness? In a meta-analysis of vocal communication of emotion, Juslin and Laukka (2003) differentiated between happiness and love–tenderness. "Happiness" included a range of positive emotional states, including cheerfulness, elation, enjoyment, and joy, whereas love–tenderness included states such as affection, love, tenderness, and passion. The meta-analysis found evidence for some degree of recognition of prosody for these two broad groups of positive emotions. Happy speech was characterized by fast speech rate, medium to high voice intensity, high pitch level, and substantial pitch variability. In contrast, tenderness typically had slow speech rate, low voice intensity, low pitch level, and little pitch variability.

Although studies have described the prosody associated with laughter in speech (Nwokah, Hsu, Davies, & Fogel, 1999) and excitement (Trouvain & Barry, 2000), there is little research comparing speech intonation among different positive emotions. Two studies using acted emotional speech have included a variety of positive emotions. Banse and Scherer (1996) examined the recognition of emotions varying in arousal. They found that elation and happiness (unlike other emotion pairs) were rarely confused with each other, suggesting that elation and happiness are two distinct emotions. Similarly, Sauter (2006) found that listeners were able to identify a range of positive emotions from inflected speech, recognizing triumph, amusement, contentment, and sensual pleasure at better-than-chance levels. Consistent with findings from nonverbal vocalizations, amusement was the best recognized of the positive emotions. These studies offer evidence that several positive emotions can be distinguished via speech prosody.

Adopting a free-naming approach, Cowie and Cornelius (2003) tested listeners' recognition of emotions using segments of spontaneous speech. Using these naturalistic stimuli, they found that listeners inferred several positive emotional states from speech inflection, including excitement, amusement, affection, love, pleasure, relaxation, and happiness. Cowie and Cornelius also noted that the emotions were typically perceived to be of fairly weak intensity, suggest-

ing that emotions expressed in speech tend to be weak to moderately strong and mixed rather than pure. They suggested that this may be because full-blown emotion expression competes for control with the cognitive systems that underpin the production of fluent speech.

Conclusions on Positive Emotions in the Voice

In infants, the early-emerging association between laughter and tickling in both human and nonhuman primate infants (Davila-Ross, Owren, & Zimmermann, 2009), and the increasing use of laughter in synchronized social games, is relatively well understood. Other vocalizations, such as gurgling and cooing, are used to tap individual differences in positive expressivity (Fox, Henderson, Rubin, Calkins, & Schmidt, 2001; Goldsmith & Rothbart, 1999; Hane et al., 2008) but have not been validated with respect to the contexts in which they occur or the manner in which they are perceived by observers. Almost nothing is known about positive vocal expressions in children between 1 and 5 years of age, although older children have been found to recognize a range of positive states from both speech and nonspeech vocalizations. To our knowledge, no work to date has assessed children's vocal production of positive emotions; research in infants includes both production and perception, but research later in the lifespan typically only examines recognition (but see Cowie & Cornelius, 2003). This raises the question of how the production of vocal signals of positive emotion, as well as their recognition, develops beyond infancy.

Adults are sensitive to a range of positive emotions in vocal signals, particularly in nonverbal vocalizations, suggesting that the voice may be a particularly important means of signaling positive affective information. Notably, amusement and relief vocalizations are well recognized and show cross-cultural consistency; for other positive emotions, such as triumph, vocalizations vary more across cultural groups. These differences highlight the importance of considering a range of distinct positive emotions when assessing cross-cultural differences and consistencies in vocal and other expressions. Some positive vocalizations—such as laughter and perhaps sighs of relief—may be fixed signals in human beings.

From childhood on, positive emotions, like negative emotions, are less easily identified from speech prosody than nonverbal vocalizations. Whether this is due to emotions expressed in speech tending to be of a weaker intensity or because the acoustic cues used in emotional communication compete with those employed in speech production is an important question for future work to address. We now turn to bodily actions that communicate positive affect.

Bodily Expressions of Positive Emotion

Although research in the domain of bodily expressions of positive emotions is limited, studies of infants, children, and adults have revealed that positive emotion is expressed through the body in various ways from early in life. We discuss two broad domains of bodily expressions of positive emotion: touch and postural cues.

A Positive Touch

In young infants, touch is affected by caregivers' responsivity during interactions. Moszkowski and Stack (2007) found that 5-month-old infants tend to use static touch (e.g., touching without moving their hands) during naturalistic interactions with their mothers. Infants use more reactive (e.g., pat, pull, grab) and soothing (e.g., stroke, finger, mouth) types of touch during periods of experimenter-requested maternal unresponsiveness (the still face). By 7 months of age, infants begin to display affectionate touch behaviors, such as patting, hugging, and kissing, which increase through 11 months (Landau, 1989). The majority of these touch behaviors are directed at the primary caregiver, suggesting that they are directed expressions of positive emotion. However, there is no evidence to date that infants of this age use specific forms of touch to communicate different types of positive emotion.

Warm touch between parent and child is associated with positive developmental outcomes in infancy. Anisfeld, Casper, Nozyce, and Cunningham (1990) randomly assigned mothers soft baby carriers ("Snugglis") designed to increase physical contact with their infants. They found that infants in the soft baby carrier condition were more likely to be securely attached at 13 months of age than were comparison children. Likewise, Weiss, Wilson, Hertenstein, and Campos (2000) found an association between "nurturing touch" and secure attachment. At older ages (5- and 6-year-olds), Oveis, Gruber, Keltner, Stamper, and Boyce (2009) found associations between warm family touch and smile intensity in children. These findings suggest that from early infancy, touch may be an important modality for communicating positive emotion that facilitates the development of secure attachment.

Touch between adults is a topic of emerging research. In a pioneering study, Hertenstein, Keltner, App, Bulleit, and Jaskolka (2006) asked whether adults could identify specific emotions from the experience of being touched by a stranger on the arm or hand, without being able to see the touch. They found that participants were able to decode emotions including love, gratitude, and sympathy via touch at better-than-chance levels (see Hertenstein & Keltner, 2010, for evidence of gender asymmetries in decoding). The researchers also examined the most commonly used types of touch for expressing different emotions, and found that love was typically signaled with stroking, gratitude was communicated with a handshake, and sympathy was expressed with a patting movement. Furthermore, participants were able to infer emotions by merely watching others communicate via touch. The finding that participants are able to decode positive emotions from being touched has since been replicated and extended to the broad state of happiness (Hertenstein, Holmes, McCullough, & Keltner, 2009).

In addition to signaling specific positive emotions, touch may also influence how well people work together. A study by Kraus, Huang, and Keltner (2010) that examined professional basketball players, found that more physical contact between players on the same team was associated with the touched individual and team performing better later in the season. This finding held even when accounting for player status, preseason expectations, and early season performance. Results of this study support the proposition that touch can facilitate social bonding and promote cooperation and performance between adults, and that touch may be a preferred modality for communicating prosocial emotions within a group.

Gestural and Postural Expressions of Positive Emotions

Infants express positive emotions through posture, gestures, and physical motion. In a frequently used temperament measure for infants and young children (Lab-TAB), positive motor activities coded include clapping, waving the arms in excitement, and banging one's hands on a table (Goldsmith & Rothbart, 1999). These patterns of movement are assumed to have a particular positive expressive value because they occur during situations designed to elicit positive emotion ("joy/pleasure episodes"). There has, however, been little systematic documentation of the proportion of infants who respond to these episodes with these types of movements, or reports on whether these movements also occur during other situations.

"Pride" is an example of a positively valenced self-conscious emotion, generally defined as the experience of positive feelings toward the self. Pride typically occurs after successful completion of a goal, and its expression involves postural and gestural, as well as facial, actions. Three-year-olds are more likely to exhibit signs of pride in response to successful completion of relatively difficult tasks compared to less difficult or failed tasks (Belsky, Domitrovich, & Crnic, 1997). Children as young as 4 years of age can accurately recognize images of pride at above-chance levels when asked whether an adult in a photo is proud, happy, or surprised (Tracy, Robins, & Lagattuta, 2005). Lewis, Takai-Kawakami, Kawakami, and Sullivan (2010) investigated pride, as indexed by behaviors such as an erect posture, smiling, and positive self-evaluation, in response to successful completion of a challenging game in Japanese and American children. The proportion of early school-age children expressing pride varied by cultural group, with markedly more American than Japanese children exhibiting signs of pride (Lewis et al., 2010). Expressions of pride, then, may vary, even in school-age children, to reflect cultural values such as individual self-expression (Dennis, Cole, Zahn-Waxler, & Mizuta, 2002; Messinger & Freedman, 1992).

There is a considerable body of work showing that pride is reliably communicated via postural cues in adults across several different cultures (for a review, see Tracy, Weidman, Cheng, & Martens, Chapter 17, this volume). Most notably, there is evidence for cross-cultural recognition of the pride expression via postural cues by individuals from a preliterate, isolated culture in Burkina Faso, West Africa, as well as by North Americans (Tracy & Robins, 2008). Both groups could reliably recognize expressions of pride, regardless of whether the displays were produced by African or American targets. The Burkinabe individuals were unlikely to have learned the pride expression through cross-cultural transmission, as their exposure to people from outside their own cultural group was very limited. Further evidence for the cross-cultural consistency of the pride display comes from a study by Tracy and Matsumoto (2008), which examined displays produced by blind athletes in response to winning Paralympic Judo matches. Photographs of participants from different nations showed that those who had won produced behaviors associated with pride expressions, including raising their arms, tilting their heads back, smiling, and expanding their chests, which is the configuration of cues recognized by observers as communicating pride (Tracy & Robins, 2007).

Aside from pride, there has been a paucity of research on gestural and postural expressions of positive emotion in children and adults. Compared to other basic emotions, happiness appears to be the most difficult emotion to recognize from whole-body expressions (de Gelder & Van den Stock, 2011), but there have been few attempts to use bodily cues to differentiate more specific positive emotions. However, one notable study found evidence for an association between gestural/postural movements and love. Gonzaga, Keltner, Londahl, and Smith (2001) examined couples in romantic relationships taking part in a series of interactions. Four different nonverbal affiliation cues (head nods, Duchenne smiles, gesticulation, and forward leans) were correlated with self-reported feelings and partner estimates of love. These findings suggest the potential of research investigating the robustness and cross-cultural validity of gestural, bodily, and facial signs of affiliative positive emotions.

Conclusions on Positive Emotions in Bodily Expressions

Touch may be a preferred modality for communicating prosocial emotions to those close to us. Infants use touch to express attachment needs to caregivers, and increased nurturing touch from caregivers is associated with secure infant attachment. In older children, warm family touch is associated with children's smile intensity. In these contexts, touch appears to reflect and support a positive emotional interplay between child and caregivers. Touch between adults predicts individuals working well together, and several prosocial positive emotions, including love, gratitude, and sympathy, can be communicated via touch.

With the exception of pride, little is known about how positive emotions can be expressed using whole-body movements. Pride is associated with a well-established set of postural cues and is consistently recognized and displayed by both children and adults across cultures. Unfortunately, studies in children have generally neglected to describe the specific ways that children express pride (e.g., erect posture may be the only postural cue) or how pride expressions change with development. Careful description of changes or continuities in pride expressions across development would provide a firm basis for continued explorations of the expression and recognition of pride in cross-cultural contexts. Investigation of pride expressions in blind individuals of various ages who do not have visual experience with pride displays represents rich ground for continued innovative research.

Positive Emotion in the Face

The smile is remarkably well recognized as a facial signature of positive emotion, with smiling expressions typically identified more easily than any other expression in studies including one category of positive emotion (see Elfenbein & Ambady, 2002, for a meta-analysis). Throughout the lifespan, smiles are caused by the zygomaticus major muscle (AU12 in the anatomically based Facial Action Coding System [FACS] and its application to infants [BabyFACS]), which pulls the lip corners sideways and slightly upward (Ekman & Friesen, 1978; Oster, 2006). There is, however, more than one way to smile. Duchenne smiles are caused by the additional action of orbicularis oculi (pars lateralis), which raises the cheeks around the eyes and, in adults, produces crow's feet (i.e., horizontal lines extending laterally from the outside corners of the eyes) (Duchenne, 1862/1990; Ekman, Davidson, & Friesen, 1990). Duchenne smiles index positive emotion, although this may be true of other smiles as well (see discussion below). Smiles may also involve lip parting and mouth opening. Mouth opening is a characteristic of the smiles of infants, children, and non-human primates, and perhaps of adults as well (Messinger & Fogel, 2007). Below we examine the literature on perceiving and producing different types of smiles across infants, children, and adults.

The Development of Positive Facial Expressions in Infancy

Infants' production of smiles begins at birth, but contrary to common belief, neonatal smiling is not caused by gas. Infant smiles are linked not to time since last feeding, as would be predicted by the gas hypothesis, but to infant behavioral states, such as active sleep (Emde & Koenig, 1969). Neonates smile during active sleep and drowsy states. In these states, around one-half of infants observed for 6 minutes exhibited bilateral Duchenne smiles, approximately one-third of which were at a moderate intensity level (Messinger et al., 2002). The relatively mature form of these smiles and their occurrence during sleep states characterized by high levels of limbic activity suggest a possible link to positive emotion (Dondi et al., 2007). While some neonatal smiles occur amid other mouthing and dimpling actions, making them harder to discern, others occur in the absence of such movements. Longer duration neonatal smiles are more likely to be recognized as smiles by naive observers, suggesting that these in particular may be perceived as expressing positive emotion (Dondi et al., 2007).

Recent research indicates that neonates also smile in awake–alert states (Cecchini, Baroni, Vito, & Lai, 2011; Dondi et al., 2007). Cecchini and colleagues (2011) found that whereas smiles during active sleep tended to occur with the mouth closed, smiles during awake periods tended to involve mouth opening. Tactile stimulation whose intensity was responsive to the infant's behavior—an unseen adult moving a finger the infant was grasping—appeared to differentially elicit open-mouth smiles, many of which also involved eye constriction (Cecchini et al., 2011). This suggests the contextual sensitivity of smiles early in life, and the possibility that open-mouth smiles are differentially reflective of arousal generated by interaction compared to other smiles.

Early positive emotion expression is social. Evidence from blind infants, for example, suggests that visually mediated social interaction is necessary to support the development of normative smiling expressions in real time and over developmental time (see Messinger & Fogel, 2007). Positive emotion itself may develop during interaction. Between 1 and 2 months of age, infants begin to engage in social smiling (Lavelli & Fogel, 2005; Oster, 1978). As infants begin smiling, their smiles tend to elicit parents' smiles (Lavelli & Fogel, 2005; Symons & Moran, 1994). The confluence of incipient positive emotion related to the initial production of the smile, together with a positive emotional response to the parent's smile, is hypothesized to create an association between the smile and the experience of positive emotion (Messinger & Fogel, 2007).

Evidence that different types of smiles convey different aspects of positive emotion in the first 6 months of life was provided by a study involving weekly observations of infants interacting with their mothers (Messinger, Fogel, & Dickson, 2001). Duchenne smiles tended to occur more than non-Duchenne smiles when the mothers were smiling, suggesting that Duchenne smiles may be associated with reciprocating positive affect. Smiles with mouth opening occurred when infants were gazing at their mothers and may reflect the exuberance associated with positive social interactions. Despite this context specificity, smiles involving eye constriction—Duchenne smiles—also tended to involve mouth opening. These combined smiles increased over the first 6 months in the context of the infant gazing at the mother's face while she was smiling, suggesting that open-mouth smiles became increasingly reliable indices of positive emotion with development. Combined open-mouth smiling with eye constriction is a common response to tickling and physical play from 6 to 12 months and appears to be an expression of intense positive emotion and arousal (Dickson, Walker, & Fogel, 2007; Fogel, Hsu, Shapiro, Nelson-Goens, & Secrist, 2006).

There is also evidence that smile strength indexes a single dimension of positive emotion intensity. In fact, Duchenne smiles with mouth opening involve a stronger smiling action than other smiles (Fogel et al., 2006). Moreover, tickling elicits stronger underlying smiles than peekaboo or pretend tickling, suggesting the importance of smile strength as an index of positive affect in infants (Fogel et al., 2006). Messinger and colleagues explored the possibility that there is a single dimension of positive affect expression in infants. They conducted automated measurements of the intensity of infant smiling, eye constriction, and mouth opening while 6-month-olds were interacting with their parent (Messinger, Mahoor, Chow, & Cohn, 2009; Messinger, Mattson, Mahoor, & Cohn, 2012). Infant smile intensity, eye constriction intensity, and degree of mouth opening were all correlated. Moreover, the intensity of each action predicted dynamic ratings of infant positive emotion made by untrained observers as the infant's video played.

Although the results of this study suggest that a single dimension can account for smile variation in young infants, smiling likely becomes more differentiated with age. Fox and Davidson (1988) found that at 10 months of age, infants used different types of smiles in different contexts. Ten-month-olds tended to respond to their mothers' approach with a Duchenne smile but responded to the approach of a stranger with a non-Duchenne smile. It is possible that the strength of the underlying smile also distinguished these responses. Alternatively, it may be that specific types of smiles with qualitatively different meanings are evident by 10 months of age in response to specific social elicitors.

The temporal sequencing of infants' smiles and gazes at their interaction partner may also create different qualitative meanings.

At 6 months, infants rarely smile and then gaze at the parent while smiling, doing so less often than one would expect by chance (Yale et al., 2003). However, approximately one-third of 8-month-olds and the majority of 12-month-olds will smile at a toy that performs an unexpected movement, such as a somersault, and then turn to smile to an adult (Parlade et al., 2009; Venezia, Messinger, Thorp, & Mundy, 2004). These anticipatory smiles, in which the smile precedes the gaze toward the adult, suggest the intentional sharing of positive affect and are associated with later parent-rated social competence (Parlade et al., 2009).

With respect to perception, Bornstein and Arterberry (2003) used a visual habituation procedure to ask how 5-month-old infants categorize smiles of different intensities. Infants' responses suggested that they perceived smiles of different intensities to be similar—that they categorized different-intensity smiles as a single expression—even when the smiles were posed by different people. Moreover, work by Kuchuk, Vibbert, and Bornstein (1986) demonstrated that 3-month-old infants were able to discriminate between smiles of differing intensity and tended to prefer more intense smiles. Interestingly, infants who were more sensitive to smiling had mothers who more often directed their infant's attention to their (the mothers') smiling faces during naturalistic observations. These results suggest that infants detect similarities between smiles of different intensities, tend to prefer stronger smiles, and that their sensitivity to differences in the intensity of smiles is dependent on experiences with their caregivers.

Smiling in Children

More is known about smiling in the first year of life—when positive emotion is relatively easily induced in a laboratory playroom—than in later infancy and childhood. Nevertheless, investigations of children's positive emotion expressions suggest continuities with the form of infant smiles. In a study by Soussignan and Schaal (1996), an unfamiliar examiner presented children between 4 and 15 years of age with pleasant and unpleasant odors. Smiles that involved lip parting or mouth opening—both Duchenne and non-Duchenne—were more likely in response to pleasant than to unpleasant

odors. By contrast, smiles involving nose wrinkling or upper lip raising (potential indices of disgust) were more likely responses to unpleasant odors. Observers were also able to ascertain correctly that both Duchenne and non-Duchenne smiles with lip parting were responses to pleasant rather than unpleasant odors. The results underline the importance of smiling involving lip parting and mouth opening as expressions of sensory enjoyment.

As with infants, social communication is key to understanding smile production in preschoolers. In children between 2 and 4 years of age, simple smiles involving neither mouth opening nor eye constriction predominate in solitary contexts (Cheyne, 1976). Open-mouth Duchenne smiling (sometimes called "broad smiles") and laughter are strongly associated, occurring at similar levels in individual 3- to 5-year-old children (Sarra & Otta, 2001). Between ages 2 and 4, boys increasingly direct open-mouth smiles to their male rather than their female peers, suggesting that this type of smiling reflects increasing sex segregation in social contact among preschoolers (Cheyne, 1976).

In early childhood, open-mouth and Duchenne smiles are associated both with experiences of success and social proximity. A set of studies by Schneider and colleagues examined preschoolers' production of smiles in experimentally manipulated games. An initial study of 3- to 6-year-olds indicated that the components of Duchenne smiles (smiling and eye constriction) were tied to social proximity; these smiles were more likely to occur while the child was playing next to the experimenter than when the experimenter was at another table (Schneider & Josephs, 1991). In a cross-sectional follow-up study, children produced stronger smiles in a game involving success and failure than in a game that did not, beginning at around 4 years of age (Schneider & Uzner, 1992). From 5 years of age, Duchenne smiles were more common when the child was successful in the game (and rewarded with a light and sound display) than when the child failed. Smiling with lip parting was more frequent in success than in failure trials at every age, suggesting the early importance of this smile configuration.

Holodynski outlines a potential role of social context in the development of smiling. Holodynski (2004) studied the expressed positive emotion of children 6 to 8 years of age. Younger children exhibited similar levels of joy across social and nonsocial contexts, whereas older children showed markedly less strong joy when alone than when accompanied by an experimenter. Although older children minimized their expressions in the solitary condition, there were no differences in the reported experience of positive emotion across conditions and ages. Holodynski argues that these results support an internalization model, in which, with development, emotional experience gradually becomes less dependent on expression. For the younger children, then, the expression of joy is simultaneously internal and social, a marker both for self and other. For older children, salient expressions of joy are not necessary for the self, but the social function of communicating happiness to others remains. Specifically, the 7- and 8-year-olds' expressions showed a "miniaturization" effect that indexed the internalization of emotion.

Adult Smiles

In adults, the aspect of positive emotional facial expression that has received the most attention from researchers is the distinction between Duchenne and non-Duchenne smiles. There is empirical support for this distinction: Ekman and colleagues (1990) found that Duchenne smiles, but not other smiles, occurred more frequently during pleasant films, and that the level of Duchenne smiling was related to subjective reports of positive emotion. Observers view Duchenne smiles as happier than non-Duchenne smiles (Miles & Johnston, 2007), and electromyographic (EMG) recordings indicate greater evidence of mimicking Duchenne than non-Duchenne smiles (Surakka & Hietanen, 1998). Duchenne smiles have also been found to be smoother in onset and more symmetrical than other smiles (Frank, Ekman, & Friesen, 1993; but see Cohn & Schmidt, 2004; Soussignan & Schaal, 1996). Intense Duchenne smiles have been shown to be specifically associated with amusement (Hess, Beaupré, & Cheung, 2002).

Although multiple studies document differences in the perception of Duchenne and non-Duchenne smiles, recent work has noted other determinants of smile perception that contextualize and challenge this distinction (reviewed in Abe, Beetham, Izard, & Abel, 2002; Niedenthal, Mermillod, Maringer, & Hess, 2010). Krumhuber and Manstead (2009) found that Duchenne smiles could be produced deliberately, and that viewers relied less on whether smiles were Duchenne or not, and more on symmetry and the duration of the smile's apex, as the basis for genuineness and amusement judgments. Although static images of Duchenne smiles were perceived as more emotionally positive than non-Duchenne smiles, video clips of Duchenne smiles were not perceived as more positive than video clips of non-Duchenne smiles. This highlights the importance of investigating the dynamics of smile production to attain a more ecologically valid understanding of positive emotional expression and perception. Several studies examining contextual influence, for example, have shown that social motivation can play a greater role than positive emotional experience in determining when and how people smile (Fernández-Dols & Ruiz-Belda, 1995; Fridlund, 1991; Kraut & Johnston, 1979).

Early research indicated that smile strength is associated with the producer's feelings of pleasure (Ekman, Friesen, & Ancoli, 1980; Hess, Kappas, McHugo, Kleck, & Lanzetta, 1989) and, in video clips, with the perceiver's ratings of enjoyment (Krumhuber & Manstead, 2009). A recent pilot study of two mothers interacting with their infants also suggests that strength of smiling—the degree of contraction of *zygomaticus major*, the muscle responsible for the central smiling action—may be a central factor in adult smiling. As with infants, smile strength was associated with the intensity of eye constriction (the Duchenne marker), and with the degree of mouth opening. Smile strength had the strongest associations with continuous ratings of positive emotion (Messinger et al., 2009). The results suggest that dynamic changes in smile strength may undergird the expression of positive emotion in some contexts, but do not rule out the potential importance of a categorical distinction between Duchenne and non-Duchenne smiles (see also Messinger et al., 2012).

The Distinction between Smiling and Laughter

Homologies have been proposed between the nonhuman primate "play face" and the facial configuration associated with human laughter, as well as between the primate bared-teeth display and the human smile (van Hooff, 1972). To ascertain whether these displays occur in similar or different behavioral contexts, behaviors associated with bared-teeth displays and play faces were coded in captive chimpanzees (Waller & Dunbar, 2005). Play faces were found to occur nearly exclusively in play situations, while bared-teeth displays were used flexibly in a range of affiliative contexts, suggesting that these signals are likely rooted in different motivational complexes. The authors argued that if these expressions share phylogenetic origins with human smiling and laughing, these should also be considered two distinct behaviors.

Although smiling and laughter may have distinct phylogenetic origins and have maintained distinct functions in chimpanzees, in some species these two displays may have converged over evolutionary time because both are used in affiliative social contexts (e.g., Preuschoft & van Hooff, 1996). Mehu (2011) conducted a naturalistic observational study of laughter and smiles in adult dyadic interactions. He found that spontaneous, but not deliberate, smiles were associated with laughter, suggesting that spontaneous smiles and laughter may share a motivational basis (see also Mehu & Dunbar, 2008a, 2008b). In fact, some theorists have suggested that in the human case, smiling and laughter both express positive states that differ in intensity (Sroufe & Waters, 1976; see also Redican, 1975). In support, tickling elicits both strong open-mouth Duchenne smiling and laughter in infants, and children's levels of open-mouth Duchenne smiling are associated with their laughter levels (Sarra & Otta, 2001). Moreover, a recent report indicates that tickling can induce laughter vocalizations in both human and nonhuman primate infants and juveniles (Davila-Ross et al., 2009).

Smiles of Different Positive Emotions

Can smiling express more differentiated emotional states than simple enjoyment or happiness? Reddy and colleagues argue that infants are already capable of expressing a type of smile expression that they describe as "shy" or "coy" (e.g., Reddy, 2000). These are smiles that occur in combination with gaze and/or head aversion, and that appear to be similar to expressions of embarrassment or shyness in older children and adults (e.g., Keltner, 1995). Draghi-Lorenz, Reddy, and Morris (2005) asked unfamiliar adults to freely label expressions in 2- to 4-month-old infants from short video clips. Two of five clips that depicted infants' smiling expressions followed by gaze and/or head aversion were predominantly labeled as shyness, suggesting that infants may be perceived as expressing shy or coy smiles. However, not all smiles with gaze and/or head aversion were perceived as coy, suggesting that these smiles may be a particular type of smile that is defined by its temporal dynamics and relationship with gaze and/or head aversion (see Yale et al., 2003).

In adults, further distinctions among smile types have been tested. Ricci-Bitti, Caterina, and Garotti (1996) studied four different types of smiles that expressed sensory pleasure, joy, and elation, and a formal-unfelt smile. They found that these were well differentiated by behavioral descriptors. Sensory pleasure smiles were characterized by closed eyes in combination with a Duchenne smile, and elation smiles were marked by the upper lid being raised. In an innovative study by Campos, Shiota, Keltner, Gonzaga, and Goetz (2012), participants produced different facial expressions when asked to pose different positive emotions. Amusement typically involved a Duchenne smile and an open mouth, the same facial actions that characterize intense positive affect expression in infants. Participants posed joy with Duchenne smiles, in which the lips were parted in half of the cases, but the mouth was open in only one-third of the cases. Contentment also involved smiling—Duchenne smiling in slightly over half the cases—in which the lips tended to be pressed together. Together, these studies suggest that some positive affective states may be signaled by physically distinct smile configurations, although they do not establish whether observers are sensitive to these distinctions.

Studies examining the recognition of smiles have tended to emphasize the role of dynamic information. In one study that directly compared the perception of static and dynamic facial expressions, Fujimura and Suzuki (2010) examined calm, excited, and joyful smiles. They found that excited and happy expressions were recognized better from dynamic stimuli, whereas calm expressions were equally well recognized from static and dynamic faces. They concluded that dynamic facial expressions may communicate a greater variety of positive states than those communicated by static presentations. Another study has found an advantage for dynamic stimuli using synthesized facial expressions (Wehrle, Kaiser, Schmidt, & Scherer, 2000). Expressions of happiness, pride, elation, and sensory pleasure were included in high- and low-intensity versions. In a forced-choice task, the dynamic stimuli were better recognized than the static stimuli, and judges did particularly well with high-intensity stimuli of the different positive emotions.

A recent study that investigated both the production and perception of smiles of spontaneous amusement, embarrassment, nervousness, and politeness further highlights the importance of temporal dynamics in smiling (Ambadar, Cohn, & Reed, 2009). Examining physical cues, as well as human judgments, the authors found that viewers are able to use not only variation in morphological features, but also the dynamic characteristics of different kinds of smiles. For example, in comparison with smiles perceived to signal politeness, smiles that were perceived by viewers as amused more often included open mouth, larger smile amplitude, larger maximum onset and offset velocity, and longer duration. Taking both morphological and dynamic features into account, viewers' judgments were directly related to the physical cues that differentiated between these expressions (see also Krumhuber, Manstead, & Kappas, 2006, on the importance of dynamic cues in smile perception). Together these findings suggest that distinct smile configurations, particularly those involving dynamic cues, may index different positive emotions.

Facial Cues beyond the Smile

In adults, several positive emotions, including relief and sensual enjoyment, may not involve smiles at all (see Sauter, 2010). Early observational research on facial expressions associated with sexual excitement described configurations similar to expressions of pain (Masters & Johnson, 1966). A recent study used an ingenious approach to examine the facial configurations of individuals experiencing sexual enjoyment (Fernández-Dols, Carrera, & Crivelli, 2011). Video clips were acquired from a website of individuals who recorded their own facial behavior while masturbating to orgasm. FACS coding confirmed a similarity between sexual excitement expressions and facial configurations of pain. However, observers are able to distinguish these expressions at greater than chance levels (Hughes & Nicholson, 2008), which suggests they are subtly different. This area of research suggests that subjectively enjoyable feelings such as sexual pleasure may involve prototypical facial expressions that do not include smiling. For additional evidence, see Gonzaga, Turner, Keltner, Campos, and Altemus's (2006) differentiation of the nonverbal displays of sexual desire and romantic love.

Facial expressions of a large set of positive emotions were investigated in a recent study by Bänziger, Mortillaro, and Scherer (2012). They recorded individuals dynamically enacting the positive emotions of amusement, pride, joy, relief, interest, pleasure, admiration, and tenderness while producing nonsense speech. Comparing across emotions and modalities, recognition rates varied greatly, but all positive emotions were best recognized from audiovisual signals. Also, all positive emotions were better recognized from visual than from auditory signals. Another study FACS-coded some of the enacted facial expressions, including pride, pleasure, and joy taken from the same stimulus set (Mortillaro, Mehu, & Scherer, 2011). They found limited differentiation of the action units involved in these different positive emotions, with no differences found between pride and joy, or between interest and pleasure. However, as the actors producing the facial stimuli were producing emotional speech, their facial movements may have been limited by the strong articulatory movements of the lower face that are involved in speech production.

In contrast to findings by Mortillaro and colleagues (2011), a recent study by Krumhuber and Scherer (2011) suggests that there may be distinct facial configurations associated with different positive emotions. The study examined the facial correlates of affect bursts (see the earlier discussion of the study by Schröder, 2003) of several negative emotions, as well as joy and relief, and the stimuli consisted of a sustained vowel to avoid coarticulation. A difference was found in the facial configurations of joy and relief, with joy often shown with the prototypical Duchenne smile configuration, while prototypical relief expressions were characterized by a low-intensity action of the lip corner puller muscle that creates smiling. They concluded that a single facial expression is insufficient to capture the many meanings of positive emotions.

Conclusions on Positive Emotions in the Face

Infants are attuned to smiles very early in life, exhibiting a preference for stronger smiles. Their sensitivity to differences in the intensity of smiles appears to be shaped by their experience with caregivers, with whom they go on to develop a system of mutual smile communication. This sets the stage for the intentional communication of positive emotion. In young children, smiling is simultaneously an internal and a social marker of enjoyment, whereas in older children smiling may increasingly be used as a means of communicating happiness to others.

In early infancy, there is evidence that both smiling and positive emotion vary along a single continuum that is indexed by the strength of smiling, which in turn is linked to the strength of the Duchenne marker (eye constriction) and mouth opening. In fact, eye constriction and mouth opening also index the intensity of the prototypical negative infant expression, the cry face (Messinger et al., 2012), suggesting these two facial actions can function to mark the intensity of both positive and negative expressions. Moreover, smiling involving eye constriction and mouth opening appear to also index enjoyment in older children.

Although it is well established that smiling is highly sensitive to social context, its relationship to felt enjoyment in adulthood is still unclear. Researchers commonly utilize categorical distinctions between Duchenne and non-Duchenne smiles, and between weaker and stronger smiles, but many are increasingly employing dynamic measures of smile intensity and trajectory. These dynamic measures distinguish spontaneous and posed smiles, and show associations with perceived enjoyment. Finally, recent research has documented facial configura-

tions of sexual enjoyment and relief that do not include smiles, highlighting the possibility that facial expressions of positive emotions in adulthood are more heterogeneous than has previously been thought.

General Conclusions

Positive Emotions across Cultures

Research on positive emotion expression has been conducted primarily in a small set of culturally similar samples. Basing our knowledge on findings from Western, and often educated, participants raises concerns about the generalizability of findings (see Henrich, Heine, & Norenzayan, 2010), and limits our understanding of differences and similarities in the nonverbal expression of positive emotions across cultures. The limited cross-cultural data available suggest that culture may play a major role in shaping signals of positive emotions (see Fogel, Toda, & Kawai, 1988; Keller & Otto, 2009; Sauter, Eisner, Ekman, & Scott, 2010), but in some research domains, including touch and smile types, work with non-Western samples is sorely lacking.

Cultures vary in their orientations to different types of positive affect. For instance, Tsai, Knutson, and Fung (2006) found that European American young adults reported that they value high-arousal positive affect, whereas Asian Americans tended to value low-arousal positive affect. One avenue through which parents and caregivers can affect positive emotional expression is by engaging, or not engaging, in particular types of play with their infants (Halberstadt & Lozada, 2011). For example, peekaboo, a game that promotes positive emotion expression with high levels of arousal, is prominent in American culture (Halberstadt & Lozada, 2011). By contrast, parents in other cultures, such as the Gusii tribe in Kenya, often engage in behaviors that discourage expressions of intense affect, including positive emotions (Richman, Miller, & LeVine, 1992).

In an exciting research program, Keller and colleagues (e.g., Keller, Borke, Lamm, Lohaus, & Yovsi, 2011) are documenting the impact of cross-cultural differences in parenting behaviors on the development of positive emotional expression. In middle-class Germans, a cultural group they characterize as more independent, mothers responded to infant vocalizations with increasing amounts of contingent visual contact and greater time spent in face-to-face play over the first months of life (Kartner, Keller, & Yovsi, 2010). By contrast, among Nso farmers in Cameroon, a cultural group characterized as more interdependent, mothers responded to infant vocalizations with more body contact and fewer face-to-face interactions (Kartner et al., 2010; Keller et al., 2011). Moreover, Wörmann, Holodynski, Kärtner, and Keller (2012) found that Northern German mothers imitated their infants' smiles more and smiled at their infants longer during mutual gazing at 12 weeks of age than did Nso mothers. While the Northern German infants demonstrated levels of social smiling and imitation comparable to those of Nso infants at 6 weeks of age, they smiled longer and imitated their mothers' smiles more often during mutual gazing at 12 weeks. These findings raise the possibility that differential responsivity to infant smiling can influence the development of smiling. Careful demonstration of socialization effects on the expression of positive emotion could suggest a mechanism for cross-cultural variability in emotional displays in multiple expressive modalities.

The degree to which the development of different positive emotions is dependent on culture-specific input will be important for future research. The results of Sauter, Eisner, Ekman, and Scott (2010) suggest that the role of culture-specific social learning may be different for different positive emotions. In their study, amusement and relief vocalizations were highly similar across the two groups, and, in particular, amusement sounds were well recognized. In contrast, triumph vocalizations were very different across the groups and not bidirectionally recognized (sensual enjoyment vocalizations also were not recognized bidirectionally, but that may have been due to differences in arousal cues in the stimuli). These findings suggest that the role of social learning is likely to vary across (positive) emotions.

Considerations for Future Work

This chapter has reviewed a wide range of research on nonverbal signals of positive

emotions in different modalities and across the lifespan. This research employs many innovative approaches. Examples include automated measurement of smile intensity of interacting infants and mothers (Messinger et al., 2012) and comparisons of the development of smiling in Northern European and African contexts (Wörmann et al., 2012). Novel approaches with adults include studies of intense emotional experiences from real life, such as blind athletes' displays of pride when winning judo matches in the Paralympic Games (Tracy & Matsumoto, 2008), and the use of a website with self-recorded video materials of individuals stimulating themselves to orgasm (Fernández-Dols et al., 2011).

This review, however, also highlights a lack of continuity. In general, research on adults has emphasized perception more than production, while developmental research includes a more even balance of these domains. In particular, the literature on positive emotion expression in infants is rich with studies of the form and context of positive expressions. Infants can easily be observed in a laboratory playroom in naturalistic play with a parent, where smiling and laughter are key behaviors. Less information is available on older children and adults, although there are some studies of positive emotional expressions in ecologically valid social situations outside the laboratory (e.g., Fernández-Dols & Ruiz-Belda, 1995; Fernández-Dols et al., 2011; Kraut & Johnston, 1979). However, few studies of infants, children, or adults ask how a given individual's production and perception of positive emotion are related.

A recent account of the role of mimicry in smiling takes theoretical steps toward bridging the gap between perception and production (Niedenthal et al., 2010). These theorists argue that judgments of the genuineness of smiles vary across individuals and cultures but cannot be explained by differences in morphology. Instead, they proposed a model of smile perception that focuses on the role of embodiment and the viewers' beliefs. Guided by the model, Maringer, Krumhuber, Fischer, and Niedenthal (2011) found that participants whose mimicry was inhibited rated the genuine-looking and fake-looking smiles as equally genuine, whereas participants whose facial movement was unconstrained differentiated between them. They argued that these results, obtained using synthesized smiles on avatars as stimuli, supported the model. Future research might test whether similar effects occur in judgments of actual human smiles, and consider the role of arousal in mimicry given the recent finding that stronger zygomatic activity is elicited in response to more highly aroused smiles (Fujimura, Sato, & Suzuki, 2010).

Although time course is clearly intrinsic to vocal signals, the dynamics of expression are likely important for all expressive modalities. The need to go beyond static morphological features and consider dynamic characteristics of facial expressions is likely true of gestural and full-body expressions of positive emotion as well. However, much work remains to be done to examine expressions across multiple channels, with only a handful of studies to date considering multimodal communication of positive emotions. Such research should ideally include information on gaze direction and its temporal relationship to other signals, to more fully integrate positive emotional expressions with the social contexts that support them.

A difficult issue in investigating the production of emotional expressions is how to describe the resultant signals. The standard set of descriptors provided by the FACS system has been crucial for our understanding of facial expressions. Standard sets of descriptors for other modalities might dramatically increase comparability across studies. However, characterizing signals such as human vocalizations is enormously complex. Although phonetic transcription can be used to code speech sounds, this system is not suitable for nonverbal vocalizations. All sounds can be measured in terms of spectrotemporal cues, but there is currently no system that provides a way of mapping the physical signal to a set of categories of vocal cues relevant to emotional communication.

Existing perception research is fractionated—studies use different sets of emotions, types of signals, (age) groups, and criteria for a signal to be "recognized," which makes it difficult to compare across studies. An alternative way to provide consistency across perception studies would be use of a standardized stimulus set, or at least the inclusion of a standard set of positive emotion descriptors. Based on the research reviewed in this chapter, a tentative suggestion may be that a key set should include happiness, sensual pleasure, relief, amusement, affection, and pride.

Finally, it is worth noting that our review suggests that different emotions may be preferentially expressed via different modalities. In a recent study, participants generated nonverbal displays of 11 emotions, including happiness, pride, love, and sympathy, using face, body, and touch (App, McIntosh, Reed, & Hertenstein, 2011). Participants favored full-body expression for pride, a facial expression for happiness, and touch for love and sympathy. The authors argue that the preferred channel of communication of different emotions is connected to their functions: The full-body expression promotes social-status emotions such as pride, facial expressions supports survival emotions, and touch is utilized for intimate emotions such as love and sympathy. The extent to which these expression–emotion pairings reflect qualitatively distinct psychological categories, as opposed to a broader class of positive emotion varying in arousal, is an exciting topic for continued study.

Acknowledgments

Disa A. Sauter is supported by Veni Grant No. 275-70-033 from the Netherlands Organization for Scientific Research. Nicole M. McDonald, Devon N. Gangi, and Daniel S. Messinger are supported by National Science Foundation Grant Nos. 0808767 and 1052736, and by National Institutes of Health Grant Nos. R01HD057284 and 1R01GM105004.

References

Abe, J., Beetham, M., Izard, C., & Abel, M. H. (2002). What do smiles mean?: An analysis in terms of differential emotions theory. In M. Abel (Ed.), *An empirical reflection on the smile* (pp. 83–109). Lewinston, NY: Edwin Mellen Press.

Ambadar, Z., Cohn, J. F., & Reed, L. I. (2009). All smiles are not created equal: Morphology and timing of smiles perceived as amused, polite, and embarrassed/nervous. *Journal of Nonverbal Behavior, 33(1)*, 17–34.

Anisfeld, E., Casper, V., Nozyce, M., & Cunningham, N. (1990). Does infant carrying promote attachment?: An experimental study of the effects of increased physical contact on the development of attachment. *Child Development, 61*(5), 1617–1627.

App, B., McIntosh, D. N., Reed, C. L., & Hertenstein, M. J. (2011). Nonverbal channel use in communication of emotion: How may depend on why. *Emotion, 11*(3), 603–617.

Banse, R., & Scherer, K. R. (1996). Acoustic profiles in vocal emotion expression. *Journal of Personality and Social Psychology, 70*, 614–636.

Bänziger, T., Mortillaro, M., & Scherer, K. R. (2012). Introducing the Geneva Multimodal expression corpus for experimental research on emotion perception. *Emotion, 12*(5), 1161–1179.

Belsky, J., Domitrovich, C., & Crnic, K. (1997). Temperament and parenting antecedents of individual differences in three-year-old boys' pride and shame reactions. *Child Development, 68*(3), 456–466.

Bornstein, M. H., & Arterberry, M. E. (2003). Recognition, discrimination and categorization of smiling by 5-month-old infants. *Developmental Science, 6*(5), 585–599.

Campos, B., Shiota, M. N., Keltner, D., Gonzaga, G. C., & Goetz, J. L. (2012). What is shared, what is different?: Core relational themes and expressive displays of eight positive emotions. *Cognition and Emotion, 27*(1), 37–52.

Cecchini, M., Baroni, E., Vito, C. D., & Lai, C. (2011). Smiling in newborns during communicative wake and active sleep. *Infant Behavior and Development, 34*(3), 417–423.

Cheyne, J. A. (1976). Development of forms and functions of smiling in preschoolers. *Child Development, 47*(3), 820–823.

Cohn, J., & Schmidt, K. (2004). The timing of facial motion in posed and spontaneous smiles. *International Journal of Wavelets, Multiresolution, 2*(2), 121–132.

Cowie, R., & Cornelius, R. R. (2003). Describing the emotional states that are expressed in speech. *Speech Communication, 40*(1–2), 5–32.

Davila-Ross, M., Owren, M. J., & Zimmermann, E. (2009). Reconstructing the evolution of laughter in great apes and humans. *Current Biology, 19*(13), 1106–1111.

de Gelder, B., & Van den Stock, J. (2011). The Bodily Expressive Action Stimulus Test (BEAST): Construction and validation of a stimulus basis for measuring perception of whole body expression of emotions. *Frontiers in Psychology, 2*, 181.

Dennis, T. A., Cole, P. M., Zahn-Waxler, C., & Mizuta, I. (2002). Self in context: Autonomy and relatedness in Japanese and U.S. mother–preschooler dyads. *Child Development, 73*(6), 1803–1817.

Dickson, K. L., Walker, H., & Fogel, A. (1997). The relationship between smile-type and play-type during parent–infant play. *Developmental Psychology, 33*(6), 925–933.

Dondi, M., Messinger, D., Colle, M., Tabasso, A., Simion, F., Dalla Barba, B., et al. (2007). A new perspective on neonatal smiling: Differences between the judgments of expert coders and naive observers. *Infancy, 12*(3), 235–255.

Draghi-Lorenz, R., Reddy, V., & Morris, P. (2005). Young infants can be perceived as shy, coy, bashful, embarrassed. *Infant and Child Development, 14*(1), 63–83.

Duchenne, G. B. (1990). *The mechanism of human facial expression* (R. A. Cuthbertson, Trans.). New York: Cambridge University Press. (Original work published 1862)

Ekman, P. (1992). An argument for basic emotions. *Cognition and Emotion, 6*, 169–200.

Ekman, P., Davidson, R. J., & Friesen, W. V. (1990). The Duchenne smile: Emotional expression and brain physiology II. *Journal of Personality and Social Psychology, 58*(2), 342–353.

Ekman, P., & Friesen, W. (1978). *The Facial Action Coding System.* Palo Alto, CA: Consulting Psychologists Press.

Ekman, P., Friesen, W. V., & Ancoli, S. (1980). Facial signs of emotional experience. *Journal of Personality and Social Psychology, 39*(6), 1125–1134.

Elfenbein, H. A., & Ambady, N. (2002). On the universality and cultural specificity of emotion recognition: A meta-analysis. *Psychological Bulletin, 128*(2), 203–235.

Emde, R. N., & Koenig, K. (1969). Neonatal smiling and rapid eye movement states. *Journal of the American Academy of Child Psychiatry, 8*, 57–67.

Fernández-Dols, J. M., Carrera, P., & Crivelli, C. (2011). Facial behavior while experiencing sexual excitement. *Journal of Nonverbal Behavior, 35*(1), 63–71.

Fernández-Dols, J. M., & Ruiz-Belda, M. A. (1995). Are smiles a sign of happiness?: Gold medal winners at the Olympic Games. *Journal of Personality and Social Psychology, 69*, 1113–1119.

Fogel, A., Hsu, H.-C., Shapiro, A. F., Nelson-Goens, G. C., & Secrist, C. (2006). Effects of normal and perturbed social play on the duration and amplitude of different types of infant smiles. *Developmental Psychology, 42*, 459–473.

Fogel, A., Toda, S., & Kawai, M. (1988). Mother–infant face-to-face interaction in Japan and the United States: A laboratory comparison using 3-month-old infants. *Developmental Psychology, 24*(3), 398–406.

Fox, N., & Davidson, R. J. (1988). Patterns of brain electrical activity during facial signs of emotion in 10 month old infants. *Developmental Psychology, 24*(2), 230–236.

Fox, N. A., Henderson, H. A., Rubin, K. H., Calkins, S. D., & Schmidt, L. A. (2001). Continuity and discontinuity of behavioral inhibition and exuberance: Psychophysiological and behavioral influences across the first four years of life. *Child Development, 72*(1), 1–21.

Frank, M. G., Ekman, P., & Friesen, W. V. (1993). Behavioral markers and recognizability of the smile of enjoyment. *Journal of Personality and Social Psychology, 64*(1), 83–93.

Franklin, B., Oller, D. K., Ramsdell, H., & Jhang, Y. S. (2011, November). *Affect identification in early infant vocalizations.* Paper presented at the American Speech–Language–Hearing Association, San Diego, CA.

Fridlund, A. J. (1991). Sociality of solitary smiling: Potentiation by an implicit audience. *Journal of Personality and Social Psychology, 60*(2), 229–240.

Fujimura, T., Sato, W., & Suzuki, N. (2010). Facial expression arousal level modulates facial mimicry. *International Journal of Psychophysiology, 76*(2), 88–92.

Fujimura, T., & Suzuki, N. (2010). Effects of dynamic information in recognising facial expressions on dimensional and categorical judgments. *Perception, 39*(4), 543–552.

Goldsmith, H. H., & Rothbart, M. K. (1999). *The Laboratory Temperament Assessment Battery* (Locomotor Version, Edition 3.1). Madison: University of Wisconsin–Madison.

Gonzaga, G. C., Keltner, D., Londahl, E. A., & Smith, M. D. (2001). Love and the commitment problem in romantic relations and friendship. *Journal of Personality and Social Psychology, 81*(2), 247–262.

Gonzaga, G. C., Turner, R. A., Keltner, D., Campos, B., & Altemus, M. (2006). Romantic love and sexual desire in close relationships. *Emotion, 6*(2), 163–179.

Halberstadt, A. G., & Lozada, F. T. (2011). Emotion development in infancy through the lens of culture. *Emotion Review, 3*(2), 158–168.

Hane, A., Fox, N. A., Henderson, H. A., & Marshall, P. J. (2008). Behavioral reactivity and approach–withdrawal bias in infancy. *Developmental Psychology, 44*(5), 1491–1496.

Hawk, S. T., Van Kleef, G. A., Fischer, A. H., & van der Schalk, J. (2009). "Worth a thousand words": Absolute and relative decoding of nonlinguistic affect vocalizations. *Emotion, 9*(3), 293–305.

Henrich, J., Heine, S. J., & Norenzayan, A. (2010). The weirdest people in the world? *Behavioural and Brain Sciences, 33*(2–3), 61–83.

Hertenstein, M. J., Holmes, R., McCullough, M., & Keltner, D. (2009). The communication of emotion via touch. *Emotion, 9*(4), 566–573.

Hertenstein, M. J., & Keltner, D. (2010). Gender and the communication of emotion via touch. *Sex Roles, 64*(1–2), 70–80.

Hertenstein, M. J., Keltner, D., App, B., Bulleit, B. A., & Jaskolka, A. R. (2006). Touch communicates distinct emotions. *Emotion, 6*(3), 528–533.

Hess, U., Beaupré, M., & Cheung, N. (2002). Who to whom and why—cultural differences and similarities in the function of smiles. In M. Abel (Ed.), *An empirical reflection on the smile* (pp. 187–216). New York: Edwin Mellen Press.

Hess, U., Kappas, A., McHugo, G. J., Kleck, R. E., & Lanzetta, J. T. (1989). An analysis of the encoding and decoding of spontaneous and posed smiles: The use of facial electromyography. *Journal of Nonverbal Behavior, 13*(2), 121–137.

Holodynski, M. (2004). The miniaturization of expression in the development of emotional self-regulation. *Developmental Psychology, 40*(1), 16–28.

Hughes, S. M., & Nicholson, S. E. (2008). Sex differences in the assessment of pain versus sexual pleasure facial expressions. Special Issue: Proceedings of the 2nd Annual Meeting of the NorthEastern Evolutionary Psychology Society. *Journal of Social, Evolutionary, and Cultural Psychology, 2*(4), 289–298

Juslin, P. N., & Laukka, P. (2003). Communication of emotions in vocal expression and music performance: Different channels, same code? *Psychological Bulletin, 129*(5), 770–814.

Kahana-Kalman, R., & Walker-Andrews, A. S. (2001). The role of person familiarity in young infants' perception of emotional expressions. *Child Development, 72*(2), 352–369.

Kartner, J., Keller, H., & Yovsi, R. D. (2010). Mother–infant interaction during the first 3 months: The emergence of culture-specific contingency patterns. *Child Development, 81*(2), 540–554.

Keller, H., Borke, J., Lamm, B., Lohaus, A., & Yovsi, R. D. (2011). Developing patterns of parenting in two cultural communities. *International Journal of Behavioral Development, 35*(3), 233–239.

Keller, H., & Otto, H. (2009). The cultural socialization of emotion regulation during infancy. *Journal of Cross-Cultural Psychology, 40*(6), 996–1011.

Keltner, D. (1995). Signs of appeasement: Evidence for the distinct displays of embarrassment, amusement, and shame. *Journal of Personality and Social Psychology, 68*(3), 441–454.

Kraus, M. W., Huang, C., & Keltner, D. (2010). Tactile communication, cooperation, and performance: An ethological study of the NBA. *Emotion, 10*(5), 745–749.

Kraut, R. E., & Johnston, R. E. (1979). Social and emotional messages of smiling: An ethological approach. *Journal of Personality and Social Psychology, 37*(9), 1539–1553.

Krumhuber, E., & Manstead, A. S. (2009). Can Duchenne smiles be feigned?: New evidence on felt and false smiles. *Emotion, 9*(6), 807–820.

Krumhuber, E., Manstead, A. S. R., & Kappas, A. (2006). Temporal aspects of facial displays in person and expression perception: The effects of smile dynamics, head-tilt, and gender. *Journal of Nonverbal Behavior, 31*(1), 39–56.

Krumhuber, E. G., & Scherer, K. R. (2011). Affect bursts: Dynamic patterns of facial expression. *Emotion, 11*(4), 825–841.

Kuchuk, A., Vibbert, M., & Bornstein, M. H. (1986). The perception of smiling and its experiential correlates in three-month-old infants. *Child Development, 57*(4), 1054–1061.

Landau, R. (1989). Affect and attachment: Kissing, hugging, and patting as attachment behaviors. *Infant Mental Health Journal, 10*(1), 59–69.

Lavelli, M., & Fogel, A. (2005). Developmental changes in the relationship between the infant's attention and emotion during early face-to-face communication: The 2-month transition. *Developmental Psychology, 41*(1), 265–280.

Lewis, M., Takai-Kawakami, K., Kawakami, K., & Sullivan, M. W. (2010). Cultural differences in emotional responses to success and failure. *International Journal of Behavioral Development, 34*(1), 53–61.

Maringer, M., Krumhuber, E. G., Fischer, A. H., & Niedenthal, P. M. (2011). Beyond smile dynamics: Mimicry and beliefs in judgments of smiles. *Emotion, 11*(1), 181–187.

Masters, W., & Johnson, V. (1966). *Human sexual response.* Boston: Little, Brown.

Mehu, M. (2011). Smiling and laughter in naturally occurring dyadic interactions: Relationship to conversation, body contacts, and displacement activities. *Human Ethology Bulletin, 26*(1), 10–28.

Mehu, M., & Dunbar, R. I. M. (2008a). Naturalistic observations of smiling and laughter in human group interactions. *Behaviour, 145*(12), 1747–1780.

Mehu, M., & Dunbar, R. I. M. (2008b). Relationship between smiling and laughter in humans *(Homo sapiens)*: Testing the power asymmetry hypothesis. *Folia Primatologica, 79*(5), 269–280.

Messinger, D., Dondi, M., Nelson-Goens, G. C., Beghi, A., Fogel, A., & Simion, F. (2002). How sleeping neonates smile. *Developmental Science, 5*(1), 48–54.

Messinger, D., & Fogel, A. (2007). The interactive development of social smiling. *Advances in Child Development and Behavior, 35,* 328–366.

Messinger, D., Fogel, A., & Dickson, K. (2001). All smiles are positive, but some smiles are more positive than others. *Developmental Psychology, 37*(5), 642–653.

Messinger, D., & Freedman, D. G. (1992). Autonomy and interdependence in Japanese and American mother–toddler dyads. *Early Development and Parenting, 1*(1), 33–38.

Messinger, D., Mahoor, M., Chow, S., & Cohn, J. F. (2009). Automated measurement of facial expression in infant–mother interaction: A pilot study. *Infancy, 14,* 285–305.

Messinger, D. S., Mattson, W. I., Mahoor, M. H., & Cohn, J. F. (2012). The eyes have it: Making positive expressions more positive and negative expressions more negative. *Emotion, 12*(3), 430–436.

Miles, L., & Johnston, L. (2007). Detecting happiness: Perceiver sensitivity to enjoyment and non-enjoyment smiles. *Journal of Nonverbal Behavior, 31*(4), 259–275.

Montague, D. P. F., & Walker-Andrews, A. S. (2001). Peekaboo: A new look at infants' perception of emotion expressions. *Developmental Psychology, 37*(6), 826–838.

Montague, D. P. F., & Walker-Andrews, A. S. (2002). Mothers, fathers, and infants: The role of person familiarity and parental involvement in infants' perception of emotion expressions. *Child Development, 73*(5), 1339–1352.

Mortillaro, M., Mehu, M., & Scherer, K. R. (2011). Subtly different positive emotions can be distinguished by their facial expressions. *Social Psychological and Personality Science, 2*(3), 262–271.

Moszkowski, R. J., & Stack, D. M. (2007). Infant touching behaviour during mother–infant face-to-face interactions. *Infant and Child Development, 16*(3), 307–319.

Niedenthal, P. M., Mermillod, M., Maringer, M., & Hess, U. (2010). The Simulation of Smiles (SIMS) model: Embodied simulation and the meaning of facial expression. *Behavioral and Brain Sciences, 33*(6), 417–433.

Nwokah, E., & Fogel, A. (1993). Laughter in mother–infant emotional communication. *Humor: International Journal of Humor Research, 6*(2),137–161.

Nwokah, E., Hsu, H., Davies, P., & Fogel, A. (1999). The integration of laughter and speech in vocal communication: A dynamic systems perspective. *Journal of Speech and Hearing Research, 42*, 880–894.

Nwokah, E. E., Hsu, H. C., Dobrowolska, O., & Fogel, A. (1994). The development of laughter in mother–infant communication: Timing parameters and temporal sequences. *Infant Behavior and Development, 17*(1), 23–35.

Oster, H. (1978). Facial expression and affect development. In M. Lewis & L. A. Rosenblum (Eds.), *The development of affect* (pp. 43–74). New York: Plenum Press.

Oster, H. (2006). *Baby FACS: Facial Action Coding System for Infants and Young Children.* Unpublished monograph and coding manual, New York University.

Oveis, C., Gruber, J., Keltner, D., Stamper, J. L., & Boyce, W. T. (2009). Smile intensity and warm touch as thin slices of child and family affective style. *Emotion, 9*(4), 544–548.

Parlade, M. V., Messinger, D. S., van Hecke, A., Kaiser, M., Delgado, C., & Mundy, P. (2009). Anticipatory smiling: Linking early affective communication and social outcome. *Infant Behavior and Development, 32*, 33–43.

Pell, M. D., Monetta, L., Paulmann, S., & Kotz, S. A. (2009). Recognizing emotions in a foreign language. *Journal of Nonverbal Behavior, 33*(2), 107–120.

Preuschoft, S., & van Hooff, J. A. (1996). Homologizing primate facial displays: A critical review of methods. *Folia Primatologica, 65*, 121–137.

Reddy, V. (2000). Coyness in early infancy. *Developmental Science, 3*(2), 186–192.

Redican, W. K. (1975). Facial expressions in nonhuman primates. In L. A. Rosenblum (Ed.), *Primate behavior: Developments in field and laboratory research* (Vol. 4, pp. 103–194). New York: Academic Press.

Ricci-Bitti, P., Caterina, R., & Garotti, P. (1996). Different behavioral markers in different smiles. In N. H. Frijda (Ed.), *Proceedings of the Eighth Conference of the International Society for Research on Emotions* (pp. 297–301). Storrs, CT: ISRE Publications.

Richman, A. L., Miller, P. M., & LeVine, R. A. (1992). Cultural and educational variations in maternal responsiveness. *Developmental Psychology, 28*(4), 614–621.

Sarra, S., & Otta, E. (2001). Different types of smiles and laughter in preschool children. *Psychological Reports, 89*(3), 547–558.

Sauter, D. (2006). *An investigation into vocal expressions of emotions: The roles of valence, culture and acoustic factors.* PhD thesis, University College London.

Sauter, D. (2010). Are positive vocalizations perceived as communicating happiness across cultural boundaries? *Communicative and Integrative Biology, 3*(5), 440–442.

Sauter, D. A., Eisner, F., Calder, A. J., & Scott, S. K. (2010). Perceptual cues in non-verbal vocal expressions of emotion. *Quarterly Journal of Experimental Psychology, 63*(11), 2251–2272.

Sauter, D. A., Eisner, F., Ekman, P., & Scott, S. K. (2010). Cross-cultural recognition of basic emotions through nonverbal emotional vocalizations. *Proceedings of the National Academy of Sciences of the United States of America, 107*(6), 2408–2412.

Sauter, D. A., Panattoni, C., & Happé, F. (2013). Children's recognition of emotions from vocal cues. *British Journal of Developmental Psychology, 31*(1), 97–113.

Sauter, D. A., & Scott, S. K. (2007). More than one kind of happiness: Can we recognize vocal expressions of different positive states? *Motivation and Emotion, 31*(3), 192–199.

Scherer, K. (1994). Affect bursts. In S. van Goozen, N. van de Poll, & J. Sergeant (Eds.), *Emotions: Essays on emotion theory* (pp. 161–196). Hillsdale: NJ: Erlbaum.

Scherer, K. R. (1986). Vocal affect expression: A review and a model for future research. *Psychological Bulletin, 99*(2), 143–165.

Scherer, K. R., Banse, R., & Wallbott, H. G. (2001).Emotion inferences from vocal expression correlate across languages and cultures. *Journal of Cross-Cultural Psychology, 32,* 76–92.

Schneider, K., & Josephs, I. (1991). The expressive and communicative functions of preschool children's smiles in an achievement-situation. *Journal of Nonverbal Behavior, 15*(3), 185–198.

Schneider, K., & Uzner, L. (1992). Preschoolers' attention and emotion in an achievement and an effect game: A longitudinal study. *Cognition and Emotion, 6*(1), 37–63.

Schröder, M. (2003). Experimental study of affect bursts. *Speech Communication, 40*(1–2), 99–116.

Simon-Thomas, E. R., Keltner, D. J., Sauter, D., Sinicropi-Yao, L., & Abramson, A. (2009). The voice conveys specific emotions: Evidence from vocal burst displays. *Emotion, 9*(6), 838–846.

Soussignan, R., & Schaal, B. (1996). Forms and social signal value of smiles associated with pleasant and unpleasant sensory experience. *Ethology, 102*(8), 1020–1041.

Sroufe, A., & Waters, E. (1976). The ontogenesis of smiling and laughter: A perspective on the organization of development in infancy. *Psychological Review, 83*(3), 173–189.

Surakka, V., & Hietanen, J. K. (1998). Facial and emotional reactions to Duchenne and non-Duchenne smiles. *International Journal of Psychophysiology, 29*(1), 23–33.

Symons, D., & Moran, G. (1994). Responsiveness and dependency are different aspects of social contingencies: An example from mother and infant smiles. *Infant Behavior and Development, 17*(2), 209–214.

Tracy, J., Robins, R., & Lagattuta, K. (2005). Can children recognize pride? *Emotion, 5*(3), 251–257.

Tracy, J. L., & Matsumoto, D. (2008). The spontaneous expression of pride and shame: Evidence for biologically innate nonverbal displays. *Proceedings of the National Academy of Sciences USA, 105*(33), 11655–11660.

Tracy, J. L., & Robins, R. W. (2007). The prototypical pride expression: Development of a nonverbal behavior coding system. *Emotion, 7*(4), 789–801.

Tracy, J. L., & Robins, R. W. (2008). The nonverbal expression of pride: Evidence for cross-cultural recognition. *Journal of Personality and Social Psychology, 94*(3), 516–530.

Trouvain, J., & Barry, W. (2000). The prosody of excitement in horse race commentaries. In R. Cowie, E. Douglas-Cowie, & M. Schröder (Eds.), *Proceedings of the International Speech Communication Association Workshop on Speech and Emotion* (pp. 86–91). Belfast, UK: Textflow.

Tsai, J. L., Knutson, B., & Fung, H. H. (2006). Cultural variation in affect valuation. *Journal of Personality and Social Psychology, 90*(2), 288–307.

van Hooff, J. (1972). A comparative approach to the phylogeny of laughter and smile. In R. Hinde (Ed.), *Nonverbal communication* (pp. 209–241). Cambridge, UK: Cambridge University Press.

Venezia, M., Messinger, D. S., Thorp, D., & Mundy, P. (2004). The development of anticipatory smiling. *Infancy, 6*(3), 397–406.

Walker-Andrews, A. S. (1997). Infants' perception of expressive behaviors: Differentiation of multimodal information. *Psychological Bulletin, 121*(3), 437–456.

Waller, B. M., & Dunbar, R. I. M. (2005). Differential behavioural effects of silent bared teeth display and relaxed open mouth display in chimpanzees (*Pan troglodytes*). *Ethology, 111*(2), 129–142.

Washburn, R. W. (1929). A study of the smiling and laughing of infants in the first year of life. *Genetic Psychology Monographs, 5*(5–6), 397–537.

Wehrle, T., Kaiser, S., Schmidt, S., & Scherer, K. R. (2000). Studying the dynamics of emotional expression using synthesized facial muscle movements. *Journal of Personality and Social Psychology, 78*(1), 105–119.

Weiss, S. J., Wilson, P., Hertenstein, M. J., & Campos, R. (2000). The tactile context of a mother's caregiving: Implications for attachment of low birth weight infants. *Infant Behavior and Development, 23*(1), 91–111.

Wörmann, V., Holodynski, M., Kärtner, J., & Keller, H. (2012). A cross-cultural comparison of the development of the social smile: A longitudinal study of maternal and infant imitation in 6- and 12-week-old infants. *Infant Behavior and Development, 35*(3), 335–347.

Yale, M. E., Messinger, D. S., & Cobo-Lewis, A. B. (2003). The temporal coordination of early infant communication. *Developmental Psychology, 39*(5), 815–824.

PART III

Social Perspectives
and Individual Differences

CHAPTER 11

Positive Emotions, Social Cognition, and Intertemporal Choice

Piercarlo Valdesolo
David DeSteno

The impact of positive emotions on social cognition has received increasing attention over the past decade. It is quite clear that the experience of such emotions influences the way we process information about the social environment. Pride, for example, has been shown automatically to cue evaluations of higher status and dominance (Tracy, Shariff, Zhao, & Heinrich, 2013); similarly, happiness has been found to impact moral decision making (Valdesolo & DeSteno, 2006) and to increase the use of stereotypical information (Bodenhausen, Kramer, & Süsser, 1994). Other chapters in this volume address a variety of specific influences, as well as mechanisms by which discrete positive emotions shape thought and behavior. Here, we focus on a narrow aspect of social cognition that we think unifies many positive emotions in terms of function, and has the potential to bridge existing theories of social cognition, person perception, and morality.

Specifically, we are interested in the influence of positive emotions on "intertemporal choice," by which we mean decisions that have different consequences as time unfolds. We propose that positive emotions function

in large part to motivate adaptive intertemporal choice, delaying immediate rewards for the possibility of long-term rewards. They do this by enhancing an individual's "social value" (defined as the value others in a social group ascribe to an individual as an interaction partner) through the motivation of behaviors and decisions that cultivate perceptions of *warmth* and *competence*—two basic dimensions of person perception (Fiske, Cuddy, & Glick, 2007). If one adopts a definition of moral systems as those characterized by cooperative and flourishing social life (cf. Haidt & Kesebir, 2010), then this perspective on positive emotions has direct implications for theories of morality and, specifically, moral emotions.

Intertemporal Choice

Humans are constantly faced with important *intertemporal choices*. Whether these involve deciding how much of a paycheck to contribute to a retirement fund, how often to visit the doctor, how to establish and maintain a healthy diet and exercise routine, or how to work through relationship problems, we are presented with decisions that on the one hand offer immediate gains, but on the other hold the potential for greater future gains. Researchers across several disciplines agree that effectively balancing these competing gains has important adaptive consequences (DeSteno, 2009; Frank, 1988; Laibson, 1997; Loewenstein, Read, & Baumeister, 2003).

How do we solve these difficult dilemmas? Rational choice models tend to locate the solution in individuals' ability to weigh consciously the corresponding options, and to make a decision that maximizes benefits. We calculate, for example, the utility we would gain from contributing a default saving rate of 3% of our salary to our 401(k) against other options, such as contributing the maximum amount that will be matched by our employer (say, 50 cents on the dollar for up to 6% of salary), or just the maximum amount allowable. Once this cost–benefit analysis has been conducted, the output informs our choice.

However, decades of research have demonstrated that fundamental biases involved in these kinds of analyses prevent rational calculus. Most importantly, the literature on temporal discounting (Ainslie, 1975; Loewenstein & Thaler, 1989) has shown how estimates of value distort over time. The value of $3,000 received today does not feel the same as $3,000 to be received 40 years from now (all else being equal). Such a bias often leads people to prefer immediate gains relative to gains that unfold over time. Spending money now would be more enjoyable than saving for retirement. Hitting the snooze button feels a lot better than getting ready for work, and we have yet to come across a heart-healthy grapefruit that smells like bacon. Now is better than later. This is the case even when future gains are potentially greater than immediate gains. This can be problematic, since so many adaptive decision-making strategies require the ability to delay immediate gratification for the sake of long-term success.

What underlies this bias? Theorizing and empirical research in psychology, neuroscience, and behavioral economics have offered one answer: Short-term rewards are preferred because of the *intuitive* appeal of immediate gratification, and long-term rewards are discounted because their appeal is rooted in more abstract and *controlled* calculations (Laibson, 1997). Now *equals* emotion. Later *equals* reason. Neuroimaging studies have supported this dual-process model of decision making, wherein intuitive and controlled systems operate in tandem and compete to determine which option in intertemporal choice paradigms people prefer (McClure, Laibson, Loewenstein, & Cohen, 2004). People who manage to save for the long term, who can pass on dessert if they are trying to lose weight, and who can suffer through the slings and arrows of fights with partners for the sake of the relationship are stifling the influence of their emotions, which scream out to buy that new iPad, order a brownie sundae, and leave that guy after the first rocky patch. It is easy to see how this explanation is rooted in the rationalist tradition of decision making. People might not always make optimal intertemporal decisions, *but when they do* it is because they have been able to suppress or ignore their emotions. How, exactly, are people able to pull off such a feat?

If you have paid attention to popular coverage of psychological research over the past several years, you are likely familiar with this answer. You might even be tempted to conclude that in solving this riddle, psychologists have finally uncovered the secret of predicting professional success, life satisfaction, and morality: It's in aisle three of your local supermarket, between the chocolate chips and the all-purpose flour. Marshmallows. Indeed, if you have not yet invested in a bag of these alluring treats, and administered the now-famous marshmallow test to all the children in your life whose future you hold dear, then you are seriously jeopardizing their careers and relationships. The task could not be simpler. Present each child with the following intertemporal choice: one marshmallow now or two marshmallows later. Can they resist temptation? Can they exert *self-control* over their deep-seated mallow-lust and sacrifice short-term pleasure for a greater long-term gain?

This capacity to exert self-control or engage in regulatory processes has been shown to predict a wide range of positive life outcomes, including academic achievement and professional success (Ayduk et al., 2000; Eigsti et al., 2006; Mischel, Shoda, & Peake, 1988; Mischel, Shoda, & Rodriguez, 1989;

Shoda, Mischel, & Peake, 1990). Indeed, self-regulation is thought to be the primary way in which controlled systems tamp down the cravings of the immediate reward system (Berns, Laibson, & Loewenstein, 2007). In the standard account, self-control is a top-down process whereby areas of the brain involved in higher-order cognitive control moderate the influence of areas of the brain involved in emotional responding. The message from decision science over the past several decades has been that if people want to become less shortsighted and start making more adaptive intertemporal decisions, they should control their emotions.

The perspective that self-control processes help stifle intuitive systems and facilitate decisions in line with higher-order reasoning has been further supported by studies that demonstrate how emotional responses to various types of moral transgressions can lead to inconsistent moral decisions (Greene, Nystrom, Engell, Darley, & Cohen, 2004; Greene, Sommerville, Nystrom, Darley, & Cohen, 2001). The well-known "trolley dilemmas" are illustrative. Participants must decide whether they would be willing to take action that would involve inflicting a direct or indirect harm on an innocent individual in order to save the lives of five others. Typically, participants are willing to inflict indirect harm to make this tradeoff (not an emotionally evocative decision), but they are not willing to inflict a direct harm (an emotionally evocative decision). This has been taken as evidence of the way in which emotions disrupt the consistent application of moral principles. Furthermore, those who are able to make consistent moral decisions across these two dilemmas show increased activity in brain areas responsible for cognitive control (Greene et al., 2001, 2004). Again, controlling and regulating emotions allow for optimal decision making.

Indeed, the ability to control emotional responding successfully and make intertemporal tradeoffs has become inextricably linked with the topic of morality in other ways as well. Many of the emotionally evocative aspects of decisions have been defined as "selfish." We desire a personal pleasure (marshmallows, sex, money) and we need to control the urge to satisfy that desire in order to act in ways that take others' perspectives, wants, and desires into account.

So self-control is not only the path to long-term success but also the path to morality. Emotion = now = selfishness. Reason = later = selflessness.

This perspective sits well within certain philosophical and religious traditions in which temperance and the ability to curb one's "animalistic" desires are next to godliness (Plato, 1949; Solomon, 1993). It does not fit so well within a growing body of research in affective science.

Emotion and Intertemporal Tradeoffs

We do not intend to argue against the importance of "self-control" (as defined in this body of work) in aiding adaptive intertemporal choice or predicting important life outcomes, and we admire the methodological elegance and predictive validity of paradigms such as the marshmallow test, as well as the utility of hypotheticals such as the trolley dilemmas. Indeed, we agree with the spirit of these lines of inquiry. Often, impulses geared toward immediate gains need to be controlled in order to act in ways that are socially acceptable, as well as conducive to our well-being. It is clear that there are decisions and stimuli in our current environments that our intuitions are ill-equipped to confront, and in these cases a healthy dose of self-control is desirable. Though a strong taste for sweets may have served our species well when calories were hard to come by, we are now better served by having the cognitive wherewithal to avoid gobbling down as many Twinkies as can fit in our grocery bags.

However, this emphasis on conscious control in models of intertemporal choice may hinge on the way decision scientists have constructed such choices. It may be that these paradigms reflect only a subset of the kinds of decisions in which humans face intertemporal tradeoffs, with important adaptive consequences. Consequently, they elicit only a subset of the kinds of emotional responses that guide decision making. As such, the emphasis these paradigms place on self-control as an index of the ability to successfully trade immediate gains for greater future gains, and the "emotion = now" conclusion that logically follows, may be an artifact of the methodology.

In decision science, the study of intertemporal choice is defined as the study of the relative value people place on payoffs that unfold at different points in time. Such theories posit that participants consciously weigh the short- and long-term value of possible actions on the way to making a choice. Studies that have investigated the role of emotions in intertemporal decisions have used choices that elicit particular types of emotional responses—such as desires for food, sex, and money—that may be uniquely focused on short-term gains. In order to draw conclusions about the relative import of emotion and conscious deliberation in promoting adaptive intertemporal outcomes, one must ask whether these choices are representative of the kinds of intertemporal dilemmas in which people typically find themselves. If they are representative, and if emotional states elicited across varied situations and by varied targets consistently motivate approach behavior toward immediate gains, it would be reasonable to conclude that regulation of emotions tends to promote long-term benefits. But do emotions always have this effect?

Such a conceptualization of the range and utility of emotional responses represents an oversimplification of the complexity of emotional states, and of their relationship to adaptive intertemporal choice. Emotions ≠ now, emotions = now *and* later. This is a fundamental error that threatens to take hold in the field of decision science. A more nuanced account reveals just how central emotions are to optimal navigation of intertemporal tradeoffs.

Before we describe the import of emotions in models of intertemporal choice, it is important to define what *we* mean by such choices. For our purposes, these choices simply hold consequences that differentially unfold over time. This is distinct from defining such choices as those that require an individual to consciously weigh two options at any given time. For example, we would define the decision of whether or not to help a friend in need as an "intertemporal choice," since it has both a potential short-term gain (to avoid incurring the cost of expending time and energy on helping) and a long-term gain (potential reciprocity, strengthening of social bond). If the adap-

tive value of the latter is greater than that of the former, processes that motivate helping would promote adaptive intertemporal choice (e.g., emotions that motivate immediate costly helping and have the consequence of ultimately strengthening a bond). In other definitions of intertemporal choice, individuals must consciously weigh the value of each consequence (e.g., spending time but strengthening a bond), then decide on a course of action. Processes that motivate the choice with the most adaptive value would promote adaptive intertemporal decisions (e.g., regulating the desire to avoid expending energy for the *expectation* of a stronger bond).

Adopting this definition, any demonstration that emotions consistently motivate behavior whose effect is to incur short-term costs and reap long-term benefits would support the role of emotion in promoting adaptive intertemporal choice. Advocates of the self-control perspective might suggest that this function is precisely what emotions are incapable of accomplishing, and that pursuit of long-term goals, including an appreciation of the adaptive importance of maintaining mutually beneficial social contacts, is the role of conscious reasoning. This is an empirical question. Is there support for the idea that distinct emotional states help accrue long-term adaptive benefits? In the coming sections we argue that emotions do this quite often, and that positive emotions play a uniquely important role in this process.

Emotions and Long-Term Social Benefits

The idea that emotions have evolved to be responsive to long-term concerns is not new. Adam Smith (1790/1976) suggested that the "moral sentiments" are essential in the formation of stable exchange relationships, which bring payoffs to the self over time. Trivers's (1971) original formulation of the processes underlying the emergence of reciprocal altruism theorized that emotions are the mediators of cooperative behavior. More recently, Frank (1988) has argued that emotions serve as commitment devices. An important part of building relationships is overcoming the worry that one will expend time and resources building a relationship, only to receive little or nothing in return. For instance, when deciding whether to enter into a social exchange or economic partnership, one must determine how likely the other person is to uphold his or her end of the bargain. Frank argues that emotions motivate individuals to engage in behaviors that commit them to incur short-term costs for the possibilities of the long-term benefits associated with mutually beneficial relationships.

All of these theories provide conceptual models for the plausibility of emotion-guided decisions that forego short-term gains and accrue long-term gains. The crux of these ideas are alive most notably in modern-day theories of functionalism (Keltner, Haidt, & Shiota, 2006), which argue that emotional states have evolved, at least in part, because they increase the probability and efficiency of adaptive responding (Barrett, Mesquita, Ochsner, & Gross, 2007; Keltner & Haidt, 1999).

Much of this past work has focused on the adaptive function of emotional states that respond to immediate concerns in the physical world. Disgust protects against exposure to, and ingestion of, potential contaminants. Fear motivates withdrawal from threats to physical safety. Anger helps remove obstacles to goal attainment. But adaptive decisions entail responding appropriately not only to the physical environment but also the social environment. The unique challenges presented from interacting with other humans have exerted strong selection pressure on the structure and function of emotional states.

Of primary importance is the ability to establish and maintain strong social networks that allow individuals to capitalize on the non-zero-sum logic of reciprocal exchange, as well as the protection and safety that group living affords. Indeed, these two long-term benefits are typically offered as rationales for the deep-seated desire to establish and maintain relationships with others (Baumeister & Leary, 1995; Campbell, 1983), as well as the serious negative consequences that accompany the lack of meaningful social connections. (Cacioppo, Hawkley, & Berntson, 2003; Williams, Case, & Govan, 2003). Emotions that motivate behavior ensuring long-term safety through these means are "functional"

in the same way as emotional states that motivate behavior geared toward immediate safety.

Given this, the question of how to embed oneself within a social network becomes imperative. How does one become a valued and important member of a community? What are the characteristics necessary to be considered a desirable interaction partner? Successfully adapting to the social environment requires developing such characteristics. A compelling, and growing, body of literature in person perception and social cognition suggests a simple answer to this question. Social value, and the adaptive benefits that accompany such status, can be secured through demonstrating *warmth* and *competence*.

Warmth and Competence as Social Value

Judgments of warmth and competence underlie our perceptions of others, driving our emotional and behavioral responses (Fiske et al., 2007). These dimensions reflect categories of sociality that are both basic and adaptive: the need to anticipate actors' intentions toward oneself (warmth: morality, trustworthiness, friendliness, kindness), and the need to anticipate actors' ability to act on their intentions (competence: efficacy, skill, creativity, competence, intelligence).

These have been identified as basic dimensions of person perception throughout much of the literature in social cognition, though they have taken on different labels depending on the particular theory. For example, Rosenberg, Nelson, and Vivekananthan (1968) instructed participants to sort into categories 64 trait words that were likely to be found in another person. These participants generated two orthogonal dimensions of person perception: *intellectual good–bad* (defined by traits such as determined, industrious, skillful, intelligent), and *social good–bad* (defined by traits such as warm, honest, helpful, sincere)—two dimensions that are strikingly similar to *warmth* and *competence*. Recent research in face perception has also demonstrated the ease and speed with which participants judge *trustworthiness* and *competence* from exposure to faces (Todorov, Pakrashi, & Oosterhof, 2009; Willis & Todorov, 2006). Again, these two dimensions overlap significantly, if not completely, with warmth and competence.

While warmth seems to be valued more than competence, communicating both warmth and competence elicits primarily admiration from others (Cuddy, Fiske, & Glick, 2008). In other words, the balance between these two dimensions of the self optimizes social value. Warmth without competence elicits pity; competence without warmth elicits envy; and contempt and disgust are felt for those who demonstrate neither (Cuddy et al., 2008). If cultivating these characteristics is the key to maintaining social value, and if social value predicts long-term well-being, then a functionalist account of emotions would predict that emotional states guide behavior and decisions in ways that shape these characteristics. Indeed, we believe that positive emotions motivate behaviors and decisions that cultivate and communicate a balance between warmth and competence.

Although, as we mentioned in the outset of this chapter, much attention in social cognition has been paid to the way that positive emotions influence information processing, less attention has been paid to the way in which the experience of positive emotions shapes the way others process information about the self. This may be a crucial component of their adaptive value.

Cultivating Warmth and Competence through Positive Emotions

While many negatively valenced emotions (anger, fear, disgust) seem geared toward removing or withdrawing the person from immediate threats to well-being, positive emotions are thought to motivate the development of "resources" whose payoffs to the self will unfold over time (Frederickson, 2001; Frederickson & Branigan, 2005). Specifically, positive emotions help people to develop four kinds of resources: social (establishing and solidifying bonds), physical (developing coordination and health), intellectual (learning and developing problem-solving skills), and psychological (cultivating resilience and goal-orientation). "Social" resources as defined here seem to map closely onto the dimension of warmth, while physical, intellectual, and psychological resources map more directly onto competence.

We believe that all of the long-term positive outcomes described by these theories ultimately contribute to an individual's social value through the cultivation of characteristics related to warmth and competence. Therefore, we suggest that the ultimate function of positive emotions is to create this value via accumulation of these resources. Conceiving of their function in this way allows modern theories of functionalism and positive emotions to synergize with decades of research in person perception and social cognition. The resources that positive emotions "broaden and build" create adaptive social value by cultivating warmth and competence. In this way, positive emotions motivate adaptive intertemporal decisions, incurring short-term costs for the long-term gains associated with the perception of these traits.

Of particular importance to theories of intertemporal choice, demonstrating warmth and honing competence often requires the delay of immediate gratification. Consider reciprocity, a crucial component of developing warmth. After receiving a benefit from another and being subsequently asked a favor in return, one might be tempted to refuse. After all, doing so would be the optimal short-term strategy—resources would have been acquired without any immediate costs. How can one resist this temptation?

Consider also perseverance, a crucial component of developing competence. When faced with the decision of whether to continue working or practicing, to turn on the television, or to take a nap, short-term logic would demand the latter. How do we resist televised marathons of *The Wire* when papers need to be written? We argue that these long-term tradeoffs are not predicted by controlled processes but by the effect of positive emotions. These states seem to be particularly effective means of achieving the same long-term goals that many decision scientists assign to self-control. If this is the case, if many of the adaptive intertemporal choices we make are mediated by the experience of positive emotional states, then this casts doubt on the simplistic dichotomy of emotion = now and reason = later that has been emphasized in much of the literature.

Evidence for the Intertemporal Function of Positive Emotions

Research into the function of discrete positive emotional states has flourished over the past decade. As evidenced by the contents of this handbook, the scope of inquiry of affective science has been broadening and building in its own right. Despite this breadth, the emotions described herein can all be described as contributing to adaptive intertemporal choice by foregoing immediate gains for the long-term social value associated with building warmth or building competence. We separate our discussion of the evidence supporting this conclusion accordingly, by first surveying the research into the states that build warmth (compassion, gratitude, love, elevation) followed by the states that build competence (pride, grit, hope, admiration/inspiration).

Positive Emotions and Warmth

The functional benefits of gratitude, compassion, and love seem to derive from their ability to increase an individual's long-term social value (and, consequently, their stability within a social group) by contributing to that individual's perceived warmth.

As suggested previously, one of the most common intertemporal choices confronted in social life involves "reciprocity"—the decision of whether or not to repay a benefit to another. The optimal short-term outcome would be to accept a benefit and not repay it. This would allow someone to capitalize on the charity of another, while incurring no costs associated with acting in kind. Of course, acting in this way carries the potential long-term cost of severing a valuable relationship and enduring the severe adaptive consequences of social ostracism, particularly if one gains a reputation as an individual who does not reciprocate (cf. Williams et al., 2003). So the decision of whether or not to reciprocate involves weighing the short-term benefits of saving energy and resources against the long-term benefits of a continued, fruitful relationship. One way to solve such an intertemporal choice would be to perform a cold calculus. Perhaps there is an intuitive, selfish desire to take a gift and run, and only our ability to

think into the future and realize that such an action would ultimately jeopardize our well-being motivates reciprocity. Perhaps it could even be a simple awareness of the social norms regarding reciprocity.

Research into the function of *gratitude* suggests otherwise. Indeed, this body of work indicates that people are actually averse to reciprocal exchange when it is perceived to be the result of calculated expectation of future benefits (Tsang, 2006; Watkins, Scheer, Ovnicek, & Kolts, 2006). Gratitude is the emotion one feels when another person has intentionally given, or attempted to give, something of value (McCullough, Kilpatrick, Emmons, & Larson, 2001; McCullough & Tsang, 2004). Theorists expect that gratitude functions to encourage an individual to reciprocate a favor, even if such reciprocity will be costly to him or her in the short term. It is also expected that, over time, this reciprocal prosocial behavior aids in building trust and, consequently, in preserving valued relationships.

Both correlational (McCullough, Emmons, & Tsang, 2002) and experimental work (Bartlett & DeSteno, 2006) support this interpretation. In the experimental research, participants were made to experience the emotional state through staged interactions in which a confederate made a costly effort to help the participant with a difficult situation (a computer malfunction). At a time removed from the initial interaction, the participant (apparently incidentally) came across the confederate trying to find help for a research project. Participants previously made to feel gratitude helped significantly more than did participants made to feel amused or affectively neutral. Importantly, the same effect was found in a subsequent study when participants were approached by a confederate with whom they had *not* previously interacted, suggesting that the motivation to reciprocate and act charitably toward others stems from the emotional response, and not alternative factors, such as a reciprocity norm governing interpersonal interactions.

Follow-up research in support of these findings shows that gratitude motivates individuals to sacrifice time and money in the context of behavioral economic games (DeSteno, Bartlett, Baumann, Williams,

& Dickens, 2010). Evidence that gratitude motivates incurring short-term costs in this context would be particularly compelling given that most models of economic decision making assume a strong, intuitive desire for short-term self-interest. Decisions favoring communal interest over individual gain are thought to derive solely from the tamping down of emotional responses geared toward immediate gratification. In line with the adaptive intertemporal function of emotional states, however, experiencing gratitude mediated increased monetary giving in the short-term even when such giving increased communal gains at the expense of individual profit.

Importantly, gratitude operates to bring about long-term benefits in the absence of any *expectation* of these benefits. That is, the tradeoff between short-term and long-term rewards is built into the adaptive logic of the emotional state. Experiencing gratitude at time 1 leads to unintended and unexpected benefits to the self at time 2. In fact, the presence of the expectation has been found to lead to the quite negative psychological state of indebtedness. Participants are most averse to gifts when they perceive that a benefactor expects something in return. With increasing expectations of return come corresponding increases in the negative state of indebtedness, as well as decreases in gratitude (Watkins et al., 2006). When reciprocity becomes calculated, when people consciously make the tradeoff between short-term and long-term benefits, rather than bind individuals together, reciprocity pulls them apart. Emotions help us optimally navigate intertemporal space where more controlled processes fail.

Of course, altruistic action does not come only in the form of reciprocity. It is often theorized to emerge from a specific other-oriented emotional response, such as *compassion* or empathic concern (Goetz, Keltner, & Simon-Thomas, 2010), that is elicited by the sight of another's distress. The adaptive logic of such costly helping behavior, however, is identical to that of reciprocity. Coming to someone else's assistance, though immediately costly, communicates the kind of interpersonal warmth others seek from interaction partners and that will ultimately contribute to one's social value through the perception of warmth.

Love serves a similar function, but in the context of romantic relationships. In the course of maintaining long-term romantic bonds, partners face the problem of deciding whether to remain committed to one another in the face of immediately appealing alternatives that pose threats to the long-term viability of the relationship (Gonzaga, Keltner, Londahl, & Smith, 2001). By motivating approach behavior through gesture, touch, or verbal communication, the processes of trust, mutual dependence, and kindness are strengthened. Through distinct facial expressions, warmth is directly communicated to a partner, increasing his or her confidence and willingness to invest personally in the relationship.

Finally, *elevation* is elicited in response to acts of virtue or great moral beauty, and motivates one's desire to become a better person and to do good deeds (Algoe & Haidt, 2009)—to emulate the warmth of the moral actor. Importantly, the effects of elevation on prosocial motivations are distinct from those of other positive emotional states such as happiness and admiration (which seem to have comparable effects on motivation to emulate *competent* others, as we discuss later).

In summary, gratitude, compassion, love, and elevation contribute to the kinds of decisions and behaviors that result in foregoing immediate gains and accruing long-term benefits. By motivating behavior that contributes to the development of perceived warmth, these emotions help one build social value.

Positive Emotions and Competence

Social value derives from not only cooperative and collaborative intent but also the ability to act successfully upon these intentions. The functional benefits of pride, grit, hope, and the cluster of admiration/inspiration seem to derive from their ability to increase individuals' long-term social value (and, consequently, their stability within a social group) by contributing to their perceived competence.

As mentioned earlier, perseverance is a crucial component of developing competence. Past research has emphasized the importance of controlled processes as explanations for how individuals resist the immediately appealing temptation of, say, taking a nap when work needs to be done. However, recent research into the function of *pride* suggests that there are other, and perhaps more effective, means of achieving long-term success.

Williams and DeSteno (2008, 2009) conducted a series of experiments in which they induced the experience of pride by providing false feedback regarding participants' performance on an ambiguous measure of cognitive ability (i.e., high performance scores and explicit praise by the experimenter). Other participants received either equally high performance scores in the absence of acclaim or no feedback at all. Supporting the view that pride motivates perseverance, proud participants worked signi?cantly longer on a subsequent onerous task, ostensibly related to the initial ability-assessing one. Moreover, levels of perseverance were directly predicted by the intensity of pride participants felt. Subsequent analyses con?rmed that increased perseverance could not be attributed to associated changes in self-esteem, self-efficacy, or general positive affect (Williams & DeSteno, 2008). These ?ndings indicate that pride leads to increased acceptance of short-term costs related to perseverance, and support the proposed role of pride in developing traits associated with competence.

A follow-up study provides an even more compelling demonstration of our theory: an empirical demonstration that *social value* increases as a function of perception of these traits. Williams and DeSteno (2009) asked participants to work in groups of three to solve a complex puzzle. They elicited pride in one participant by giving private acclaim for her ability on a prior task that ostensibly measured skills relevant to solving the puzzle. It was expected that proud individuals would later take on a dominant leadership role in working on the puzzle and, importantly, would also be perceived as more likable by their partners. Con?rming this view, proud participants were viewed as the most dominant members of the groups and were more liked by their counterparts. Furthermore, this increased social attractiveness of the proud participants was not simply a result of their increased efforts on the task, as effort alone did not predict liking. The increased liking

of proud participants was driven by the perceived social value of a competent interaction partner. In other words, the experience of pride seems to motivate behaviors that increase an individual's value or status in the eyes of others.

The relationship between pride and perceptions of status has been further supported by research examining observers' reactions to nonverbal expressions of pride, attesting to the function of the emotional state as a marker of competence-based social value (see Shariff & Tracy, 2009).

Research into the function of states such as grit and hope suggests that these emotions operate according to a similar adaptive logic. Duckworth, Peterson, Matthews, and Kelly (2007) define "grit" as passion and perseverance for long-term goals—an emotion that motivates the sustained and focused application of effort over time. "Hope" has been defined as a combination of understanding how to achieve long-term goals and the desire to realize those goals (Snyder, 2002). While pride's influence on perseverance results from positive feedback regarding an ability, grit and hope seem to motivate perseverance even in the face of adversity, failure, and plateaus in progress. In other words, even when the immediate benefits of withdrawing effort from an activity are high, both physically and psychologically, these states motivate the incursion of short-term costs for long-term gains in skills and abilities. These findings are particularly compelling demonstrations of the adaptive intertemporal tradeoffs motivated by these competence-relevant positive emotions.

Finally, admiration and inspiration are elicited in response to witnessing acts of great skill or ability, and motivate the desire to emulate the target and to succeed (Haidt & Seder, 2009). The adaptive function of these states, again, is rooted in the benefits of individuals learning culturally valued skills or abilities from high-status others and the motivation to pursue these long-term goals (Algoe & Haidt, 2009).

In summary, pride, grit, hope, and the cluster of admiration/inspiration contribute to the kinds of decisions and behaviors that result in forgoing immediate gains and accruing long-term benefits. Through contributing to one's perceived competence, these emotions help to create social value.

Implications for Theories of Morality

It seems that humans are capable of experiencing a range of positive emotional states that are not geared toward approaching immediate gains. Models of intertemporal choice that insist intuitively appealing options are shortsighted may result from a lack of appreciation of this range—a function of the kinds of choices that participants typically face in decision science paradigms. This is not to say that self-regulation does not play a role in fostering adaptive behavior; it certainly does. However, by solidifying individuals' status in social networks through the cultivation of warmth and competence, specific positive emotions also represent response systems that motivate short-term sacrifices and long-term gains.

Adopting this view of the function of positive emotions and their relationship to social cognition has interesting implications for theories of morality. First, it casts aside simplistic theories of morality arguing that selfishness *equals* now, which *equals* emotion, by demonstrating that a range of emotional states (those that cultivate warmth) operate to stifle self-interest and focus us on the immediate well-being of others. It also sheds new light on what might be considered self-interested emotions (those that cultivate competence). Emotions such as pride and grit, though they do focus on developing individual skills and abilities, might also indirectly contribute to long-term collective well-being as a result of their effects on the collective capabilities of groups. If one adopts a definition of morality that places primary import on the ultimate flourishing of groups (cf. Haidt & Kesebir, 2010), then these competence-based emotions might also fall within the moral realm. Moral emotions have been defined as those "that are linked to the interests or welfare either of society as a whole or at least of persons other than the judge or agent" (Haidt, 2003, p. 853). Are emotional states that motivate individuals to incur short-term costs for the sake of developing individual skills and abilities still linked to the welfare of others? How might emotions that seem to motivate self-interested pursuits ultimately contribute to other-interest as well?

The idea that societies flourish when individuals pursue their own interests is not new, of course. Psychologists, particularly those interested in the function of social emotions, have long cited Adam Smith's *The Theory of Moral Sentiments* (1790/1976) as a reference attesting to the ubiquity of other-interested positive emotions, such as compassion, empathy, love, and gratitude, in social life. This is counterintuitive because Adam Smith is best known, primarily in *The Wealth of Nations* (1776/1937), for his advocacy of the pursuit of immediate self-interest as the key to flourishing societies. His theorizing on the power of free markets suggests that it is precisely the drive for self-interest through which societies advance. This idea was captured in Smith's metaphor of the *invisible hand*: Collective well-being is best achieved by groups of individuals who pursue their own advancement without concern for others. The engine of this process is *specialization*. Focusing individuals' efforts on skills/domains in which they have a comparative advantage ultimately benefits a community by maximizing the collective capabilities of group members, allowing for a potentially wider and richer distribution of resources, as well as a competitive advantage relative to other groups. Consequently, having motivations and emotions that foster such an end may ultimately benefit the community by enhancing the collective competence of a population.

We believe that Smith is right about the collective value created by self-focused motivational states, such as the competence-based positive emotions we have described in this chapter. Indeed, we agree with the sentiment that "by pursuing his own interest he frequently promotes that of the society more effectually than when he really intends to promote it" (Smith, 1776/1937, p. 423). By this reasoning, even competence-based positive emotions might be considered "moral emotions" according to some current and popular definitions.

We make this claim cautiously, however, because, on balance, academics interested in human nature have emphasized the import of self-interest to a much greater degree than that of other-interest, and we hesitate to perpetuate that mistake further. In the study of positive and moral emotions, however, the opposite mistake threatens to take hold. It is neither surprising nor particularly controversial to argue for the moral importance of other-interested emotions to those who study the likes of emotions that appear in this handbook. But it is indeed a departure to argue for the moral importance of competence-based emotions, as doing so would seem to corroborate the kinds of self-interested views of human nature against which emotion researchers have sought to argue.

Those who might worry about championing the moral value of self-focused emotions need not worry. Social value, and therefore collective value, cannot be achieved through the honing of competence alone. Specialization only pays off when a market defined by the free-flowing *exchange* of resources has been established. In other words, societies flourish when composed of individuals who (1) maximize their individual potential in terms of skills/abilities and (2) are willing to exchange those resources with others. What drives this willingness? Smith (1776/1937, p. 14) initially offered a strong answer: "It is not from the benevolence of the butcher, brewer or baker that we should expect our dinner, but from a regard for their self-interest." On this we disagree. It is not solely through regard for their own interest that people in groups should expect their dinner—it is *also* through the benevolence of the butcher, brewer and baker.

A critical insight provided by sociobiology and functional accounts of emotion has been the adaptive value of other-interested emotional states—those that cultivate perceptions of warmth. If competence-based emotions motivate behaviors that contribute to specialization, then warmth-based emotions motivate behaviors that contribute to the desire to exchange the fruits of such specialization. A balance of these motivations maximizes long-term well-being. Societies composed of individuals with the intentions to act warmly toward others, as well as the capacity to act on those intentions, will best achieve long-term collective well-being. Theories arguing for the importance of competence without warmth ignore the social functions of other-interested emotional states (mediating the emergence of reciprocal altruism; cf. Trivers, 1971); those arguing for the importance of warmth without competence ignore the importance of the process through which individual resources contribute to collective value. From this per-

spective, then, it is no wonder that perceivers prefer people who are both warm and competent: These are the kinds of individuals who ultimately contribute to the flourishing of social groups.

Though Smith does indeed acknowledge that "how selfish 'soever man may be supposed, there are evidently some principles in his nature, which interest him in the fortune of others" (Smith 1790/1976, p. 9), he falls short of demonstrating how these principles of nature contribute meaningfully to societal flourishing. Indeed, it has been tempting for some philosophers, economists, and decision scientists to conclude from this lack of a functional argument that these other-interested motivations compromise collective well-being by distracting focus from self-interested pursuits. But competence needs warmth in order to translate social value into collective value. Other-interested motivations solidify social groups by establishing and maintaining mutually beneficial relationships, and by providing the proximal mechanisms that motivate exchange of resources that individuals have accrued. The positive emotions that motivate cultivation of both these traits are essential in the ultimate creation of flourishing societies and, consequently, can be considered moral emotions (cf. Valdesolo & DeSteno, 2011).

Conclusion

There is no question that positive emotions motivate the incursion of short-term costs for the sake of long-term gains and deserve a more prominent role in theories of intertemporal choice. Whether manifested as putting oneself in harm's way to help someone in danger or shooting 1,000 free throws after a long practice, these states are by no means shortsighted in adaptive value.

Why? If positive emotions broaden and build, then it makes sense that they would do so in a way that ultimately contributes to an individual's well-being. If well-being has in large part been determined by one's ability to become embedded in a stable social group, then these emotions should contribute meaningfully to that end. By cultivating warmth and competence, the two basic dimensions of person perception—the dimensions by which the character and value of all individuals are judged—positive emotions accomplish exactly that.

References

Ainslie, G. (1975). Specious reward: A behavioral theory of impulsiveness and impulse control. *Psychological Bulletin, 82*(4), 463–496.

Algoe, S. B., & Haidt, J. (2009). Witnessing excellence in action: The "other-praising"emotions of elevation, gratitude, and admiration. *Journal of Positive Psychology, 4*(2), 105–127.

Ayduk, O., Mendoza-Denton, R., Mischel, W., Downey, G., Peake, P. K., & Rodriguez, M. (2000). Regulating the interpersonal self: Strategic self-regulation for coping with rejection sensitivity. *Journal of Personality and Social Psychology, 79*(5), 776–792.

Barrett, L. F., Mesquita, B., Ochsner, K. N., & Gross, J. J. (2007). The experience of emotion. *Annual Review of Psychology, 58,* 373–403.

Bartlett, M. Y., & DeSteno, D. (2006). Gratitude and prosocial behavior helping when it costs you. *Psychological Science, 17*(4), 319–325.

Baumeister, R. F., & Leary, M. R. (1995). The need to belong: Desire for interpersonal attachments as a fundamental human motivation. *Psychological Bulletin, 117*(3), 497–529.

Berns, G. S., Laibson, D., & Loewenstein, G. (2007). Intertemporal choice—toward an integrative framework. *Trends in Cognitive Sciences, 11,* 482–488.

Bodenhausen, G. V., Kramer, G. P., & Süsser, K. (1994). Happiness and stereotypic thinking in social judgment. *Journal of Personality and Social Psychology, 66*(4), 621–632.

Cacioppo, J. T., Hawkley, L. C., & Berntson, G. G. (2003). The anatomy of loneliness. *Current Directions in Psychological Science, 12*(3), 71–74.

Campbell, D. T. (1983). The two distinct routes beyond kin selection to ultrasociality: Implications for the humanities and social sciences. In D. Bridgeman (Ed.), *The nature of prosocial development: Theories and strategies* (pp. 11–39). New York: Academic Press.

Cuddy, A. J., Fiske, S. T., & Glick, P. (2008). Warmth and competence as universal dimensions of social perception: The stereotype content model and the BIAS map. *Advances in Experimental Social Psychology, 40,* 61–149.

DeSteno, D. (2009). Social emotions and intertemporal choice: "Hot" mechanisms for building social and economic capital. *Current Directions in Psychological Science, 18*(5), 280–284.

DeSteno, D., Bartlett, M. Y., Baumann, J., Williams, L. A., & Dickens, L. (2010). Gratitude as moral sentiment: Emotion-guided cooperation in economic exchange. *Emotion, 10*(2), 289–293.

Duckworth, A. L., Peterson, C., Matthews, M. D., & Kelly, D. R. (2007). Grit: Perseverance and passion for long-term goals. *Journal of Personality and Social Psychology, 92*(6), 1087–1101.

Eigsti, I. M., Zayas, V., Mischel, W., Shoda, Y., Ayduk, O., Dadlani, M. B., et al. (2006). Predicting cognitive control from preschool to late adolescence and young adulthood. *Psychological Science, 17*(6), 478–484.

Fiske, S. T., Cuddy, A. J., & Glick, P. (2007). Universal dimensions of social cognition: Warmth and competence. *Trends in Cognitive Sciences, 11*(2), 77–83.

Frank, R. H. (1988). *Passions within reason: The strategic role of the emotions.* New York: Norton.

Fredrickson, B. L. (2001). The role of positive emotions in positive psychology: The broaden-and-build theory of positive emotions. *American Psychologist, 56*(3), 218–226.

Fredrickson, B. L., & Branigan, C. (2005). Positive emotions broaden the scope of attention and thought–action repertoires. *Cognition and Emotion, 19*(3), 313–332.

Goetz, J. L., Keltner, D., & Simon-Thomas, E. (2010). Compassion: An evolutionary analysis and empirical review. *Psychological Bulletin, 136*(3), 351–374.

Gonzaga, G. C., Keltner, D., Londahl, E. A., & Smith, M. D. (2001). Love and the commitment problem in romantic relations and friendship. *Journal of Personality and Social Psychology, 81*(2), 247–262.

Greene, J. D., Nystrom, L. E., Engell, A. D., Darley, J. M., & Cohen, J. D. (2004). The neural bases of cognitive conflict and control in moral judgment. *Neuron, 44*(2), 389–400.

Greene, J. D., Sommerville, R. B., Nystrom, L. E., Darley, J. M., & Cohen, J. D. (2001). An fMRI investigation of emotional engagement in moral judgment. *Science, 293,* 2105–2108.

Haidt, J. (2003). The moral emotions. In R. J. Davidson, K. R. Scherer, & H. H. Goldsmith (Eds.), *Handbook of affective sciences* (pp. 852–870). Oxford, UK: Oxford University Press.

Haidt, J., & Kesebir, S. (2010). Morality. In S. T. Fiske, D. T. Gilbert, & G. Lindzey (Eds.), *Handbook of social psychology* (5th ed., pp. 797–832). Hoboken, NJ: Wiley.

Haidt, J., & Seder, P. (2009). Admiration/awe. In D. Sander & K. Scherer (Eds.), *Oxford companion to emotion and the affective sciences* (pp. 4–5). New York: Oxford University Press.

Keltner, D., & Haidt, J. (1999). Social functions of emotions at four levels of analysis. *Cognition and Emotion, 13*(5), 505–521.

Keltner, D., Haidt, J., & Shiota, M. N. (2006). Social functionalism and the evolution of emotions. In M. Schaller, J. A. Simpson, & D. T. Kenrick (Eds.), *Evolution and social psychology* (pp. 115–142). New York: Psychology Press.

Laibson, D. (1997). Golden eggs and hyperbolic discounting. *Quarterly Journal of Economics, 112*(2), 443–478.

Loewenstein, G., Read, D., & Baumeister, R. (Eds.). (2003). *Time and decision: Economic and psychological perspectives on intertemporal choice.* New York: Russell Sage Foundation.

Loewenstein, G., & Thaler, R. H. (1989). Anomalies: Intertemporal choice. *Journal of Economic Perspectives, 3*(4), 181–193.

McClure, S. M., Laibson, D. I., Loewenstein, G., & Cohen, J. D. (2004). Separate neural systems value immediate and delayed monetary rewards. *Science, 306,* 503–507.

McCullough, M. E., Emmons, R. A., & Tsang, J. A. (2002). The grateful disposition: A conceptual and empirical topography. *Journal of Personality and Social Psychology, 82*(1), 112–127.

McCullough, M. E., Kilpatrick, S. D., Emmons, R. A., & Larson, D. B. (2001). Is gratitude a moral affect? *Psychological Bulletin, 127*(2), 249–266.

McCullough, M. E., & Tsang, J. A. (2004). Parent of the virtues?: The prosocial contours of gratitude. In R. A. Emmons & M. E. McCullough (Eds.), *The psychology of gratitude* (pp. 123–144). New York: Oxford University Press.

Mischel, W., Shoda, Y., & Peake, P. K. (1988). The nature of adolescent competencies predicted by preschool delay of gratification. *Journal of Personality and Social Psychology, 54*(4), 687–696.

Mischel, W., Shoda, Y., & Rodriguez, M. (1989). Delay of gratification in children. *Science, 244,* 933–938.

Plato. (1949). *Timaeus* (B. Jowett, Trans.). Indianapolis, IN: Bobbs Merrill. (Original work published 4th century B.C.)

Rosenberg, S., Nelson, C., & Vivekananthan, P. S. (1968). A multidimensional approach to the structure of personality impressions. *Journal of Personality and Social Psychology, 9,* 283–294.

Shariff, A. F., & Tracy, J. L. (2009). Knowing who's boss: Implicit perceptions of status from the nonverbal expression of pride. *Emotion, 9*(5), 631–639.

Shoda, Y., Mischel, W., & Peake, P. K. (1990). Predicting adolescent cognitive and self-regulatory competencies from preschool delay of gratification: Identifying diagnostic conditions. *Developmental Psychology, 26*(6), 978–986.

Smith, A. (1937). *The wealth of nations.* New York: Modern Library. (Original work published 1776)

Smith, A. (1976). *The theory of moral sentiments.* Oxford, UK: Clarendon Press. (Original work published 1790)

Snyder, C. R. (2002). Hope theory: Rainbows in the mind. *Psychological Inquiry, 13*(4), 249–275.

Solomon, R. C. (1993). The philosophy of emotions. In M. Lewis & J. Haviland (Eds.), *Handbook of emotions* (pp. 3–15). New York: Guilford Press.

Todorov, A., Pakrashi, M., & Oosterhof, N. N. (2009). Evaluating faces on trustworthiness after minimal time exposure. *Social Cognition, 27*(6), 813–833.

Tracy, J. L., Shariff, A. F., Zhao, W., & Henrich, J. (2013). Cross-cultural evidence that the nonverbal expression of pride is an automatic status signal. *Journal of Experimental Psychology: General, 142*(1), 163–180.

Trivers, R. L. (1971). The evolution of reciprocal altruism. *Quarterly Review of Biology, 46,* 35–57.

Tsang, J. A. (2006). The effects of helper intention on gratitude and indebtedness. *Motivation and Emotion, 30*(3), 198–204.

Valdesolo, P., & DeSteno, D. (2006). Manipulations of emotional context shape moral judgment. *Psychological Science, 17*(6), 476–477.

Valdesolo, P., & DeSteno, D. (2011). The virtue

in vice: Short-sightedness in the study of moral emotions. *Emotion Review, 3*(3), 276–277.

Watkins, P., Scheer, J., Ovnicek, M., & Kolts, R. (2006). The debt of gratitude: Dissociating gratitude and indebtedness. *Cognition and Emotion, 20*(2), 217–241.

Williams, K. D., Case, T. I., & Govan, C. L. (2003). Impact of ostracism on social judgments and decisions: Explicit and implicit responses. In J. P. Forgas, K. D. Williams, & W. von Hippel (Eds.), *Social judgments: Implicit and explicit processes* (Sydney Symposium of Social Psychology Series, Vol. 5,

pp. 325–342). New York: Cambridge University Press.

Williams, L. A., & DeSteno, D. (2008). Pride and perseverance: The motivational role of pride. *Journal of Personality and Social Psychology, 94*(6), 1007–1017.

Williams, L. A., & DeSteno, D. (2009). Pride: Adaptive social emotion or seventh sin? *Psychological Science, 20*(3), 284–288.

Willis, J., & Todorov, A. (2006). First impressions: Making up your mind after a 100-ms exposure to a face. *Psychological Science, 17*(7), 592–598.

■ ■ ■ ■ ■ ■ ■ ■ ■

CHAPTER 12

Positive Emotions in Close Relationships

Claire I. Yee
Gian C. Gonzaga
Shelly L. Gable

Strong emotional experiences are part and parcel of close relationships. On the positive side they motivate initial attraction and bonding, solidify commitment between partners, and help defend relationships against external threats (e.g., Algoe, 2012; Gonzaga, Keltner, Londahl, & Smith, 2001). On the negative side they can expose cracks and faults in the bond, lead to vicious cycles of negativity and blame, and may even play a key role in relationship dissolution (Christensen & Heavey, 1990; Heavey, Christensen, & Malamuth, 1995). Theorists have even proposed that emotions evolved, in large part, to help us regulate our connections with others and navigate our social world (e.g., Frank, 1988; Nesse, 1990; Keltner & Haidt, 1999; Keltner & Kring, 1998; Tooby & Cosmides, 1990). With this in mind, it is not surprising that the study of emotions in relationships has long been a pillar of social psychology and relationship science.

However, the study of emotions in relationships has been somewhat lopsided. A majority of the work on emotions in relationships has focused on the problematic consequences of negative emotion (for a review, see Fredrickson, 1998). This may be driven in large part by the vast empirical attention paid to relationship conflict, which elicits negative emotions at a much greater rate than positive emotions. Perhaps best known is the finding that the display of contempt is a powerful predictor of later relationship dissolution (Levenson & Gottman, 1983). However, evidence that anger can escalate conflict (Allred, 2000), and that anxiety in rejection sensitivity can perpetuate self-fulfilling prophecies of poor relationship outcomes (Downey, Freitas, Michaelis, & Khouri, 1998), has had considerable impact on the field as well.

While the volume of research is significantly smaller, there is growing interest in the impact of positive emotions on relationships as well. Positive emotions are not merely the opposite or absence of negative emotions, and as we demonstrate, they have distinct implications for relational processes. The extant research suggests that positive emotions have powerful and unique impacts on close relationships, and are therefore critical for understanding how these relationships begin, grow, and are successfully maintained. Researchers have focused their efforts on the broad ways in which positive emotions serve relational functions, on the ways that established intrapersonal functions of positive emotion carry over into interpersonal contexts, and on particular positive emotions that may have evolved specifically to support close relationships, such as love and gratitude. Although the relational impact of negative emotions cannot be ignored, the experience and sharing of positive emotions may be even more critical to relationship success.

The Social Functions of Emotions

While many aspects of William James's (1884) question "What is an emotion?" are still the topic of much debate, most researchers agree that emotions help promote adaptive, fitness-enhancing responses to important features of the environment (e.g., Ekman, 1992; Frijda & Mesquita, 1994; Izard, 1977; Lazarus, 1991; Nesse & Ellsworth, 2009; Plutchik, 1980; Russell, 2003; Scherer, 2009; Tooby & Cosmides, 2008; for a review, see Shiota, Chapter 3, this volume). According to many of these theorists, emotional responses help individuals manage specific kinds of adaptive problems, such as acquiring food, avoiding predation, and producing offspring. Various components of emotional responding, such as facial, postural, and vocal expressions, physiological changes, modulation of perception and cognition, action tendencies, and overt behaviors, may be recruited to help support fulfillment of the emotion's function in this regard. Some aspects of emotional responding are inherently social. For example, the expressive display of an emotion rapidly communicates one's internal state to others and can provide information about one's likely subsequent actions.

Still, early functional accounts of emotions tended to emphasize the immediate survival value of negative emotions, such as fear and disgust, experienced in response to threats in the environment (e.g., Ekman, 1992; Lazarus, 1991; Plutchik, 1980). For example, fear has been conceptualized as an emotion elicited by physical threats to the self, particularly from predators, and promoting a flexible constellation of expressive (e.g., silence or cries for help), physiological (e.g., changes in heart rate, blood pressure), cognitive (e.g., altered visual field), and

behavioral responses (e.g., freezing, flight) that increase the chance of surviving this particular event (Levenson, 1999; Tooby & Cosmides, 2008). Disgust seems designed to protect the individual from threats of contamination or disease, such as rotting food and infected conspecifics (Rozin & Fallon, 1987; Schaller & Duncan, 2007). Both fear and disgust are thought to have enhanced adaptive fitness by coordinating responses that helped our ancestors avoid or escape from threats to their survival.

Functional accounts of emotions such as anger and sadness began to acknowledge the importance of conspecifics as crucial, emotion-eliciting elements in our environment. For example, anger has been conceptualized as an emotional response to demeaning offenses from others (e.g., Lazarus, 1991), and sadness as a response to the loss of a loved one (e.g., Averill, 1968; Keller & Nesse, 2006). In each of these cases the function of the emotion is still intrapersonal, in the sense that the emotional response is thought to give the individual experiencing that emotion a direct fitness advantage, such as by compelling a concession from others (e.g., Van Kleef, De Dreu, & Manstead, 2004), or by evoking others' immediate caregiving and concern (Hendriks, Croon, & Vingerhoets, 2010).

More recently, emotion theorists have explored the possibility that our ongoing relationships with others make crucial contributions to human fitness in their own right. This notion reaches beyond recognition of individual people as emotion-eliciting agents, to the recognition that relationships themselves serve important roles in passing on one's genes. Humans survive by forming and maintaining a plethora of relationships: cooperative alliances, friendships, and mating partnerships. Important activities of life—finding resources, avoiding threats, producing and raising offspring—are often performed by multiple people in close alliance rather than by individuals alone (Ainsworth, 1989; Buss, 1994; Caporael & Brewer, 1995; de Waal, 1996; Shaver, Hazan, & Bradshaw, 1988; Trivers, 1972). All of these potential benefits require extended, interdependent relations with others in a dyadic or group context.

From an interpersonal or social-function perspective, emotions are a crucial element in navigating the distinct set of threats and opportunities that such relationships present (Barrett & Campos, 1987; Ekman, 1992; Frijda & Mesquita, 1994; James, 1884; Keltner & Haidt, 1999; Lazarus, 1991; Lutz & White, 1986; Tooby & Cosmides, 1990). Specifically, emotions facilitate close relationships by helping us identify appropriate relationship partners, maintain a relationship once it is formed, and coordinate action between relationship partners (Barrett & Campos, 1987; Keltner & Haidt, 1999; Keltner & Kring, 1998; Nesse, 1990). In this sense the social functions of emotions are indirect, supporting the close relationships that more directly benefit our individual fitness, yet powerful nonetheless.

This functional lens has been used to examine how negative emotions may actually benefit relationships. For example, jealousy can help individuals to protect monogamous relationships in the presence of a relationship threat, by increasing one's attention to the actions of a partner and any attractive rivals, and increasing the likelihood that one will defend the relationship from an interloper (Buss, Larsen, Westen, & Semmelroth, 1992; Daly, Wilson, & Weghorst, 1982). Similarly, guilt and embarrassment have both been conceptualized as unpleasant but highly functional emotion states that facilitate relationship-repair behavior after one has erred or transgressed (e.g., Keltner & Buswell, 1997; Tangney, Miller, Flicker, & Barlow, 1996).

However, positive emotions' unique focus on opportunities renders them particularly well suited to making the most of the opportunities relationships offer (Shiota, Campos, Keltner, & Hertenstein, 2004). For instance, relationships require identifying and investing in potentially beneficial partners. The experience of positive emotion helps an individual identify a current interaction partner as worthy of further investment. Amusement and joy can identify potential friends or ingroup members, or provide information to the individual about the partner's affiliative intentions. Sexual desire helps an individual identify potential romantic partners who might contribute health, good genes, and resources to future offspring (Buss, 1989). Positive emotions also serve as rewards for behaviors that help maintain relationships, as well as promoting greater

depth in the relationship. For example, an infant's smile elicits positive interaction from a caregiver, acting as an important reward and encouraging further investment in the parent–offspring relationship (Bower, 1977; Emde, Katz, &Thorpe, 1978). Positive emotions also help coordinate action between individuals, whether raising offspring or pursuing resources together. For example, while mostly studied in the context of parent–offspring relationships (e.g., secondary intersubjectivity; Butterworth & Jarrett, 1991), specific emotions such as amusement and awe may facilitate group-level interactions by helping one take others' perspectives and comprehend one's role as a member of a larger group.

Recognizing the importance of relationships for an individual's fitness provides a context for understanding the functionality and importance of positive emotions, where approaches emphasizing intrapersonal functions have struggled. Conversely, recognizing the more direct adaptive functions of positive emotions, and the specific kinds of benefits they may confer on the individual, can also inform research on the implications of positive emotion for close relationships. In the next section we discuss several specific theories regarding the functions of positive emotions. While these theories were originally developed to explain functionality from an intrapersonal perspective, evidence suggests that each is also quite useful in considering the implications of positive emotions for close relationships.

Functions of Positive Emotions: Major Theories and Application to Relationships

Despite the recognition, discussed earlier, that positive emotions may be distinctly suited to serving social functions, theories specifically addressing the functions of positive emotions have tended to emphasize direct benefits to the individual. However, when considered in a social context, many of these same theoretical perspectives can shed light on the roles of positive emotions in initiating and maintaining relationships as well. In this section we consider how several of the most influential perspectives on the functions of positive emotions can provide a rich theoretical background to understanding the implications of positive emotions for close relationships. After a short explanation of each theory in terms of the effects of positive emotion on an individual, we consider how the same processes might play out in a relationship.

Broaden-and-Build Theory

In her influential broaden-and-build theory, Fredrickson (1998, 2001; see also Tugade, Devlin, & Fredrickson, Chapter 2, this volume) proposed that positive emotions serve different, but equally important, functions compared to negative emotions. By this account, positive emotions do not merely signal the absence of threat in the environment, satiety, or safety. Instead, positive emotions actively promote broadening of attentional scope and build cognitive, behavioral, and social resources. Whereas negative emotions are designed to deal with threats, positive emotions are designed to help us take advantage of opportunities. The response tendencies associated with positive emotions do more than point out these opportunities; each component of a positive emotional response can be recruited to facilitate an individual's pursuit of that opportunity to the fullest. Positive emotions allow an individual to process information from the environment in more global, innovative, flexible, and creative ways (e.g., Fredrickson & Branigan, 2005; Isen, Daubman, & Nowicki, 1987)—the "broaden" effect in the theory's name. This increases the likelihood that opportunities and potential benefits in the environment will be detected and effectively pursued. These opportunities may be material, informational, or even social; in each case, a likely consequence will be a "building" of the resource for future use.

In relational terms, the attentional breadth promoted by positive emotion can help build stronger relationships. For example, whereas a negative emotion such as anger tends to narrow one's focus to why one's partner is to blame in a conflict (Keltner, Ellsworth, & Edwards, 1993), positive emotion may expand one's focus to include the partner's perspective, and promote appreciation of the relationship itself as an overarching goal. Positive emotions may also support relationships by altering perceptions of self and partner. For example, in a study of first-

semester college students, reports of positive emotions were found to be associated with greater feelings of self–other overlap between the participants and their roommates (Waugh & Fredrickson, 2006). Thus, the ways in which positive emotions change the individual can bleed over into perceptions of relationships with close others.

The "Undoing" Effect of Positive Emotions

Positive emotions can help "undo" the impact of negative emotions. In the moment, experimentally induced positive emotions have been found to help people return more rapidly to a neutral state after experiencing a negative emotion (e.g., Fredrickson & Levenson, 1998). At the trait level, this same process can have longer-term effects on an individual's ability to cope with stress. "Resilience" has been defined as the ability to recover quickly and fully from stressful experiences or difficult times (Block & Block, 1980; Lazarus, 1993). Resilient individuals are more likely to use positive emotions in coping with stressful events, which helps them to minimize the psychological and physiological impact of such situations (Tugade & Fredrickson, 2004). Moreover, the experience of positive emotions after a highly stressful negative event (e.g., the attacks of September 11, 2001), has been found to predict both decreased likelihood of developing depression and increased growth in postcrisis psychological resources (Fredrickson, Tugade, Waugh, & Larkin, 2003).

Considering that relationships are themselves a source of stress, this undoing function of positive emotion also has important relational implications. Research suggests that partners in satisfying, long-lasting marriages are characterized by their ability to regulate negative emotions during conflict, as indicated by relatively mild physiological arousal and emotional behavior (Gottman & Levenson, 1992). Couples who display short moments of positive emotion during conflict are less likely to suffer negative relational consequences (Carstensen, Gottman, & Levenson, 1995). The impact of these bursts of positive affect may result, in part, from individual-level down-regulation of physiological arousal associated with expressing a positive emotion (Yuan, McCarthy,

Holley, & Levenson, 2010). Yuan and colleagues found that during a 15-minute conversation about a source of marital conflict, 20-second periods of physiological downregulation from high to low arousal were typically accompanied by an increase in positive emotional behavior. Thus, positive emotions may help to limit the damage negative emotions can do in inevitable relationship conflicts, while helping couples avoid runaway negative emotion spirals that can be devastating to a relationship.

Approach Motivation

An alternative theoretical perspective emphasizes the distinction between a proposed neurological approach motivation system and a separate avoidance system. Examples of this general perspective include Carver and Scheier's (1998) conceptualization of the behavioral approach system (BAS) and the behavioral inhibition system (BIS), as well as Cacioppo, Gardner, and Bernston's (1997) proposal of two distinct systems for approaching appetitive stimuli and avoiding aversive stimuli. Within each of these traditions, activation of the approach system promotes moving the individual forward to engage proactively with some target in the environment. Although the overlap between approach motivation and positive emotion is not complete (see the rich work on anger as a high-approach emotion; e.g., Carver & Harmon-Jones, 2009), approach motivation has offered a useful theoretical perspective for predicting a wide range of effects of positive emotion.

Shelly Gable (2006) has posited the concepts of approach and avoidance social goals, broadening the approach–avoid distinction to include goals for relationships. In this model, "approachable" outcomes include intimacy and growth of close relationships, whereas avoidance goals include avoidance of conflict and rejection. One's natural inclination toward approach or avoidance social goals has been found to affect relationship interactions. A focus on approach outcomes could strengthen relationships over time by helping partners perceive more benefits within the relationship than those who focus on avoiding relationship threats. For example, Strachman and Gable (2006) found that participants with

strong approach goals are more likely to recall neutral social interactions in a positive light. Positive emotions may also play an important mediating role in helping individuals achieve approach-related relationship outcomes. In a series of studies, Impett and colleagues (2010) found that those with high approach goals reported more positive emotions, as did their partners. Positive emotions, in turn, predicted increased relationship satisfaction and perception of closeness with one's partner.

Upward Spirals of Positive Emotion and Well-Being

Finally, positive emotions can trigger upward spirals linking psychological and relational well-being. Again, the "upward spiral" concept was first articulated as an individual-level process. Because positive emotions (1) help individuals build creative and innovative solutions to environmental challenges, (2) facilitate recovery from the ill effects of negative emotions, and (3) increase psychological resilience, they help individuals to develop a greater set of resources to deal with both challenges and opportunities in the environment. This feeds the individual's confidence and well-being, promoting the experience of more positive emotion (and conceivably less negative emotion). In turn, this facilitates even more innovation and creativity, faster recovery from stressors, and greater resilience, which then lead to even more positive emotions, and so forth, in an upward spiral.

Recent work suggests that there are also dyadic upward spirals that benefit close relationships. When individuals experience successes or other positive events in their lives, they are likely to share those events with close others, a process known as "capitalization" (Langston, 1994). The mere process of sharing positive events with others has been found to increase the positive emotions and psychological well-being derived from these events beyond what can be accounted for by the events themselves (Gable, Reis, Impett, & Asher, 2004). Importantly, the partner's response can further enhance the benefits of capitalization. When a partner responds to positive news in an active (e.g., engaged and interested) and constructive (i.e., building on the positive event) manner, positive event disclosure leads to even greater positive affect, psychological well-being, and higher relationship satisfaction (Gable, Gonzaga, & Strachman, 2006).

One of the most powerful positive responses a partner can offer during capitalization is to demonstrate pride in the accomplishments of the discloser. Although pride has traditionally been viewed as a self-promoting positive emotion (Tracy & Robins, 2004), here it fuels a positive interaction between partners, increasing the discloser's well-being and positive affect, presumably making the discloser more likely to respond to the partner's good news in an active and constructive manner in the future (Gable, Gonzaga, et al., 2006). Thus, positive emotions not only lead to intrapsychic upward spirals but, they can also be a key component in interpersonal upward spirals of well-being, in which partners feed each other's positive affect and well-being to the benefit of each, and of the relationship.

Relationship-Specific Positive Emotions

This broad theoretical background sets the stage for functional accounts of specific positive emotions. Indeed, like discrete negative emotions, there is increasing and compelling evidence that discrete positive emotions serve specific and important relational functions. Positive emotions, at their core, are critical elements in initiating, building, and maintaining our interpersonal bonds. In this section we highlight two specific examples of positive emotions that are inherently relationship-focused in terms of the kinds of opportunities they target: love and gratitude. First, we frame the challenges and opportunities that individuals have in initiating, growing, and maintaining relationships. Second, we review the relevant research on each of these emotions, and how different components of the emotion help individuals take advantage of relational opportunities. Finally, we explore implications of this work for future study of the individual states.

Love

In all relationships, couples face what is known as the commitment problem. Long-term, monogamous relationships offer myriad benefits: reproductive opportunity, increased opportunity for alliance formation, more efficient distribution of labor, and social support during difficult times. To gain these benefits, an individual must resist the temptations of attractive alternatives that may appeal in the moment but pose obvious threats to the relationship (Frank, 1988). Romantic jealousy, extramarital affairs, and divorce all point to the potential dangers of attractive alternatives and to the powerful psychology that has evolved to deal with these threats (Buss, 1988, Buss & Shackelford, 1997; Daly & Wilson, 1988; Daly et al., 1982). Moreover, many cultural practices that have developed to promote commitment not only legally bind two individuals together but also often make the commitment public to others, in theory discouraging interlopers and rallying the support of the social network to help the bond succeed: Wedding vows are spoken in front of others, marriage is a legal agreement in most cultures, rings are a signal both to the spouses and to others that a commitment has been made.

The momentary experience of love, which many consider to be the prototypical emotional experience (Fehr, 1988), facilitates commitment between intimates in a number of important ways. Broadly, the feeling of close connectedness that helps define love promotes approach toward a partner and creates distance from attractive alternatives. Indeed, the literal behavior of leaning in toward a partner is a key component of the expressive display of love (Gonzaga et al., 2001). Moreover, the experience of love is positively related to other approach-oriented emotional states, such as desire, sympathy, and happiness, and relates to other behaviors that promote approach, such as shared activity (Gonzaga et al., 2001). In these ways, love promotes approach toward a specific other, increasing the likelihood of a stronger psychological bond, while decreasing the likelihood of developing a bond with another.

Research on the neurobiology of love finds that the experience of passionate love, both short term and over the longer term, is linked to activation in brain areas that are key components of the reward and approach systems, such as the ventral tegmental area, which is rich with dopamine receptors

(Bartels & Zeki, 2000; Ortigue, Bianchi-Demichelli, Hamilton, & Grafton, 2007; Xu et al., 2011). In addition, as the relationship matures, areas of the brain implicated in attachment are also activated by the experience of passionate love, such as the globus pallidus, substantia, nigra, and raphe nucleus, among others (Acevedo, Aron, Fisher, & Brown, 2012). Consistent activation of these areas in relation to the romantic partner likely associates the partner with the physiological rewards that cascade from these brain systems, which means that an individual will not only feel the reward in the partner's presence but also actively seek the partner out to experience these rewards.

These findings suggest that behavioral approach motivation brought on by the experience of love is the result of coordination among several key systems, including activation in neural areas linked to approach and attachment, the subjective experience of approach-related emotions that accompany love, outward expression of love literally bringing partners closer together, and other behavioral expressions resulting in more time spent with each other rather than with alternatives. Importantly, these processes are partner-specific, enhancing growth in that relationship relative to other relationships and solidifying commitment between the two partners.

In addition, the expressive component of love plays a key role in solidifying commitment by communicating the internal experience of love- and commitment-related motivations to both romantic partners and others. In the early stages of a relationship, an expressive display of love demonstrates willingness to consider and pursue an intimate relationship (Buss, 1988). As a relationship matures and grows, expressive display can promote and protect commitment in many ways, from assuring the partner of commitment during uncertain times to initiating intimate interactions. In addition, the expression of love between two individuals is a clear indicator to potential alternatives of commitment to the partner.

During moment-to-moment interactions, love is signaled by a set of four affiliation cues: Duchenne smiles, positive gesticulation, affirmative head nods, and leaning toward the partner (Gonzaga et al., 2001; Gonzaga, Turner, Keltner, Campos, & Alte-

mus, 2006). These same expressive cues have also been linked to states closely related to the experience of love, such as psychological closeness, interpersonal warmth, openness, and approach (e.g., J. F. Andersen, Andersen, & Jensen, 1977; P. A. Andersen, 1985; Beier & Sternberg, 1977; McGinley, McGinley, & Nicholas, 1978; Mehrabian, 1971). Importantly, love is encoded into these cues (i.e., they are related to self-reports of love) and the display of these cues is decoded by the partner as love (i.e., they predict partner assessments of how much one is feeling love). Thus, these behaviors are reliable indicators of the momentary experience of love between romantic partners. The display of affiliation cues predicts several indicators of relational health, including self-perceptions of trust, playful criticism, and mutual influence on life goals (Gonzaga et al., 2001), but does not predict intimate feelings and behavior tangential to commitment, such as sexual satisfaction and expression of sexual attraction during teasing (Gonzaga et al., 2006).

Beyond the overt expression of love, the experience of love changes an individual's cognitive processing in ways that support the maintenance of long term relationships, by removing or minimizing threats posed by attractive alternatives. For example, Maner, Rouby, and Gonzaga (2008) showed that participants induced to feel love reduced their attention to attractive alternatives, even at a preconscious stage of processing. In this way, the experience of love appears to remove threats to the relationship even before an individual becomes aware that there are attractive alternatives in the environment.

Once the existence of an attractive alternative enters into consciousness, love can still facilitate cognitive strategies to minimize the threat. In one experiment, Gonzaga, Haselton, Smurda, Davies, and Poore (2008) demonstrated that love promotes successful suppression of thoughts about attractive alternatives. After an experimental task eliciting love or sexual desire for the participant's own romantic partner, participants were shown photos of attractive alternatives. After receiving instruction to suppress thoughts of the attractive alternative, participants in the desire and neutral control conditions experienced the typical rebound effect, in which attempt to suppress thoughts of the alternative partner actually leads to increased thoughts of that person. In the love condition, however, instruction to suppress thoughts of the alternative effectively reduced the number of subsequent thoughts, thereby reversing the typical rebound effect. Moreover, participants in the love condition later recalled fewer details about the attractive alternative during a free recall task than did participants in the other conditions; this effect was specific to details about the alternative's attractiveness per se (e.g., had a good body), and did not generalize to details unrelated to attractivenss (e.g., wearing a white sweater). Thus, the effect of love on attention and memory seemed to address threats to the relationship specifically.

These effects extend beyond attention and memory to how people process information. Consistent with broaden-and-build theory, Forster, Ozelsel, and Epstude (2010) demonstrated that the experience of love promotes future-oriented, global, and holistic cognitive processing, whereas sexual desire elicits more detail-oriented processing. This suggests that love helps individuals see the big picture of a relationship rather than focusing on details. Love also enhances creative thinking and expansive thought, potentially allowing individuals to broaden their cognitive resources, as well as securing the relationship itself (Forster, Ozelsel, & Epstude, 2009). Thus, the experience of love may have psychological benefits beyond the maintenance of the relationship.

In our earlier discussion we emphasized love between romantic partners, which presents certain kinds of challenges and opportunities for the relationship. There are multiple kinds of intimate relationships, however, and researchers have proposed that different shades of love may have arisen to support the challenges and opportunities of each relationship type and role (Shaver, Morgan, & Wu, 1996). For example, *attachment love* encourages an individual to trust and accept help from a caregiver, most typically a parent, but alternatively another family member, romantic partner, or close friend (Ainsworth, 1989; Shiota, Keltner, & John, 2006). In contrast, nurturant love is thought to promote caring for relationship partners, most typically one's own children and young kin, that generalizes to others displaying cues of youthfulness and/or vulnerability (Hildebrandt & Fitzgerald, 1979). Preliminary evidence already points to some diverging effects of these two types of love. For example, in one study, participants induced to feel either attachment or nurturant love were then asked to indicate the extent to which they were convinced by a lengthy and detailed, but objectively weak, persuasive message (Griskevicius, Shiota, & Neufeld, 2010). Participants in the attachment love condition were more easily persuaded by the weak message, possibly reflecting an overall sense of trust in others and transfer of responsibility away from the self. In contrast, participants in the nurturant love condition showed reduced persuasion by the weak message compared to neutral control, consistent with increased vigilance. The extent of overlap and difference among various kinds of love is far from fully understood, and we hope it will be the focus of much future research.

Gratitude

Whereas love helps us solve the problem of committing to an established long-term relationship, gratitude may help us to identify and stay close to others who will likely provide us with support and resources in the future. One can maintain a relationship with someone who is able to provide useful benefits via a strategy known as "reciprocal altruism." This strategy relies on multiple transactions between two people, in which a benefit to one comes at a cost to the other but is later repaid in kind (Trivers, 1971). Gratitude experienced by the recipient of a benefit may help to promote balance in such relationships by motivating the recipient to repay the benefactor. The act of reciprocation can even encourage the original benefactor to act in a prosocial manner in the future. From this perspective, gratitude is seen as an integral part of the cycle of exchange relationships (McCullough, Kilpatrick, Emmons, & Larson, 2001).

Whereas this description emphasizes the immediate response to a benefit, Fredrickson (2004) proposes that gratitude may expand the recipient's focus beyond the present situation, broadening the view of both the benefactor and the potential opportunities a relationship with the benefactor might offer in the future. In their "find–remind–bind" theory of gratitude, Algoe, Haidt, and Gable (2008) propose that gratitude helps us identify and hold onto individuals who are attentive to our needs. While acknowledgment and repayment of the gift are important in the experience of gratitude, this perspective suggests that behavioral inclinations should focus primarily on creating a lasting relationship with the benefactor. For example, instead of repaying the benefactor in kind, a recipient might seek to repay the benefactor in more abstract ways that extend and deepen their relationship. This conceptualization addresses the role of gratitude in communal relationships, in which partners act from a commitment to meet the needs of both partners rather than in an exchange relationship, in which equal services are traded back and forth (Clark & Mills, 1993).

Although this view of gratitude is relatively new, research begun to address specific ways in which gratitude supports the initiation and maintenance of communal relationships. From this perspective, one important factor in gratitude-eliciting situations is the recognition of an especially responsive action or gift (Algoe et al., 2008). Perceptions of responsiveness are vital to creating intimacy in close relationships (Reis, Clark, & Holmes, 2004). A responsive gesture signals that another person cares about, understands, and approves of the recipient. In a study of sororities with a tradition of gift giving to younger members, Algoe and colleagues (2008) found that the main predictor of the recipient's gratitude was the perceived thoughtfulness of the gift, which was more important than cost, value, and how surprising the gift was. Algoe and colleagues argue that gratitude is uniquely elicited by perceptions of thoughtfulness because of the important opportunity a thoughtful gift signals. This opportunity is a potential communal relationship, which Clark and Mills (1993) differentiate from an exchange relationship in terms of the level of security each provides.

Among the cognitive effects of gratitude, researchers have found that individuals feeling gratitude compared to joy in a relived experience task were more likely to recall positive traits of the benefactor or helper (Algoe & Haidt, 2009; Watkins, Scheer, Ovnicke, & Kolts, 2006). In another study, using hypothetical scenarios to elicit gratitude, Weinstein, DeHaan, and Ryan (2010) found that participants reported greater liking and perceived closeness to the hypothetical helpers. Thus, gratitude broadens the recipient's focus beyond the immediate benefit when thinking of the benefactor and also enhances perception of relationship quality.

Participants recalling a time they felt gratitude report a desire to acknowledge the benefactor's actions (Algoe & Haidt, 2009), and to repay the benefactor (Campos, Shiota, Keltner, Gonzaga, & Goetz, 2013). This repayment can come not only in the form of an exchange of services (Bartlett & DeSteno, 2006), but also in more abstract forms, such as time, loyalty, or adoration (Algoe & Haidt, 2009; Watkins et al., 2006). Recent studies have shown that repayment often focuses on the needs of the benefactor; thus, reciprocating the benefactor's perceived responsiveness to individual needs appears to be the important element of the repayment (Bartlett, Condon, Cruz, Baumann, & DeSteno, 2012). This supports the idea that gratitude is meant to broaden and strengthen an important future communal relationship rather than simply even the score between a benefactor and recipient.

In addition to promoting new close relationships, gratitude is theorized to support the strengthening of existing relationships. The study of sororities discussed earlier revealed that recipients' feelings of gratitude predicted degree of integration within the sorority community as a whole, as well as both the recipient's and benefactor's feelings of closeness in the relationship (Algoe et al., 2008). In order to look at how gratitude functions in already-close relationships, Algoe, Gable, and Maisel (2010) asked romantic couples to report thoughtful acts they conceived and actually did for their partners over the course of 2 weeks. They found that each partner's report of feeling gratitude predicted increased perception of relationship closeness by *both* partners the following day. Thus, gratitude can also serve as a "booster shot" for long-term relationships, reminding the individual of an existing partner's responsiveness. These studies support the roles gratitude may play in both the formation of new communal relationships, by helping to identify responsive partners, and the maintenance of close relationships, by signaling the value of already-responsive partners.

Conclusions and Future Directions

Emotions serve important adaptive functions, helping individuals to acquire opportunities and avoid threats. Although the individual can handle some opportunities and threats effectively, a crucial part of an individual's success relies on close, interdependent relationships with others. Positive emotions are not only uniquely suited to helping individuals take advantage of the opportunities that relationships present but also are critical for finding and maintaining the relationships themselves.

Much research on positive emotions in relationships has started with theories about the functions of emotion for the individual, and generalizing these to the relationship context. An interesting future direction might be to consider what unique properties of emotions might emerge from the process of two individuals interacting with each other. For instance, above and beyond what is currently known about joy, could the shared experience of joy by two individuals give rise to behaviors or physiological changes that would not be observed in a single individual? Could such a process help in coordinating the emotions and goals of individuals in a relationship?

A separate area of research, equally understudied, might ask how positive emotions play out across different kinds of relationships, and in the same relationships over time. Are certain emotions, such as pride or gratitude, more appropriate in some relationships than in others? Based on the proposed function of gratitude, discussed earlier, we might predict that gratitude is more important in nonkin relationships lacking a biological imperative for commitment, which must be built and maintained over time. Is there a natural time course for positive emotions within relationships? Do some emotions become obsolete as the relationship progresses, only to be replaced by others? Such developments might reflect changes in the importance of different opportunities across the lifespan. Both of these sets of questions consider emotions themselves to

be inherently social—an area where much work remains to be done.

References

Acevedo, B. P., Aron, A., Fisher, H. E., Brown, L. L. (2012). Neural correlates of long-term intense romantic love. *Social Cognitive and Affective Neuroscience, 7*(2), 145–159.

Ainsworth, M. D. S. (1989). Attachments beyond infancy. *American Psychologist, 44,* 709–716.

Algoe, S. B. (2012). Find, remind, and bind: The functions of gratitude in everyday relationships. *Social and Personality Psychology Compass, 6*(6), 455–469.

Algoe, S. B., Gable, S. L., & Maisel, N. C. (2010). It's the little things: Everyday gratitude as a booster shot for romantic relationships. *Personal Relationships, 17*(2), 217–233.

Algoe, S. B., & Haidt, J. (2009). Witnessing excellence in action: The "other-praising" emotions of elevation, gratitude, and admiration. *Journal of Positive Psychology, 4*(2), 105–127.

Algoe, S. B., Haidt, J., & Gable, S. L. (2008). Beyond reciprocity: Gratitude and relationships in everyday life. *Emotion, 8*(3), 425–429.

Allred, K. G. (2000). Anger and retaliation in conflict: The role of attribution. In M. Deutsch & P. T. Coleman (Eds.), *The handbook of conflict resolution: Theory and practice* (pp. 236–255). San Francisco: Jossey-Bass.

Andersen, J. F., Andersen, P. A., & Jensen, A. D. (1979). The measurement of nonverbal immediacy. *Journal of Communication Research, 7,* 153–180.

Andersen, P. A. (1985). Nonverbal intimacy in interpersonal communication. In A. W. Siegman & S. Feldstein (Eds.), *Multichannel integrations of nonverbal behavior* (pp. 1–36). Hillsdale, NJ: Erlbaum.

Averill, J. R. (1968). Grief: Its nature and significance. *Psychological Bulletin, 70,* 721–748.

Barrett, K. C., & Campos, J. J. (1987). Perspectives on emotional development II: A functionalist approach to emotions. In J. D. Osofsky (Ed.), *Handbook of infant development* (2nd ed., pp. 558–578). New York: Wiley.

Bartels, A., & Zeki, S. (2000). The neural basis of romantic love. *NeuroReport, 11*(17), 3829–3834.

Bartlett, M. Y., Condon, P., Cruz, J., Baumann, J., & DeSteno, D. (2012). Gratitude: Prompting behaviors that build relationships. *Cognition and Emotion, 26*(1), 2–13.

Bartlett, M. Y., & DeSteno, D. (2006). Gratitude and prosocial behavior: Helping when it costs you. *Psychological Science, 17*, 319–325.

Beier, E. G., & Sternberg, D. P. (1977). Marital communication: Subtle cues between newlyweds. *Journal of Human Communication, 27*, 92–97.

Block, J. H., & Block, J. (1980). The role of ego-control and ego-resiliency in the origination of behavior. In W. A. Collings (Ed.), *The Minnesota Symposia on Child Psychology* (Vol. 13, pp. 39–101). Hillsdale, NJ: Erlbaum.

Bower, T. G. (1977). *A primer of infant development.* San Francisco: Freeman.

Buss, D. M. (1988). The evolution of intrasexual competition: Tactics of mate attraction. *Journal of Personality and Social Psychology, 54*(4), 616–628.

Buss, D. M. (1989). Sex differences in human mate preferences: Evolutionary hypotheses tested in 37 countries. *Behavioral and Brain Sciences, 12*, 1–49.

Buss, D. M. (1994). *The evolution of desire: Strategies of human mating.* New York: Basic Books.

Buss, D. M., Larsen, R. J., Westen, D., & Semmelroth, J. (1992). Sex differences in jealousy: Evolution, physiology, and psychology. *Psychological Science, 3*(4), 251–255.

Buss, D. M., & Shackelford, T. K. (1997). From vigilance to violence: Mate retention tactics in married couples. *Journal of Personality and Social Psychology, 72*(2), 346–361.

Butterworth, G., & Jarrett, N. (1991). What minds have in common is space: Spatial mechanisms serving joint visual attention in infancy. *British Journal of Developmental Psychology, 9*, 55–72.

Cacioppo, J. T., Gardner, W. L., & Berntson, G. G. (1997). Beyond bipolar conceptualizations and measures: The case of attitudes and evaluative space. *Personality and Social Psychology Review, 1*, 3–25.

Campos, B., Shiota, M. N., Keltner, D., Gonzaga, G. C., & Goetz, J. L. (2013). What is shared, what is different?: Core relational themes and expressive displays of eight positive emotions. *Cognition and Emotion, 27*, 37–52.

Caporael, L. R., & Brewer, M. B. (1995). Hierarchical evolutionary theory: There is an alternative, and it's not creationism. *Psychological Inquiry, 6*, 31–34.

Carstensen, L. L., Gottman, J. M., & Levenson, R. W. (1995). Emotional behavior in long-term marriage. *Psychology and Aging,* 10, 140–149.

Carver, C. S., & Harmon-Jones, E. (2009). Anger is an approach-related affect: Evidence and implications. *Psychological Bulletin, 135*, 183–204.

Carver, C. S., & Scheier, M. F. (1998). *On the self regulation of behavior.* New York: Cambridge University Press.

Christensen, A., & Heavey, C. L. (1990). Gender and social structure in the demand/withdraw pattern of marital conflict. *Journal of Personality and Social Psychology, 59*, 73–81.

Clark, M. S., & Mills, J. (1993). The difference between communal and exchange relationships: What it is and what it is not. *Personality and Social Psychology Bulletin, 19*(6), 684–691.

Daly, M., & Wilson, M. (1988). *Homicide.* Hawthorne, NY: de Gruyter.

Daly, M., Wilson, M., & Weghorst, S. J. (1982). Male sexual jealousy. *Ethology and Sociobiology, 3*(1), 11–27.

de Waal, F. B. M. (1996). *Good natured.* Cambridge, MA: Harvard University Press.

Downey, G., Freitas, A. L., Michaelis, B., & Khouri, H. (1998). The self-fulfilling prophecy in close relationships: Rejection sensitivity and rejection by romantic partners. *Journal of Personality and Social Psychology, 75*, 545–560.

Ekman, P. (1992). An argument for basic emotions. *Cognition and Emotion, 6*, 169–200.

Emde, R. N., Katz, E. L., & Thorpe, J. K. (1978). Emotional expression in infancy: II. Early deviations in Down's syndrome. In M. Lewis & L. Rosenblum (Eds.), *The development of affect* (pp. 351–360). New York: Plenum Press.

Fehr, B. (1988). Prototype analysis of the concepts of love and commitment. *Journal of Personality and Social Psychology, 55*(4), 557–579.

Forster, J., Ozelsel, A., & Epstude, K. (2009). Why love has wings and sex has not: how reminders of love and sex influence creative and analytic thinking. *Personality and Social Psychology Bulletin, 35*, 1479–1491.

Forster, J., Ozelsel, A., & Epstude, K. (2010). How love and lust change people's perception of relationship partners. *Journal of Experimental Social Psychology, 46*, 237–246.

Frank, R. H. (1988). *Passions within reason: The strategic role of the emotions.* New York: Norton.

Fredrickson, B. L. (1998). What good are positive emotions? *Review of General Psychology,* 2, 300–319.

Fredrickson, B. L. (2001). The role of positive emotion in psychology: The broaden-and-build theory of positive emotions. *American Psychologist, 56,* 218–226.

Fredrickson, B. L. (2004). Gratitude, like other positive emotions, broadens and builds. In R. A. Emmons & M. E. McCullough (Eds.), *The psychology of gratitude* (pp. 145–166). New York: Oxford University Press.

Fredrickson, B. L., & Branigan, C. (2005). Positive emotions broaden the scope of attention and thought–action repertoires. *Cognition and Emotion, 19,* 313–332.

Fredrickson, B. L., & Levenson, R. W. (1998). Positive emotions speed recovery from the cardiovascular sequelae of negative emotions. *Cognition and Emotion, 12,* 191–220.

Fredrickson, B. L., Tugade, M. M., Waugh, C. E., Larkin, G. R. (2003). What good are positive emotions in crises?: A prospective study of resilience and emotions following the terrorist attacks on the United States on September 11th, 2001. *Journal of Personality and Social Psychology, 84*(2), 365–376.

Frijda, N. H., & Mesquita, B. (1994). The social roles and functions of emotions. In S. Kitayama & H. Marcus (Eds.), *Emotion and culture: Empirical studies of mutual influenced.* (pp. 51–87). Washington, DC: American Psychological Association.

Gable, S. L. (2006). Approach and avoidance social motives and goals. *Journal of Personality, 74,* 175–222.

Gable, S. L., Gonzaga, C. E., & Strachman, A. (2006). Will you be there for me when things go right?: Supportive responses to positive event disclosures. *Journal of Personality and Social Psychology, 91*(5), 904–917.

Gable, S. L., Reis, H. T., Impett, E. A., & Asher, E. R. (2004). What do you do when things go right?: The intrapersonal and interpersonal benefits of sharing positive events. *Journal of Personality and Social Psychology, 87*(2), 228–245.

Gonzaga, G. C., Haselton, M. G., Smurda, J., Davies, M. S., & Poore, J. C. (2008). Love, desire, and the suppression of thoughts of romantic alternatives. *Evolution and Human Behavior, 29,* 119–126.

Gonzaga, G. C., Keltner, D., Londahl, E. A., & Smith, M. D. (2001). Love and the commitment problem in romantic relationships and friendship. *Journal of Personality and Social Psychology, 81,* 247–262.

Gonzaga, G. C., Turner, R. A., Keltner, D., Campos, B., & Altemus, M. (2006). Romantic love and sexual desire in close relationships. *Emotion, 6*(2), 163–179.

Gottman, J. M., & Levenson, R. W. (1992). Marital processes predictive of later dissolution: Behavior, physiology, and health. *Journal of Personality and Social Psychology, 63,* 221–233.

Griskevicius, V., Shiota, M. N., & Neufeld, S. L. (2010). Influence of different positive emotions on persuasion processing: A functional evolutionary approach. *Emotion, 10,* 190–206.

Heavey, C. L., Christensen, A., & Malamuth, N. M. (1995). The longitudinal impact of demand and withdraw during marital conflict. *Journal of Consulting and Clinical Psychology, 63,* 797–801.

Hendricks, M. C. P., Croon, M. A., & Vingerhoets, J. J. M. (2010). Social reactions to adult crying: The help-soliciting function of tears. *Journal of Social Psychology, 148,* 22–42.

Hildebrandt, K. A., & Fitzgerald, H. E. (1979). Adults' perceptions of infant sex and cuteness. *Sex Roles, 5,* 471–481.

Impett, E. A., Gordon, A. M., Kogan, A., Oveis, C., Gable, S. L., & Keltner, D. (2010). Moving toward more perfect unions: Daily and long-term consequences of approach and avoidance goals in romantic relationships. *Journal of Personality and Social Psychology, 99*(6), 948–963.

Isen, A. M., Daubman, K. A., & Nowicki, G. P. (1987). Positive affect facilitates creative problem solving. *Journal of Personality and Social Psychology, 52,* 1122–1131.

Izard, C. E. (1977). *Human emotion.* New York: Plenum Press.

James, W. (1884). What is an emotion? *Mind, 9,* 188–205.

Keller, M. C., & Nesse, R. M. (2006). The evolutionary significance of depressive symptoms: Different adverse situations lead to different depressive symptom patterns. *Journal of Personality and Social Psychology, 91,* 316–330.

Keltner, D., & Buswell, B. N. (1997). Embarrassment: Its distinct form and appeasement functions. *Psychological Bulletin, 122,* 250–270.

Keltner, D., Ellsworth, P. C., & Edwards, K. (1993). Beyond simple pessimism: Effects of sadness and anger on social perception. *Jour-*

nal of Personality and Social Psychology, 64, 740–752.

Keltner, D., & Haidt, J. (1999). Social functions of emotions at four levels of analysis. Cognition and Emotion, 13, 505–521.

Keltner, D., & Kring, A. M. (1998). Emotion, social function, and psychopathology. Review of General Psychology, 2, 320–342.

Langston, C. A. (1994). Capitalizing on and coping with daily-life events: Expressive responses to positive events. Journal of Personality and Social Psychology, 67, 1112–1125.

Lazarus, R. S. (1991). Emotion and adaptation. New York: Oxford University Press.

Lazarus, R. S. (1993). From psychological stress to the emotions: A history of changing outlooks. Annual Review of Psychology, 44, 1–22.

Levenson, R. W. (1999). The intrapersonal functions of emotion. Cognition and Emotion, 13, 481–504.

Levenson, R. W., & Gottman, J. M. (1983). Marital interaction: Physiological linkage and affective exchange. Journal of Personality and Social Psychology, 45, 587–597.

Lutz, C. A., & White, G. (1986). The anthropology of emotion. Annual Review of Anthropology, 15, 405–436.

Maner, J. K., Rouby, D. A., & Gonzaga, C. E. (2008). Automatic inattention to attractive alternatives: The evolved psychology of relationship maintenance. Evolution and Human Behavior, 29(5), 343–349.

McCullough, M. E., Kilpatrick, S. D., Emmons, R. A., & Larson, D. B. (2001). Is gratitude a moral affect? Psychological Bulletin, 127(2), 249–266.

McGinley, H., McGinley, P., & Nicholas, K. (1978). Smiling, body position, and interpersonal attraction. Bulletin of the Psychonomic Society, 12, 21–24.

Mehrabian, A. (1971). Verbal and nonverbal interactions of strangers in a waiting situation. Journal of Experimental Research in Personality, 5, 127–138.

Nesse, R. M. (1990). Evolutionary explanations of emotions. Human Nature, 1(3), 261–289.

Nesse, R. M., & Ellsworth, P. C. (2009). Evolution, emotions, and emotional disorders. American Psychologist, 64(2), 129–139.

Ortigue, S., Bianchi-Demicheli, F., Hamilton, A. F., & Grafton, S. T. (2007). The neural basis of love as a subliminal prime: An event-related functional magnetic resonance imaging study.

Journal of Cognitive Neuroscience, 19(7), 1218–1230.

Plutchik, R. (1980). Emotion: A psychoevolutionary synthesis. New York: Harper & Row.

Reis, H. T., Clark, M. S., & Holmes, J. G. (2004). Perceived partner responsiveness as an organizing construct in the study of intimacy and closeness. In D. J. Mashek & A. Aron (Eds.), Handbook of closeness and intimacy (pp. 27–52). Mahwah, NJ: Erlbaum.

Rozin, P., & Fallon, A. E. (1987). A perspective on disgust. Psychological Review, 94(1), 23–41.

Russell, J. A. (2003). Core affect and the psychological construction of emotion. Psychological Review, 110, 145–172.

Schaller, M., & Duncan, L. A. (2007). The behavioral immune system: Its evolution and social psychological implications. In J. P. Forgas, M. G. Haselton, & W. von Hippel (Eds.), Evolution and the social mind: Evolutionary psychology and social cognition (pp. 293–307). New York: Psychology Press.

Scherer, K. R. (2009). The dynamic architecture of emotion: Evidence for the component process model. Cognition and Emotion, 23(7), 1307–1351.

Shaver, P., Hazan, C., & Bradshaw, D. (1988). Love as attachment: The integration of three behavioral systems. In R. Sternberg & M. Barnes (Eds.), The anatomy of love (pp. 68–99). New Haven, CT: Yale University Press.

Shaver, P., Morgan, H. J., & Wu, S. (1996). Is love a basic emotion? Personal Relationships, 3, 81–96.

Shiota, M. N., Campos, B., Keltner, D., & Hertenstein, M. J. (2004). Positive emotion and the regulation of interpersonal relationships. In P. Philippot & R. S. Feldman (Eds), The regulation of emotion (pp. 127–155). Mahwah, NJ: Erlbaum.

Shiota, M. N., Keltner, D., & John, O. P. (2006). Positive emotion dispositions differentially associated with the Big Five personality and attachment style. Journal of Positive Psychology, 1, 61–71.

Strachman, A., & Gable, S. L. (2006). What you want (and don't want) affects what you see (and don't see): Avoidance social goals and social events. Personality and Social Psychology Bulletin, 32, 1446–1458.

Tangney, J. P., Miller, R. S., Flicker, L., & Barlow, D. H. (1996). Are shame, guilt, and embarrassment distinct emotions? *Journal of Personality and Social Psychology, 70,* 1256–1279.

Tooby, J., & Cosmides, L. (1990). The past explains the present: Emotional adaptations and the structure of ancestral environments. *Ethology and Sociobiology, 11,* 375–424.

Tooby, J., & Cosmides, L. (2008). The evolutionary psychology of the emotions and their relationship to internal regulatory variables. In M. Lewis, J. M. Haviland-Jones, & L. F. Barrett (Eds.), *Handbook of emotions* (3rd ed.,pp. 114–137). New York: Guilford Press.

Tracy, J. L., & Robins, R. W. (2004). Putting the self into self-conscious emotions: A theoretical model. *Psychological Inquiry, 14,* 57–62.

Trivers, R. L. (1971). The evolution of reciprocal altruism. *Quarterly Review of Biology, 46,* 35–57.

Trivers, R. L. (1972). Parental investment and sexual selection. In B. Campbell (Ed.), *Sexual selection and the descent of man—1871–1971* (pp. 136–179). Chicago: Aldine-Atherton.

Tugade, M. M., & Fredrickson, B. L. (2004). Resilient individuals use positive emotions to bounce back from negative emotional experience. *Journal of Personality and Social Psychology, 88*(2), 320–333.

Van Kleef, G. A., De Dreu, C. K. W., & Manstead, A. S. R. (2004). The interpersonal effects of anger and happiness in negotiations. *Journal of Personality and Social Psychology, 86,* 57–76.

Watkins, P. C., Scheer, J., Ovnicke, M., & Kolts, R. (2006). The debt of gratitude: Dissociating gratitude and indebtedness. *Cognition and Emotion, 20,* 217–241.

Waugh, C. E., & Fredrickson, B. L. (2006). Nice to know you: Positive emotions, self-other overlap, and complex understanding in the formation of a new relationship. *Journal of Positive Psychology, 1*(2), 93–106.

Weinstein, N., DeHaan, C. R., & Ryan, R. M. (2010). Attributing autonomous versus introjected motivation to helpers and the recipient experience: Effects on gratitude, attitudes, and well-being. *Motivation and Emotion, 34*(4), 418–431.

Xu, X., Aron, A., Brown, L., Cao, G., Feng, T., & Weng, X. (2011). Reward and motivation systems: A brain mapping study of early-stage intense romantic love in Chinese participants. *Human Brain Mapping, 32,* 249–257.

Yuan, J. W., McCarthy, M., Holley, S. R., & Levenson, R. W. (2010). Physiological downregulation and positive emotion in marital interaction. *Emotion, 10*(4), 467–474.

CHAPTER 13

Traversing Affective Boundaries

Examining Cultural Norms for Positive Emotions

Chelsea Mitamura
Janxin Leu
Belinda Campos
Chelsea Boccagno
Michele M. Tugade

Cultures differ in how they understand, recognize, and experience positive emotions. Although most individuals strive to be happy (Diener, 2000), there is considerable cultural variation in the manner in which happiness is valued and experienced. A rapidly expanding literature reveals substantial variability between and within cultures in how people appraise, experience, express, regulate, and perceive emotion (e.g., Chang, Tugade, & Asakawa, 2006; D'Andrade, 1984; Elfenbein & Ambady, 2002, 2003; Ellsworth, 1994; Kitayama, Duffy, & Uchida, 2007; Kitayama, Mesquita, & Karasawa, 2006; Lutz, 1988; Mesquita & Leu, 2007; Nisbett & Cohen, 1996; Tsai, Knutson, & Fung, 2006). As globalization and technological progress bring together individuals from diverse cultural contexts, there is also growing appreciation of culture's role in shaping emotional experience. Lessons learned from research on these implications of culture are yielding a more comprehensive scientific understanding of human emotions, including positive emotions.

This chapter examines the current research on cultural influences in positive emotions. We first discuss important theoretical approaches to the study of culture and emotion. Next, we review empirical research that reveals how positive emotions (their meaning, expression, regulation, and function) are shaped by culture. Finally, we discuss challenges in the study of positive emotions and culture, and consider future directions for this area of research. Our overall aim in this chapter is to illuminate the ways in which cultural variability shapes the experience and meaning of positive emotions.

Theories of Culture and Emotions

Currently, the most influential theories of emotion are built on a conception of the individual as an independent, self-directed entity, whose behavior is largely a consequence of internal traits, motives, and values. While this concept of the "independent self" and the psychological phenomena linked to the self might characterize individuals from a Western European cultural background, it applies less readily to members of other cultures. Moreover, dominant models of emotion typically conceptualize the stimuli that elicit emotions as independent of each other, with properties that make them either desirable or undesirable, but not both. This conceptual approach reflects a Western, Aristotelian philosophical perspective that differs in important ways from the philosophical principles on which other cultures are founded. In this section we review theories positing relationships between these core cultural differences and the experience and meaning of positive emotions.

Individualism–Collectivism and Affect Valuation Theory

Affect valuation theory (AVT) posits that, especially when studying implications of culture for emotion, it is important to distinguish between two distinct aspects of affect. The first, "ideal affect," is the affect that people would like to feel—a goal. The second, "actual affect," is the affect that people actually feel—a state of being. The research literature on emotions offers widely differing perspectives on whether emotions are primarily universal versus culturally constructed. An AVT perspective may help to reconcile these differing accounts. According to recent analyses, studies examining the physiological and behavioral aspects of emotions, and/or reports of the frequency and intensity of subjective emotional experience, primarily emphasize actual affect; in contrast, studies examining the emotional practices in which people engage may be tapping ideal affect (Tsai et al., 2006).

Actual affect has typically been the focus of studies used to support a more universal model of emotional experience, whereas ideal affect may show a more culturally differentiated pattern. For example, in a study testing the predictive validity of AVT, Tsai and colleagues (2006) found that actual and ideal affect (as measured via a questionnaire with separate sets of items for desired and actual emotional experience) were two distinct factors. Furthermore, variability in actual positive emotion was predicted primarily by individual differences in personality variables, such as Extraversion and Neuroticism, with no significant effect of culture, whereas cultural differences in ideal affect were pronounced. Specifically,

European Americans and Asian Americans reported valuing high-activation positive affect (e.g., excitement) more highly than did Hong Kong Chinese. In contrast, Hong Kong Chinese reported valuing low-activation positive affect (e.g., calm) more highly than did European Americans. Overall, Tsai and colleagues' findings suggested that actual affect is shaped more strongly by inherited temperament, whereas ideal affect is shaped more strongly by cultural factors.

The cultural shaping of ideal affect communicates "unwritten codes" or "display rules" that govern the manner in which emotions should be felt and expressed through modeling, social consequences, and other socialization mechanisms (e.g., Ekman & Friesen, 1969; Izard, 1980; Saarni, 1999). Different rules may be internalized as a function of an individual's culture, gender, or family background (Ekman & Friesen, 1975). The socialization of ideal affect can be detected very early in the lifespan (Tsai, 2007). Research suggests that even preschool-age children learn ideal affect through cultural products, such as children's storybooks (Tsai, Louie, Chen, & Uchida, 2007).

One key aspect of culture with strong implications for ideal affect is the distinction between "individualism," the perception that the self and its well-being are independent from other people, and "collectivism," the perception that the self is defined in large part by one's relationships and group memberships (Markus & Kitayama, 1991). For example, whereas members of individualist cultures such as the United States and Canada tend to emphasize personal achievements in evaluating their own happiness (Uchida, Norasakkunkit, & Kitayama, 2004), members of more collectivist cultures, including Asian and Latino cultures, are likely to emphasize group harmony and relationship status over individual needs as determinants of happiness (Diener & Suh, 2003; Uchida et al., 2004). A culture's relative emphasis on individualism versus collectivism can have important implications for what kinds of positive emotion are valued. In one study, European American preschool children preferred excited (vs. calm) smiles and activities, and perceived an excited (vs. calm) smile as happier than did Taiwanese Chinese preschoolers (Tsai et al., 2007).

This is consistent with adult media representations of happiness, with American best-sellers containing more excited and arousing content in their books than Taiwanese best-sellers, and American women displaying more excited smiles compared to Chinese women in equivalent magazines (Tsai & Wong, 2007). These findings suggest that cultural differences in ideal affect become evident very early and persist through adulthood.

It is important to note, however, that not all collectivist cultures display the same patterns of ideal affect (Ruby, Falk, Heine, Villa, & Silberstein, 2012). Mexican culture, for example, has a cultural script of *simpatía* that emphasizes promoting group harmony through the open expression of positive emotion (Triandis, Marin, Lisansky, & Betancourt, 1984). In one study, Ruby and colleagues (2012) compared individuals from East Asia and Mexico, and found that Mexican participants showed a preference for high-activation (e.g., excited, enthusiastic, elated) over low-activation (e.g., calm, "at rest," serene) positive emotions, whereas Chinese participants showed the opposite pattern. In another important study asking whether Latin American and East Asian differences extended from ideal affect to actual subjective experience and physiological reactivity, Soto, Levenson, and Ebling (2005) found that Mexican Americans reported experiencing significantly more emotion following an acoustic startle task than did Chinese Americans; this cultural difference did not extend to physiology. These findings suggest that the differential emphasis on expression of emotion between Mexican and Asian cultures (i.e., open vs. subdued expression of emotion, respectively) reflects cultural influence rather than biological differences between cultural groups.

That there is variation between Mexican and Asian cultures in preference for and expression of positive emotions is noteworthy for two reasons. First, it indicates that there is more than one cultural script for promoting interdependent relationships. Misunderstandings regarding the meaning of emotional behavior can occur not only between individualist and collectivist cultural groups but also between two distinct collectivist cultures (e.g., Mexican and Asian). Second, at least two distinct types of collectivism exist. This calls into question the unintended consequences that might arise when researchers focus primarily on differences between the United States (to represent individualism) and East Asian countries (to represent collectivism) in studying the impact of culture on emotion. That is, considering that collectivism manifests in different forms, an exclusive East–West focus can result in too-narrow conclusions about the implications of individualism and collectivism (Cohen, 2007).

Linear versus Dialectical Epistemologies

Moving beyond the implications of self-concept, Nisbett (2003) has suggested that Westerners and Easterners think about, interpret, and see the world differently in a variety of ways. Emotion theorists would extend this view and posit that members of these different cultures may also *feel* and *experience* emotions differently. Some differences in emotion are thought to reflect the influence of ancient Western and East Asian philosophies (Peng & Nisbett, 1999). Ancient Greek philosophers endorsed the law of identity (if *A* is true, then *A* is always true), the law of contradiction (*A* cannot equal not-*A*), and the law of the excluded middle (everything is either true or false). In contrast, East Asian philosophers in ancient times emphasized the principle of holism (everything in the universe is related), the principle of change (the universe is constantly changing), and the principle of contradiction (two sides of an apparent contradiction can *both* be true). These philosophies have had long-lasting impact on thought, affect, and behavior, reinforced by the institutionalization of these principles in all aspects of life—law, science, language, education, media, and so forth.

These philosophical differences can be seen in Western and Eastern cultural "scripts" for emotion—cultural norms that influence how people expect emotions to be experienced and regulated (Miyamoto & Ryff, 2011). Research indicates, for instance, that in Western cultures, the dominant emotion script presumes that people maximize positive emotions and minimize negative emotions (Kitayama & Markus, 1999). Western scripts for emotion also emphasize that positive and negative emotions are opposing constructs, not to be experienced simultaneously (Russell & Carroll, 1999). Interestingly, this epistemological approach extends to cultural contexts that are both Western and collectivist. For example, Latin American cultures also have emotion scripts that emphasize maximizing positive emotions and minimizing negative emotions (Triandis et al., 1984). In contrast, East Asian emotion scripts based on dialectical reasoning emphasize a "middle way," experiencing a balance between positive and negative emotions, or even experiencing positive and negative emotions simultaneously (e.g., Bagozzi, Wong, & Yi, 1999; Shiota, Campos, Gonzaga, Keltner, & Peng, 2010). In these ways, the distinction between linear and dialectical epistemologies might suggest culture-specific styles of affective responding.

Broaden-and-Build Theory: New Directions for Culture and Positive Emotion?

Incorporating cultural perspectives into the study of affect has the potential to expand our understanding of the functions of positive emotions. Broaden-and-build theory (Fredrickson, 1998) articulates the complementary function and effects of positive emotions, suggesting that positive emotions serve to "broaden" an individual's thought–action repertoire, which subsequently enables the individual to abandon automatic behavioral scripts and to pursue innovative, unscripted courses of thought and behavior. These novel courses of thought and behavior help "build" social, physical, intellectual, and psychological resources that extend beyond the duration of the positive emotions themselves. Fredrickson points to joy, interest, contentment, and love as four major positive emotion families that may help to build various kinds of resources.

Fredrickson speculates that "joy," the term used to capture emotions such as happiness and exhilaration, and "interest," sharing conceptual space with curiosity, intrigue, excitement and wonder, lead an individual to engage in extended exploration and play. Whereas exploration exposes an individual to experiences and information otherwise undiscovered, increasing his or her knowledge base, in play an individual can potentially bolster his or her range of physical,

social, and intellectual skills (Fredrickson, 1998). "Contentment," also conceptualized as tranquility or serenity, prompts an individual to appreciate his or her current life circumstances and experience a sense of connectedness to the world. Contentment can lead an individual to incorporate recent events and achievements into the self-concept and consequently expand his or her worldview and self-complexity. Finally, "love" of all kinds induces other positive emotions and their benefits, as well as building social support (Fredrickson, 1998).

Research suggests that positive emotions may lead to expansion of attentional focus and creativity, improved understanding of complex situations, and engagement in a broader range of actions than previously accessible. Furthermore, positive emotions may function to counter negative emotions, which narrow an individual's thought–action repertoire (Fredrickson, 1998). This proposal is referred to as the "undoing hypothesis," which predicts that positive emotions reestablish autonomic quiescence following negative emotional arousal, and potentially restore more flexible thinking (Fredrickson & Levenson, 1998; Fredrickson, Tugade, Waugh, & Larkin, 2003; Tugade & Fredrickson, 2007). For example, research demonstrates that people who view a positive film, thereby inducing a positive emotional experience, recover faster from negative emotional arousal than those who view a sad or neutral film (Fredrickson & Levenson, 1998).

A question remains: Are the functions and benefits of positive emotions consistent across cultures? Positive emotions, like all individual experiences, may be intrinsically tied to the norms and values to which an individual adheres. They may therefore serve different functions across different cultures and peoples. In the section that follows, we build on these theories of positive emotions and discuss how culture shapes the meaning, expression, and function of positive emotions.

Cultural Contexts Shape Positive Emotions

Cultural contexts profoundly shape positive emotions. As the values, norms, and practices of diverse communities vary, so do the meaning, expression, and functional implications of positive emotions. From a cognitive-appraisal perspective, emotions are responses to perceived threats and opportunities in the environment that implicate the psychological self (Lazarus, 1991). To the extent that these perceptions and the psychological self differ across cultures, so do positive emotions. In this section, research presenting systematic comparisons across cultural contexts is reviewed to support the argument that positive emotions are powerfully culturally constructed.

Cultural Variability in the Experience of Positive Emotion

Models of agency (e.g., disjoint vs. conjoint agency) have been applied to understand how cultures can differ in the actual experience of emotions, as well as in ideal affect (Uchida, Townsend, Markus, & Bergsieker, 2009). Uchida and colleagues (2009) suggest that North American contexts reflect a disjoint agency model, such that emotions are experienced "within people" and individually through internal self-reflection. In this cultural context, one's emotions are personal and separate from those of others (e.g., "I feel joy"). In contrast, Japanese cultural contexts reflect a relational or conjoint agency model, such that emotional experiences are experienced "between people" and evaluated based on the relationship between others and the self. Here, emotions inherently involve others (e.g., "I would like to share my happiness with others"; Uchida et al., 2009). These findings elaborate on the individualism–collectivism distinction, such that in American cultural contexts, emotions are understood as self-focused, whereas in Japanese cultural contexts they are relationship-focused.

Cultural Variability in the Meaning of Positive Emotion

Consider the positive emotion of happiness, which signals the moral primacy of autonomy in individualist, Western cultural contexts, where selfhood is celebrated as independent and unique from others (Markus & Kitayama, 1991). Among middle-class European Americans, the expression of positive feelings is associated with individual success and fundamental self-worth (Heine, Lehman, Markus, & Kitayama, 1999; Kitayama, Markus, & Kurokawa, 2000). Excitement, an emotion marked by high arousal and a pleasant valence, reflects a Judeo-Christian ideal (Tsai, 2007).

In contrast, positive emotions are not conceptualized as unequivocally good in many East Asian cultural contexts, situated within the philosophical traditions of Buddhism, Confucianism, and Daoism. Buddhists believe that pure pleasantness either leads to suffering in the long run or is impossible to obtain. The Daoist concept of yin–yang suggests that positive emotions are, in part, inherently bad. These beliefs may create a psychological tendency to be cautious toward positive emotions. This perspective is illustrated by a famous Chinese folktale. In the story, a farmer experiences losses and gains (his horse runs away, only to return with a wild horse, only to cause his son to break his leg in trying to tame the wild horse, only to save his son from army conscription, etc.). The moral of the story is that not only can one never tell whether an event is good or bad, but also one should guard against extreme feelings—even positive ones. Implications are evident in the conceptual networks surrounding positive emotion in East Asian versus Western cultures. For example, Japanese are more likely than European Americans to associate happiness with negative social consequences, such as jealousy in others and disharmony in social relationships (Uchida & Kitayama, 2009).

Cultural Variability in Emotion Expression and Regulation

In individualist, Western cultural contexts, where positive emotions are viewed as unequivocally good, a strategy of hedonic emotion regulation (i.e., savoring and maximizing positive emotions) seems functional and appropriate. Indeed, this is also the case in collectivist Western cultural contexts, specifically, Latin American cultures, where expressing strong positive emotion in the service of relationships is encouraged (Triandis et al., 1984). For example, Holloway, Waldrip, and Ickes (2009) found that same-sex dyadic interactions including at least one Latino participant contained more expressions of positive emotion, and were subjectively reported as having a higher quality, than dyads in which both members were European American and/or African American. In contrast, positive emotions carry negative connotations in many East Asian cultural contexts, and a strategy of emotion moderation (i.e., balancing positive emotions) appears to be more common (Leu et al., 2010; Miyamoto & Ma, 2011). For example, using retrospective memory procedures, East Asians recalled engaging in hedonic emotion regulation less often than Westerners, even after researchers controlled for their initial emotional reactions. In other studies, these differences were found to be mediated by beliefs that positive emotions may have negative consequences (Miyamoto & Ma, 2011).

Recruiting negative emotions to balance positive ones may be one regulatory strategy to obtain the goal of emotion moderation. Empirical evidence for this idea can be found in research on "dialectical emotions," or emotions that are simultaneously positive and negative (Bagozzi et al., 1999). Many cross-national surveys have observed a negative correlation between positive and negative emotions among Western samples (i.e., "I feel either happy or sad"), whereas in East Asian samples, there is either no correlation, a positive correlation (i.e., "I feel both happy and sad"), or a smaller negative correlation (Bagozzi et al., 1999; Schimmack, Oishi, & Diener, 2002). For example, in multiple studies, Asians report equal levels of pleasant and unpleasant feelings, in contrast to North Americans, who report more positive emotions (Kitayama et al., 2000; Mesquita & Karasawa, 2002).

Experimental evidence suggests that these cultural differences are driven by variability in the appraised meaning of positive events but not negative events. For example, Leu and colleagues (2010) demonstrated that in positive, but not negative, situations, the correlation between positive and negative emotions was more negative among European Americans than among Chinese or Japanese participants. Similarly, Miyamoto, Uchida, and Ellsworth (2010) indicated that Japanese participants reported more simultaneous positive and negative emotions than did European Americans, but only in positive situations. These data suggest that in positive situations, Asians may "find the bad

in the good" more often than do European Americans.

Cultural Variability in the Function of Positive Emotions

Both established and recent findings suggest further cultural variability in the function of positive emotions relative to well-being and health. When deciding how satisfied they are, people in nations characterized as individualistic consult their feelings; pleasant emotions predict higher life satisfaction in cross-national surveys (Diener, 2000; Suh, Diener, Oishi, & Triandis, 1998). However, in nations characterized as collectivistic, pleasant emotions are not as predictive of subjective well-being; instead, appraisals of family and friends play a stronger role. For example, in one study, Kitayama and colleagues (2000) found that the reported frequency of general positive emotions (e.g., calm, elated) was most closely associated with the reported frequency of interpersonally engaged positive emotions (e.g., friendly feelings) in Japan, but with the reported frequency of interpersonally disengaged positive emotions (e.g., pride) in the United States. Moreover, Americans reported higher frequency of experience for positive emotions than for negative emotions, whereas among Japanese reports were higher for engaged emotions than for disengaged emotions. These findings reflect the central importance of feeling positive for Americans, and of feeling interpersonally connected for Japanese.

Cultural differences in the meaning of positive emotions may have implications for their functional relevance to health. Leu, Wang, and Koo (2011) surveyed over 600 European American, immigrant Asian, and Asian American college students to investigate how positive and negative emotions are related to mental health. They found that increased positive emotions were directly related to decreases in depression symptoms among European Americans, but not among immigrant Asians. Furthermore, the influence of perceived stress on depression was partially explained by intensity of positive feelings only among European Americans (Leu et al., 2011); no correlation was found among immigrant Asians. Negative emotions predicted poorer mental health to a similar extent in all three groups, suggesting that there may be greater cultural variability relative to health implications of positive emotions' effects than those of negative emotions.

These findings also raise questions about the cross-cultural generalizability of other findings that involve positive emotion and mental health. For example, studies of the protective effects of positive emotions against depression (Fredrickson et al., 2003) have been conducted on almost exclusively Western samples. Recent work suggests that cultural variability in the *meaning* of positive emotions may have implications for physical health, beyond the implications of the emotions themselves. Studies with Latin American samples suggest that these cultures' emphasis on open expression of positive emotion has favorable mental and physical health implications. For example, one study comparing Mexican American and European American patients with schizophrenia found that family warmth—an element of *simpatía*—was a protective factor against schizophrenia relapse for Mexican Americans (Lopez et al., 2004). Another study that assessed the relationship between positive emotion and onset of frailty (e.g., impaired strength, endurance, and balance) in older Mexican Americans found that high baseline positive affect was associated with a 3% reduction in risk of frailty 7 years later (Ostir, Ottenbacher, & Markides, 2004).

In contrast, using data from two nationally-representative surveys of Japanese and Americans, Miyamoto and Ryff (2011) found that dialectical emotions were associated with fewer physical symptoms in Japan but not in the United States. Whereas "pure" positive emotions seem to predict better health outcomes in Western populations, this study suggests that the balance of positive and negative emotions is more associated with physical health among Japanese. Taken together, these studies suggest that cultural scripts around the value of positive emotions may be of clinical relevance.

Interpreting Cultural Differences as Variability in Socialization

An important consideration is how we interpret the underlying causes of cultural differences in emotion. Variability in emotion may be attributed to differing socialization practices, or to inherent racial or ethnic differences. Although the two are conflated in most studies, there are notable exceptions. In one study, Asian Canadian college students who were shown Canadian primes reported fewer dialectical emotions than those who were shown Asian primes (Perunovic, Heller, & Rafaeli, 2007). In the survey of positive emotions and depression symptoms described earlier (Leu et al., 2011), the results for Asian Americans fell between those of European Americans and immigrant Asians: The correlation between positive emotions and depression was negative, but smaller than that among European Americans. Both findings suggest that cultural socialization and context are more important than race per se in explaining cultural differences in emotion.

Cultural differences in the meaning, expression, and function of positive emotions may reflect cultural variability in what kinds of events are perceived as threats and opportunities. A positive event may signal threat to East Asians, yet trigger unequivocal happiness in many European Americans (Leu et al., 2009; Miyamoto et al., 2010). "Good" feelings are associated with interpersonally engaged emotions among Japanese but with disengaged emotions among European Americans (Kitayama et al., 2000). Whereas positive feelings predict fewer depression symptoms among European Americans, these are uncorrelated among immigrant Asians (Leu et al., 2011). Instead, mixed emotions predict better physical health among Japanese (Miyamoto & Ryff, 2011). These examples provide initial evidence that positive emotions are, by nature, culturally constructed and therefore variable in their meaning, expression, and function given differences (e.g., East Asian versus Western) in self-construal, values, norms, and practices.

Cultural Variability in the Determination of "Happiness"

Happiness is generally considered, across cultures, to be a desirable state. Culture affects the way people evaluate their life satisfaction or "happiness" by influencing the definition, nature, meaning, and pursuit of happiness, as well how happiness influences evaluation of the self (Diener, Scollon, Oishi, Dzokoto, & Suh, 2000; Lu & Gilmour, 2004). For example, happiness can be defined in terms of a mental state of satisfaction or contentment, positive feelings/emotions, a harmonious homeostasis, achievement and hope, and/or freedom from ill-being.

Implications of Linear versus Dialectical Epistemology

Happiness can be conceptualized as single-sided, with only positive elements, or as dialectical, dynamically interdependent with unhappiness (Lu & Gilmour, 2004). Americans conceptualize positive and negative emotions as opposites, which could account for their mutually exclusive nature in Western societies (Miyamoto et al., 2010). In Eastern cultures people are taught to accept constant situational and emotional change and contradiction, to accept negative emotions alongside positive emotions (Heine et al., 1999). As noted earlier, positive and negative emotions are highly correlated and can occur simultaneously in Eastern cultures, but they are found to be negatively or uncorrelated in Western cultures (Bagozzi et al., 1999; Miyamoto et al., 2010; Uchida & Kitayama, 2009).

Similarly, in Eastern cultures, happiness is believed to be dialectical in nature—with the positive inherently comes the negative. The two opposing entities give one another meaning and are naturally intertwined. When prompted to describe happiness, Americans focus on its positive aspects, whereas Japanese people typically refer to both positive and negative aspects (Miyamoto & Ma, 2011). In Western cultures people are encouraged to maximize positivity of the self, as well as positive emotions, and to minimize negative emotions (Miyamoto et al., 2010). As noted earlier, ideal positive affect and happiness are much lower in arousal and intensity in Eastern cultures than in Western cultures (Tsai et al., 2006).

It is unsurprising, then, that previous research has found cultural differences in savoring (up-regulation, maintenance) versus dampening (down-regulation) of positive emotions (Miyamoto & Ma, 2011). Whereas people from Western cultures strive to savor and maintain their positive emotions, and to stave off negative emotions as long as possible, people from Eastern cultures do not function in the same way. For example, Japa-

nese people are more likely to try to dampen their positive emotions following a personal success, and report fear of troubling others and dialectical beliefs as the main impetuses for their behavior. European Americans, on the other hand, are more likely to try to find activities to increase or maintain their positive emotions (Miyamoto & Ma, 2011).

Do people in all cultures recruit positive emotions in coping with negative experiences? Happiness is associated with greater self-control, self-regulatory, and coping abilities in European samples (Fredrickson & Joiner, 2002). Yet happiness may not help buffer against negative experiences and tendencies in Eastern cultures in the same way it does in Western cultures. For example, whereas happy European Americans were less likely to ruminate and therefore experience depressive symptoms than unhappy European Americans in one study, this effect did not hold for Asian Americans. Importantly, however, rumination and depressive symptoms were associated with less psychological harm for Asian Americans than for European Americans (Tsai, Chang, Sanna, & Herringshaw, 2011).

Because of their differing values, it follows that Eastern and Western cultures recruit positive emotions differently to cope with a stressor. Whereas people from Western cultures value positive emotions and see them as a factor that successfully decreases negative emotions (associated with the stressor), people from Eastern cultures hold a more dialectical perspective. In believing that with the positive there inevitably comes the opposing negative, and vice versa, people from Eastern cultures need not necessarily recruit positive emotions to cope with a stressor. For example, Japanese people do not evaluate unhappiness in the same, purely negative way as Americans; rather, they associate unhappiness with more nonnegative attributes (Uchida & Kitayama, 2009). The goal is not to minimize the negative but to attain contentment and harmonious balance.

Implications of Individualism–Collectivism

In North American countries with individualistic views, happiness is typically viewed as infinite, attainable, and internally experienced. In collectivistic cultures, such as

Japan, however, happiness is more relational and includes myriad social and external factors and resides in shared experiences with other people. This has a number of implications for how people assess and experience happiness. When people judge their level of happiness rather than looking at their life in terms of individual elements and events, they tend to look to a specific cue or piece of information that appears comprehensively to sum up their life state (Suh & Oishi, 2002). Culture influences the most chronically salient cue. In individualist cultures, this cue is typically an internal attribute. In collectivist cultures, this cue is typically a social element of the self (e.g., other people's evaluations of the self). For example, Suh and colleagues (1998) found that the more individualistic the society, the more individuals based life satisfaction judgments on relevant internal emotions.

Furthermore, the way people pursue happiness differs depending on their definition of happiness, cultural values, and norms. In Eastern, collectivist cultures, happiness is conceptualized in terms of positive feelings imbued within a harmonious pattern of social relations, achievement in work, and contentment with life (Lu & Shih, 1997). People therefore find happiness in conforming to social norms and fulfilling relational obligations. Although people in Eastern cultures do value morally disciplined personal striving, it is thought that a meaningful life and fate should be received and welcomed with appreciation whatever its cause (Lu & Gilmour, 2004). In Western cultures, on the other hand, happiness is conceptualized primarily as an individual achievement toward which one has a personal responsibility to strive (Lu & Gilmour, 2004). Thus, people in Western cultures place greater value on the endeavor to control their social surroundings and utilize personal freedom to fulfill their potential and desires (Lu & Gilmour, 2004). Western cultures stress the universal possibility of happiness, and imagine happiness as attainable for everybody (Uchida & Kitayama, 2009).

Conclusions and Future Directions

As this review has demonstrated, the study of cultural norms for positive emotions is a growing area of research. Still, there are several challenges for this line of scholarly inquiry. One of the biggest challenges in cultural research and human emotions is the lack of diversity in participant samples. As with most of the studies in cultural psychology (Cohen, 2007), research on positive emotions thus far has focused almost exclusively on individuals with East Asian and European American cultural orientations. Many research findings describe response patterns from one kind of collectivist context (i.e., East Asian, usually Chinese or Japanese), with the assumption that such patterns hold true in other collectivist contexts as well (Ruby et al., 2012). This methodological approach can limit our understanding of how positive emotions vary.

A second challenge lies in the fact that culture is fluid, ever-changing, and dynamic rather than static (Matsumoto, 1990). Categorizing cultures as "collectivistic" versus "individualistic" is useful as a heuristic but may paint an incomplete picture because no single culture is purely collectivistic or purely individualistic. A more contemporary view of cultural relations reveals that culture is more complex than previously thought (Matsumoto, 1990). As cultures continue to evolve it is necessary that research progress with these changes.

A third challenge involves finding affective terms to describe accurately the pleasant hedonic experiences across different cultural groups. Words are idiosyncratic to languages, and as such, the emotion constructs they capture are not equivalent across cultures. For example, "happiness" has a buoyant meaning in English, referring to a high-arousal, exuberant experience. In Hindi, *sukhi* is a similar term; however, it refers to the low-arousal, pleasant affective experience of peace and happiness. In Kenya, for the Kipsigis, "happiness" occurs "when nothing is bothering you" and therefore has a quiet, calm connotation. Although subjective happiness is inherent in all three definitions, interpretation of these terms could lead researchers to make assumptions about happiness that are not culturally valid (Mesquita & Frijda, 1992).

A growing body of compelling research on positive emotions and culture has begun to emerge. Future studies can increase understanding of the role of culture in shaping positive emotions by placing greater emphasis on possible pathways of influence. Under what conditions—cultural or situational—are different positive emotions likely to arise? In addition, future studies can provide insight by expanding research beyond subjective experience. By examining cognitive appraisals, expressive and regulatory behavior, as well as social consequences, one can gain insight into the broader positive emotion process.

References

Bagozzi, R. P., Wong, N. Y., & Yi, Y. (1999). The role of culture and gender in the relationship between positive and negative affect. *Cognition and Emotion, 13*(6), 641–672.

Chang , E. C., Tugade, M. M., & Asakawa, K. (2006). Stress, appraisals, and coping among Asian Americans: Lazarus and Folkman's model and beyond. In C. Scott & P. T. Wong (Eds.), *Handbook of multicultural perspectives on stress and coping* (pp. 439–455). Dallas, TX: Spring Publications.

Cohen, D. (2007). Methods in cultural psychology. In S. Kitayama & D. Cohen (Eds.), *Handbook of cultural psychology* (pp.196–236). New York: Guilford Press.

D'Andrade, R. G. (1984). Cultural meaning systems. In R. A. Shweder & R. A. LeVine (Eds.), *Culture theory: Essays on mind, self and emotion* (pp. 88–119). Cambridge, UK: Cambridge University Press.

Diener, E. (2000). Subjective well-being: The science of happiness and a proposal for a national index. *American Psychologist, 55*(1), 34–43.

Diener, E., Scollon, C. K. N., Oishi, S., Dzokoto, V., & Suh, E. M. (2000). Positivity and the construction of life satisfaction judgments: Global happiness is not the sum of its parts. *Journal of Happiness Studies, 1*, 159–176.

Diener, E., & Suh, E. (2003). National differences in subjective well-being. In D. Kahneman, E. Diener, & N. Schwarz (Eds.), *Wellbeing: The foundations of hedonic psychology* (pp. 434–450). New York: Russell Sage Foundation.

Ekman, P., & Friesen, W. V. (1969). The repertoire of nonverbal behavior: Categories, origins, usage, and coding. *Semiotica, 1*, 49–98.

Ekman, P., & Friesen, W. V. (1975). *Unmasking the face: A Guide to recognizing emotions from facial cues*. Englewood Cliffs, NJ: Prentice Hall.

Elfenbein, H. A., & Ambady, N. (2002). On the universality and cultural specificity of emotion recognition: A meta-analysis. *Psychological Bulletin, 128*(2), 203–235.

Elfenbein, H. A., & Ambady, N. (2003). When familiarity breeds accuracy: Cultural exposure and facial emotion recognition. *Journal of Personality and Social Psychology, 85*(2), 276–290.

Ellsworth, P. C. (1994). Sense, culture, and sensibility. In S. Kitayama & H. R. Markus (Eds.), *Emotion and culture: Empirical studies of mutual influence* (pp. 23–50). Washington, DC: American Psychological Association.

Fredrickson, B. L. (1998). What good are positive emotions? *Review of General Psychology, 2*, 300–319.

Fredrickson, B. L., & Joiner, T. (2002). Positive emotions trigger upward spirals toward emotional well-being. *Psychological Science, 13*, 172–175.

Fredrickson, B. L., & Levenson, R. W. (1998). Positive emotions speed recovery from the cardiovascular sequelae of negative emotions. *Cognition and Emotion, 12*, 191–220.

Fredrickson, B. L., Tugade, M. M., Waugh, C. E., & Larkin, G. R. (2003). What good are positive emotions in crisis?: A prospective study of resilience and emotions following the terrorist attacks on the United States on September 11th, 2001. *Journal of Personality and Social Psychology, 84*, 365–376.

Heine, S. J., Lehman, D. R., Markus, H. R., & Kitayama, S. (1999). Is there a universal need for positive self-regard? *Psychological Review, 106*(4), 766–794.

Holloway, R. A., Waldrip, A. M., & Ickes, W. (2009). Evidence that a *simpático* self-schema accounts for differences in the self-concepts and social behavior of Latinos versus Whites (and Blacks). *Journal of Personality and Social Psychology, 96*, 1012–1028.

Izard, C. (1980). *Maximally Discriminative Facial Movement Coding (MAX)*. Newark: University of Delaware Press.

Kitayama, S., Duffy, S., & Uchida, Y. (2007). Self as cultural mode of being. In S. Kitayama & D. Cohen (Eds.), *Handbook of cultural psychology* (pp. 136–174). New York: Guilford Press.

Kitayama, S., & Markus, H. R. (1999). Yin and yang of the Japanese self: The cultural psychology of personality coherence. In D. Cervone & Y. Shoda (Eds.), *The coherence of personality:*

Social-cognitive bases of personality consistency, variability, and organization (pp. 242–302). New York: Guilford Press.

Kitayama, S., Markus, H. R., & Kurokawa, M. (2000). Culture, emotion, and well-being: Good feelings in Japan and the United States. *Cognition and Emotion, 14*(1), 93–124.

Kitayama, S., Mesquita, B., & Karasawa, M. (2006). Cultural affordances and emotional experience: Socially engaging and disengaging emotions in Japan and the United States. *Journal of Personality and Social Psychology, 91*(5), 890–903.

Lazarus, R. S. (1991). Progress on a cognitive-motivational–relational theory of emotion. *American Psychologist, 46*(8), 819–834.

Leu, J., Mesquita, B., Ellsworth, P. C., Zhang, Z., Huijuan, Y., Buchtel, E., et al. (2010). Situational differences in dialectical emotions: Boundary conditions in a cultural comparison of North Americans and East Asians. *Cognition and Emotion, 24*, 419–435.

Leu, J., Wang, J., & Koo, K. (2011). Are positive emotions just as "positive" across cultures? *Emotion, 11*(4), 994–999.

Lopez, S. R., Hipke, K. N., Polo, A. J., Jenkins, J. H., Karno, M., Vaughn, C., et al. (2004). Ethnicity, expressed emotion, attributions, and course of schizophrenia: Family warmth matters. *Journal of Abnormal Psychology, 113*, 428–439.

Lu, L., & Gilmour, R. (2004). Culture and conceptions of happiness: Individual oriented and social oriented SWB. *Journal of Happiness Studies, 5*(3), 269–291.

Lu, L., & Shih, J. B. (1997). Sources of happiness: A qualitative approach. *Journal of Social Psychology, 137*, 181–187.

Lutz, C. (1988). *Unnatural emotions: Everyday sentiments on a Micronesian atoll and their challenge to Western theory.* Chicago: University of Chicago Press.

Markus, H. R., & Kitayama, S. (1991). Culture and the self: Implications for cognition, emotion, and motivation. *Psychological Review, 98*(2), 224–253.

Matsumoto, D. (1990). Cultural similarities and differences in display rules. *Motivation and Emotion, 14*(3), 195–214.

Mesquita, B., & Frijda, N. H. (1992). Cultural variations in emotions: A review. *Psychological Bulletin, 112*(2), 179–204.

Mesquita, B., & Karasawa, M. (2002). Different emotional lives. *Cognition and Emotion, 16*(1), 127–141.

Mesquita, B., & Leu, J. (2007). The cultural psychology of emotion. In S. Kitayama & D. Cohen (Eds.), *Handbook of cultural psychology* (pp. 734–759). New York: Guilford Press.

Miyamoto, Y., & Ma, X. (2011). Dampening or savoring positive emotions: A dialectical cultural script guides emotion regulation. *Emotion, 11*(6), 1346–1357.

Miyamoto, Y., & Ryff, C. (2011). Cultural differences in the dialectical and non-dialectical emotional styles and their implications for health. *Cognition and Emotion, 25*(1), 22–39.

Miyamoto, Y., Uchida, Y., & Ellsworth, P. C. (2010). Culture and mixed emotions: Co-occurrence of positive and negative emotions in Japan and the United States. *Emotion, 10*, 404–415.

Nisbett, R. E. (2003). *The geography of thought: How Asians and Westerners think differently—and why.* New York: Free Press.

Nisbett, R. E., & Cohen, D. (1996). *Culture of honor: The psychology of violence in the South.* Boulder, CO: Westview Press.

Ostir, G. V., Ottenbacher, K. J., & Markides, K. S. (2004). Onset of frailty in older adults and the protective role of positive affect. *Psychology and Aging, 19*, 402–408.

Peng, K., & Nisbett, R. E. (1999). Culture, dialectics, and reasoning about contradiction. *American Psychologist, 54*(9), 741–754.

Perunovic, W. Q. E., Heller, D., & Rafaeli, E. (2007). Within-person changes in the structure of emotion: The role of cultural identification and language. *Psychological Science, 18*, 607–613.

Ruby, M. B., Falk, C. F., Heine, S. J., Villa, C., & Silberstein, O. (2012). Not all collectivisms are equal: Opposing preferences for ideal affect between East Asians and Mexicans. *Emotion, 12*(6), 1206–1209.

Russell, J. A., & Carroll, J. M. (1999). On the bipolarity of positive and negative affect. *Psychological Bulletin, 125*, 3–30.

Saarni, C. (1999). The development of emotional competence. *Journal of Psychology, 12*, 234–245.

Schimmack, U., Oishi, O., & Diener, E. (2002). Cultural influences on the relation between pleasant emotions and unpleasant emotions: Asian dialectic philosophies or individualism-collectivism. *Cognition and Emotion, 16*(6), 705–719.

Shiota, M. N., Campos, B., Gonzaga, G. C., Keltner, D., & Peng, K. (2010). I love you but . . . : Cultural differences in emotional complexity during interaction with a romantic partner. *Cognition and Emotion, 24*, 786–799.

Soto, J. A., Levenson, R. W., & Ebling, R. (2005). Cultures of moderation and expression: Emotional experience, behavior, and physiology in Chinese Americans and Mexican Americans. *Emotion, 5*, 154–165.

Suh, E., Diener, E., Oishi, S., & Triandis, H. C. (1998). The shifting basis of life satisfaction judgments across cultures: Emotions versus norms. *Journal of Personality and Social Psychology, 74*(2), 482–493.

Suh, E. M., & Oishi, S. (2002). Subjective well-being across cultures. *Online Readings in Psychology and Culture, 10*(1).

Triandis, H. C., Marin, G., Lisansky, J., & Betancourt, H. (1984). *Simpatía* as a cultural script of Hispanics. *Journal of Personality and Social Psychology, 47*, 1363–1375.

Tsai, J., Knutson, B., & Fung, H. (2006). Cultural variation in affect valuation. *Journal of Personality and Social Psychology, 90*, 288–307.

Tsai, J. L. (2007). Ideal affect: Cultural causes and behavioral consequences. *Perspectives on Psychological Science, 2*, 242–259.

Tsai, J. L., Louie, J., Chen, E. E., & Uchida, Y. (2007). Learning what feelings to desire: Socialization of ideal affect through children's storybooks. *Personality and Social Psychology Bulletin, 33*, 17–30.

Tsai, J. L., & Wong, Y. (2007). *Socialization of ideal affect through magazines.* Unpublished manuscript.

Tsai, W., Chang, E. C., Sanna, L. J., & Herringshaw, A. J. (2011). An examination of happiness as a buffer of the rumination–adjustment link: Ethnic differences between European and Asian American students. *Asian American Journal of Psychology, 2*(3), 168–180.

Tugade, M. M., & Fredrickson, B. L. (2007). Regulation of positive emotions: Emotion regulation strategies that promote resilience. *Journal of Happiness Studies, 8*(3), 311–333.

Uchida, Y., & Kitayama, S. (2009). Happiness and unhappiness in East and West: Themes and variations. *Emotion, 9*, 441–456.

Uchida, Y., Norasakkunkit, V., & Kitayama, S. (2004). Cultural constructions of happiness: Theory and empirical evidence. *Journal of Happiness Studies, 5*(3), 223–239.

Uchida, Y., Townsend, S. S., Markus, H. R., & Bergsieker, H. B. (2009). Emotions as within or between people?: Cultural variation in lay theories of emotion expression and inference. *Personality and Social Psychology Bulletin, 35*(11), 1427–1439.

CHAPTER 14

Vive la Différence

The Ability to Differentiate Positive Emotional Experience and Well-Being

Leslie D. Kirby
Michele M. Tugade
Jannay Morrow
Anthony H. Ahrens
Craig A. Smith

Bob and Jane are sending their oldest child, Sam, off to college. Years of hard work and planning are behind them, and Sam has been accepted into a prestigious university, even earning a full scholarship. They buy bedding and a dorm fridge, negotiate and ultimately agree to let Sam take the TV from her room, and now the big day has finally arrived. They have unloaded everything into the small dorm room, met Sam's new roommate, and helped Sam unpack and get everything set up. They say an emotional good-bye to Sam, and head back to their car.

As they are leaving the dorm, a campus newspaper reporter asks if he can briefly interview them for an article on move-in day. "How's everyone feeling?" the reporter asks. Jane replies, teary-eyed, "Well, I'm very excited for Sam. She has a lot of wonderful opportunities here, and she's eager about starting this new aspect of her life. We're also very proud of her. She worked very hard, and it's nice to see that her efforts were rewarded, not only getting in here, but winning a scholarship as well. Of course, we are going to miss her. It's going to be like a hole in the family, and I'm probably going to be texting her constantly. I know she'll be fine, though. She's

got great social skills and she's a really interesting person with a diverse background, so I know she'll make friends quickly. And we left a copy of her favorite movie, *Bambi*, to remind her of home when she feels sad. I am dreading the car ride home, though—it's going to be so quiet!" The reporter then turns to Bob, who's also teary-eyed, but Bob's response is somewhat different. "I'm okay, I guess," he says, and continues to move toward his car.

As this example illustrates, people differ widely in the degree to which they tend to, and perhaps are able to, subjectively differentiate their personal emotional experience. For some people, like Jane, their ability to differentiate is very high, and they report numerous distinct emotional states, even in response to the same event. Others, like Bob, do not go much beyond a general sense that things are "fine" or "not good." The issue we explore in this chapter is whether these individual differences are psychologically meaningful, and whether subjective emotional differentiation, particularly the ability to differentiate among positive emotions, is linked to individual differences in well-being. We review theoretical reasons for expecting that the ability to differentiate one's emotional experience will be associated with well-being. Then we briefly review related empirical literatures suggesting that such a link may actually exist. Next we review existing evidence that more directly examines whether the differentiation of subjective emotional experience is related to health and well-being. Noting that much of this work has focused on the ability to differentiate either emotional experience in general or negative emotional experience, we consider the possibility that the ability to differentiate among distinct positive emotions may be uniquely related to well-being. We describe our initial efforts to develop a self-report measure of the tendency to differentiate one's positive emotional experience, and present preliminary evidence that the individual differences captured by this measure are related to well-being. Finally, we discuss prospects for future research in this area.

Why Might the Ability to Differentiate Emotional Experience Matter?

Theoretically, there is good reason to expect that the ability to differentiate one's emotional experiences would be positively associated with well-being. Among contemporary and recent emotion theorists (e.g., Ekman, 1984; Frijda, 1986; Izard, 1977; Lazarus, 1991; Plutchik, 1980) there is considerable consensus that emotions are largely adaptive responses to the perceived environmental demands confronting an individual, with emotion serving, in part, as a signal system that contributes to self-regulation (e.g., Frijda & Swagerman, 1987; Simon, 1967). Different emotions are thought to be elicited by circumstances having different types of adaptational relevance. The emotional response acts as a compelling signal to call the person's attention to his or her circumstances, while the distinctive feeling state conveys considerable information about the nature of those circumstances. The motivational urges and physiological activities associated with the emotion motivate and physically prepare the person to respond. As an example, in fear, the compelling subjec-

tive feeling alerts the person that he or she is in a potentially dangerous situation, and the associated motivational urges and physiological changes push the person toward heightened vigilance, while preparing him or her potentially to flee.

If, in fact, one key function of emotion is to serve as an important self-regulatory signal system, then it stands to reason that, all else being equal, individuals who are better able to identify and interpret the signals provided by emotions (high differentiators) should be adaptationally advantaged relative to individuals who are less able to identify and interpret these signals (low differentiators). The literatures on alexithymia and emotional intelligence both lend support, albeit somewhat indirectly, for this proposition.

Alexithymia

Working from a deficit model, the literature on alexithymia suggests that individuals who are characterized, in part, by very low ability to differentiate their emotional states experience a wide array of difficulties. The very name of the condition—*a* (without) *lexi* (words) *thymia* (feelings): without words for feelings—alludes to a core symptom displayed by individuals with this condition, namely, extreme trouble in describing their emotional states (e.g., Sifneos, 1973). More broadly, alexithymia is described as a syndrome in which individuals are characterized as having difficulty identifying and distinguishing among feelings and bodily sensations, difficulty describing emotions, reduced levels of daydreaming and imaginative thought, and a propensity for nonpsychological, externally oriented thinking (e.g., Bagby, Parker, & Taylor, 1994). As one might expect, these deficits interfere with one's ability to regulate emotions, and individuals diagnosed with alexithymia often dwell on, misinterpret, and amplify the physiological sensations that accompany emotional arousal (Taylor, Bagby, & Parker, 1997).

As a result, individuals with alexithymia demonstrate an array of physical, emotional, and social problems. These include elevated levels of depression (Taylor & Bagby, 2004), as well as overrepresentation in populations seeking treatment for conditions with potential psychosomatic components, such as chronic pain (e.g., Lumley, 2004). In addition, individuals with alexithymia often experience a host of interpersonal problems: They demonstrate poor attachment to others, social avoidance, and difficulty handling interpersonal conflict and emotionally tense situations (e.g., Vanheule, Vandenbergen, Verhaeghe & Desmet, 2010). Finally, alexithymia may place individuals at risk for an early death. In a study of middle-aged men, Kauhanen, Kaplan, Cohen, Julkunen, and Salonen (1996) found that even after controlling for a wide variety of potentially confounding factors (e.g., health behaviors, physiological risk factors, socioeconomic and marital status, depressive symptoms, and perceived health), individuals with the highest levels of alexithymic symptoms had a significantly higher risk of all-cause death, and especially death from accident, injury, or violence, than individuals with low levels of alexithymic symptoms.

The deficits and negative outcomes exhibited by individuals with alexithymia certainly suggest that inability to differentiate one's emotional experience is costly. However, the syndromal nature of alexithymia makes this evidence somewhat indirect, as it is difficult to isolate the contributions to poor functioning of the person's low emotion-differentiation abilities from those of their nonimaginative and externally oriented cognitive styles.

Emotional Intelligence

Conversely, working from a skills perspective, "emotional intelligence," which represents the ability to perceive, understand, use, and manage or regulate emotions (Mayer & Salovey, 1997; Mayer, Salovey, & Caruso, 2002), has been associated with heightened well-being. For instance, scores on the Mayer–Salovey–Caruso Emotional Intelligence Test (MSCEIT; Mayer & Salovey, 1997) are positively related to several aspects of psychological well-being (Ryff, 1989), including mastery, personal growth, positive relations with others, purpose in life, and self-acceptance (Brackett & Mayer, 2003). These findings are supported by a comprehensive meta-analysis of the existing literature on emotional intelligence that documented clear and consistent associations

between emotional intelligence and indicators of mental, psychosomatic, and physical health (Martins, Ramalho, & Morin, 2010). Recent research also indicates that emotional intelligence acts as a buffer against state-level stress in both laboratory and real-world settings (Görgens-Ekermans & Brand, 2012; Mikolajczak, Petrides, Coumans, & Luminet, 2009). Together, the accumulation of data indicates that having the ability to understand, perceive, and manage emotions effectively is related to important benefits in the domains of psychological well-being and health.

These results are highly suggestive because clarity about the emotion(s) one is experiencing at any given time is often described as a core feature of emotional intelligence (e.g., Mayer, Salovey & Caruso, 2004). Thus, emotional intelligence includes, in part, the ability to differentiate one's emotional experience. It is difficult to navigate one's social world if one does not know which emotion one is experiencing, and there are several indications that clarity about one's feelings is directly associated with well-being (e.g., Fernández-Berrocal, Alcaide, Extremera, & Pizarro, 2006; Shulman & Hemenover, 2006). However, the emotional intelligence construct is inherently multidimensional and includes other abilities that also contribute to well-being, including the ability to manage negative emotions and accurately perceive emotions in others (Mayer & Salovey, 1997). The multidimensional nature of emotional intelligence makes this literature somewhat inconclusive regarding the specific contribution of emotion differentiation to well-being, and more direct evidence is needed.

Evidence Relating the Ability to Differentiate Emotions and Well-Being

Beyond the literatures on alexithymia and emotional intelligence, emerging evidence suggests more specifically that people who are better at differentiating their emotional states, in fact, regulate their emotions better and tend to experience higher levels of well-being. For instance, Barrett, Gross, Christensen, and Benvenuto (2001) used experience sampling methods to examine the relations between emotion differentiation and emotion regulation. In a daily diary, participants rated their emotional reactions in terms of nine emotions—five negative and four positive—in response to the most intense emotional event of the day on each of 14 days. In addition, they completed a questionnaire regarding their use of a range of regulation strategies to manage both their positive and negative emotions over a 2-week period. The investigators computed separate indices of differentiation for each participant's positive and negative emotions by intercorrelating the negative emotions on the one hand, and the positive emotions on the other, over the 14 rating occasions. They found that increased differentiation among the negative emotions (lower average intercorrelations across occasions) was associated with use of a broader range of regulation strategies for negative emotions, especially as the intensity of the negative emotions increased. Corresponding relations were not observed for differentiation of positive emotions in predicting the use of regulation strategies for managing positive emotions. The authors hypothesized that this was because positive emotions require less regulation than negative ones. The relationship between differentiation of positive emotions and use of strategies to regulate negative emotions was not tested, and efficacy of the various regulation strategies in managing negative emotions was not assessed.

Focusing only on the differentiation of negative emotional experience, Kashdan, Ferssizidis, Collins, and Muraven (2010) provided more direct evidence that individuals who differentiate their negative emotions may manage those emotions more effectively. To measure differentiation, they computed an average intraclass correlation among several negative emotions reported via experience sampling methods for each participant (Shrout & Fliess, 1979; Tugade, Fredrickson, & Barrett, 2004). Using this index, they found that underage social drinkers who reported more differentiated negative emotional experiences consumed less alcohol in response to intense negative emotions than did those who reported less differentiated negative emotional experiences.

Using a self-report measure of emotional complexity, which the authors define as comprising both emotional differentiation as we are considering it in this chapter and the degree to which the person experiences a broad range of emotions in daily life, Kang and Shaver (2004) found that their Emotional Differentiation subscale was positively related to several different measures of interpersonal adjustment. Their measure focuses on emotional differentiation in general and does not assess the degree to which individuals differentiate positive versus negative emotional experience.

These findings lend more direct support to the notion that ability to differentiate one's emotional experiences per se contributes to both effective self-regulation and positive outcomes. Research by Carstensen and colleagues (e.g., 2011; Carstensen, Pasupathi, Mayr, & Nesselroade, 2000) indicates that the relationship between general emotion differentiation/complexity and health and well-being hold up across the lifespan.

However, the implication of ability to differentiate *positive* emotional experience for self-regulation, health, and well-being outcomes has not been examined in most studies. Barrett and colleagues (2001) did examine positive emotion differentiation but did not investigate whether it was associated with regulation of negative emotions (which they considered more adaptationally important than regulation of positive emotions), and Kashdan and colleagues (2010) only examined differentiation of negative emotions. Kang and Shaver (2004) measured emotion differentiation across both positive and negative emotions using a single scale, and the studies by Carstensen and colleagues (2000, 2011) also examined a combined index of differentiation of positive and negative emotions. Thus, although evidence is mounting that the ability to differentiate one's emotional experiences in general, or negative emotional experiences in particular, is relevant to well-being, the potential contribution of the ability to regulate positive emotions has largely been neglected. Below, we consider whether this neglect is justified, or whether it is likely that the specific ability to regulate positive emotions is related to well-being.

Why Ability to Differentiate Positive Emotions Should Matter

Given that the ability to differentiate both negative emotional experience and emotional experience in general has been associated with well-being, there are a number of reasons to expect that the ability to differentiate positive emotional experience should also be associated with well-being, possibly in ways that extend beyond the links between ability to differentiate negative emotions and well-being.

First, empirical research increasingly suggests that humans are equipped to experience a range of positive emotions, serving a variety of adaptive functions (see Smith, Tong, & Ellsworth, Chapter 1, this volume). This research supports a prerequisite condition for any unique effects of ability to differentiate positive emotional experience: If there is little "real" differentiation of positive emotions to begin with, then the ability to recognize and appreciate differentiation among positive emotions is unlikely to be important. Although traditional theories often have proposed that positive emotional experience consists of happiness or joy, possibly interest and/or surprise, and little else (e.g., Ekman, 1984; Izard, 1977; Tomkins, 1962), evidence is mounting that a diverse range of positive emotions, including (but not limited to) happiness, pride, gratitude, challenge/determination, hope, interest, awe, tranquility, love, and compassion, may each serve distinctive adaptational functions (e.g., Griskevicius, Shiota, & Nowlis, 2010; Keltner & Haidt, 2003; Smith, 1991). For instance, whereas both happiness and pride are proposed, in part, to reinforce success, gratitude and compassion are both thought to motivate prosocial behavior, albeit in different ways, and hope and challenge are thought to motivate perseverance and sustained commitment in the face of difficulty (e.g., Smith et al., Chapter 1, this volume).

It is further notable that in line with proposals made by Watson and Tellegen (1985) and Cacioppo, Larsen, Smith, and Bernston (2004), the motivational functions served by positive emotions are often different in kind from those served by negative emotions. This is true both of the specific motivational functions served by particular positive emotions, and the broader motivational functions served by positive emotions more generally. First, whereas negative emotions tend to serve self-protective functions, such as avoiding harm when one is fearful, or disengaging from hopeless situations and soliciting help when one is sad; positive emotions tend to serve more appetitive functions, such as motivating perseverance when one is challenged, and rewarding success when one feels pride, as noted earlier. That positive emotions have motivational functions that are fundamentally different in kind than those of negative emotions increases the likelihood that the ability to differentiate positive emotions contributes to well-being in ways distinct from the contribution of the ability to differentiate negative ones.

Second, as described in the broaden-and-build theory of positive emotion (Fredrickson, 1998, 2001), positive emotions often play important roles in the management and control of negative emotions. For example, research shows that positive emotion can play an important role in "undoing" the effects of negative emotion once the conditions eliciting the negative emotion have passed and the effects of the negative emotions are no longer needed or desirable (Fredrickson & Levenson, 1998; Fredrickson, Mancuso, Branigan, & Tugade, 2000). Negative emotions involve a narrowing of thought–action repertoires, accompanied by physiological changes to prepare the body to contend with the emotion-eliciting circumstances. According to the broaden-and-build theory, once the threatening situation has passed, positive emotions broaden the thought–action repertoire, and this should "undo" the physiological changes associated with the negative emotion. Thus, positive emotions have the unique ability to speed recovery from negative emotional arousal (Fredrickson & Levenson, 1998) and attenuate the cognitive vigilance associated with negative emotions. This is especially important because significant physical costs associated with sustained negative emotion (e.g., wear-and-tear on the body, compromised immune system functioning) can be associated with subsequent vulnerability to stress and illness (McEwen, 1998). In addition, if the narrowed scope of attention associated with negative emotion lingers, it can inhibit subsequent learning and creativity.

Both of the previous lines of consideration point to the conclusion that positive emotions play roles in coping, adaptation, and adjustment, just as negative emotions do, although the roles served by positive emotions seem both different from and complementary to those served by negative emotions. Indeed, the work on the broaden-and-build theory suggests that positive emotions contribute in important ways to the regulation of negative emotions (Tugade, 2011; Tugade & Fredrickson, 2004, 2007). Adding further support to this perspective, strategies that increase positive emotion in the midst of distress (e.g., positive reappraisal) are associated with emotion regulation and psychological well-being (Folkman, 1997; Folkman & Moskowitz, 2000; Shiota, 2006; Shiota & Levenson, 2012; Tugade & Fredrickson, 2004). Thus, just as the ability to differentiate negative experience is related to well-being, so too is the ability to differentiate positive experience. At present, very little research directly examines this hypothesis; however, the evidence that does exist is highly suggestive.

First, in an experience-sampling study, Tugade, Fredrickson, and Barrett (2004) found that their measure of positive emotional differentiation was related to participants' characteristic coping styles. Participants reported their momentary emotional experience at randomly chosen periods, 10 times per day, for a total of 28 days. Positive emotion differentiation was determined for each participant by computing an average intraclass correlation (Shrout & Fleiss, 1979) among positive emotion terms: amusement, happiness, interest, joy, and pride. Participants also completed measures of coping and cognitive styles. Those who differentiated positive emotions more were found to be more engaged in the coping process, and cognitively were less likely to use heuristics to guide their coping behaviors, and were instead more likely to think through their behavioral options before acting.

In a similar vein, Ahrens and McIntosh (2009) found that, in responding to hypothetical scenarios, participants who report more highly intercorrelated levels of gratitude, pride, happiness, and relief, thus differentiating emotions less, score both higher in fear of emotions and lower in one aspect of mindfulness, acceptance without judgment. These relations have numerous health implications. Fear of emotion and lower mindfulness are in turn associated with a variety of mental health problems, including posttraumatic stress disorder (PTSD; Lang et al., 2012; Price, Monson, Callahan, & Rodriguez, 2006), generalized anxiety disorder (Roemer et al., 2009; Turk, Heimberg, Luterek, Mennin, & Fresco, 2005), and bor-

derline personality disorder (Sauer & Baer, 2012; Yen, Zlotnick, & Costello, 2002). The Ahrens and McIntosh (2009) finding suggests that lack of differentiation among positive emotions may also be associated with such disorders. Thus, although preliminary, the available data and theory suggest that examining the adaptational implications of individual differences in the differentiation of positive emotional experience is well worth pursuing.

The DOPES: A New Measure of Ability to Differentiate Positive Emotional Experience

An important gap in this area of research is a valid and reliable measure of individual differences in the tendency to distinguish among different positive emotional experiences. With the exception of the Differentiation subscale of the measure developed by Kang and Shaver (2004), which comprises general statements regarding individuals' general tendency to distinguish among different feelings they experience (e.g., "I am aware of the subtle differences between feelings I have"), previous measures of emotion differentiation have relied on experience-sampling methods (e.g., Barrett et al., 2001; Tugade et al., 2004). This approach offers an important advantage in that the measures are based on participants' actual emotional experiences as they unfold over time, revealing unique patterns of emotional experience within each individual. However, this approach also has considerable limitations. First, because the experiences sampled are those that arise spontaneously in respondents' lives, the set of experiences can vary greatly from individual to individual, rendering the scores difficult to compare across individuals. There would be considerable utility in differentiation scores derived from a common set of experiences. Second, the experience-sampling methodology is expensive and difficult to implement. Thus, this methodology greatly limits the range of studies in which a measure of positive emotion differentiation might be employed.

To address these issues, we have begun work on the development and validation of a measure of the degree to which individuals differentiate among several positive emotions in their own emotional experiences. We call this individual-difference measure the Differentiation of Positive Emotion Scale (DOPES).

Overview of the Measure

In designing this measure, we chose to assess respondents' emotions across multiple situations (e.g., Tugade et al., 2004), as opposed to asking them general questions about their emotional response styles (e.g., Kang & Shaver, 2004). We believed that the former approach would more clearly capture respondents' actual emotional reactions rather than their beliefs about emotions, and would therefore provide a more valid measure. At the same time, we wanted respondents to describe their responses to a common set of experiences, to maximize the comparability of the resulting scores from individual to individual. To combine these aims, the DOPES asks individuals to indicate their imagined emotional reactions to a common set of emotion-eliciting events, each of which is designed to elicit the experience of a different positive emotion.

Specifically, respondents are asked to imagine themselves in eight different vignettes designed to elicit happiness, pride, gratitude, interest, hope, challenge/determination, awe or contentment. For example, the vignette designed to elicit interest involves settling in to listen to a lecture one has looked forward to for a long time, whereas the vignette for pride involves being recognized for taking the lead on a group project that is extremely well received (a preliminary version of the DOPES, used in Study 1, included vignettes specific to student life; the vignettes in the current DOPES version, used in Studies 2 and 3, are included in Appendix 14.1). For each vignette, respondents are asked to rate their imagined emotional responses in terms of each of the eight targeted emotions. The degree of emotion differentiation for each respondent is quantified by intercorrelating the ratings for each emotion scale across the eight vignettes, then computing the mean intercorrelation. To normalize the distribution of the resulting scores, this average correlation is subjected to an r-to-z transformation. Higher mean intercorrelations reflect *lower* levels of differentiation because they indicate that the emotion ratings covary strongly across the vignettes. Therefore, to provide an index in which increasing scores reflect greater emotion differentiation, the sign of the scores is reversed by subtracting the z-transformed mean intercorrelations from a constant. We have used "2" as the constant because this typically produces differentiation indexes in which resulting scores have a positive sign.

Study 1: Multisite Undergraduate Study

As part of a larger study examining several aspects of differentiation of positive emotional experience, participants completed a battery of individual-difference measures that included the following:

- A preliminary version of the DOPES.
- The Appraisal Styles Inventory (ASI; Smith & Kirby, 2013), which assesses appraisal styles across situations for the appraisal components described by Smith and Lazarus (1990), including Motivational Relevance, Motivational Congruence, Self-Accountability, Other-Accountability, Problem-Focused Coping Potential, Emotion-Focused Coping Potential, and Future Expectancy; it includes subscales to assess these appraisal styles in general, and separately across negative and positive situations.
- A modified version of the COPE (Carver, Scheier, & Weintraub, 1989), which includes subscales assessing a wide variety of coping strategies, including Self-Isolation, Denial, Active Coping, and Acceptance.
- The Trait Meta-Mood Scale (TMMS; Salovey, Mayer, Goldman, Turvey, & Palfai, 1995), a commonly used as a measure of emotional intelligence, which includes subscales to assess Mood Repair, Clarity of Emotion, and Attention to Emotion.
- The Short Form–36 Health Survey which measures functional health and well-being (SF-36, Version 2; Ware, Kosinski, & Dewey, 2000), and includes subscales assessing Social Functioning, Mental Health, Bodily Pain, Interference with Physical Activities, and General Health.

This initial survey was conducted on student samples at two different universities, with a total $N = 281$ (60% female). The average age was 18.64 years ($SD = 0.88$), with a range of 17–22 years.

In this sample the mean between-emotion correlations from which DOPES scores are derived ranged from −.11 to +.90, with a mean of +.15. Cronbach's alpha, based on the 28 intercorrelations among emotions that are averaged into the final score, was .87.

As an initial step toward validating this new measure, correlations between DOPES scores and the subscales of the ASI, COPE, TMMS, and SF-36 were examined. Given the existing work on emotion differentiation, reviewed earlier, we anticipated that higher levels of emotion differentiation would be associated with higher levels of adaptive appraisal and coping styles, emotional intelligence, health, and well-being. Several small, but statistically significant, correlations emerged from this analysis, and all were consistent with these predictions, although as noted below, a number of predicted correlations did not approach statistical significance.

Appraisal Style

The DOPES was positively correlated with appraisals of motivational congruence in positive situations ($r = .14$, $p < .05$), which is the tendency to perceive positive situations as having positive aspects, or things that the individual wants. It was also negatively correlated with perceived incongruence in negative situations ($r = −.29$, $p < .001$), which is the tendency to perceive negative situations as having things that the individual does not want. Thus, across both positive and negative situations, individuals showing high levels of positive emotion differentiation were prone to see their circumstances as more in line with their goals than were others. The DOPES was not significantly related to other dimensions of appraisal style.

COPE

The DOPES was negatively correlated with Self-Isolation ($r = −.17$, $p < .01$) and marginally negatively correlated with Denial ($r = −.10$, $p = .10$), two forms of coping that tend to be associated with poor outcomes when used habitually. DOPES scores were not significantly correlated with Active Coping ($r = −.02$, nonsignificant [ns]) or Acceptance ($r = −.04$, ns).

TMMS

The DOPES was marginally positively correlated with the Mood Repair and Clarity subscales of the TMMS (both r's = .11, $p = .06$), but not the Attention subscale ($r = −.03$, ns). Of the three, the correlation with Clarity is of particular interest because clarity regarding one's emotional state and the tendency to differentiate among one's emotional responses are thought to be closely related.

SF-36

The DOPES was significantly related to the Social Functioning subscale ($r = .13$, $p < .05$), and marginally positively correlated with the Mental Health subscale ($r = .12$, $p = .06$) of the SF-36. In addition, it was negatively correlated with the SF-36 subscales assessing Bodily Pain ($r = −.17$, $p < .01$) and the degree to which one's health interferes with one's physical activities ($r = −.14$, $p < .05$). The DOPES was not reliably associated with the General Health subscale of the SF-36 ($r = .04$, ns). The correlations with Mental Health and Social Functioning provide some direct evidence that differentiation of positive experience, as assessed by the DOPES, is associated with psychological well-being. The findings regarding health outcomes echo those frequently observed for alexithymia (e.g., Lumley, 2004), in which relative inability to describe one's emotions is more strongly associated with conditions having a psychosomatic or behavioral component, such as pain or limitation to functioning, than with direct indicators of physical health.

Although small, these initial correlations are quite promising. They suggest that the DOPES taps into the differentiation of positive emotion as intended, and that such differentiation is related to well-being and health, as theoretically predicted. Subsequent studies have further refined the DOPES and examined its reliability and validity.

Study 2: Community Sample

A follow-up study used a slightly revised version of the DOPES, designed to make the vignettes less student-focused and more applicable to a general population, in order to expand examination of the reliability and validity of the DOPES into a community sample. In this study, participants were recruited via an e-mail inviting them to participate in an online survey. E-mails were sent to several community groups (e.g., churches, temples, social groups) in the greater Poughkeepsie, New York area; postings were listed on Craigslist (community/volunteers section) in several metropolitan areas in the Northeast (Hudson Valley, New York City, northern New Jersey, and Washington, D.C.); and postings were also listed on *backpage.com* in major metropolitan areas across the eastern United States (New York City, Nashville, Washington, D.C., New Jersey, Baltimore, Philadelphia, Birmingham, Atlanta, Boston, Virginia Beach, and Delaware). This study included 127 respondents (60% female), with an average age of 31.7 years ($SD = 11.6$), and a range in age from 17 to 65. Ninety-seven percent of the sample had at least some college education, and 42% had a bachelor's degree or higher. The reliability of the DOPES in this sample (Cronbach's alpha based on the 28 intercorrelations between specific positive emotions) was .93.

As with the initial study, this study examined the DOPES in relation to the COPE and the TMMS. Instead of the SF-36, the Pennebaker Inventory of Limbic Languidness (PILL; Pennebaker, 1982) was used to assess health. Participants also reported on positive and negative affect (Positive and Negative Affect Schedule [PANAS]; Watson & Clark, 1994); satisfaction with life (Diener, Emmons, Larsen, & Griffin, 1985), and resilience (Block & Kremen, 1996). The ASI was not assessed.

COPE

As in Study 1, the DOPES was negatively correlated with Denial ($r = -.34$, $p < .001$). Due to a survey error, self-isolation was not examined in this study. However, unlike the initial study, correlations of the DOPES with Active Coping ($r = .20$, $p < .05$) and Acceptance ($r = .19$, $p < .05$) both reached significance. These correlations all suggest that greater tendency to differentiate among one's positive experiences is associated with a tendency toward healthy, adaptive coping.

TMMS

Unlike the first study, in this study the DOPES was not reliably associated with any of the three subscales of the TMMS (Attention: $r = .15$, $p = .11$; Mood Repair: $r = -.001$, *ns*; Clarity: $r = .11$, *ns*).

Other Outcomes

The PILL was not significantly associated with the DOPES ($r = .05$, *ns*; compare with the General Health dimension of the SF-36 in the previous study). DOPES scores also were not significantly correlated with Positive Affect, Negative Affect, Satisfaction with Life, or Resilience.

Study 3: Experience Sampling Study

Finally, a student sample was used to compare individual differences in positive emotion differentiation, as measured by the DOPES, with a measure of positive differentiation obtained through experience sampling methods, similar to those used by Barrett and colleagues (2001) and Tugade and colleagues (2004). In this study, participants ($N = 152$, 42 males, 110 females; mean age = 19.21 years, $SD = 1.56$, with an age range of 17–29 years) reported to the laboratory, where they individually completed a set of measures, including the revised DOPES used in Study 2, Center for Epidemiologic Studies—Depression scale (CES-D) measure of depressive symptomatology (Radloff, 1977), NEO Personality Inventory—Neuroticism scale (Costa & McCrae, 1985), and Affective Control Scale (Williams, Chambless, & Ahrens, 1997). Participants were then given a Palm Pilot which, for the next 7 days, alerted participants four times a day. At each of these times, they answered a variety of questions, including momentary reporting on a subset of DOPES emotions (happiness, gratitude, contentment, and pride). Of the 152 participants, 135 completed at least half of the Palm Pilot surveys and were therefore included in the analyses involving momentary assessments.

Cronbach's alpha reliability of the DOPES in this study was .89. The DOPES was significantly negatively correlated with CES-D scores ($r = -.17$, $p < .05$) and with both Fear of Depression ($r = -.25$, $p < .01$) and Fear of Anxiety ($r = -.17$, $p < .05$) subscales of the Affect Control Scale, as well as the overall Fear of Emotion score ($r = -.21$, $p = .01$). The DOPES was also negatively correlated with the Neuroticism subscale of the NEO ($r = -.18$, $p < .05$). Most importantly, the DOPES was significantly correlated with the experience-sampling-based measure of positive emotion differentiation ($r = .19$, $p < .05$).

These data indicate that differentiation in positive emotional responses to the hypothetical situations in the DOPES predicts differentiation of emotional responses to actual events—thereby providing initial evidence of the DOPES's validity. Furthermore, the results of this study provide additional evidence that positive emotional differentiation, as captured by the DOPES, is associated with well-being, as reflected in negative correlations with both depressive symptoms and neuroticism, as well as indicators of fear of negative emotion.

Preliminary Conclusions and Future Directions

The results of these three studies must be viewed as preliminary, but they are nonetheless promising. In addition to providing some initial evidence for the DOPES's validity, they also indicate that differentiation of positive emotional experience is associated with psychological well-being and highly worthy of further study. The correlations observed between the DOPES and criterion measures were small and did not always replicate across samples, but the thrust of the observed correlations was clear: In every case in which a statistically significant correlation was observed, it supported the hypothesis that greater tendency to differentiate one's positive emotional experiences is associated with higher psychological well-being, and processes believed to promote well-being (e.g., appraisal and coping styles; social functioning).

Given these initial results, it is important to continue efforts to develop and validate the DOPES as a measure of positive emotional differentiation, and we are pursuing such efforts. For instance, we are currently investigating the degree to which our initial vignettes were successful at normatively and selectively inducing their intended emo-

tions. We suspect that some of the current vignettes are not as selective in the emotions they normatively elicit as we intended, and that by revising these vignettes to improve their selectivity, we will produce a more valid, psychometrically stronger measure of positive emotional differentiation. We intend to use this improved measure in a series of validation studies in which, across samples, we include a common battery of measures related to emotional intelligence, alexithymia, and appraisal and coping styles, among others. In this way we can more systematically assess the strength and stability of the relations of the DOPES to other constructs and establish both its predictive and discriminant validity.

Another key item on our research agenda is to compare positive emotion differentiation, as assessed by the DOPES, with negative emotion differentiation, as assessed by a (to be developed) corresponding measure of negative emotion differentiation. As noted earlier, there is mounting evidence that negative emotion differentiation is associated with well-being. To this body of evidence we have now added evidence that positive emotion differentiation is also associated with well-being. A key question to pursue is whether these two relations reflect a simple, unidimensional relation between emotion differentiation and adjustment (as Kang & Shaver, 2004, might argue), or whether positive and negative emotion differentiation contribute to well-being in distinct and at least partially nonredundant ways. We suspect the latter, but this remains to be seen.

Conclusions

In this chapter we have made the case that the ability to differentiate one's emotional experiences—to identify and describe the emotions one is experiencing with clarity and specificity—is a skill highly relevant to psychological well-being. In reviewing the existing literature, we have discussed evidence that both alexithymia and emotional intelligence, broader-level individual differences that include the ability (or lack thereof) to differentiate emotional experiences, are clearly related to well-being. In addition, we have documented more direct evidence indicating that ability to differentiate negative emotions, or emotional states in general, is related to adjustment.

To these findings we have added initial evidence that the ability to differentiate positive emotional experience is also related to psychological well-being, and we have introduced a promising new measure of the tendency to differentiate positive experiences. Future research should build on this start and further examine the relations between positive emotional differentiation and adjustment. As this work progresses, one important issue to address, which thus far is absent from the literature on emotional differentiation, is the set of mechanisms by which the ability to differentiate one's emotional experiences (both positive and negative) contributes to positive well-being. By exploring such mechanisms, it is likely that we will find ways to improve these abilities in individuals who currently lack them and, by so doing, potentially help them improve the quality of their lives.

APPENDIX 14.1. Differentiation of Positive Emotions Scale (DOPES)

Instructions

For the next set of questions, you will see brief descriptions of hypothetical situations. Each situation is followed by a series of questions. For each situation, try to imagine yourself in the situation as vividly as you can. If such a situation happened to you, how do you think you would be feeling while you were in this situation? When you are imagining yourself in the situation as vividly as you can, please answer the questions that follow each description to rate your feelings. When you have answered all the questions for one situation, you should go on to the next situation, until you have imagined yourself in all eight situations. There are no right or wrong answers. Please try to answer every question as best you can, and make it true for you.

Vignettes

Awe

You are walking up a hill through thick woods. It was raining earlier, but the rain stopped a short time ago, and the sun is now shining. All of a sudden, you come to a clearing near the top of the hill and enter a beautiful meadow filled with wildflowers and butterflies. A clear stream is running through the meadow, and there is a rainbow in the sky. Off in the distance you can see the snow-capped peaks of a nearby mountain range.

Challenge/Determination

You have been spending a fair bit of time trying to solve a difficult problem that is part of an important project on which you have been working. So far you have been unable to solve the problem, but you believe that a solution is possible and you know that if you keep at it, you will be able to solve the problem and make the project a success.

Contentment

After working very hard for several weeks, you are finally able to take some time off. Right now you are relaxing on the beach. There is a nice breeze, you have a drink, and you are relishing the knowledge that there's nothing at all you need to be doing right now.

Gratitude

You are walking around in a strange city and suddenly realize that you are lost. As you are standing at a street corner, intensely studying your map to try to figure out where you are, someone comes up to you and asks you in a friendly way where you are trying to go. After you answer, this person says that he or she is headed that way and suggests that you go together. Within a few minutes this person has taken you to your destination, having pointed out some interesting sights along the way.

Happiness

You're at a party on Saturday night in honor of your friend's wedding anniversary. You're with a group of close friends and family members, and the atmosphere is festive. You generally like special occasions like this when everyone comes together to have fun. Everyone, including you, is laughing and dancing, and having a great time.

Hope

Things in your life have been somewhat difficult lately, but you are optimistic about what lies ahead. You know that there are new opportunities available to help things get better, and they seem promising. You trust that things will be better soon. You are looking forward to good things to come and a bright future ahead. You are thinking about the positive change that can happen.

Interest

A public figure that you admire has come to town, and you have the opportunity to hear this person speak. You are out for the evening to attend the talk. It is on a topic you have wanted to know more about for a long time. You have settled into your chair. The speaker, who has just been introduced, is beginning the presentation.

Pride

You have been working very hard on a group project. The rest of your group members have been contributing, but you have gone the extra distance for the project. You know that the project wouldn't be nearly as good had you not worked so hard. Your group has just presented the project and it is extremely well received. As your group is receiving praise for an excellent job, a member of your group speaks up and indicates that the group owes its success to you, that you really pulled the project together. The other members of the group start spontaneously applauding you and your efforts.

Scale

Please indicate on the following scale the extent to which you would feel the following if you were in this situation:

1-----2-----3-----4-----5-----6-----7-----8-----9
not at all   moderately   extremely much

Ratings are then obtained, using the previous scale, for each of the following items: interested/curious; proud; hopeful; happy; grateful; awed; challenged/determined/motivated; content/satisfied.

Administration

Instructions are presented individually on the first page (or screen) of the questionnaire. Each vignette is then presented on a separate page/screen followed by all eight emotion ratings for each vignette. Although listed here alphabetically, vignettes are presented in random order when used in studies.

References

Ahrens, A. H., & McIntosh, E. (2009). [Positive emotion intercorrelations and fear of emotion]. Unpublished raw data.

Bagby, R. M., Parker, J. D., & Taylor, G. J. (1994). The twenty-item Toronto Alexithymia Scale–I: Item selection and cross-validation of the factor structure. *Journal of Psychosomatic Research, 38,* 23–32.

Barrett, L. F., Gross, J., Christensen, T. C., & Benvenuto, M. (2001). Knowing what you're feeling and knowing what to do about it: Mapping the relation between emotion differentiation and emotion regulation. *Cognition and Emotion, 15,* 713–724.

Block, J., & Kremen, A. M. (1996). IQ and ego-resiliency: Conceptual and empirical connections and separateness. *Journal of Personality and Social Psychology, 70,* 349–361.

Brackett, M. A., & Mayer, J. D. (2003). Convergent, discriminant, and incremental validity of competing measures of emotional intelligence. *Personality and Social Psychology Bulletin, 29,* 1147–1158.

Cacioppo, J. T., Larsen, J. T., Smith, N. K., & Bernston, G. G. (2004). The affect system: What lurks below the surface of feelings? In A. S. R. Manstead, N. H. Frijda, & A. H. Fischer (Eds.), *Feelings and emotions: The Amsterdam conference* (pp. 223–242). New York: Cambridge University Press.

Carstensen, L. L., Pasupathi, M., Mayr, U., & Nesselroade, J. R. (2000). Emotional experience in everyday life across the adult life span. *Journal of Personality and Social Psychology, 79,* 644–655.

Carstensen, L. L., Turan, B., Scheibe, S., Ram, N., Ersner-Hershfield, H., Samanez-Larkin, G. R., et al. (2011). Emotional experience improves with age: Evidence based on over 10 years of experience sampling. *Psychology and Aging, 26,* 21–23.

Carver, C. S., Scheier, M. F., & Weintraub, J. K. (1989). Assessing coping strategies: A theoretically based approach. *Journal of Personality and Social Psychology, 56,* 267–283.

Costa, P. T., & McCrae, R. R. (1985). *The NEO Personality Inventory manual.* Odessa, FL: Psychological Assessment Resources.

Diener, E., Emmons, R. A., Larsen, R. J., & Griffin, S. (1985). The Satisfaction with Life Scale. *Journal of Personality Assessment, 49,* 71–75.

Ekman, P. (1984). Expression and the nature of emotion. In K.R. Scherer & P. Ekman (Eds.), *Approaches to emotion* (pp. 319–343). Hillsdale, NJ: Erlbaum.

Fernández-Berrocal, P., Alcaide, R., Extremera, N., & Pizarro, D. (2006). The role of emotional intelligence in anxiety and depression among adolescents. *Individual Differences Research, 4*, 16–27.

Folkman, S. (1997). Positive psychological states and coping with severe stress. *Social Science and Medicine, 45*, 1207–1221.

Folkman, S., & Moskowitz, J. T. (2000). Stress, positive emotion, and coping. *Current Directions in Psychological Science, 9*, 115–118.

Fredrickson, B. L. (1998). What good are positive emotions? [Special issue]. *Review of General Psychology, 2*, 300–319

Fredrickson, B. L. (2001). The role of positive emotions in positive psychology: The broaden-and-build theory of positive emotions. *American Psychologist, 56*, 218–226.

Fredrickson, B. L., & Levenson, R. W. (1998). Positive emotions speed recovery from the cardiovascular sequelae of negative emotions. *Cognition and Emotion, 12*, 191–220.

Fredrickson, B. L., Mancuso, R. A., Branigan, C., & Tugade, M. M. (2000). The undoing effect of positive emotions. *Motivation and Emotion, 24*, 237–258.

Frijda, N. H. (1986). *The emotions*. New York: Cambridge University Press.

Frijda, N. H., & Swagerman, J. (1987). Can computers feel?: Theory and design of an emotional system. *Cognition and Emotion, 1*, 235–257.

Görgens-Ekermans, G. G., & Brand, T. T. (2012). Emotional intelligence as a moderator in the stress–burnout relationship: A questionnaire study on nurses. *Journal of Clinical Nursing, 21*, 2275–2285.

Griskevicius, V., Shiota, M. N., & Nowlis, S. M. (2010). The many shades of rose-colored glasses: An evolutionary approach to the influence of different positive emotions. *Journal of Consumer Research, 37*, 238–250.

Izard, C. E. (1977). *Human emotions*. New York: Plenum Press.

Kang, S. M., & Shaver, P. R. (2004). Individual differences in emotional complexity: Their psychological implications. *Journal of Personality, 72*, 687–726.

Kashdan, T. B., Ferssizidis, P., Collins, R. L., & Muraven, M. (2010). Emotion differentiation as resilience against excessive alcohol use an ecological momentary assessment in underage social drinkers. *Psychological Science, 21*, 1341–1347.

Kauhanen, J., Kaplan, G. A., Cohen, R. D., Julkunen, J., & Salonen, J. (1996). Alexithymia and risk of death in middle-aged men. *Journal of Psychosomatic Research, 41*, 541–549.

Keltner, D., & Haidt, J. (2003). Approaching awe, a moral, spiritual, and aesthetic emotion. *Cognition and Emotion 17*, 297–314.

Lang, A. J., Strauss, J. L., Bomyea, J., Bormann, J. E., Hickman, S. D., Good, R. C., et al. (2012). The theoretical and empirical basis for meditation as an intervention for PTSD. *Behavior Modification, 36*, 759–786.

Lazarus, R. S. (1991). *Emotion and adaptation*. New York: Oxford University Press.

Lumley, M. (2004). Alexithymia, emotional disclosure, and health: A program of research. *Journal of Personality, 72*, 1271–1300.

Martins, A., Ramalho, N., & Morin, E. (2010). A comprehensive meta-analysis of the relationship between emotional intelligence and health. *Personality and Individual Differences, 49*, 554–564.

Mayer, J. D., & Salovey, P. (1997). What is emotional intelligence? In P. Salovey & D. Sluyter (Eds.), *Emotional development and emotional intelligence: Educational implications* (pp. 3–31). New York: Basic Books.

Mayer, J. D., Salovey, P., & Caruso, D. (2002). *Mayer–Salovey–Caruso Emotional Intelligence Test user's manual*. Toronto: Multi-Health Systems.

Mayer, J. D., Salovey, P., & Caruso, D. R. (2004). Emotional intelligence: Theory, findings, implications. *Psychological Inquiry, 15*, 197–215.

McEwen, B. S. (1998). Protective and damaging effects of stress mediators. *New England Journal of Medicine, 388*, 171–179.

Mikolajczak, M., Petrides, K. V., Coumans, N., & Luminet, O. (2009). An experimental investigation of the moderating effects of trait emotional intelligence on laboratory-induced stress. *International Journal of Clinical and Health Psychology, 9*, 355–477.

Pennebaker, J. W. (1982). *The psychology of physical symptoms*. New York: Springer-Verlag.

Plutchik, R. (1980). *Emotion: A psychoevolutionary synthesis*. New York: Harper & Row.

Price, J. L., Monson, C. M., Callahan, K., & Rodriguez, B. F. (2006). The role of emotional functioning in military-related PTSD and its treatment. *Journal of Anxiety Disorders, 20*, 661–674.

Radloff, L. S. (1977). The CES-D Scale: A self-report depression scale for research in the general population. *Applied Psychological Measurement, 1*, 385–401.

Roemer, L., Lee, J. K., Salters-Pedneault, K., Erisman, S. M., Orsillo, S. M, & Mennin, D. (2009). Mindfulness and emotion regulation difficulties in generalized anxiety disorder: Preliminary evidence for independent and overlapping contributions. *Behavior Therapy, 40*, 142–154.

Ryff, C. D. (1989). Happiness is everything, or is it?: Explorations on the meaning of psychological well-being. *Journal of Personality and Social Psychology, 57*, 1069–1081.

Salovey, P., Mayer, J. D., Goldman, S. L., Turvey, C., & Palfai, T. P. (1995). Emotional attention, clarity, and mood repair: Exploring emotional intelligence using the Trait Meta-Mood Scale. In J. W. Pennebaker (Ed.), *Emotion, disclosure and health* (pp. 125–154). Washington, DC: American Psychological Association.

Sauer, S. E., & Baer, R. A. (2012). Ruminative and mindful self-focused attention in borderline personality disorder. *Personality Disorders: Theory, Research, and Treatement 3*, 233–441.

Shiota, M. N. (2006). Silver linings and candles in the dark: Differences among positive coping strategies in predicting subjective well-being. *Emotion, 6*, 335–339.

Shiota, M. N., & Levenson, R. W. (2012). Turn down the volume or change the channel?: Emotional effects of detached versus positive reappraisal. *Journal of Personality and Social Psychology, 103*, 416–429.

Shrout, P. E., & Fleiss, J. L. (1979). Intraclass correlations: Uses in assessing rater reliability. *Psychological Bulletin, 86*, 420–428.

Shulman, T. E., & Hemenover, S. H. (2006). Is dispositional emotional intelligence synonymous with personality? *Self and Identity, 5*, 147–171.

Sifneos, P. E. (1973). The prevalence of "alexithymic" characteristics in psychosomatic patients. *Psychotherapy and Psychosomatics, 22*, 255–262.

Simon, H. A. (1967). Motivational and emotional controls of cognition. *Psychological Review, 74*, 29–39.

Smith, C. A. (1991). The self, appraisal, and coping. In C. R. Snyder & D. R. Forsyth (Eds.), *Handbook of social and clinical psychology: The health perspective* (pp. 116–137). New York: Pergamon Press.

Smith, C. A., & Kirby, L. D. (2013). *From state to trait and back: Introducing a multidimensional measure of appraisal style.* Manuscript submitted for publication.

Smith, C. A., & Lazarus, R. S. (1990). Emotion and adaptation. In L. A. Pervin (Ed.), *Handbook of personality theory and research* (pp. 609–637). New York: Guilford Press.

Taylor, G. J., & Bagby, R. M. (2004). New trends in alexithymia research. *Psychotherapy and Psychosomatics, 73*, 68–77.

Taylor, G. J., Bagby, R. M., & Parker, J. D. A. (1997). *Disorders of affect regulation: Alexithymia in medical and psychiatric illness.* New York: Cambridge University Press.

Tomkins, S. S. (1962). *Affect, imagery, consciousness: Vol. 1. The positive affects.* New York: Springer-Verlag.

Tugade, M. M. (2011). Positive emotions, coping, and resilience. In S. Folkman (Ed.), *Oxford handbook of stress, health, and coping* (pp. 186–199). New York: Oxford University Press.

Tugade, M. M., & Fredrickson, B. L. (2004). Resilient individuals use positive emotions to bounce back from negative emotional experiences. *Journal of Personality and Social Psychology, 86*, 320–333.

Tugade, M. M., & Fredrickson, B. L. (2007). Regulation of positive emotions: Emotion regulation strategies that promote resilience [Special issue]. *Journal of Happiness Studies, 8*, 311–333.

Tugade, M. M., Fredrickson, B. L., & Barrett, L. F. (2004). Psychological resilience and emotional granularity: Examining the benefits of positive emotions on emotion regulation and health. *Journal of Personality, 72*, 1161–1190.

Turk, C. L., Heimberg, R. G., Luterek, J. A., Mennin, D. S., & Fresco, D. M. (2005). Emotion dysregulation in generalized anxiety disorder: A comparison with social anxiety disorder. *Cognitive Therapy and Research, 29*, 89–106.

Vanheule, S., Vandenbergen, J., Verhaeghe, P., & Desmet, M. (2010). Interpersonal problems in alexithymia: A study in three primary care groups. *Psychology and Psychotherapy: Theory, Research and Practice, 83*, 351–362.

Ware, J. E., Kosinski, M., & Dewey, J. E. (2000). *How to score Version 2 of the SF-36 Health Survey (standard and acute forms).* Lincoln, RI: Quality Metric, Inc.

Watson, D., & Clark, L. A. (1994). *The PANAS-

X: *Manual for the Positive and Negative Affect Schedule—Expanded Form*. Unpublished manuscript, University of Iowa.

Watson, D., & Tellegen, A. (1985). Toward a consensual structure of mood. *Psychological Bulletin, 98,* 219–235.

Williams, K. E., Chambless, D. L., & Ahrens, A. H. (1997). Are emotions frightening?: An extension of the fear of fear construct. *Behaviour Research and Therapy, 35,* 239–248.

Yen, S., Zlotnick, C., & Costello, E. (2002). Affect regulation in women with borderline personality disorder traits. *Journal of Nervous and Mental Disease, 190,* 693–696.

CHAPTER 15

Positive Emotions across the Adult Life Span

Joseph A. Mikels
Andrew E. Reed
Lauren N. Hardy
Corinna E. Löckenhoff

Quick, think of the typical older person. What comes to mind? If you were to answer "feeble, gray hair, slow, hard of hearing," and maybe "wise," then you would be conveying the predominantly negative stereotypes of later life that exist within U.S. culture (Hummert, 2011) and across the world (Löckenhoff et al., 2009). To some extent, such pessimistic views present an accurate portrayal of age-related declines in physical, sensory, and cognitive abilities (for reviews, see, e.g., Birren & Schaie, 2006; Craik & Salthouse, 2008). Given the pervasiveness of such losses, one might expect to find a similar downward trajectory in the emotional lives and social relationships of older individuals. However, counter to such expectations, it has become increasingly clear that healthy aging is associated with stable or improved socioemotional well-being (see Carstensen, Mikels, & Mather, 2006; Charles & Carstensen, 2010; Scheibe & Carstensen, 2010). To provide the reader with a better understanding of this apparent paradox, this chapter reviews theoretical explanations, considers underlying emotion regulatory mechanisms, and explores practical implications for the lives of older adults.

We begin with a review of age trajectories in various aspects of well-being and consider competing theoretical accounts of such effects. Next, we examine age differences in emotion regulatory strategies, with particular emphasis on the "positivity effect," an age-related tendency to shift processing resources away from negatively valenced material, toward the positive (Carstensen & Mikels, 2005; Mather & Carstensen, 2005). After reviewing evidence for age differences in specific aspects of emotion regulation, we consider practical implications for interpersonal relationships, decision making, and—ultimately—longevity. We conclude by identifying open questions and contextualizing age differences in positive emotions within the broader framework of life-span development.

Age Differences in Positive Emotions and Emotional Well-Being

Psychological well-being has been conceptualized in terms of life satisfaction, negative and positive affectivity, and the absence of psychopathology (Diener, Suh, Lucas, & Smith, 1999). A review of the extant literature reveals convergent age trajectories across these aspects of well-being. With regard to life satisfaction, early cross-sectional studies indicated that despite age-related declines in income and increased rates of widowhood, well-being remained stable and relatively high through middle age and into later life (for a review, see Diener et al., 1999). Subsequent longitudinal research found that life satisfaction increases until ages 65–70, at which point there is a decline (Mroczek & Spiro, 2005). However, this late life decline appears to be due to proximity to death, not chronological age per se (also see Gerstorf et al., 2010). Thus, as measured by life satisfaction, well-being appears generally to increase with healthy aging.

Similar patterns have been observed for trajectories of positive and negative affect. In both cross-sectional and longitudinal studies, older adults report lower levels of negative affect and relatively stable levels of positive affect relative to younger adults (Carstensen, Pasupathi, Mayr, & Nesselroade, 2000; Carstensen et al., 2011; Charles, Reynolds, & Gatz, 2001; Mroczek & Kolarz, 1998). Importantly, these patterns are consistent across methodologies and have been observed in retrospective ratings of average emotional states (Charles et al., 2001), as well as everyday emotional experiences assessed via experience sampling (Carstensen et al., 2000, 2011). Such consistencies indicate that age-related changes in the tracking and recall of one's emotional experiences cannot account for the observed improvements in affect. Moreover, results are not limited to temporary mood states but also are found at the level of dispositional emotions: Large-scale longitudinal studies and comprehensive meta-analyses have documented age-related increases in emotional stability and decreases in the propensity to experience negative emotions (Roberts, Walton, & Viechtbauer, 2006; Terracciano, McCrae, Brant, & Costa, 2005).

Epidemiological evidence also suggests that psychopathology declines with age, with the exception of dementia and other neurological conditions specific to later life. In a nationally representative U.S. sample, the prevalence of anxiety, mood, and substance abuse disorders was found to be significantly lower among those age 60 and older compared to younger age groups (Kes-

sler et al., 2005). Similarly, in the National Health Interview Survey, the one-month prevalence of serious psychological distress was significantly higher in midlife than in old age (age 65 and over; Centers for Disease Control and Prevention [CDC], 2006).

In summary, despite the numerous losses that occur in later life, advanced age appears to be associated with stable or even improved levels of emotional well-being, positive emotions, and mental health. Although there is general consensus about the size and direction of this effect, there is less agreement about the underlying mechanisms.

Theoretical Perspectives

Over the past few decades, competing theoretical explanations for age-related patterns in emotional well-being have been proposed (see Table 15.1). These theories vary in not only the specific mechanisms proposed to underlie age effects but also the degree to which they conceptualize age-related functional losses as a contributing factor.

At one end of the spectrum, it has been argued that sustained well-being in late life is a direct consequence of declines in cognitive and neural functioning. Cacioppo, Berntson, Bechara, Tranel, and Hawkley (2011) suggest that age-related limitations in the reactivity of affective brain circuits, especially in the amygdala, may account for decreased negative affect in advanced age. Similarly, Labouvie-Vief's (2003) dynamic integration theory (DIT; Labouvie-Vief, Grühn, & Studer, 2010) contends that emotional and cognitive functioning are inextricably linked. According to DIT, positive emotional development reflects a dynamic balance between "optimization" (i.e., a hedonic emphasis on positive emotions) and "differentiation" (i.e., the ability to tolerate mixed and negative emotions to maintain a realistic view of the world and the self). Age-related limitations in cognitive resources are thought to shift this balance toward optimization, which is less cognitively demanding than differentiation.

Life-span developmental frameworks, such as Baltes's model of selective optimization with compensation (SOC; Baltes, 1997; Baltes & Baltes, 1990), take a more optimistic stance. According to the SOC model, age-related losses in various areas of functioning

TABLE 15.1. Theoretical Models of Adult Life-Span Emotional Development

Theory	Abbreviation	Primary mechanism	Developmental outcome
Aging brain model (Cacioppo)	ABM	Selective age-related neural degradation in systems processing negative stimuli	Dampened emotional response to and memory for negative stimuli
Dynamic integration theory (Labouvie-Vief)	DIT	Age-related limitations in cognitive resources	Shift in dynamic balance from affect differentiation toward optimization
Selective optimization with compensation (Baltes)	SOC	With advancing age, developmental losses outweigh gains across multiple areas of functioning	Increased selectivity in goal pursuit and devotion of resources to goal pursuit; use of compensatory strategies to counteract losses
Selective optimization and compensation with emotion regulation (Urry & Gross)	SOC-ER	Age-related shifts in internal and external resources	Selection and optimization of emotion regulatory strategies that draw on resources which are enhanced or preserved with age
Motivational theory of lifespan development (Heckhausen)	MTL	Age-related losses in primary control (i.e., control over environment)	Increased reliance on internal secondary control mechanisms over primary control mechanisms
Socioemotional selectivity theory (Carstensen)	SST	Age-related shifts in goals as a result of limitations in future time perspective	Prioritization of emotionally meaningful present-oriented goals over information-related future-oriented goals
Strength and vulnerability integration (Charles)	SAVI	Age-related shifts in the balance of emotion regulatory strengths and vulnerabilities	Prioritization of antecedent- over response-focused strategies; impaired coping with extended and intense negative experiences

lead individuals to be more selective in their goal pursuit, optimizing personally relevant goals while employing compensatory strategies in other aspects of life. Thus, successful functioning and emotional well-being can be maintained despite compounding losses. In a recent extension of this model (selective optimization and compensation with emotion regulation, SOC-ER), Urry and Gross (2010) have argued that in advanced age, individuals selectively engage in regulatory strategies that draw on resources that are well preserved with age.

In a similar vein, the motivational theory of life-span development (MTL; Heckhausen, Wrosch, & Schulz, 2010) argues that "primary control," the ability to exert active control over one's physical and social environment, peaks in midlife and declines in old age. In contrast, secondary control mechanisms aimed at emotion regulation

and goal adjustment are thought to remain viable into advanced old age. Both the SOC and MTL frameworks emphasize the active role of older adults in responding to functional losses with emotion regulatory strategies and flexible goal adjustment. Nevertheless, these theories consider age-related declines in functional capacity as a driving force of age differences in emotions.

Socioemotional selectivity theory (SST), in contrast, emphasizes age-associated changes in future time horizons and their implications for motivational priorities and emotional experience (Carstensen, 2006; Carstensen, Isaacowitz, & Charles, 1999). Specifically, the theory proposes that when future time horizons are perceived as expansive, as is typical in youth, individuals prioritize future-oriented goals such as information acquisition and the development of extended social networks. As time horizons narrow and one's future time is perceived as more limited, as is typical in older age, individuals focus on goals that are relevant to the present moment. This motivational shift is thought to lead to a prioritization of positively valenced and emotionally meaningful experiences.

Finally, in an effort to integrate existing theories into a broader theoretical framework, Charles's (2010) strength and vulnerability integration (SAVI) model argues that from an emotion regulatory point of view, aging is associated with both strengths (e.g., life experience, shifts in time horizons and goal priorities) and weaknesses (i.e., reduced physiological flexibility). This model further posits that older adults fare better in situations in which attentional strategies, reappraisal, or situation selection are feasible, but respond less favorably to situations involving sustained negative arousal.

Table 15.1 summarizes the proposed mechanisms and developmental outcomes in each of the theoretical explanations. To evaluate their relative merit, we proceed by reviewing the evidence for age differences in the strategic processing of emotional information, as well as other types of emotion regulatory strategies.

Age Differences in Emotion Regulation and the Age-Related Positivity Effect

The broad term "emotion regulation" encompasses a variety of strategies aimed at altering emotional states to align better with personal goals and priorities. Importantly, emotion regulatory goals are not always "prohedonic" (i.e., aimed at maximizing positive emotions). In some situations, individuals may follow contrahedonic motivations and purposely elicit or maintain negative states, for instance, to motivate effortful performance (Tamir, Chiu, & Gross, 2007) or to gain self-knowledge (Labouvie-Vief et al., 2010). As noted earlier, SST proposes an age-related shift from future-oriented goals toward goals aimed at optimizing the present moment. Consistent with this notion, evidence from a large-scale experience sampling study suggests that the relative balance between pro- and contrahedonic goals shifts with age, such that contrahedonic motivations are most prevalent in adolescence,

whereas prohedonic motivations dominate in old age (Riediger, Schmiedek, Wagner, & Lindenberger, 2009).

Emotion regulatory strategies can be broadly classified according to the stage of the emotion generation process that is targeted (Gross, 1998; Urry & Gross, 2010). Early on, people may actively select or avoid specific emotion-generating situations (*situation selection*). Once a given situation is encountered, people may try to change the situation (*situation modification*), or direct their attention toward favorable aspects of the situation (*attentional deployment*). At later stages of the emotion generation cycle, individuals may modify their appraisal of the situation (*cognitive change*). Finally, once a given emotion has been elicited, people may attempt to change its subjective experience or external expression (*response modulation*; Opitz, Gross, & Urry, 2012; Urry & Gross, 2010).

To date, the literature on emotional aging has focused disproportionately on the early stages of the emotion regulatory process. The most striking evidence for age-related shifts comes from research examining "motivated cognition," that is, the strategic allocation of processing resources to support desired outcomes or emotional states (Mather & Carstensen, 2005). Although some aspects of cognitive functioning remain stable or improve with age (e.g., crystallized intelligence and implicit memory), effortful and deliberative processing abilities generally decline across the adult life span (Craik et al., 2008). However, several early studies indicated that older adults remember emotional material better than other types of material (Carstensen & Turk-Charles, 1994; Fung & Carstensen, 2003; Hashtroudi, Johnson, & Chrosniak, 1990). Older adults' focus on emotionally salient information may reflect, in part, a strategic shift toward affect-rich and experience-based processing modes that are relatively spared from cognitive decline (Peters, Diefenbach, Hess, & Vastfjäll, 2007).

Crucially, age groups differ not only in their emphasis on emotional material in general but also their relative emphasis on positive relative to negative material. While there is long-standing evidence for a cognitive processing bias toward negative material among younger adults (for reviews, see Baumeister, Bratslavsky, Finkenauer, & Vohs, 2001; Rozin & Royzman, 2001), this pattern does not extend across the entire life span (Carstensen et al., 2006; Carstensen & Mikels, 2005; Mather & Carstensen, 2005). Instead, the allocation of processing resources appears to shift with age toward positive relative to negative information, a pattern termed the "age-related positivity effect" (Carstensen & Mikels, 2005).

Over the past decade, the positivity effect has been observed across a wide range of methods and stimulus types. In studies examining attentional deployment, both dot-probe tasks and eye-tracking technologies show an age-related focus toward positive and/or away from negative material (Allard & Isaacowitz, 2008; Bannerman & Regner, 2011; Isaacowitz & Choi, 2011; Isaacowitz, Wadlinger, Goren, & Wilson, 2006a, 2006b; Knight et al., 2007; Mather & Carstensen, 2003). The positivity effect has also been found in working memory (Mikels, Larkin, Reuter-Lorenz, & Carstensen, 2005) and memory for emotionally salient scenes, facial expressions, and words (Charles, Mather, & Carstensen, 2003, Chung, 2010; Grady, Hongwanishkul, Keightley, Lee, & Hasher, 2007; Grühn, Scheibe, & Baltes, 2007; Kensinger, 2008; Langeslag & van Strien, 2009; Leigland, Schulz, & Janowsky, 2004; Spaniol, Voss, & Grady, 2008; but see, e.g., Denburg, Buchanan, Tranel, & Adolphs, 2003; Grühn, Smith, & Baltes, 2005), as well as for autobiographical memory (Kennedy, Mather, & Carstensen, 2004; Ready, Weinberger, & Jones, 2007; Schlagman, Schulz, & Kvavilashvili, 2006), and false memory (Fernandes, Ross, Wiegand, & Schryer, 2008).

Corresponding patterns emerge at the neural level. Specifically, neural reactivity to negative stimuli appears to be lower among older adults, whereas reactivity to positive stimuli does not change with age. Convergent evidence for such effects comes from electroencephalographic (EEG) studies examining event-related potentials (Kisley, Wood, & Burrows, 2007), as well as functional magnetic resonance imaging (fMRI) studies examining the activation of subcortical emotional circuits including the amygdala (Mather et al., 2004). At first glance, the selective dampening of responses to negative material is consistent with accounts based on selective deterioration in the neural circuits supporting negative affect (Cacioppo et al., 2011). However, neural degradation and decline may not be the primary mechanism. In fact, recent evidence suggests that the positivity effect depends on better, not worse, cognitive functioning. Mather and Knight (2005) found that the memory bias toward positive material was limited to older adults who scored higher on a measure of cognitive control. Moreover, in divided attention tasks, in which cognitive resources are occupied by a competing task, older adults do not show a positivity effect (Mather & Knight, 2005) or even focus on the negative (Knight et al., 2007).

Furthermore, consistent with the notion that the positivity effect serves an emotion regulatory function, older adults spend more time looking at positive stimuli after a negative mood induction, whereas younger adults look more at negative, mood-congruent stimuli in this situation (Isaacowitz, Toner, Goren, & Wilson, 2008). Looking toward positive and away from negative stimuli leads to more positive moods—but only for older adults with higher levels of attentional functioning (Isaacowitz, Toner, & Neupert, 2009). In fact, attentional deployment may be a particularly effective emotion regulatory strategy for older adults. When focusing attention away from a negative film clip and toward positive memories, older adults showed a larger drop in negative emotions than did their younger counterparts (Phillips, Henry, Hosie, & Milne, 2008). In summary, there is consistent support for the view that the positivity effect represents a form of motivated cognition driven by age-related shifts toward prohedonic emotion regulatory strategies.

Compared to the rich research record on age-related shifts in the deployment of processing resources, much less is known about *situation selection and modification*, although mounting evidence suggests that the age-related positivity effect extends to the earliest stages of the emotion regulation cycle. In groundbreaking work using narrative vignettes, Blanchard-Fields, Jahnke, and Camp (1995; for a review, see Blanchard-Fields, 2007), found that older adults avoided situations that might elicit negative emotions to a greater extent than did younger adults.

Rovenpor, Skogsberg, and Isaacowitz (2013) recently extended these findings to a laboratory setting. They allowed older and younger adults to choose among multiple affective streams consisting of video clips and reading material that varied in emotional valence. Age differences were limited to participants with high emotion regulatory efficacy, but within that group, older adults chose *less* negative material (relative to neutral and positive material), whereas younger adults chose *more* negative material. This finding is not only consistent with an age-related emphasis on prohedonic goals, but it also suggests that successful emotion regulation depends on perceived resources in the form of emotion regulatory efficacy.

Evidence for age differences in *situation modification* is similarly limited, but recent findings suggest that age groups differ in the construction of temporal sequences of emotional events. When asked to view a series of positive, negative, and neutral images, younger adults constructed improving sequences that saved the best images for last, whereas older adults constructed spreading sequences that avoided prolonged clusters of negative images (Löckenhoff, Reed, & Maresca, 2012). These findings are consistent with the SAVI model, which suggests that older adults avoid sustained emotional arousal because it prevents a threat to homeostasis (Charles, 2010), and also support SST insofar as a preference for spreading sequences was found to be associated with more limited future time horizons (Löckenhoff et al., 2012).

Taken together, the literature offers consistent evidence of age-related stability or improvement in antecedent-focused forms of emotion regulation. In comparison, research on age differences in the later stages of emotion regulation is much more limited. From a theoretical point of view, SOC-ER and SAVI proponents would agree that age-related decrements in effortful processing and physiological resilience may limit older adults' use of response-focused emotion regulatory strategies (Charles, 2010; Urry & Gross, 2010). Empirical evidence, however, reveals a more complex pattern.

With regard to *cognitive change strategies,* older adults report using cognitive reappraisal more frequently than do younger adults (John & Gross, 2004), but recent evidence suggests that reappraisal is more effective in younger age groups (Urry & Gross, 2010). In part, age differences in the benefits of cognitive reappraisal may depend on the specific type of strategy that is employed. In particular, older adults are less adept than younger adults at using strategies that rely on emotional detachment from the current situation but superior at reappraising situations in a more positive manner (Shiota & Levenson, 2009).

Evidence for age differences in *response modulation* is similarly mixed. When stimuli are age-appropriate, older adults' self-reported and physiological emotional responses are at least as strong as those of younger adults (Kunzmann & Grühn, 2005; Kunzmann & Richter, 2009; Magai, Consedine, Krivoshekova, Kudadjie-Gyamfi, & McPherson, 2006). Thus, observed age effects are not well explained by age decrements in emotional reactivity or emotion regulatory load. Also, age effects appear to differ depending on whether modulatory strategies target outward expression as opposed to interior states. Research with younger adults has found that the suppression of emotional behaviors and expressions can take a toll on subjective well-being and social relationships (Butler et al., 2003). Given older adults' prioritization of prohedonic goals, one would expect to see an age-related decrease in such strategies, and the literature generally supports this idea (John & Gross, 2004). However, when older adults are asked to actively suppress or amplify their emotional expressions, they do so just as effectively as their younger counterparts (Kunzmann, Kupperbusch, & Levenson, 2005; Phillips et al., 2008; Shiota & Levenson, 2009). Thus, age differences in the use of expressive modulation are likely to reflect proactive preferences rather than passive losses in the necessary skills. Older adults also perform as well as younger adults in modulating internal affective states (Scheibe & Blanchard-Fields, 2009), and this type of emotion modulation appears to be less cognitively depleting for older than for younger adults: When instructed to down-regulate their feelings after viewing a disgust-inducing video, younger adults showed reduced working memory performance, whereas older adults did not (Scheibe & Blanchard-Fields, 2009).

In summary, the literature suggests that most emotion regulatory skills are preserved across the life span. Older adults are not only well equipped to manage their emotions, but, consistent with SST, they are more likely to pursue prohedonic goals aimed at reducing negative or fostering positive states. In support of the SAVI and SOC-ER models, older adults appear to rely more heavily on attentional deployment than younger adults, and they may select and structure emotional experience in a way that avoids prolonged negative emotions. At the same time, there is little evidence that age differences in emotion regulation are driven by age-related cognitive losses. The positivity effect relies on active control mechanisms, and some aspects of emotion regulation actually appear to be *less* resource intensive for older relative to younger adults. In combination, age differences in emotion regulatory motivations and mechanisms provide a plausible account for the preservation of emotional well-being into the later years.

Implications for Successful Functioning

Thus far, this review has focused on basic laboratory studies, but age-related shifts in emotion regulatory strategies may have practical implications for successful functioning in a variety of life domains. In the following sections we illustrate such effects with regard to social relationships, decision making, and—ultimately—longevity.

Relationships

Across the life span, perceived social support and a strong social network are important predictors of mental and physical well-being (Stephens, Alpass, Towers, & Stevenson, 2011). Consistent with an age-related emphasis on situation selection, SST suggests that older individuals restructure their social contacts to create tight-knit networks of familiar social partners that are conducive to emotionally meaningful and positively valenced interactions (Carstensen, 2006; Carstensen et al., 1999). Empirical evidence for such effects comes from a variety of sources. In studies of social partner preferences, older adults and those with limited time horizons were found to prefer close and famil-

iar social partners over novel social partners (Fredrickson & Carstensen, 1990; Fung & Carstensen, 2004; Fung, Carstensen, & Lutz, 1999). Also, older adults' actual social networks are smaller and contain a greater proportion of close social partners than do the networks of younger adults (Lang & Carstensen, 2002). Importantly, age differences in network characteristics appear to be due to a process of active pruning rather than passive loss. In a longitudinal study of older adults' social networks, perceived closeness to death was associated with a deliberate discontinuation of peripheral social relationships, whereas relationships with close relatives and life partners were selectively strengthened (Lang, 2000).

Older adults are not only selective about their social networks but also the types of interactions in which they engage. When asked to develop solutions for hypothetical problem scenarios, older adults are more likely than their younger counterparts to avoid interpersonal conflicts (Blanchard-Fields, 2007; Blanchard-Fields et al., 1995). In the same vein, daily diary and actual dyadic interaction studies examining exposure and reactivity to interpersonal tensions revealed that older adults used more avoidant and less confrontational strategies than their younger counterparts, resulting in more positive emotions (Birditt & Fingerman, 2005; Birditt, Fingerman, & Almeida, 2005; Lefkowitz & Fingerman, 2003). In concrete terms, whereas younger adults were more likely to actively exit confrontations or raise their voices, older adults were more likely simply to "do nothing" (Birditt & Fingerman, 2005).

When avoidant strategies are not possible, older adults may actively infuse the situation with positive affect. In a laboratory study in which couples were asked to discuss a topic of mutual conflict, older, compared to middle-aged, couples were more likely to express affection or temporarily switch to a more favorable topic (Carstensen, Gottman, & Levenson, 1995; Levenson, Carstensen, Gottman, 1994). Nevertheless, recent evidence suggests that age-related reductions in interpersonal tensions are limited to situations in which conflict can be avoided; actual confrontations are found to be equally upsetting for adults of all ages (Charles, Piazza, Luong, & Almeida, 2009).

Consistent with an age-related emphasis on prohedonic motivation, age differences in interpersonal strategies appear to benefit emotional well-being. Older adults with small and close-knit social networks report lower interpersonal strain (Lang & Carstensen, 2002), and older adults' use of avoidant strategies is associated with lower interpersonal tension and greater relationship satisfaction (Birditt & Fingerman, 2005; Birditt et al., 2005; Lefkowitz & Fingerman, 2003). In general, advanced age is associated with better marriages, greater perceived social support, and less interpersonal conflict than in younger age (Fingerman & Charles, 2010).

Despite the obvious emotional benefits, older adults' tendency to avoid conflict and reappraise interactions in positive terms also carries certain risks because it may prevent a realistic assessment of relationship concerns. For instance, when discussing a disagreement with their spouses, older adults were more likely than middle-aged adults to view their spouse's behavior as positive, even when independent observers did not (Story et al., 2007). A similar tension between potential benefits and detriments of age differences in emotion regulatory strategies is seen in the context of decision making.

Decision Making

Older adults are often charged with the task of making crucial, complex decisions in domains such as retirement investment, health care, and prescription drug coverage. Recent findings indicate that such decisions require both emotional and cognitive capacities (see, e.g., Kahneman, 2003; Slovic, Peters, Finucane, & MacGregor, 2005). Thus, although much of the research on aging and decision making has focused on cognitive decline (Sanfey & Hastie, 2000), age-related changes in affective processing and emotion regulatory strategies are likely to play a role as well. For example, older adults' tendency to avoid decisions (Dror, Katona, & Mungur, 1998), to delegate decisions (Finucane et al., 2002; Meyer, Russo, & Talbot, 1995), and to rely on simplified decision rules (Johnson, 1990, 1993) is typically interpreted as a consequence of age-related limitation in cognitive resources. However, such patterns may also reflect a

form of situation selection because they limit exposure to emotionally aversive tradeoffs that are part and parcel of complex decision making (Luce, Payne, & Bettman, 2000).

Similarly, older adults have been observed to seek out and examine less information before making decisions than their younger counterparts (for a review, see Mata & Nunes, 2010). In part, this likely reflects age-related deficits in the ability to manipulate large amounts of information. Indeed, older adults show deficits in information comprehension and in the integration of information across situations (e.g., Finucane, Mertz, Slovic, & Schmidt, 2005; Finucane et al., 2002). However, age-related decrements in information seeking do not affect all types of information equally. Instead, the observed age pattern is consistent with motivated resource deployment and the age-related positivity effect. In particular, when older and younger adults are presented with tabular arrays of decision options, older adults review and recall more positive versus negative information than do younger adults (Löckenhoff & Carstensen, 2007, 2008; Mather, Knight, & McCaffrey, 2005). Consistent with SST, a greater focus on positive choice attributes is associated with limited future time horizons (Löckenhoff & Carstensen, 2007). Similarly, when presented with a choice among everyday items (e.g., a pen, a mug) and asked explicitly to evaluate the options, older adults list a greater number of positive versus negative attributes than do younger adults (Kim, Healey, Goldstein, Hasher, & Wiprzycka, 2008).

In further support for an age-related positivity effect in judgment and decision making, age groups differentially display one of the most robust biases in human decision making: the "framing effect" (i.e., the phenomenon whereby superficial differences in the description of a given choice substantially alter people's preferences). For instance, risk seeking is typically found to be greater when alternatives are described as losses versus gains, underscoring the impact of negative losses on younger adults (Kahneman & Tversky, 2000). Recent evidence indicates that, in contrast to younger adults, older adults do not show risk seeking in loss frames, which suggests that losses are less impactful for older adults (Mikels & Reed,

2009). Furthermore, whereas younger adults respond equally to gains and losses, older adults show reduced responses to losses, and intact neural and affective responses to gains (Samanez-Larkin et al., 2007). Also, consistent with this general pattern, older relative to younger adults were found to be more responsive to health messages when they were framed in positive versus negative terms (Shamaskin, Mikels, & Reed, 2010).

In decision making, as in social relationships, age differences in the processing and regulation of emotions may have beneficial *and* detrimental consequences. Consistent with an age-related prioritization of prohedonic goals, older adults' emphasis on positive choice characteristics is associated with more positive emotional experiences during the decision-making process (Löckenhoff & Carstensen, 2008), more favorable recall of past choices (Löckenhoff & Carstensen, 2007, 2008; Mather & Johnson, 2000), and greater choice satisfaction (Kim et al., 2008). Moreover, relying on emotion-focused decision-making styles may help older adults to make objectively better decisions because, relative to deliberative decision strategies, intuitive processing is comparatively well preserved with age (Queen & Hess, 2010). Consistent with this idea, older adults made better decisions in hypothetical health care scenarios when focusing on their emotional reactions versus the actual details, whereas younger adults showed the opposite pattern (Mikels et al., 2010). Thus, reliance on emotion and intuition may offer older adults a path toward sound and satisfactory choices. However, exclusive reliance on this type of processing may sometimes lead to flawed decisions (Gilovich, Griffin, & Kahneman, 2002). Moreover, the age-related positivity effect could put older adults at risk of overlooking critical disadvantages of decision options, and may make them more susceptible to fraud and false advertising (Löckenhoff & Carstensen, 2004).

Positivity and Increased Longevity

Ultimately, the age-related emphasis on positive emotions and emotional well-being may confer significant benefits in terms of longevity. A long research tradition examining personality predictors of longevity indicates that emotional stability and optimism are associated with lower mortality in both healthy populations and patient samples (Maruta, Colligan, Malinchoc, & Offord, 2000; Novotny et al., 2010; Terracciano, Löckenhoff, Zonderman, Ferrucci, & Costa, 2008; see also Moskowitz & Saslow, Chapter 24, this volume). The benefits of positive affect are not limited to dispositions. In a sample of nuns, the proportion of positive emotional content in written biographies composed in the early 20s predicted survival up to six decades later (Danner, Snowdon, & Friesen, 2001). Similar effects are found for everyday emotional experiences. Carstensen and colleagues (2011) followed adults of different ages across a 13-year span. Those individuals who experienced more positive versus negative emotions were more likely to survive. Importantly, the experience of positive emotions predicted longevity above and beyond age, sex, and ethnicity. Finally, there is mounting evidence that positive attitudes toward the aging process are associated with enhanced longevity. In a series of studies, Levy and colleagues (Levy & Myers, 2005; Levy, Slade, Kunkel, & Kasl, 2002; Levy, Slade, May, & Caracciolo, 2006) have found that individuals with more positive attitudes toward their own aging process experienced better health outcomes and lower mortality.

Taken together, these findings suggest that while positivity benefits health and longevity across the life span, it may take on particular relevance in advanced age as individuals face various health challenges and confront negative societal stereotypes about the aging process. Future research is needed to examine the specific mechanisms by which age differences in emotion regulatory strategies may translate into better physical health.

Directions for Future Research

This review of the literature indicates that despite age-related losses across many domains of functioning, positive emotions and emotional well-being remain stable or even show improvement well into advanced old age. Although a variety of theoretical explanations of these effects has been proposed, well-preserved emotion-regulatory skills and the selective use of specific processing strategies appear to play key roles. In general, the pattern of results is consistent with a proactive shift toward prohedonic goals driven by age-related limitations in future time horizons. In contrast, there is little evidence that the observed age trajectories are the result of neural or cognitive deficits, although—consistent with SAVI—adaptive responses to vulnerabilities in other aspects of functioning may be a contributing factor.

Apart from their theoretical relevance, age differences in emotion regulatory strategies have important practical implications. In this chapter, we have illustrated such effects in the contexts of interpersonal relationships, decision making, and longevity, but other domains of functioning may be affected as well. As discussed earlier, age-related shifts in emotional processing may have both beneficial and detrimental effects on successful functioning. Targeted interventions to address potential vulnerabilities of older populations are needed, but, to date, important gaps in the research record hamper their development.

First, it is critical to understand the extent to which older adults are aware of age-related shifts in emotion regulatory strategies, and the degree to which such strategies can be modulated by instructional manipulations. With regard to the positivity effect, initial evidence is quite promising. Two studies suggest that whereas younger adults are not aware of the positivity effect, older adults have some insight into its existence. For example, when asked to take the perspective of another person in retelling a story, older adults used a greater proportion of positive versus negative words when taking the perspective of an older compared to younger target person. In contrast, the emotional content of younger adults' responses was not affected by the age of the target person (Sullivan, Mikels, & Carstensen, 2010). Similarly, Löckenhoff and Carstensen (2008) found that older adults reviewed a greater proportion of positive information than did younger adults when making decisions for themselves or another older person, but equal proportions of positive and negative material when deciding for a younger person. Younger adults, in contrast, did not modulate their search patterns across target persons.

Importantly, older adults are not only aware of the positivity effect, but they are also able to reduce their focus on the positive in response to situational demands. The positivity effect in autobiographical memory (Kennedy et al., 2004) and pre-decisional information search (Löckenhoff & Carstensen, 2007) is eliminated if instructional manipulations elicit information-seeking as opposed to emotion regulatory goals. Notably, in two studies that failed to find evidence for an age-related positivity effect, participants were informed in advance that their retention of the presented material would be assessed (Denburg et al., 2003; Grühn et al., 2005), likely activating information-seeking goals. In combination, these results suggest that age differences in emotion regulatory strategies can be modulated in response to situational demands, and that older adults may be at least partially aware of their emotional biases. To date, however, such findings remain limited to the attentional deployment stage of the emotion regulatory process, representing another important gap in the research record.

Few studies of age differences in emotion regulation have clearly differentiated among different stages of regulation. Whereas some studies use wording that could apply equally to all types of emotion regulation (Gross et al., 1997), others focus only on select types. In recent years, the information-processing stage of emotion regulation has received disproportionate attention, because research on the age-related positivity effect has dominated the field (Scheibe & Carstensen, 2010). Although this body of work is critical in many ways, it may be equally worthwhile to direct attention to both earlier and later stages of the emotion generation process. In doing so, the process model of emotion regulation (Gross, 1998; Urry & Gross, 2010) can serve as a guide to categorize specific regulatory strategies within a general framework. Particularly important gaps in the literature concern situation selection and modification. Also, affective forecasting skills, which are a key prerequisite for selecting emotionally satisfying situations, constitute an important avenue for future research (Löckenhoff, 2011; Nielsen, Knutson, & Carstensen, 2008; Scheibe, Mata, & Carstensen, 2010).

When examining age differences in various emotion regulatory strategies, it is also critical to differentiate between older adults' preferences for a given strategy and their ability to implement that strategy successfully. As exemplified by age patterns in the modulation of emotional expressions (John & Gross, 2004), the finding that older adults do not typically rely on a certain strategy need not imply that they are unable to use that strategy when prompted to do so (Kunzmann et al., 2005). A better understanding of divergent age trajectories in emotion regulatory *skills* versus *preferences* would provide key insights into the underlying mechanisms.

Finally, future studies should examine the universality of age trajectories in emotional well-being and regulatory strategies. Following SST, one would expect that age-related limitations in time horizons and the associated emphasis on emotional meaning are found regardless of cultural context. However, in individualistic U.S. cultures, the pursuit of emotionally meaningful goals is likely to coincide with the optimization of personal well-being. Conceivably, differential patterns may emerge for interdependent cultures where the well-being of the group takes priority. Consistent with this idea, the positivity effect in attention and memory in older Chinese participants was found to be less pronounced among those whose self-concepts were more interdependent than among those who were more independent (Fung, Isaacowitz, Lu, & Li, 2010). At the same time, cross-cultural differences in emotion regulatory strategies and priorities need to be differentiated from culture-specific interpretations of emotional stimuli. For instance, a study examining memory for emotional images in younger versus older Koreans found a positivity effect, but only when cultural and age differences in valence ratings were taken into account (Kwon, Scheibe, Samanez-Larkin, Tsai, & Carstensen, 2009). Clearly, further research examining a wider range of cultures, using culturally appropriate stimuli, and covering a more comprehensive range of emotion regulatory strategies, is needed.

In conclusion, while studies of age differences in cognitive skills and physical prowess may paint a rather bleak picture of the later years, age trajectories of positive emotions and emotional well-being offer a more optimistic outlook, emphasizing stability or even age-related improvement. Once the remaining gaps in the literature have been closed and a better understanding of the underlying mechanisms has been acquired, it may be possible to leverage the emotion regulatory strategies typically employed by older adults to offer younger populations an early glimpse at the serenity and balance of late life. Given the associations between positivity and lower mortality, this approach holds the promise of not only happier but also longer lives.

References

Allard, E. S., & Isaacowitz, D. M. (2008). Are preferences in emotional processing affected by distraction?: Examining the age-related positivity effect in visual fixation within a dual-task paradigm. *Aging, Neuropsychology, and Cognition, 15,* 725–743.

Baltes, P. B. (1997). On the incomplete architecture of human ontogeny: Selection, optimization, and compensation as foundation of developmental theory. *American Psychologist, 52,* 366–380.

Baltes, P. B., & Baltes, M. M. (1990). Selective optimization with compensation. In P. B. Baltes & M. M. Baltes (Ed), *Successful aging: Perspectives from the behavioral sciences* (pp. 1–34). New York: Cambridge University Press.

Bannerman, R. L., & Regner, P. (2011). Binocular rivalry: A window into emotional processing in aging. *Psychology and Aging, 26*(2), 372–380.

Baumeister, R. F., Bratslavsky, E., Finkenauer, C., & Vohs, K. D. (2001). Bad is stronger than good. *Review of General Psychology, 5,* 323–373.

Birditt, K. S., & Fingerman, K. L. (2005). Do we get better at picking our battles?: Age group differences in descriptions of behavioral reactions to interpersonal tensions. *Journals of Gerontology B: Psychological Sciences, 60*(3), 121–128.

Birditt, K. S., Fingerman, K. L., & Almeida, D. M. (2005). Age differences in exposure and reactions to interpersonal tensions: A daily diary study. *Psychology and Aging, 20,* 330–340.

Birren, J., & Schaie, K. (2006). *Handbook of the psychology of aging* (6th ed.). Amsterdam: Elsevier.

Blanchard-Fields, F. (2007). Everyday problem

solving and emotion: An adult developmental perspective. *Current Directions in Psychological Science, 16,* 26–31.

Blanchard-Fields, F., Jahnke, H. C., & Camp, C. (1995). Age differences in problem-solving style: The role of emotional salience. *Psychology and Aging, 10*(2), 173–180.

Butler, E. A., Egloff, B., Wilhelm, F. H., Smith, N. C., Erickson, E. A., & Gross, J. J. (2003). The social consequences of expressive suppression. *Emotion, 3*(1), 48–67.

Cacioppo, J. T., Berntson, G. G., Bechara, A., Tranel, D., & Hawkley, L. C. (2011). Could an aging brain contribute to subjective well-being?: The value added by a social neuroscience perspective. In A. Todorov, S. T. Fiske, & D. A. Prentice (Eds.), *Social neuroscience: Toward understanding the underpinnings of the social mind* (pp. 249–262). New York: Oxford University Press.

Carstensen, L. L. (2006). The influence of a sense of time on human development. *Science, 312,* 1913–1915.

Carstensen, L. L., Gottman, J. M., & Levenson, R. W. (1995). Emotional behavior in long-term marriage. *Psychology and Aging, 10*(1), 140–149.

Carstensen, L. L., Isaacowitz, D. M., & Charles, S. T. (1999). Taking time seriously: A theory of socioemotional selectivity. *American Psychologist, 54,* 165–181.

Carstensen, L. L., & Mikels, J. A. (2005). At the intersection of emotion and cognition: Aging and the positivity effect. *Current Direction Psychological Science, 14*(3), 117–121.

Carstensen, L. L., Mikels, J. A., & Mather, M. (2006). Aging and the intersection of cognition, motivation and emotion. In J. E. Birren & K. W., Schaie (Eds.), *Handbook of the psychology of aging* (pp. 343–362). San Diego, CA: Academic Press.

Carstensen, L. L., Pasupathi, M., Mayr, U., & Nesselroade, J. R. (2000). Emotional experience in everyday life across the adult life span. *Journal of Personality and Social Psychology, 79,* 644–655.

Carstensen, L. L., Turan, B., Scheibe, S., Ram, N., Ersner-Hershfeld, H., Samanez-Larkin, G. R., et al. (2011). Emotional experience improves with age: Evidence based on over 10 years of experience sampling. *Psychology and Aging, 26*(1), 21–33.

Carstensen, L. L., & Turk-Charles, S. (1994). The salience of emotion across the adult life span. *Psychology and Aging, 9*(2), 259–264.

Centers for Disease Control and Prevention (CDC). (2006). Early release of selected estimates based on data from the January–June 2006 National Health Interview Survey. Retrieved from *www.cdc.gov/nchs/data/nhis/earlyrelease/200612_13.pdf.*

Charles, S. T. (2010). Strength and vulnerability integration: A model of emotional well-being across adulthood. *Psychological Bulletin, 136*(6), 1068–1091.

Charles, S. T., & Carstensen, L. L. (2010). Social and emotional aging. *Annual Review of Psychology, 61,* 383–409.

Charles, S. T., Mather, M., & Carstensen, L. L. (2003). Aging and emotional memory: The forgettable nature of negative images for older adults. *Journal of Experimental Psychology, 132,* 310–324.

Charles, S. T., Piazza, J. R., Luong, G., & Almeida, D. A. (2009). Now you see it, now you don't: Age differences in affective reactivity to social tensions. *Psychology and Aging, 24*(3), 645–653.

Charles, S. T., Reynolds, C. A., & Gatz, M. (2001). Age-related differences and change in positive and negative affect over 23 years. *Journal of Personality and Social Psychology, 80,* 136–151.

Chung, C. (2010). Effects of view of life and selection bias on emotional memory in old age. *GeroPsych: The Journal of Gerontopsychology and Geriatric Psychiatry, 23*(3), 161–168.

Craik, F. I. M., & Salthouse, T. A. (2008). *The handbook of aging and cognition* (3rd ed.) New York: Psychology Press.

Danner, D. D., Snowdon, D. A., & Friesen, W. V. (2001). Positive emotions in early life and longevity: Findings from the nun study. *Journal of Personality and Social Psychology, 80*(5), 804–813.

Denburg, N. L., Buchanan, T. W., Tranel, D., & Adolphs, R. (2003). Evidence for preserved emotional memory in normal older persons. *Emotion, 3,* 239–253.

Diener, E., Suh, E. M., Lucas, R. E., & Smith, H. L. (1999). Subjective well-being: Three decades of progress. *Psychological Bulletin, 125,* 276–302.

Dror, I. E., Katona, M., & Mungur, K. (1998). Age differences in decision making: To take a risk or not? *Gerontology, 44*(2), 67–71.

Fernandes, M., Ross, M., Wiegand, M., & Schryer, E. (2008). Are the memories of older adults positively biased? *Psychology and Aging, 23,* 297–306.

Fingerman, K. L., & Charles, S. T. (2010). It takes two to tango: Why older people have the best relationships. *Current Directions in Psychological Science, 19*(3), 172–176.

Finucane, M. L., Mertz, C. K., Slovic, P., & Schmidt, E. S. (2005). Task complexity and older adults' decision-making competence. *Psychology and Aging, 20*(1), 71–84.

Finucane, M. L., Slovic, P., Hibbard, J. H., Peters, E., Mertz, C. K., & MacGregor, D. G. (2002). Aging and decision-making competence: An analysis of comprehension and consistency skills in older versus younger adults considering health-plan options. *Journal of Behavioral Decision Making, 15*(2), 141–164.

Fredrickson, B. L., & Carstensen, L. L. (1990). Choosing social partners: How old age and anticipated endings make people more selective. *Psychology and Aging, 5*(3), 335–347.

Fung, H. H., & Carstensen, L. L. (2003). Sending memorable messages to the old: Age differences in preferences and memory for advertisements. *Journal of Personality and Social Psychology, 85*(1), 163–178.

Fung, H. H., & Carstensen, L. L. (2004). Motivational changes in response to blocked goals and foreshortened time: Testing alternatives to socioemotional selectivity theory. *Psychology and Aging, 19*(1), 68–78.

Fung, H. H., Carstensen, L. L., & Lutz, A. M. (1999). Influence of time on social preferences: Implications for life-span development. *Psychology and Aging, 14*(4), 595–604.

Fung, H. H., Isaacowitz, D. M., Lu, A. Y., & Li, T. (2010). Interdependent self-construal moderates age-related negativity reduction effect in memory and visual attention. *Psychology and Aging, 25*, 321–329.

Gerstorf, D., Ram, N., Mayraz, G., Hidajat, M., Lindenberger, U., Wagner, G. G., et al. (2010). Late-life decline in well-being across adulthood in Germany, the UK, and the US: Something is seriously wrong at the end of life. *Psychology and Aging, 25*(2), 477–485.

Gilovich, T., Griffin, D., & Kahneman, D. (Eds.). (2002). *Heuristics and biases: The psychology of intuitive judgment.* New York: Cambridge University Press.

Grady, C. L., Hongwanishkul, D., Keightley, M., Lee, W., & Hasher, L. (2007). The effect of age on memory for emotional faces. *Neuropsychology, 21*(3), 371–380.

Gross, J. J. (1998). Antecedent- and response-focused emotion regulation: Divergent consequences for experience, expression, and physiology. *Journal of Personality and Social Psychology, 74*(1), 224–237.

Gross, J. J., Carstensen, L. L., Pasupathi, M., Tsai, J., Skorpen, C. G., & Hsu, A. Y. C. (1997). Emotion and aging: Experience, expression, and control. *Psychology and Aging, 12*, 590–599.

Grühn, D., Scheibe, S., & Baltes, P. B. (2007). Reduced negativity effect in older adults' memory for emotional pictures: The heterogeneity list paradigm. *Psychology and Aging, 22*, 644–649.

Grühn, D., Smith, J., & Baltes, P. B. (2005). No aging bias favoring memory for positive material: Evidence from a heterogeneity-homogeneity list paradigm using emotionally toned words. *Psychology and Aging, 20*, 579–588.

Hashtroudi, S., Johnson, M. K., & Chrosniak, L. D. (1990). Aging and qualitative characteristics of memories for perceived and imagined complex events. *Psychology and Aging, 5*, 119–126.

Heckhausen, J., Wrosch, C., & Schulz, R. (2010). A motivational theory of life-span development. *Psychological Review, 117*(1), 32–60.

Hummert, M. L. (2011). Age stereotypes and aging. In K. W. Schaie & S. L. Willis (Eds.), *Handbook of the psychology of aging* (pp. 249–262). San Diego, CA: Academic Press.

Isaacowitz, D. M., & Choi, Y. (2011). Looking, feeling, and doing: Are there age differences in attention, mood, and behavioral responses to skin cancer information? *Health Psychology, 30*(10), 1–11.

Isaacowitz, D. M., Toner, K., Goren, D., & Wilson, H. (2008). Looking while unhappy: Mood congruent gaze in young adults, positive gaze in older adults. *Psychological Science, 19*, 848–853.

Isaacowitz, D. M., Toner, K., & Neupert, S. D. (2009). Use of gaze for real-time mood regulation: Effects of age and attentional functioning. *Psychology and Aging, 24*, 989–994.

Isaacowitz, D. M., Wadlinger, H. A., Goren, D., & Wilson, H. R. (2006a). Is there an age-related positivity effect in visual attention?: A comparison of two methodologies. *Emotion, 6*, 511–516.

Isaacowitz, D. M., Wadlinger, H. A., Goren, D., & Wilson, H. R. (2006b). Selective preference in visual fixation away from negative images in old age?: An eye tracking study. *Psychology and Aging, 21*(1), 40–48.

John, O. P., & Gross, J. J. (2004). Healthy and unhealthy emotion regulation: Personality processes, individual differences, and life span development. *Journal of Personality, 72*(6), 1301–1333.

Johnson, M. M. S. (1990). Age differences in decision making: A process methodology for examining strategic information processing. *Journal of Gerontology Psychological Sciences, 45*(2), 75–78.

Johnson, M. M. S. (1993). Thinking about strategies during, before, and after making a decision. *Psychology and Aging, 8,* 231–241.

Kahneman, D. (2003). A perspective on judgment and choice: Mapping bounded rationality. *American Psychologist, 58*(9), 697–720.

Kahneman, D., & Tversky, A. (2000). *Choices, values, and frames.* New York: Cambridge University Press.

Kennedy, Q., Mather, M., & Carstensen, L. L. (2004). The role of motivation in the age-related positivity effect in autobiographical memory. *Psychological Science, 15,* 208–214.

Kensinger, E. A. (2008). Age differences in memory for arousing and non-arousing emotional words. *Journals of Gerontology B: Psychological Sciences, 63,* 13–18.

Kessler, R. C., Berglund, P., Demler, O., Jin, R., Merikangas, K. R., & Walters, E. E. (2005). Lifetime prevalence and age-of-onset distributions of DSM-IV disorders in the National Comorbidity Survey Replication. *Archives of General Psychiatry, 62*(7), 768–768.

Kim, S., Healey, M. K., Goldstein, D., Hasher, L., & Wiprzycka, U. J. (2008). Age differences in choice satisfaction: A positivity effect in decision making. *Psychology and Aging, 23,* 33–38.

Kisley, M. A., Wood, S., & Burrows, C. L. (2007). Looking at the sunny side of life: Age-related change in an event-related potential measure of the negativity bias. *Psychological Science, 18*(9), 838–843.

Knight, M., Seymour, T. L., Gaunt, J. T., Baker, C., Nesmith, K., & Mather, M. (2007). Aging and goal-directed emotional attention: Distraction reverses emotional biases. *Emotion, 7,* 705–714.

Kunzmann, U., & Grühn, D. (2005). Age differences in emotional reactivity: The sample case of sadness. *Psychology and Aging, 20,* 47–59.

Kunzmann, U., Kupperbusch, C. S., & Levenson, R. W. (2005). Behavioral inhibition and amplification during emotional arousal: A comparison of two age groups. *Psychology and Aging, 20*(1), 144–158.

Kunzmann, U., & Richter, D. (2009). Emotional reactivity across the adult life span: The cognitive pragmatics make a difference. *Psychology and Aging, 24*(4), 879–889.

Kwon, Y., Scheibe, S., Samanez-Larkin, G. R., Tsai, J. L., & Carstensen, L. L. (2009). Replicating the positivity effect in picture memory in Koreans: Evidence for cross-cultural generalizability. *Psychology and Aging, 24,* 748–754.

Labouvie-Vief, G. (2003). Dynamic integration: Affect, cognition, and the self in adulthood. *Current Directions in Psychological Science, 12*(6), 201–206.

Labouvie-Vief, G., Grühn, D., & Studer, J. (2010). Dynamic integration of emotion and cognition: Equilibrium regulation in development and aging. In M. E. Lamb, A. M. Freund, & R. M. Lerner (Eds.), *The handbook of life-span development: Vol 2. Social and emotional development* (pp. 79–115). Hoboken, NJ: Wiley.

Lang, F. R. (2000). Endings and continuity of social relationships: Maximizing intrinsic benefits within personal networks when feeling near to death. *Journal of Social and Personal Relationships, 17*(2), 155–182.

Lang, F. R., & Carstensen, L. L. (2002). Time counts: Future time perspective, goals, and social relationships. *Psychology and Aging, 17*(1), 125–139.

Langeslag, S. J. E., & van Strien, J. W. (2009). Aging and emotional memory: The co-occurrence of neurophysiological and behavioral positivity effects. *Emotion, 9,* 369–377.

Lefkowitz, E. S., & Fingerman, K. L. (2003). Positive and negative emotional feelings and behaviors in mother–daughter ties in late life. *Journal of Family Psychology, 17*(4), 607–617.

Leigland, L. A., Schulz, L. E., & Janowsky, J. S. (2004). Age related changes in emotional memory. *Neurobiology of Aging, 25,* 1117–1124.

Levenson, R. W., Carstensen, L. L., & Gottman, J. M. (1994). Influence of age and gender on affect, physiology, and their interrelations: a study of long-term marriages. *Journal of Personality and Social Psychology, 67*(1), 56–68.

Levy, B. R., & Myers, L. M. (2005). Relationship between respiratory mortality and self-perceptions of aging. *Psychology and Health, 20*(5), 553–564.

Levy, B. R., Slade, M. D., Kunkel, S. R., & Kasl,

S. V. (2002). Longevity increased by positive self-perceptions of aging. *Journal of Personality and Social Psychology, 83,* 261–270.

Levy, B. R., Slade, M. D., May, J., & Caracciolo, E. A. (2006). Physical recovery after acute myocardial infarction: Positive age self-stereotypes as a resource. *International Journal of Aging and Human Development, 62*(4), 285–301.

Löckenhoff, C. E. (2011). Age, time, and decision making: From processing speed to global time horizons. *Annals of the New York Academy of Sciences, 1235,* 44–56.

Löckenhoff, C. E., & Carstensen, L. L. (2004). Socioemotional selectivity theory, aging, and health: The increasingly delicate balance between regulating emotions and making tough choices. *Journal of Personality, 72*(6), 1395–1424.

Löckenhoff, C. E., & Carstensen, L. (2007). Aging, emotion, and health-related decision strategies: Motivational manipulation can reduce age differences. *Psychology and Aging, 22*(1), 134–146.

Löckenhoff, C. E., & Carstensen, L. L., (2008). Decision strategies in health care choices for self and others: Older but not younger adults make adjustments for the age of the decision target. *Journals of Gerontology B: Psychological Sciences, 63*(2), 106–109.

Löckenhoff, C. E., De Fruyt, F., Terracciano, A., McCrae, R. R., De Bolle, M., Costa, P. T., et al. (2009). Perceptions of aging across 26 cultures and their culture-level associates. *Psychology and Aging, 24*(4), 941–954.

Löckenhoff, C. E., Reed, A. E., & Maresca, S. N. (2012). Who saves the best for last: Age differences in decisions about affective sequences. *Psychology and Aging, 27*(4), 840–848.

Luce, M. F., Payne, J. W., & Bettman, J. R. (2000). Coping with unfavorable attribute values in choice. *Organizational Behavior and Human Decision Processes, 81*(2), 274–299.

Magai, C., Consedine, N. S., Krivoshekova, Y. S., Kudadjie-Gyamfi, E., & McPherson, R. (2006). Emotion experience and expression across the adult life span: Insights from a multimodal assessment study. *Psychology and Aging, 21*(2), 303–317.

Maruta, T., Colligan, R. C., Malinchoc, M., & Offord, K. P. (2000). Optimists vs pessimists: Survival rate among medical patients over a 30-year period. *Mayo Clinic Proceedings, 75*(2), 140–143.

Mata, R., & Nunes, L. (2010). When less is enough: Cognitive aging, information search, and decision quality in consumer choice. *Psychology and Aging, 25*(2), 289–298.

Mather, M., Canli, T., English, T., Whitfield, S., Wais, P., Ochsner, K., et al. (2004). Amygdala responses to emotionally valenced stimuli in older and younger adults. *Psychological Science, 15*(4), 259–263.

Mather, M., & Carstensen, L. L. (2003). Aging and attentional biases for emotional faces. *Psychological Science, 14,* 409–415.

Mather, M., & Carstensen, L. L. (2005). Aging and motivated cognition: The positivity effect in attention and memory. *Trends in Cognitive Sciences, 9,* 496–502.

Mather, M., & Johnson, M. K. (2000). Choice-supportive source monitoring: Do our decisions seem better to us as we age? *Psychology and Aging, 15*(4), 596–606.

Mather, M., & Knight, M. (2005). Goal-directed memory: The role of cognitive control in older adults' emotional memory. *Psychology and Aging, 20*(4), 554–570.

Mather, M., Knight, M. R., & McCaffrey, M. (2005). The allure of the alignable: younger and older adults' false memories of choice features. *Journal of Experimental Psychology: General, 134*(1), 38–51.

Meyer, B. J. F., Russo, C., & Talbot, A. (1995). Discourse comprehension and problem solving: Decisions about the treatment of breast cancer by women across the life span. *Psychology and Aging, 10*(1), 84–103.

Mikels, J. A., Larkin, G. R., Reuter-Lorenz, P. A., & Carstensen, L. L. (2005). Divergent trajectories in the aging mind: Changes in working memory for affective versus visual information with age. *Psychology and Aging, 20,* 542–553.

Mikels, J. A., Löckenhoff, C. E., Maglio, S. J., Goldstein, M. K., Garber, A., & Carstensen, L. L. (2010). Following your heart or your head: Focusing on emotions versus information differentially influences the decisions of younger and older adults. *Journal of Experimental Psychology: Applied, 16*(1), 87–95.

Mikels, J. A., & Reed, A. E. (2009). Monetary losses do not loom large for older adults: Evidence for a more balanced framing effect in older adults. *Journals of Gerontology B: Psychological Sciences, 64,* 457–460.

Mroczek, D. K., & Kolarz, C. M. (1998). The effect of age on positive and negative affect: A developmental perspective on happiness. *Journal of Personality Social Psychology, 75*(5), 1333–1349.

Mroczek, D. K., & Spiro, A. (2005). Change in life satisfaction over 20 years during adulthood: findings from the VA Normative Aging Study. *Journal of Personality and Social Psychology, 88*(1), 189–202.

Nielsen, L., Knutson, B., & Carstensen, L. L. (2008). Affect dynamics, affective forecasting, and aging. *Emotion, 8*(3), 318–330.

Novotny, P., Colligan, R. C., Szydlo, D. W., Clark, M. M., Rausch, S., Wampfler, J., et al. (2010). A pessimistic explanatory style is prognostic for poor lung cancer survival. *Journal of Thoracic Oncology, 5*(3), 326–332.

Opitz, P. C., Gross, J. J., & Urry, H. L. (2012). Selection, optimization, and compensation in the domain of emotion regulation: Applications to adolescence, older age, and major depressive disorder. *Social and Personality Psychology Compass, 6*(2), 142–155.

Peters, E., Diefenbach, M. A., Hess, T. M., & Västfjäll, D. (2008). Age differences in dual information-processing modes: Implications for cancer decision making. *Cancer, 113*(12, Suppl.), 3556–3567.

Phillips, L. H., Henry, J. D., Hosie, J. A., & Milne, A. B. (2008). Effective regulation of the experience and expression of negative affect in old age. *Journals of Gerontology: Psychological Sciences B: Psychological Sciences, 63*(3), P138–P145.

Queen, T. L., & Hess, T. M. (2010). Age differences in the effects of conscious and unconscious thought in decision making. *Psychology and Aging, 25*(2), 251–261.

Ready, R. E., Weinberger, M. I., & Jones, K. M., (2007). How happy have you felt lately?: Two diary studies of emotion recall in older and younger adults. *Cognition and Emotion, 21*(4), 728–757.

Riediger, M., Schmiedek, F., Wagner, G., & Lindenberger, U. (2009). Seeking pleasure and seeking pain: Differences in prohedonic and contra-hedonic motivation from adolescence to old age. *Psychological Science, 20,* 1529–1535.

Roberts, B. W., Walton, K. E., & Viechtbauer, W. (2006). Patterns of mean-level change in personality traits across the life course: A meta-analysis of longitudinal studies. *Psychological Bulletin, 132*(1), 1–25.

Rovenpor, D., Skogsberg, N., & Isaacowitz, D. M. (2013). The choices we make: An examination of situation selection in younger and older adults. *Psychology and Aging, 28*(2), 365–376.

Rozin, P., & Royzman, E. B. (2001). Negativity bias, negativity dominance, and contagion. *Personality and Social Psychology Review, 5*(4), 296–320.

Samanez-Larkin, G. R., Gibbs, S. B., Khanna, K., Nielsen, L., Carstensen, L. L., & Knutson, B. (2007). Anticipation of monetary gain but not loss in healthy older adults. *Nature Neuroscience, 10*(6), 787–791.

Sanfey, A. G., & Hastie, R. (2000). Judgment and decision making across the adult life span: A tutorial review of psychological research. In D. C. Park & N. Schwarz (Eds.), *Cognitive aging: A primer* (pp. 253–273). New York: Psychology Press.

Scheibe, S., & Blanchard-Fields, F. (2009). Effects of regulating emotions on cognitive performance: What is costly for young adults is not so costly for older adults. *Psychology and Aging, 24*(1), 217–223.

Scheibe, S., & Carstensen, L. L. (2010). Emotional aging: Recent findings and future trends. *Journals of Gerontology B: Psychological Sciences, 65,* 135–144.

Scheibe, S., Mata, R., & Carstensen, L. L. (2010). Age differences in affective forecasting and experienced emotion surrounding the 2008 US presidential election. *Cognition and Emotion, 25*(6), 1029–1044.

Schlagman, S., Schulz, J., & Kvavilashvili, L. (2006). A content analysis of involuntary autobiographical memories: Examining the positivity effect in old age. *Memory, 14,* 161–175.

Shamaskin, A. M., Mikels, J. A., & Reed, A. E. (2010). Getting the message across: Age differences in the positive and negative framing of health care messages. *Psychology and Aging, 25*(3), 746–751.

Shiota, M. N., & Levenson, R. W. (2009). Effects of aging on experimentally instructed detached reappraisal, positive reappraisal, and emotional behavior suppression. *Psychology and Aging, 24,* 890–900.

Slovic, P., Peters, E., Finucane, M. L., & MacGregor, D. G., (2005). Affect, risk, and decision making. *Health Psychology, 24*(4), 35–40.

Spaniol, J., Voss, A., & Grady, C. L. (2008). Aging and emotional memory: Cognitive mechanisms underlying the positivity effect. *Psychology and Aging, 23*(4), 859–872.

Stephens, C., Alpass, F., Towers, A., & Stevenson, B. (2011). The effects of types of social networks, perceived social support, and loneliness on the health of older people: Accounting for the social context. *Journal of Aging and Health, 23*(6), 887–911.

Story, T. N., Berg, C. A., Smith, T. W., Beveridge, R., Henry, N. M., & Pearce, G. (2007). Age, marital satisfaction, and optimism as predictors of positive sentiment override in middle-aged and older married couples. *Psychology and Aging, 22*(4), 719–727.

Sullivan, S. J., Mikels, J. A., & Carstensen, L. L. (2010). You never lose the ages you've been: Affective perspective taking in older adults. *Psychology and Aging, 25*(1), 229–234.

Tamir, M., Chiu, C. Y., & Gross, J. J. (2007). Business or pleasure?: Utilitarian versus hedonic considerations in emotion regulation. *Emotion, 7*(3), 546–554.

Terracciano, A., Löckenhoff, C. E., Zonderman, A. B., Ferrucci, L., & Costa, P. T. (2008). Personality predictors of longevity: Activity, emotional stability, and conscientiousness. *Psychosomatic Medicine, 70*(6), 621–627.

Terracciano, A., McCrae, R. R., Brant, L. J., & Costa, P. T. (2005). Hierarchical linear modeling analyses of the NEO-PI-R scales in the Baltimore Longitudinal Study of Aging. *Psychology and Aging, 20*(3), 493–506.

Urry, H. L., & Gross, J. J. (2010). Emotion regulation in older age. *Current Directions in Psychological Science, 19*(6), 352–357.

PART IV

Select Positive Emotions

CHAPTER 16

■ ■ ■ ■ ■ ■ ■ ■

Finding Happiness

Tailoring Positive Activities for Optimal Well-Being Benefits

S. Katherine Nelson
Sonja Lyubomirsky

We all live with the objective of being happy;
our lives are all different and yet the same.
—ANNE FRANK

No matter how different people's lives—whether due to age, gender, culture, or life experience—the desire for happiness is widespread. Across cultures, the majority of people include happiness as one of their primary goals in life (Diener, 2000), and many seek ways to render themselves happier (Bergsma, 2008). Not surprisingly, the secrets of how to become happier and live a more fulfilling life have been topics of philosophical and lay interest for many years (Kesebir & Diener, 2008). However, the route to happiness may be different for each individual. With recent developments in the field of positive psychology, the question of how to become happier has become a topic of growing scientific interest (Lyubomirsky & Layous, 2013; Lyubomirsky, Sheldon, & Schkade, 2005; Seligman, Steen, Park, & Peterson, 2005), but few have examined how individuals may differ in their pursuit of happiness. That being so, Anne Frank's recognition of the commonalities and differences in people's lives, as well as in the pur-

suit of happiness itself, points to important new directions for research.

What Is Happiness?

Researchers have been theorizing about happiness for more than three decades (Diener, 1984; Diener, Suh, Lucas, & Smith, 1999; Ryan & Deci, 2001; Ryff, 1989). Traditionally, theorists have distinguished between hedonic and eudaimonic well-being, suggesting that the former is associated with the pursuit of pleasure and the latter with following meaningful goals and finding purpose in life (Ryan & Deci, 2001). Recent work, however, suggests that this distinction represents not two different types of happiness but two different ways of pursuing it (Kashdan, Biswas-Diener, & King, 2008). Other researchers have also recognized the need to examine several dimensions of well-being (Kashdan & Steger, 2011), and to consider multiple ways to conceptualize its structure (Busseri & Sadava, 2011). Thus, a comprehensive definition of well-being includes not only subjective well-being but also meaning and purpose in life.

Subjective well-being is most frequently described as comprising an affective component (i.e., the experience of relatively frequent positive and relatively infrequent negative emotions) and a cognitive component (i.e., life satisfaction or the overall evaluation of a person's life) (Diener, 1984; Diener et al., 1999). Thus, a "happy" person is one who reports frequent positive emotions, infrequent negative emotions, and high life satisfaction. In this chapter, we use the terms *happiness* and *subjective well-being* interchangeably.

Other theories emphasize the importance of meaning and purpose in understanding well-being (Ryff, 1989; Steger, 2009). Individuals who report having meaning in life are those who see significance in their lives and have the capacity to view their own life purpose or mission (Steger, 2009). Although meaning in life is strongly correlated with overall well-being (Steger, Kashdan, Sullivan, & Lorentz, 2008), research suggests that the two constructs are not selfsame (Steger & Kashdan, 2007). Thus, including assessments of meaning in addition to assessments of subjective happiness may substantively add to scientists' understanding of well-being.

In this chapter, our focus is on experimental intervention studies, in which participants are prompted to engage in a positive activity over time; almost all such studies use either measures of overall happiness or its two components (i.e., mood/emotions and life satisfaction) as outcome variables. However, because of the importance of meaning in life as a related construct, we also sometimes refer to *meaning in life*, depending on the research being described.

Is It Possible and Desirable to Become Happier?

Research indicates that people's happiness levels are stable across time—and therefore not amenable to improvement—due to genetic factors (Lykken & Tellegen, 1996; Nes, Roysamb, Tambs, Harris, & Reichborn-Kjennerud, 2006), personality influences (Diener & Lucas, 1999; McCrae

& Costa, 1990), and inevitable hedonic adaptation to positive and negative life experiences (Frederick & Loewenstein, 1999; Lyubomirsky, 2011). Despite these reasons for pessimism, other work provides evidence that happiness can indeed sustainably change for the better. For example, happiness is not always stable across a person's lifetime (Fujita & Diener, 2005), and personality can change over time, even after age 30 (Helson, Jones, & Kwan, 2002; Roberts, Walton, & Viechtbauer, 2006). In addition, studies have shown that well-being can be improved via lifestyle changes (e.g., exercise, nutrition; Walsh, 2011), and by engaging in positive activities, such as performing acts of kindness, becoming more grateful, or practicing optimism (see Sin & Lyubomirsky, 2009, for a meta-analytic review).

In their sustainable happiness model, Lyubomirsky, Sheldon, and Schkade (2005) integrated past research findings to argue that although more than half of population differences in happiness are due to genetics, personality, and life circumstances, a large portion are likely accounted for by people's intentional activities; that is, how people think (e.g., whether they think positively or gratefully) and what they do (e.g., whether they perform acts of kindness or forgiveness) in their daily lives can play a large role in how happy they are. In summary, the sustainable happiness model suggests that people have a fair amount of control over their happiness.

Supporting the sustainable happiness model, one study followed students over the course of 12 weeks and asked them to track positive changes in their lives—both those that entailed beginning new activities (e.g., pursuing an important new goal) and those that entailed improvements in their life circumstances (e.g., obtaining a new roommate). The results revealed that activity changes are associated with bigger and longer-lasting increases in happiness than circumstantial changes (Sheldon & Lyubomirsky, 2006a). Also providing evidence for the sustainable happiness model are numerous studies in which participants are instructed to engage in a positive activity, such as performing acts of kindness or writing gratitude letters. A recent meta-analysis of the benefits of positive interventions revealed that such activities typically show a moderate effect size (mean $r = .30$; Sin & Lyubomirsky, 2009), suggesting that performing them leads to robust improvements in well-being.

Just because people can improve their happiness, however, does not mean that they should. Is the pursuit of happiness a desirable and advisable goal? In a meta-analysis of 225 studies, happiness was found to precede, correlate with, and cause many beneficial outcomes, including more prosocial behavior, more satisfying relationships with others, better health, and superior job performance (Lyubomirsky, King, & Diener, 2005). Thus, a large and persuasive body of work suggests that being happy not only makes the individual feel good but it also benefits him or her, his or her family, and the community in myriad ways. Other research, however, has revealed that happiness may have a "dark side" (Gruber, Mauss, & Tamir, 2011). For example, in one study, valuing happiness was associated with disappointment and decreased, rather than increased, well-being (Mauss, Tamir, Anderson, & Savino 2011). These findings suggest that when designing experiments to test which activities or practices promote well-being, researchers should strive to direct their participants' efforts and attention on the particular activities (e.g., practicing acts of kindness) and not on the value of becoming happier.

Happiness-Increasing Positive Activity Interventions

The question of how people can improve their personal well-being is the focus of both great public and scientific interest. *Amazon.com* boasts more than 6,000 titles under the categories of happiness and self-help, with titles such as *Every Day a Friday: How to Be Happier 7 Days a Week* and *The 18 Rules of Happiness: How to Be Happy.* Unfortunately, many trade books that boast secrets to happiness are not grounded in scientific evidence or theory, and do not draw on the growing research on strategies that people can use to enhance their well-being (Sin & Lyubomirsky, 2009). For example, positive activities such as counting blessings (Emmons & McCullough, 2003; Lyubomirsky, Sheldon, & Schkade, 2005; Shel-

don & Lyubomirsky, 2006b), visualizing a bright future (Boehm, Lyubomirsky, & Sheldon, 2011; King, 2001; Layous, Nelson, & Lyubomirsky, 2013; Lyubomirsky, Dickerhoof, Boehm, & Sheldon, 2011; Sheldon & Lyubomirsky, 2006b), performing acts of kindness (Lyubomirsky, Sheldon, & Schkade, 2005; Sheldon, Boehm, & Lyubomirsky, 2012), and writing letters of gratitude (Boehm et al., 2011; Lyubomirsky et al., 2011; Seligman et al., 2005) have been found to improve well-being in multiple randomized controlled intervention studies.

How and Why Do Positive Activity Interventions Work?

An important goal of research on positive activity interventions is not only to establish that particular activities are successful in increasing well-being but also to uncover how and why these activities work, as well as the optimal conditions for their success. In other words, what activities work best, under what conditions, and for whom? Accordingly, we describe below a number of important factors that mediate and moderate the effectiveness of positive activities to enhance well-being.

Mediators of Intervention Effectiveness

Understanding the underlying mechanisms that lead positive activities to improve well-being successfully—that is, the "why" question—is an important goal of positive activity research. If researchers can identify precisely why happiness activities are effective, they will gain a better scientific understanding of the determinants of happiness, as well as the tools to design more successful activities to improve well-being. To date, studies have provided preliminary support for three mediators underlying the effectiveness of happiness-enhancing activities— increased positive emotions, more positive reactions from others, and increased need satisfaction.

Positive Emotions. Positive emotions are an important component of happiness; people who experience more frequent positive emotions report higher subjective well-being (Fredrickson & Joiner, 2002). Furthermore, theory suggests that the more positive emotions an individual experiences after a positive life change, the more likely his or her well-being boost will last (Lyubomirsky, 2011). Hence, not surprisingly, positive emotions are likely to play an important role in positive activities.

Two studies found support for positive emotions as a mechanism by which positive activities promote well-being. In one study, participants who practiced gratitude or optimism became happier over time, and this effect was mediated by their ability to derive positive emotions from their daily experiences and to find those experiences satisfying (Lyubomirsky & Dickerhoof, 2010). In another study, participants who received social support for performing acts of kindness became happier over a 9-week period, and this effect was mediated by their enjoyment of the activity (Sin, Della Porta, & Lyubomirsky, 2011). These findings suggest that the more that practicing happiness strategies (e.g., expressing gratitude to family members) leads people to derive joy and satisfaction from their daily experiences (e.g., enjoying spending time with family), the more likely those strategies are to foster happiness. Thus, the ability of positive activities to increase and sustain positive emotions successfully is an important factor in determining and sustaining later well-being.

Positive Reactions from Others. The degree to which an individual receives positive reactions from others after performing positive activities is another important mediator of intervention effectiveness. In one study, performing acts of kindness increased participants' happiness via their perception that others were grateful for their kindnesses (Tkach, 2006). Future studies should further examine positive feedback from others as a potential mediator for other positive activities. For example, experiencing positive reactions from the recipients of a gratitude letter may mediate the link between that activity and enhanced well-being.

Need Satisfaction. Self-determination theory suggests that the fulfillment of innate psychological needs is necessary to achieve optimal well-being (Deci & Ryan, 2000). The three basic needs are *autonomy* (i.e., feeling that one's actions are under one's control), *relatedness* (i.e., feeling close and

connected to others), and *competence* (i.e., feeling effective and skilled). Feelings of need satisfaction have been related to well-being and performance across many contexts (Deci & Ryan, 2008; Ryan & Deci, 2008; Sheldon, 2004), as well as to more positive affect and less negative affect (Sheldon, Elliott, Kim, & Kasser, 2001).

A few studies have shown that increases in need satisfaction lead to subsequent increases in subjective well-being (Niemiec, Ryan, & Deci, 2009; Sheldon & Elliot, 1999). These findings suggest that positive activities may improve people's well-being by increasing their feelings of need satisfaction. Indeed, one experiment found that the effect of expressing gratitude or optimism on improvements in well-being was mediated by feelings of autonomy and relatedness, but not competence (Boehm & Lyubomirsky, 2011). Another study found that doing acts of kindness fostered feelings of autonomy (Sin et al., 2011), and these bolstered feelings mediated increases in happiness.

Moderators of Intervention Effectiveness

Timing. In multiple studies, the timing with which positive activities are practiced has been found to be an important moderator of the activities' effectiveness. In a gratitude intervention (Lyubomirsky, Sheldon, & Schkade, 2005), participants were instructed to count their blessings either three times or one time each week. Interestingly, only participants who counted their blessings once a week showed significantly larger gains in well-being than the control group. Participants who counted their blessings only once per week may have found the activity more meaningful and rewarding, whereas participants who counted their blessings multiple times per week may have grown bored with the activity or had trouble generating new aspects of their lives for which to be grateful.

In another test of the importance of timing, students were instructed to perform five acts of kindness, all in one day (e.g., all on Monday) or on any day of the week (Lyubomirsky, Sheldon, & Schkade, 2005). Participants who performed all five acts of kindness in one day became happier over the course of the intervention, but participants who spread their kindnesses out across the week did not show any changes. Those who carried out all five kindnesses in a single day may have obtained a relatively larger and more salient burst of positive emotions from those activities, and this burst may have set into motion an upward spiral, such that feeling joyful or fulfilled on Monday may have enhanced their work productivity or a close relationship on the same day, which may have generated yet more positive emotions on Tuesday, and so on (cf. Fredrickson & Joiner, 2002).

As evidenced by these two studies, timing positive activities in ways that generate the greatest boost in positive emotion and minimize boredom is critical when striving to optimize well-being. Future studies would do well to test how varied timing and frequency of practice may influence the effectiveness of other positive activities. For example, does practicing optimistic thinking deliver the biggest rewards when done once a day, once a week, or only when one is feeling low? Similarly, due to the stress surrounding life transitions (e.g., moving away from home or having a baby), investigators may seek to establish the costs and benefits of timing the practice of optimism activities around these transitions.

Variety. Just as spicing up a physical exercise routine yields better fitness results, instilling variety into the practice of positive activities leads to superior results with respect to happiness. In two studies, Sheldon and colleagues (2012) demonstrated the influence of variety on activity effectiveness. In the first study, participants who reported greater variety in a recent circumstantial or activity life change showed the biggest gains in positive emotions. In a second study, a 10-week acts of kindness intervention, those who varied their acts of kindness showed increases in well-being over the course of the intervention, whereas those instructed to do the same acts each week actually became less happy (Sheldon et al., 2012). These findings illustrate that individuals can inject variety into their efforts in pursuing happiness by changing up a particular positive strategy. Another way to introduce variety into one's positive practices is to engage in different types of happiness-increasing activities— serially or simultaneously. Indeed, research with large, diverse samples shows that peo-

ple typically practice up to eight activities at a given time to improve well-being (Parks, Della Porta, Pierce, Zilca, & Lyubomirsky, 2012).

Motivation and Effort. Undoubtedly, individuals who are motivated to become happier and who muster effort toward that goal benefit more from happiness activities. For example, in one study, participants self-selected into either a "happiness activity" study (and, presumably, were motivated to become happier) or into a "cognitive exercises" study (and, presumably, were relatively not motivated to seek happiness) (Lyubomirsky et al., 2011). Participants who were motivated to become happier showed greater increases in well-being when performing positive activities (which involved expressing gratitude or optimism) relative to control activities. In addition, participants who put more effort into the positive activities (as judged by independent raters) showed greater increases in well-being.

Consistent with research on the role of effort, studies have also demonstrated that individuals who persevere in practicing positive activities are also more likely to demonstrate well-being benefits (Cohn & Fredrickson, 2010; Sheldon & Lyubomirsky, 2006b). In one study, participants who continued to practice a happiness activity (which involved meditation) after the study was complete— thus exhibiting more effort—showed sustained increases in well-being for up to 18 months (Cohn & Fredrickson, 2010).

Person–Activity Fit. Not all happiness-increasing activities benefit every person to the same degree. One factor that may influence the extent to which an individual becomes happier as a result of a particular activity involves the degree to which that activity matches his or her personality, goals, interests, and values. For example, introverts may benefit relatively more from a reflective activity (e.g., counting blessings), whereas extraverts may benefit relatively more from a social activity (e.g., performing acts of kindness). We have come to define this idea as "person–activity fit" (Lyubomirsky, 2008; Lyubomirsky, Sheldon, & Schkade, 2005). Greater fit has been found to be associated with greater benefit from the activity (Sin et al., 2011). For example, in one study, students who reported higher social responsibility derived relatively greater well-being gains from performing acts of kindness (Nelson, Layous, Oberle, Schonert-Reichl, & Lyubomirsky, 2012).

In another test of person–activity fit, participants were asked to complete a positive activity based on their previous activity preferences. Compared to individuals randomly assigned to positive activities, those who were matched to an activity based on their preferences reported greater increases in subjective well-being (Schueller, 2011). Similarly, another study found that participants whose assigned happiness-increasing strategy fit their personality (i.e., they enjoyed it, and it felt natural to them) reported greater increases in well-being than did those who practiced an ill-fitting happiness activity or a control activity (Dickerhoof, 2007). These findings support the hypothesis that person–activity fit is a key moderator of activity effectiveness.

Summary

In summary, a significant amount of work on the underlying mediators and moderators of activity effectiveness has uncovered many "secrets" to becoming happier. Findings from these studies reveal that the most successful practitioners of happiness-increasing activities are those who are motivated to become happier and put effort into that goal. Furthermore, successful activities are those that increase positive emotions and fulfill psychological needs, are practiced with optimal timing to minimize boredom, and, finally, infuse variety into one's life and daily pursuits.

Tailoring Positive Activities for Specific Populations: Population–Activity Fit

Although a considerable amount of research has examined the underlying mediators and moderators of the effectiveness of happiness activities, surprisingly little has tried to understand whether certain activities may be more or less beneficial for different groups of people. One recent review emphasized the importance of context (e.g., whether an individual is in a happy or troubled relationship) in determining whether

strategies such as forgiveness, kindness, optimism, and positive attributions will be beneficial to his or her well-being (McNulty & Fincham, 2012). Given that not everyone responds equally well to particular positive activities, an important new research direction to uncover the role of context in happiness interventions involves understanding how special groups or populations of individuals respond to positive activities.

Although a "population–activity fit" approach has yet to be applied to understanding the success of positive activities, this approach has been prominent in psychotherapy research for decades (Kazdin & Blase, 2011). In 1967, a clinical researcher posed the following key question: "*What* treatment, by *whom* is most effective for *this* individual with *that* specific problem and under *which* set of circumstances?" (Paul, 1967, p. 111). More recently, researchers have noted the value of understanding "moderator profiles"—that is, identifying which individuals are at risk for mental health conditions and who responds best to certain kinds of treatment—as a way to prevent mental illness (Atkins & Frazier, 2011; Shoham & Insel, 2011). Mirroring this approach, understanding which individuals respond better to positive activities is critical because it will help researchers to tailor particular strategies to particular groups of individuals, and allow the general public to better select and implement the most optimal strategies for themselves.

Using a population–activity fit approach to identify group-level moderators of activity effectiveness, we describe below several groups likely to benefit from further research and analysis. With respect to these groups, future investigators could ask three questions:

1. How do these groups respond to positive activities in general?
2. Do these groups benefit from particular activities more than others?
3. Can specific activities be tailored to better fit particular groups?

For example, in the case of people suffering from depression, research could first examine whether positive activities in general can effectively improve well-being in this population, then determine whether certain activities (e.g., practicing gratitude) are a better fit than other activities. Finally, researchers could test the best ways to implement the successful activities with depressed individuals (e.g., practicing gratitude by counting blessings vs. writing letters).

Children and Adolescents

Although subjective well-being among children and adolescents relates to important academic (Suldo, Thalji, & Ferron, 2011), emotional (Schmid et al., 2011), and social (Richards & Huppert, 2011) outcomes, surprisingly little work has been conducted on positive psychological constructs in this population. A recent content analysis of the literature in school psychology revealed a striking imbalance: Of the 1,168 articles reviewed, happiness was the topic of four articles, optimism was the topic of three, and purpose/meaning in life was the topic of none (Froh, Huebner, Youssef, & Conte, 2011).

Despite the limited work in this area, some studies do suggest that children and adolescents may obtain well-being benefits from positive activities (Froh, Kashdan, Ozinkowski, & Miller, 2009; Froh, Sefick, & Emmons, 2008; Gilham, Reivich, Jaycox, & Seligman, 1995; Layous, Nelson, Oberle, Schonert-Reichl, & Lyubomirsky, 2012). For example, several experiments have demonstrated that children and youth may benefit from expressing gratitude. In one study, children ages 11–14 were instructed either to count their blessings daily for 2 weeks or to complete a control activity. Those children who counted their blessings reported more gratitude, optimism, and life satisfaction, and less negative affect, relative to a hassles control group (Froh et al., 2008). Similarly, another study found that children and adolescents ages 8–19 who were low in positive affect and wrote letters of gratitude to people in their lives showed relatively greater gratitude and positive affect immediately following the activity, as well as 2 months later (Froh et al., 2009).

Children and adolescents have also been found to benefit from a variety of other positive activities designed to raise well-being. In one study, fourth- and fifth-grade students were instructed either to perform three acts of kindness or to visit three places during the week (Layous et al., 2012). Children who performed acts of kindness became happier and more popular over the course of the study, as compared to children who visited three places. In a study of 16- to 17-year-old adolescents, those who engaged in simple, self-directed positive activities (i.e., visits, acts of kindness, and gratitude letters) for 3 weeks improved in well-being and maintained this improvement after a 3-week follow-up (Haworth et al., 2013). Finally, another study found that adolescents who were encouraged to use their character strengths in their daily lives, to learn new strengths, and to recognize strengths in others demonstrated greater improvements in life satisfaction relative to those who were not encouraged (Proctor et al., 2011).

Although the literature is limited, these studies suggest that positive activities are beneficial for children and adolescents. However, much more work is needed. For example, research that suggests optimism significantly contributes to adolescents' well-being (Oberle, Schonert-Reichl, & Zumbo, 2011), as well as the fact that children are often asked about future events and activities (e.g., "What do you want to be when you grow up?"), supports the idea that positive activities designed to promote optimism may be especially fitting for this age group. Future investigators should continue striving to understand the underlying mechanisms involved in the effectiveness of positive activities in children and adolescents, as well as whether some activities are more effective than others. For example, because of its social nature, the visit activity (Layous et al., 2012) may be an appropriate fit for children at a time in their lives when they are forming friendships, learning social skills, and developing their identities. Given the numerous benefits of well-being specific to these age groups (e.g., academic achievement) (Richards & Huppert, 2011; Schmid et al., 2011; Suldo et al., 2011), understanding ways to improve the happiness of children and adolescents is an important avenue for future research.

Older Adults

Just as pursuing well-being is important for young children and adolescents, it is important for older adults. Although older adults have been found on average to be happier than their younger peers (e.g., Carstensen et al., 2011; Mroczek & Spiro, 2005; Williams et al., 2006), studies have indicated several critical areas of need in this population. In one investigation of older adult women, for example, older age was associated with lower levels of purpose in life, personal growth, and positive relationships, and poor health in this age group was associated with more depression and anxiety (Heidrich, 1993). A longitudinal study of adults over age 60 found increases in depressive symptoms over a 6-year period (Dunne, Wrosch, & Miller, 2011). The prevalence of illness, health problems, and loss of loved ones among older adults, and the numerous benefits of well-being for health and social relationships (Lyubomirsky, King, & Diener, 2005) highlight the need for designing well-being activities for this age group.

Furthermore, research suggests that successful methods of pursuing happiness in older adults may differ from those of other age groups. For example, one study queried a variety of age groups about aspects of life essential for well-being (Ryff, 1989). Although all age groups endorsed good relationships and the pursuit of enjoyable activities as important for well-being, younger adults focused more on self-knowledge, competence, and self-acceptance, whereas older adults focused more on positive coping with change (see also Carstensen, Isaacowitz, & Charles, 1999). Similarly, older adults have been found to experience less personal growth and autonomy, but more mastery, than other age groups (Ryff, 1991). Finally, Oswald and colleagues (2007) found that older adults' (ages 75–89) perceptions of their living situations is an important factor predicting their well-being. Participants who lived in more accessible homes, who viewed their home as purposeful and meaningful, and had a greater sense of internal control reported relatively greater well-being. These findings suggest that positive activities may function differently in this age group. For example, activities that target coping may be better suited for older adults, and activities that promote self-knowledge or acceptance (e.g., affirming personal values and characteristics) may be better suited for younger adults. Other successful, positive activities for older adults could promote meaningful and purposeful use of their homes—for example, by designating a space for a personal hobby or interest (e.g., crafts) and encouraging meaningful engagement with that hobby. Finally, older adults may be able to enjoy meaning and personal growth by redirecting attention to and helping a younger generation. For example, rather than focusing on personal achievements and success at the end of their careers, they may find growth and purpose by mentoring younger colleagues.

Although very few positive activity interventions have been conducted with older adults, the limited work in this area suggests that positive activities can successfully improve their well-being. In a classic study in a nursing home, older adults who were given a plant to care for and reminded of their personal choice and responsibility in their everyday lives demonstrated greater gains in well-being relative to control participants whose plants were cared for by staff members (Langer & Rodin, 1976). Furthermore, in a 14-week intervention, women ages 56–80, who reviewed areas of their lives (e.g., love, goals, turning points) with respect to their past, present, and future, showed significant increases in psychological well-being relative to controls (Arkoff, Meredith, & Dubanoski, 2004). Future studies should continue to establish the effectiveness of positive activities that primarily have been tested on young and middle-aged adults, to increase the well-being of older adults. In addition, particular attention should be directed to determining the most effective activities for this population. For example, as individuals approach the end of their lives, expressing gratitude for loved ones may be a better-fitting activity than envisioning a bright future.

Individuals with Depression and Anxiety

Individuals suffering from depression or anxiety may derive considerable benefit from the practice of well-being-enhancing activities. Indeed, recent literature has highlighted the importance of positive activities as a possible way to alleviate depression and encourage depressed individuals to live more fulfilling lives, beyond the point of languishing (Layous, Chancellor, Lyubomirsky, Wang, & Doraiswamy, 2011; Sin, Della Porta, & Lyubomirsky, 2011).

Two areas of research provide support for the effectiveness of positive activities for individuals suffering from depression. First, studies have suggested that positive activities not only improve well-being, but they are also capable of ameliorating depressive symptoms. For example, a recent meta-analysis found that positive psychology exercises can successfully reduce depressive symptoms in individuals with a range of symptom levels ($r = .31$; Sin & Lyubomirsky, 2009).

Second, positive activity intervention studies have successfully improved well-being in individuals suffering from mild depression (Seligman et al., 2005; Seligman, Rashid, & Parks, 2006). In one study, relative to controls, moderately depressed participants instructed to write and deliver a gratitude letter demonstrated gains in happiness and decreased depressive symptoms immediately afterward, and maintained these improvements at 1-month follow-up. In the same study, participants who kept track of three good things or used their signature strengths in new ways maintained improvements in happiness and reduced depressive symptoms, relative to those in the control group, for up to 6 months (Seligman et al., 2005). In a second intervention, patients suffering from mild-to-moderate depression performed different positive psychology exercises (i.e., using signature strengths, counting blessings, writing a gratitude letter, practicing active/constructive responding, and savoring) each week for 6 weeks. Patients reported decreased depressive symptoms for up to 1 year, relative to controls (Seligman et al., 2006).

Preliminary evidence suggests that individuals suffering from depression may respond differently to various positive activities. In one study, dysphoric individuals were instructed to write letters of gratitude to people whom they had never properly thanked. Surprisingly, the gratitude activity decreased well-being in this group (Sin, Della Porta, & Lyubomirsky, 2011), possibly because participants felt bad about not having expressed gratitude earlier to these individuals, or because the letters were challenging to compose. Another study tested the effects of expressing gratitude on individuals with depressive personality styles (i.e., high self-criticism and neediness). In

this intervention, self-critics responded well to the gratitude exercise, but needy individuals reported decreased subsequent well-being (Sergeant & Mongrain, 2011), possibly because the exercises reminded needy individuals of their need for approval from others. These findings highlight the importance of testing different types of activities among different groups to determine which activities work best and which ones may actually be detrimental to well-being (cf. McNulty & Fincham, 2012). Whereas gratitude activities typically improve well-being in the general population (Emmons & McCullough, 2003), it may not be advisable to recommend a gratitude activity to someone suffering from depression or dysphoria. On the other hand, researchers may be able to tailor certain types of gratitude activities for a depressed population. For example, depressed individuals may benefit from the relatively undemanding gratitude task of counting their blessings, compared to writing a gratitude letter, which requires much more effort and deliberation, as well as a frank appraisal of their close relationships.

Another study examined the effect of the practice of optimism and self-compassion among individuals vulnerable to depression (i.e., those high in self-criticism and low in connectedness). Overall, both the optimism and self-compassion manipulations led to relatively greater increases in happiness and decreases in depressive symptoms. Interestingly, however, the results revealed that individuals with low connectedness benefited more from practicing self-compassion than optimism, perhaps because this activity fulfilled their need to generate compassionate feelings toward themselves. Conversely, those high in self-criticism benefited more from practicing optimism than self-compassion, possibly due to the ability of the optimism exercise to curtail cycles of rumination (Shapira & Mongrain, 2010). These findings further demonstrate that depressed individuals respond differently to different types of positive activities, suggesting the need for tailored interventions based on individual circumstances, symptoms, and areas of weakness.

Research suggests that positive activities may also be beneficial to individuals suffering from anxiety. In one study, patients with affective disorders (i.e., major depression, panic disorder, social phobia, generalized anxiety disorder, and obsessive–compulsive disorder) were assigned to complete well-being therapy, in which they kept a diary of the positive events in their daily lives, or cognitive-behavioral therapy (CBT). Participants in both conditions demonstrated improvements, but those who completed well-being therapy showed greater decreases in anxiety and increases in contentment (Fava, Rafanelli, Cazzaro, Conti, & Grandi, 1998). Similarly, another study, which compared CBT to a combination of CBT and well-being therapy among patients with generalized anxiety disorder, found that the combination of CBT and well-being therapy led to significantly greater improvements in psychological well-being and reductions in anxiety than did CBT alone (Fava et al., 2005).

Given the growing rates of depression and anxiety in the United States (Kessler, Chiu, Demler, & Walters, 2005), as well as the high cost of treatment (Watkins et al., 2009; Witten, 2002), positive activities may be an easy, accessible, nonstigmatizing, and low-cost method to alleviate depression and anxiety. The research in this area is promising and suggests that positive activities can decrease depressive and anxiety symptoms, and improve well-being. However, much more work is needed to understand fully how anxious, depressed, or dysphoric individuals respond to various positive activities—especially as some appear to be detrimental to their well-being.

Individuals with Physical Illness

Individuals with physical health problems or who have received a recent diagnosis may also have much to gain from happiness-enhancing activities. Recent research has linked cancer diagnosis to detriments in mental health, mood, and psychological well-being (Costanzo, Ryff, & Singer, 2009), suggesting a clear need for well-being interventions for patients with impending or recent serious diagnoses. Indeed, improving patients' happiness has implications for not only their psychological well-being but also their health prognosis (Lyubomirsky, King, & Diener, 2005). A meta-analysis revealed that well-being positively impacts short-term health outcomes ($r = .15$), long-term health

outcomes ($r = .11$), and disease or symptom control ($r = .13$) (Howell, Kern, & Lyubomirsky, 2007). Thus, although most of the data are correlational, improving the well-being of individuals with health problems may not only make them feel better in general and help them cope better with their illness but may also have salutary effects on the very physical health issues they are facing.

Cross-sectional studies of patients highlight the importance of interventions in this area. One such study found that greater uncertainty, thought intrusions, and avoidance, as well as less talk about cancer, were associated with greater depression and lower well-being among cancer survivors (Cordova, Cunningham, Carlson, & Andrykowski, 2001). Accordingly, researchers designing strategies to improve this population's well-being may consider activities that involve patients talking about the cancer diagnosis or engaging with their cancer treatment to decrease avoidance.

Studies by health psychologists also provide evidence that positive activities may be beneficial for individuals suffering from brain injury (Bédard et al., 2003), breast cancer (Antoni et al., 2001), chronic fatigue (Surway, Roberts, & Silver, 2005), and rheumatoid arthritis (Zautra et al., 2008). For example, in one study, patients receiving treatment for breast cancer participated in a 10-week stress management program (Antoni et al., 2001). This program reduced the prevalence of depression, and increased benefit finding and optimism regarding the diagnosis. In particular, the intervention was most successful for women low in optimism at baseline. In another study, patients who had suffered a traumatic brain injury participated in a 12-week mindfulness-based stress reduction program at least 1 year following the injury. Participants in the treatment group demonstrated improvements in quality of life and decreases in depressive symptoms relative to control participants (Bédard et al., 2003).

The majority of interventions in this area have focused on cultivating mindfulness (Bédard et al., 2003; Surway et al., 2005; Zautra et al., 2008). However, some evidence suggests that other positive psychology-based interventions (Huffman et al., 2011) and meaning interventions (Lee, Cohen, Edgar, Laizner, & Gagnon, 2006) may be successful among this population. Given the many changes that typically occur in an individual's life following a grave diagnosis, engaging in activities that foster meaning in life may be particularly helpful to patients coping with these changes. Indeed, one study found that a meaning-making intervention successfully improved cancer patients' self-esteem, optimism, and self-efficacy following a diagnosis (Lee et al., 2006).

Although a growing number of studies suggest that positive activities can improve the well-being of patients with a variety of medical problems, much more research is needed in this area. Future investigators should continue to examine the relative effect of a variety of positive activities on patients' well-being. Finally, given the diversity of health conditions and treatment options, researchers would do well to test potential moderators of intervention effectiveness among different patient groups, including illness type. For example, cancer patients may respond well to activities designed to enhance meaning in life, whereas cardiovascular disease patients may respond better to activities designed to reduce stress.

Victims of Trauma and Abuse

Ameliorating adverse outcomes following trauma and abuse is an important focus of both psychological research and clinical practice. Many people are resilient in the face of trauma (Bonanno, Galea, Bucciarelli, & Vlahov, 2006), and positive activities may be one way to bolster resilience. Support for the effectiveness of engaging in positive activities by victims of trauma and abuse comes from a variety of sources. First, evidence suggests that disclosive writing about a traumatic experience leads to beneficial outcomes for health, reduce physiological markers of stress, and alleviate self-reported emotional distress, negative affect, and depression (Pennebaker, 1997). This writing paradigm has been used as a basis for several positive activities designed to improve well-being (e.g., King, 2001).

Second, forgiveness activities have been found to be effective in improving the well-being of individuals impacted by trauma or abuse. In one study, women who had suffered spousal emotional abuse were assigned either to a forgiveness therapy group or a control group. Participants in the forgiveness therapy group experienced greater reductions in depression, anxiety, and stress symptoms, and improved self-esteem, forgiveness, environmental mastery, and ability to find meaning in suffering (Reed & Enright, 2006). Similarly, female survivors of childhood sexual trauma who participated in a forgiveness intervention demonstrated increases in forgiveness and hope, as well as decreases in anxiety and depression, relative to those in a control group (Freedman & Enright, 1996).

Although the forgiveness interventions in each of these studies were administered one-on-one and more closely resemble therapy, they provide preliminary support for the use of forgiveness activities as an effective strategy to improve well-being in this group. Likewise, a recent meta-analysis found that forgiveness activities can effectively promote self-esteem, positive affect, and forgiveness, as well as reduce negative affect (Lundahl, Taylor, Stevenson, & Roberts, 2008). Future work could determine the effectiveness of forgiveness activities when self-administered, and hence, more convenient and accessible, and less costly and time-consuming to practice.

Forgiveness has been associated with greater prosocial orientation, increased feelings of relatedness toward others (even to those beyond the target of the wrongdoing), and increased philanthropic behavior (Karremans, Van Lange, & Holland, 2005). These findings indicate that forgiving one's offender may be one way to generate an upward spiral toward greater well-being and recovery from wrongdoing. However, other research suggests that individuals may not always benefit from forgiveness. For example, one study of newlywed couples found that the tendency to express forgiveness was associated with stable levels of psychological and physical aggression during the first 4 years of marriage, whereas less forgiving attitudes were associated with declines in such aggression (McNulty, 2011). Similarly, an investigation of women at a domestic violence shelter found that more forgiving women were more likely to return to their abusive partner (Gordon, Burton, & Porter, 2004). Thus, it remains important to consider the type of abuse, and whether that abuse is ongoing, before recommending a forgiveness activity. Forgiveness may be a good fit for people who are trying to move on from their trauma, who no longer have contact with their abuser, or whose targets of forgiveness have learned or are learning their lesson, but could be potentially harmful if the act of forgiveness has the result of pardoning the targets for their wrongdoing.

Activities designed to cultivate meaning after trauma may also be particularly beneficial for sufferers of trauma and abuse. Meaning in life has been positively related to well-being in the general population (Steger et al., 2008), and the ability to find meaning after trauma has been identified as one of the mechanisms by which trauma sufferers may be able to experience positive outcomes and posttraumatic growth (Helgeson, Reynolds, & Tomich, 2006; Park & Ai, 2006).

Developing positive activities to cultivate meaning in life is a new direction in positive psychology. Preliminary evidence suggests that people who focus on aspects of their lives that bring meaning (e.g., by focusing on their most important values) can successfully improve their well-being and boost life meaning (Nelson, Fuller, Choi, & Lyubomirsky, 2013). Surprisingly, however, no studies have attempted to enhance life meaning among trauma victims, despite considerable evidence supporting the benefits of posttraumatic meaning making (e.g., Helgeson et al., 2006). Thus, researchers may want to examine how positive activities can promote meaning in life and happiness among people who have experienced trauma, and whether particular types of interventions are optimal in this population. For example, future studies could investigate whether activities such as visualizing a bright future, writing letters of gratitude, or performing acts of kindness are appropriate for individuals in this context. Envisioning an optimistic future, given past troubles, may help trauma sufferers take steps toward moving forward. In addition, writing letters of gratitude specifically to those who helped them weather a difficult time, and helping others with their troubles, may aid them in taking the focus off of themselves and their tribulations.

Individuals from Different Cultures

There are many reasons to believe that the pursuit of happiness may function differently across cultures. Members of individualist cultures tend to emphasize independence and autonomy over the needs of the larger group, whereas those from collectivist cultures exhibit a stronger emphasis on maintaining social harmony and obligation to the group (Triandis, 1995). These cultural differences also carry over to the ways people make well-being judgments. People from individualist cultures have been found to ground their life satisfaction more in intrapersonal than in interpersonal factors, whereas those from collectivist cultures do the reverse (Suh, Diener, Oishi, & Triandis, 1998). Moreover, cultural background appears to moderate the determinants of well-being—for example, self-esteem is more important to the well-being of people in individualist cultures than to those in collectivist cultures (Diener & Diener, 1995). Thus, norms in collectivist cultures may be less supportive of self-expression, self-improvement, and the pursuit of individual goals. These observations and findings suggest that traditional, individually focused happiness activities may be less effective for people belonging to collectivist cultures than for those in individualist cultures.

A few studies provide support for these claims. For example, in one experiment, Anglo Americans and foreign-born Asian Americans were assigned to practice optimism or gratitude, or to a control activity. Although all participants in the optimism and gratitude conditions demonstrated gains in well-being, these gains were larger for Anglo Americans than for Asian Americans (Boehm et al., 2011). Similarly, a study with college students living in the United States and South Korea found that practicing acts of kindness led to greater gains in well-being in the U.S. sample than in the South Korean sample (Della Porta, 2012).

Investigators should continue to examine cultural differences in response to positive activities. One possible research direction is suggested by a study that surveyed participants from 27 nations on their orientations to seeking happiness. The results revealed three clusters of happiness-seeking orientations: those who seek happiness via pleasure and engagement (e.g., France, Germany, and Ireland); those who seek happiness via engagement and meaning (e.g., United States, South Africa, Israel, and South

Korea); and those who do not endorse these ways of seeking happiness (e.g., Finland, Italy, and the United Kingdom) (Park, Peterson, & Ruch, 2009). These cultural distinctions provide a theoretical framework for testing different types of happiness activities among cultural groups. For example, studies could compare activities designed to cultivate meaning (e.g., taking pictures of and reflecting on meaningful pursuits and individuals in one's life), with activities targeting pleasure (e.g., engaging in activities for pure fun) among individuals in these three different clusters. This type of research is essential to understand better how individuals from different cultures respond to positive activities.

Military Personnel and Their Families

Soldiers and their families must cope with a variety of unique stressors, including those involving deployment, relocation, and managing postcombat stress. To help healthy soldiers and their families cope with the adversity and challenges associated with military life, the U.S. military recently launched an initiative to focus on comprehensive soldier fitness (Casey, 2011). An important characteristic of this program involves prevention; it was specifically created to help military personnel cultivate positive emotions and to build resilience and emotion regulation skills to prevent the development of mental health problems. The ability to build these skills is incredibly important. The numerous benefits of positive emotions include more flexible responses in the face of threat, better problem-solving skills, faster wound healing, increased physical health, and longer lives (Brown, Ryan, & Creswell, 2007; Lyubomirsky, King, & Diener, 2005; Pressman & Cohen, 2005). Thus, cultivating positive emotions is likely to be particularly beneficial in managing the many challenges facing military personnel (Algoe & Fredrickson, 2011).

Psychologists are currently empirically testing the success of various programs being implemented in the U.S. military as part of the comprehensive soldier fitness program. For example, one study examined the effect of resilience training on sergeants. This program includes many components of commonly practiced positive activities, such as cultivating gratitude, as well as identifying and using signature strengths. Although the findings are preliminary, initial evaluations of the program were highly positive (Reivich, Seligman, & McBride, 2011), suggesting that these strategies may be an effective method to improve the well-being of military personnel.

Given the unique situation of soldiers and their families, their needs for positive activities and well-being may be very different from those of the general population. For example, they may particularly benefit from activities designed to target stress (e.g., meditation) or build interpersonal relationships (e.g., practicing gratitude or kindness). However, research has yet to test these activities among members of the military and their families. Given the magnitude of potential benefits to be gained, such tests should be a priority for future research.

Final Thoughts and Conclusions

In summary, research on positive activities has come a long way in providing a scientific foundation for a variety of techniques that people can implement to improve their personal well-being. Recent studies on the mediators and moderators of activity effectiveness have also advanced the scientific understanding of how and why these activities are successful. However, much remains to be learned about the mechanisms by which positive activities "work" to make people happier. In this chapter, we have been especially concerned with the question of how to apply research on happiness-increasing practices to the unique personalities, needs, and resources of specific populations. Our review of the relevant research in this area suggests that different circumstances may call for different types of positive activities, tailored to fit each specific person, situation, and time (Schwartz & Sharpe, 2010). Future studies should strive to understand better the ways to deliver positive activities to obtain the most beneficial outcomes. To borrow again from mental health research, studies should aim to answer the question: "*What* [activity] . . . is most effective for *this* individual with *that* specific problem and under *which* set of circumstances" (Paul, 1967, p. 111, original emphasis).

References

Algoe, S. B., & Fredrickson, B. L. (2011). Emotional fitness and the movement of affective science from lab to field. *American Psychologist, 66*, 35–42.

Antoni, M. H., Lehman, J. M., Kilbourn, K. M., Boyers, A. E., Culver, J. L., Alferi, S. M., et al. (2001). Cognitive-behavioral stress management intervention decreases the prevalence of depression and enhances benefit finding among women under treatment for early-stage breast cancer. *Health Psychology, 20*, 20–32.

Arkoff, A., Meredith, G. M., & Dubanoski, J. P. (2004). Gains in well-being achieved through retrospective-proactive life review by independent older women. *Journal of Humanistic Psychology, 44*, 204–214.

Atkins, M. S., & Frazier, S. L. (2011). Expanding the toolkit or changing the paradigm: Are we ready for a public health approach to mental health? *Perspectives on Psychological Science, 6*, 483–487.

Bédard, M., Felteau, M., Mazmanian, D., Fedyk, K., Klein, R., Richardson, J., et al. (2003). Pilot evaluation of a mindfulness-based intervention to improve quality of life among individuals who sustained traumatic brain injuries. *Disability and Rehabilitation, 25*, 722–731.

Bergsma, A. (2008). Do self-help books help? *Journal of Happiness Studies, 9*, 341–360.

Boehm, J. K., & Lyubomirsky, S. (2011). [Feelings of autonomy and relatedness mediate the effectiveness of positive activities on well-being]. Unpublished raw data.

Boehm, J. K., Lyubomirsky, S., & Sheldon, K. M. (2011). A longitudinal experimental study comparing the effectiveness of happiness-enhancing strategies in Anglo Americans and Asian Americans. *Cognition and Emotion, 25*, 1263–1272.

Bonanno, G. A., Galea, S., Bucciarelli, A., & Vlahov, D. (2006). Psychological resilience after disaster: New York City in the aftermath of the September 11th terrorist attack. *Psychological Science, 17*, 181–186.

Brown, K. W., Ryan, R. M., & Creswell, J. D. (2007). Mindfulness: Theoretical foundations and evidence for its salutary effects. *Psychological Inquiry, 18*, 211–237.

Busseri, M. A., & Sadava, S. W. (2011). A review of the tripartite structure of subjective well-being: Implications for conceptualization, operationalization, analysis, and synthesis. *Personality and Social Psychology Review, 15*, 290–314.

Carstensen, L. L., Isaacowitz, D. M., & Charles, S. T. (1999). Taking time seriously: A theory of socioemotional selectivity. *American Psychologist, 54*, 165–181.

Carstensen, L. L., Turan, B., Scheibe, S., Ram, N., Ersner-Hershfield, H., Samanez-Larkin, G. R., et al. (2011). Emotional experience improves with age: Evidence based on over 10 years of experience sampling. *Psychology and Aging, 26*, 21–33.

Casey, G. W. (2011). Comprehensive soldier fitness: A vision for psychological resilience in the U.S. Army. *American Psychologist, 66*, 1–3.

Cohn, M. A., & Fredrickson, B. L. (2010). In search of durable positive psychology interventions: Predictors and consequences of long-term positive behavior change. *Journal of Positive Psychology, 5*, 355–366.

Cordova, M. J., Cunningham, L. L. C., Carlson, C. R., & Andrykowski, M. A. (2001). Social constraints, cognitive processing, and adjustment to breast cancer. *Journal of Consulting and Clinical Psychology, 69*, 706–711.

Costanzo, E. S., Ryff, C. D., & Singer, B. H. (2009). Psychosocial adjustment among cancer survivors: Findings from a national survey of health and well-being. *Health Psychology, 28*, 147–156.

Deci, E. L., & Ryan, R. M. (2000). The "what" and "why" of goal pursuits: Human needs and the self-determination theory of behavior. *Psychological Inquiry, 11*, 227–268.

Deci, E. L., & Ryan, R. M. (2008). Self-determination theory: A macrotheory of human motivation, development, and health. *Canadian Psychology, 49*, 182–185.

Della Porta, M. D. (2012). Enhancing the effects of happiness-boosting activities: The role of autonomy support in an experimental longitudinal intervention. *Dissertation Abstracts International B: Sciences and Engineering, 73*, 3518646.

Dickerhoof, R. (2007). Expressing optimism and gratitude: A longitudinal investigation of cognitive strategies to increase well-being. *Dissertation Abstracts International B: Sciences and Engineering, 68*, 4174.

Diener, E. (1984). Subjective well-being. *Psychological Bulletin, 95*, 542–575.

Diener, E. (2000). Subjective well-being: The science of happiness and a proposal for a national index. *American Psychologist, 55*, 34–43.

Diener, E., & Diener, M. (1995). Cross-cultural correlates of life satisfaction and self-esteem. *Journal of Personality and Social Psychology, 68,* 653–663.

Diener, E., & Lucas, R. E. (1999). Personality and subjective well-being. In D. Kahneman, E., Diener, & N. Schwarz (Eds.), *Well-being: The foundations of hedonic psychology* (pp. 213–229). New York: Russell Sage Foundation.

Diener, E., Suh, E. M., Lucas, R. E., & Smith, H. L. (1999). Subjective well-being: Three decades of progress. *Psychological Bulletin, 125,* 276–302.

Dunne, E., Wrosch, C., & Miller, G. E. (2011). Goal disengagement, functional disability, and depressive symptoms in old age. *Health Psychology, 30,* 763–770.

Emmons, R. A., & McCullough, M. E. (2003). Counting blessings versus burdens: An experimental investigation of gratitude and subjective well-being in daily life. *Journal of Personality and Social Psychology, 84,* 377–389.

Fava, G. A., Rafanelli, C., Cazzaro, M., Conti, S., & Grandi, S. (1998). Well-being therapy: A novel psychotherapeutic approach for residual symptoms of affective disorders. *Psychological Medicine, 28,* 475–480.

Fava, G. A., Ruini, C., Rafanelli, C., Finos, L., Salmaso, L., Mangelli, L., et al. (2005). Well-being therapy of generalized anxiety disorder. *Psychotherapy and Psychosomatics, 74,* 26–30.

Frederick, S., & Loewenstein, G. (1999). Hedonic adaptation. In D. Kahneman, E., Diener, & N. Schwarz (Eds.), *Well-being: The foundations of hedonic psychology* (pp. 302–329). New York: Russell Sage Foundation.

Fredrickson, B. L., & Joiner, T. (2002). Positive emotions trigger upward spirals toward emotional well-being. *Psychological Science, 13,* 172–175.

Freedman, S. R., & Enright, R. D. (1996). Forgiveness as an intervention goal with incest survivors. *Journal of Consulting and Clinical Psychology, 64,* 983–992.

Froh, J. H., Huebner, E. S., Youssef, A. J., & Conte, V. (2011). Acknowledging and appreciating the full spectrum of the human condition: School psychology's (limited) focus on positive psychological functioning. *Psychology in the Schools, 48,* 110–123.

Froh, J. J., Kashdan, T. B., Ozimkowski, K. M., & Miller, N. (2009). Who benefits the most from a gratitude intervention in children and adolescents?: Examining positive affect as a moderator. *Journal of Positive Psychology, 4,* 408–422.

Froh, J. J., Sefick, W. J., & Emmons, R. A. (2008). Counting blessings in early adolescents: An experimental study of gratitude and subjective well-being. *Journal of School Psychology, 46,* 213–233.

Fujita, F., & Diener, E. (2005). Life satisfaction set point: Stability and change. *Journal of Personality and Social Psychology, 88,* 158–164.

Gilham, J. E., Reivich, K. J., Jaycox, L. H., & Seligman, M. E. P. (1995). Prevention of depressive symptoms in schoolchildren: Two-year follow-up. *Psychological Science, 6,* 343–351.

Gordon, K. C., Burton, S., & Porter, L. (2004). Predicting the intentions of women in domestic violence shelters to return to partners: Does forgiveness play a role? *Journal of Family Psychology, 18,* 331–338.

Gruber, J., Mauss, I. B., & Tamir, M. (2011). A dark side of happiness?: How, when, and why happiness is not always good. *Perspectives on Psychological Science, 6,* 222–233.

Haworth, C., Nelson, S. K., Layous, K., Jacobs Bao, K., Lyubomirsky, S., & Plomin, R. (2013). *The Twins Wellbeing Intervention Study (TWIST): Results of a genetically sensitive online intervention.* Manuscript in preparation.

Heidrich, S. M. (1993). The relationship between physical health and psychological well-being in elderly women: A developmental perspective. *Research in Nursing and Health, 16,* 123–130.

Helgeson, V. S., Reynolds, K. A., & Tomich, P. L. (2006). A meta-analytic review of benefit finding and growth. *Journal of Consulting and Clinical Psychology, 74,* 797–816.

Helson, R., Jones, C., & Kwan, V. S. Y. (2002). Personality can change over 40 years of adulthood: Hierarchical linear modeling analyses of two longitudinal samples. *Journal of Personality and Social Psychology, 83,* 752–766.

Howell, R. T., Kern, M. L., & Lyubomirsky, S. (2007). Health benefits: Meta-analytically determining the impact of well-being on objective health outcomes. *Health Psychology Review, 1,* 83–136.

Huffman, J. C., Mastromauro, C. A., Boehm, J. K., Seabrook, R., Fricchione, G. L., Denninger, J. W., et al. (2011). Development of a positive psychology intervention for patients with acute cardiovascular disease. *Heart International, 6,* 47–54.

Karremans, J. C., Van Lange, P. A. M., & Holland, R. W. (2005). Forgiveness and its associations with prosocial thinking, feeling, and doing beyond the relationship with the offender. *Personality and Social Psychology Bulletin, 31,* 1315–1326.

Kashdan, T. B., Biswas-Diener, R., & King, L. A. (2008). Reconsidering happiness: The costs of distinguishing between hedonics and eudaimonia. *Journal of Positive Psychology, 3,* 219–233.

Kashdan, T. B., & Steger, M. F. (2011). Challenges, pitfalls, and aspirations for positive psychology. In K. M. Sheldon, T. B., Kashdan, & M. F. Steger (Eds.), *Designing positive psychology: Taking stock and moving forward* (pp. 9–21). New York: Oxford University Press.

Kazdin, A. E., & Blase, S. L. (2011). Interventions and models of their delivery to reduce the burden of mental illness: Reply to commentaries. *Perspectives on Psychological Science, 6,* 507–510.

Kesebir, P., & Diener, E. (2008). In pursuit of happiness: Empirical answers to philosophical questions. *Perspectives on Psychological Science, 3,* 117–125.

Kessler, R. C., Chiu, W. T., Demler, O., & Walters, E. E. (2005). Prevalence, severity, and comorbidity of twelve-month DSM-IV disorders in the National Comorbidity Survey Replication (NCS-R). *Archives of General Psychiatry, 62,* 617–627.

King, L. A. (2001). The health benefits of writing about life goals. *Personality and Social Psychology Bulletin, 27,* 798–807.

Langer, E. J., & Rodin, J. (1976). The effects of choice and enhanced personal responsibility for the aged: A field experiment in an institutional setting. *Journal of Personality and Social Psychology, 34,* 191–198.

Layous, K., Chancellor, J., Lyubomirsky, S., Wang, L., & Doraiswamy, P. M. (2011). Delivering happiness: Translating positive psychology intervention research for treating major and minor depressive disorders. *Journal of Alternative and Complementary Medicine, 17,* 675–683.

Layous, K., Nelson, S. K., & Lyubomirsky, S. (2013). What is the optimal way to deliver a positive activity intervention? The case of writing about one's best possible selves. *Journal of Happiness Studies, 14,* 635–654.

Layous, K., Nelson, S. K., Oberle, E., Schonert-Reichl, K., & Lyubomirsky, S. (2012). Kindness counts: Prompting prosocial behavior in preadolescents boosts peer acceptance and well-being. *PLOS ONE, 7,* e51380.

Lee, V., Cohen, S. R., Edgar, L., Laizner, A. M., & Gagnon, A. J. (2006). Meaning-making intervention during breast or colorectal cancer treatment improves self-esteem, optimism, and self-efficacy. *Social Science and Medicine, 62,* 3133–3145.

Lundahl, B. W., Taylor, M. J., Stevenson, R., & Roberts, K. D. (2008). Process-based forgiveness intervention: A meta-analytic review. *Research on Social Work Practice, 18,* 465–478.

Lykken, D. & Tellegen, A. (1996). Happiness is a stochastic phenomenon. *Psychological Science, 7,* 186–189.

Lyubomirsky, S. (2008). *The how of happiness: A scientific approach to getting the life you want.* New York: Penguin Press.

Lyubomirsky, S. (2011). Hedonic adaptation to positive and negative experiences. In S. Folkman (Ed.), *Oxford handbook of stress, health, and coping* (pp. 200–224). New York: Oxford University Press.

Lyubomirsky, S., & Dickerhoof, R. (2010). A construal approach to increasing happiness. In J. P. Tangney & J. E. Maddux (Eds.), *Social psychological foundations of clinical psychology* (pp. 229–244). New York: Guilford Press.

Lyubomirsky, S., Dickerhoof, R., Boehm, J. K., & Sheldon, K. M. (2011). Becoming happier takes both a will and a proper way: An experimental longitudinal intervention to boost well-being. *Emotion, 11,* 391–402.

Lyubomirsky, S., King, L. A., & Diener, E. (2005). The benefits of frequent positive affect. *Psychological Bulletin, 131,* 803–855.

Lyubomirsky, S., & Layous, K. (2013). How do simple positive activities increase well-being? *Current Directions in Psychological Science, 22,* 57–62.

Lyubomirsky, S., Sheldon, K., & Schkade, D. (2005). Pursuing happiness: The architecture of sustainable change. *Review of General Psychology, 9,* 111–131.

Mauss, I. B., Tamir, M., Anderson, C. L., & Savino, N. S. (2011). Can seeking happiness make people unhappy?: Paradoxical effects of valuing happiness. *Emotion, 11,* 807–815.

McCrae, R. R., & Costa, P. T. (1990). *Personality in adulthood.* New York: Guilford Press.

McNulty, J. K. (2011). The dark side of forgiveness: The tendency to forgive predicts continued psychological and physical aggression in marriage. *Personality and Social Psychology Bulletin, 37,* 770–783.

McNulty, J. K., & Fincham, F. D. (2012). Beyond positive psychology?: Toward a contextual view of psychological processes and well-being. *American Psychologist, 67*(2), 101–110.

Mroczek, D. K., & Spiro, A., III. (2005). Change in life satisfaction during adulthood: Findings from the Veterans Affairs Normative Aging Study. *Journal of Personality and Social Psychology, 88,* 189–202.

Nelson, S. K., Fuller, J. A. K., Choi, I., & Lyubomirsky, S. (2013). *Beyond self-protection: Self-affirmation benefits well-being.* Manuscript submitted for publication.

Nelson, S. K., Layous, K., Oberle, E., Lyubomirsky, S., & Schonert-Reichl, K. A. (2012, January). *An acts of kindness intervention among school-age children.* Poster presented at the annual meeting for the Society for Personality and Social Psychology, San Diego, CA.

Nes, R. B., Roysamb, E., Tambs, K., Harris, J. R., & Reichborn-Kjennerud, T. (2006). Subjective well-being: Genetic and environmental contributions to stability and change. *Psychological Medicine, 36,* 1033–1042.

Niemic, C. P., Ryan, R. M., & Deci, E. L. (2009). The path taken: Consequences of attaining intrinsic and extrinsic aspirations in post-college life. *Journal of Research in Personality, 43,* 291–306.

Oberle, E., Schonert-Reichl, K. A., & Zumbo, B. D. (2011). Life satisfaction in early adolescence: Personal, neighborhood, school, family, and peer influences. *Journal of Youth and Adolescence, 40,* 889–901.

Oswald, F., Wahl, H. W., Schilling, O., Nygren, C., Fange, A., Sixsmith, A., et al. (2007). Relationships between housing and healthy aging in very old age. *Gerontologist, 47,* 96–107.

Park, C. L., & Ai, A. L. (2006). Meaning making and growth: New directions for research on survivors of trauma. *Journal of Loss and Trauma, 11,* 389–407.

Park, N., Peterson, C., & Ruch, W. (2009). Orientations to happiness and life satisfaction in twenty-seven nations. *Journal of Positive Psychology, 4,* 273–279.

Parks, A. C., Della Porta, M. D., Pierce, R. S., Zilca, R., & Lyubomirsky, S. (2012). Pursuing happiness in everyday life: The characteristics and behaviors of online happiness seekers. *Emotion, 12*(6), 1222–1234.

Paul, G. L. (1967). Strategy of outcome research in psychotherapy. *Journal of Consulting Psychology, 31,* 109–118.

Pennebaker, J. W. (1997). Writing about emotional experiences as a therapeutic process. *Psychological Science, 8,* 162–166.

Pressman, S. D., & Cohen, S. (2005). Does positive affect influence health? *Psychological Bulletin, 131,* 925–971.

Proctor, C., Tsukayama, E., Wood, A. M., Maltby, J., Eades, J. F., & Linley, P. A. (2011). Strengths gym: The impact of a character strengths-based intervention on the life satisfaction and well-being of adolescents. *Journal of Positive Psychology, 6,* 377–388.

Reed, G. L., & Enright, R. D. (2006). The effects of forgiveness therapy on depression, anxiety, and posttraumatic stress for women after spousal emotional abuse. *Journal of Consulting and Clinical Psychology, 74,* 920–929.

Reivich, K. J., Seligman, M. E. P., & McBride, S. (2011). Master resilience training in the U.S. Army. *American Psychologist, 66,* 25–34.

Richards, M., & Huppert, F. A. (2011). Do positive children become positive adults?: Evidence from a longitudinal birth cohort study. *Journal of Positive Psychology, 6,* 75–87.

Roberts, B. W., Walton, K. E., & Viechtbauer, W. (2006). Patterns of mean-level change in personality traits across the life course: A meta-analysis of longitudinal studies. *Psychological Bulletin, 132,* 1–25.

Ryan, R. M., & Deci, E. L. (2001). On happiness and human potentials: A review of research on hedonic and eudaimonic well-being. *Annual Review of Psychology, 52,* 141–166.

Ryan, R. M., & Deci, E. L. (2008). Self-determination theory and the role of basic psychological needs in personality and the organization of behavior. In O. P. John, R. W. Robins, & L. A. Pervin (Eds.), *Handbook of personality psychology: Theory and research* (3rd ed., pp. 654–678). New York: Guilford Press.

Ryff, C. D. (1989). Happiness is everything, or is it?: Explorations on the meaning of psychological well-being. *Journal of Personality and Social Psychology, 57,* 1069–1081.

Ryff, C. D. (1991). Possible selves in adulthood and old age: A tale of shifting horizons. *Psychology and Aging, 6,* 286–295.

Schmid, K. L., Phelps, E., Kiely, M. K., Napolitano, C. M., Boyd, M. J., & Lerner, R. M. (2011). The role of adolescents' hopeful futures in predicting positive and negative developmental trajectories: Findings from the 4-H study of positive youth development. *Journal of Positive Psychology, 6,* 45–56.

Schueller, S. M. (2011). To each his own well-being boosting intervention: Using preference to guide selection. *Journal of Positive Psychology, 6,* 300–313.

Schwartz, B., & Sharpe, K. (2010). *Practical wisdom: The right way to do the right thing.* New York: Riverhead.

Seligman, M. E. P., Rashid, T., & Parks, A. C. (2006). Positive psychotherapy. *American Psychologist, 61,* 774–788.

Seligman, M. E. P., Steen, T. A., Park, N., & Peterson, C. (2005). Positive psychology progress: Empirical validation of interventions. *Personality and Individual Differences, 49,* 368–373.

Sergeant, S., & Mongrain, M. (2011). Are positive psychology exercises helpful for people with depressive personality styles? *Journal of Positive Psychology, 6,* 260–272.

Shapira, L. B., & Mongrain, M. (2010). The benefits of self-compassion and optimism exercises for individuals vulnerable to depression. *Journal of Positive Psychology, 5,* 377–389.

Sheldon, K. M. (2004). *Optimal human being: An integrated multi-level perspective.* Mahwah, NJ: Erlbaum.

Sheldon, K. M., Boehm, J. K., & Lyubomirsky, S. (2012). Variety is the spice of happiness: The hedonic adaptation prevention (HAP) model. In S. David, I. Boniwell, & A. Conley Ayers (Eds.), *Oxford handbook of happiness* (pp. 901–914). Oxford, UK: Oxford University Press.

Sheldon, K. M., & Elliot, A. J. (1999). Goal striving, need-satisfaction, and longitudinal well-being: The Self-Concordance Model. *Journal of Personality and Social Psychology, 76,* 482–497.

Sheldon, K. M., Elliot, A. J., Kim, Y., & Kasser, T. (2001). What is satisfying about satisfying events?: Testing 10 candidate psychological needs. *Journal of Personality and Social Psychology, 80,* 325–329.

Sheldon, K. M., & Lyubomirsky, S. (2006a). Achieving sustainable increases in happiness: Change your actions, not your circumstances. *Journal of Happiness Studies, 7,* 55–86.

Sheldon, K. M., & Lyubomirsky, S. (2006b). How to increase and sustain positive emotion:

The effects of expressing gratitude and visualizing best possible selves. *Journal of Positive Psychology, 1,* 73–82.

Shoham, V., & Insel, T. R. (2011). Rebooting for whom?: Portfolios, technology, and personalized intervention. *Perspectives on Psychological Science, 6,* 478–482.

Sin, N. L., Della Porta, M. D., & Lyubomirsky, S. (2011). Tailoring positive psychology interventions to treat depressed individuals. In S. I. Donaldson, M. Csikszentmihalyi, & J. Nakamura (Eds.), *Applied positive psychology: Improving everyday life, health, schools, work, and society* (pp. 79–96). New York: Routledge.

Sin, N. L., & Lyubomirsky, S. (2009). Enhancing well-being and alleviating depressive symptoms with positive psychology interventions: A practice-friendly meta-analysis. *Journal of Clinical Psychology: In Session, 65,* 467–487.

Steger, M. F. (2009). Meaning in life. In S. J. Lopez (Ed.), *Oxford handbook of positive psychology* (2nd ed., pp. 679–687). Oxford, UK: Oxford University Press.

Steger, M. F., & Kashdan, T. B. (2007). Stability and specificity of meaning in life and life satisfaction over one year. *Journal of Happiness Studies, 8,* 161–179.

Steger, M. F., Kashdan, T. B., Sullivan, B. A., & Lorentz, D. (2008). Understanding the search for meaning in life: Personality, cognitive style, and the dynamic between seeking and experiencing meaning. *Journal of Research in Personality, 42,* 660–678.

Suh, E. M., Diener, E., Oishi, S., & Triandis, H. C. (1998). The shifting basis of life satisfaction judgments across cultures: Emotions versus norms. *Journal of Personality and Social Psychology, 74,* 482–493.

Suldo, S., Thalji, A., & Ferron, J. (2011). Longitudinal academic outcomes predicted by early adolescents' subjective well-being, psychopathology, and mental health status yielded from a dual factor model. *Journal of Positive Psychology, 6,* 17–30.

Surway, C., Roberts, J., & Silver, A. (2005). The effect of mindfulness training on mood and measures of fatigue, activity, and quality of life in patients with chronic fatigue syndrome on a hospital waiting list: A series of exploratory studies. *Behavioural and Cognitive Psychotherapy, 33,* 103–109.

Tkach, C. T. (2006). Unlocking the treasury of human kindness: Enduring improvements in mood, happiness, and self-evaluations. *Dissertation Abstracts International B: Sciences and Engineering, 67,* 603.

Triandis, H. C. (1995). *Individualism and collectivism.* Boulder, CO: Westview Press.

Walsh, R. (2011). Lifestyle and mental health. *American Psychologist, 66,* 579–592.

Watkins, K. E., Burnam, M. A., Orlando, M., Escarce, J. J., Huskamp, H. A., & Goldman, H. H. (2009). The health value and cost of care for major depression. *Value in Health, 12,* 65–72.

Williams, L. M., Brown, K. J., Palmer, D., Liddell, B. J., Kemp, A. H., Olivieri, G., et al. (2006). The mellow years?: Neural basis of improving emotional stability over age. *Journal of Neuroscience, 26,* 6422–6430.

Witten, H.-U. (2002). Generalized anxiety disorder: Prevalence, burden, and cost to society. *Depression and Anxiety, 16,* 162–171.

Zautra, A. J., Davis, M. C., Reich, J. W., Nicassario, P., Tennen, H., Finan, P., et al. (2008). Comparison of cognitive behavioral and mindfulness meditation interventions on adaptation to rheumatoid arthritis for patients with and without history of recurrent depression. *Journal of Consulting and Clinical Psychology, 76,* 408–421.

■ ■ ■ ■ ■ ■ ■ ■ ■

CHAPTER 17

Pride

The Fundamental Emotion of Success, Power, and Status

Jessica L. Tracy
Aaron C. Weidman
Joey T. Cheng
Jason P. Martens

When explaining the need for a "positive psychology" movement, Mihalyi Csikszentmihalyi, one of the field's founders, drew on his experiences as a child during World War II:

> I noticed with surprise how many of the adults I had known as successful and self-confident became helpless and dispirited . . . yet there were a few who kept their integrity and purpose despite the surrounding chaos. . . . What sources of strength were these people drawing on? (Seligman & Csikszentmihalyi, 2000, p. 6)

Apparently, Csikszentmihalyi was inspired by the everyday feelings of success, confidence, and self-purpose that shaped the lives of the adults surrounding him. His observation of these emotions, and the ability of certain individuals to maintain them in the face of intensely traumatic external events, motivated him to promote a new subfield of psychological science. Thus, it is somewhat ironic that the very feelings that led Csikszentmihalyi to found the field, feelings that correspond closely to *pride,* have, to date, received considerably less attention from

positive psychologists than emotions such as happiness, compassion, and gratitude—positive emotions that not only feel good, but also appear to be *good for us* and those around us. Unlike those emotions, pride is not a purely "positive" emotion, in the sense of having an unambiguous positive impact on psychological well-being, mental health, and relationships. In fact, a growing body of research indicates that pride comprises two distinct facets, one of which has deleterious effects on well-being, mental health, and interpersonal functioning. However, if we define "positive emotions" as those that are positively valenced and pleasurable to experience, then pride certainly merits inclusion in the category.

Furthermore, despite an absence of research by positive psychologists, pride has received a great of psychological research attention in recent years. Based on a PsycINFO search for articles with keywords *pride* or *proud*, there have been three distinct periods of research on pride since 1980 (see Figure 17.1). Prior to 1990, psychologists paid little attention to pride, producing an average of only 2.9 pride-related papers

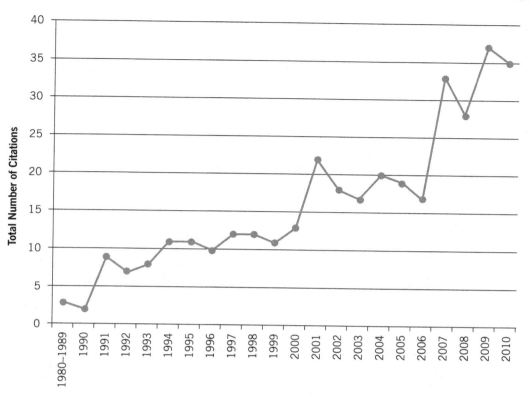

FIGURE 17.1. History of psychological research on pride, 1980–2010, based on a PsycINFO keyword search.

per year. The 1990s saw interest rise, with an average of 9.3 pride papers per year, likely fostered by the emergence of self-conscious emotion research more broadly—exemplified by Tangney and Fischer's (1995) comprehensive volume on the topic. However, most self-conscious emotion research in the 1990s focused on the negatively valenced emotions of guilt and shame; notably, there was no chapter in the 1995 volume dedicated to pride, and only three out of 20 chapters mentioned it. It was not until the past decade that a major surge in pride research occurred, with an average of 23.3 articles per year, each year since 2000.

We are pleased by this recent surge because, as we argue in this chapter, pride is a unique and important positive emotion that differs from other positive states (e.g., happiness, contentedness, excitement) and therefore needs to be studied as a distinct entity. Here, we review findings suggesting that pride is (1) an evolved part of human nature,

(2) unique from other positive emotions, and (3) functional primarily in the social, interpersonal domain. In taking this perspective, we draw on a larger movement in emotion research that emphasizes the evolutionary history and contemporary functions of discrete positive emotions (as opposed to treating positive affect as a single dimensional construct; e.g., Bartlett & DeSteno, 2006; Fredrickson, 1998; Griskevicius, Shiota, & Neufeld, 2010; Keltner, Haidt, & Shiota, 2006; Tracy & Robins, 2007c). Below, we first discuss research on the psychological structure of pride, which demonstrates that pride is a complex and not entirely positive emotion. We then review research showing that pride, like other evolved emotions, is associated with a distinct, universally recognized nonverbal expression. Consistent with this evolutionary approach, we next review findings on the development and neuroscience of pride, then discuss emerging work that addresses the question of why

pride evolved, and what functions it serves. Finally, we conclude with several current directions in pride research, each of which moves beyond questions about what pride is and why people experience it, toward questions of pride's impact on the social world. In our view, these directions are exciting both for their suggestion that pride is critical to a range of social processes, and because they take for granted that pride is a distinct and fundamental emotion that plays an important role in social life.

The Psychological Structure of Pride

Scholars have taken note of pride's dual-faceted nature for over a millennium; its dark or "sinful" side, in particular, has been cautioned against by religious scholars and philosophers ranging from Aristotle and Lao Tzu to Thomas Aquinas and the Dalai Lama (see Tracy, Shariff, & Cheng, 2010). Partly on the basis of these accounts, emotion researchers have postulated distinct "authentic," or "beta pride," and "hubristic," or "alpha pride," components of the emotion (Lewis, 2000; Tracy & Robins, 2004a; Tangney, Wagner, & Gramzow, 1989); several lines of research support this account (Tracy & Robins, 2007c). First, when asked to think about and list words relevant to pride, research participants consistently generate two very different categories of concepts, which empirically form two separate clusters of semantic meaning. The first cluster (labeled "authentic pride") includes words such as *accomplished* and *confident*, and fits with the prosocial, achievement-oriented conceptualization of pride. The second cluster (labeled "hubristic pride") includes words such as *arrogant* and *conceited*, and fits with a more self-aggrandizing, egotistical conceptualization (Tracy & Robins, 2007c). A very similar two-cluster pattern also emerged in a recent study examining semantic conceptualizations of pride in Mainland China, among university student participants who generated pride words indigenously in Chinese (Shi et al., 2013). This cross-cultural replication suggests that the tendency to make conceptual distinctions between authentic and hubristic pride is not likely to be an artifact of Western culture, but rather may reflect pride's universal structure.

The second piece of evidence supporting the dual-faceted structure of pride comes from studies that asked participants to rate their subjective feelings during an actual pride experience, or the feelings that describe their general dispositional tendency to feel pride (i.e., trait pride). Across several studies, factor analyses of participants' ratings consistently revealed two relatively independent factors, which closely parallel the two semantic clusters. Subsequent analyses demonstrated that the two pride factors are not artifacts of a tendency to group together good versus bad, activated versus deactivated, or trait versus state words (Tracy & Robins, 2007c). These factor-analytic findings have also been replicated in Mainland China and South Korea, using both indigenously derived pride-related words (in Chinese and Korean) and translated versions of the English words found to represent authentic and hubristic pride in the U.S. (Shi et al., 2013). Chinese and Korean cultures tend to emphasize collectivistic, interdependent self-construals, and to downplay self-enhancing emotions in favor of those that are more self-derogating (Heine, Lehman, Markus, & Kitayama, 1999; Markus & Kitayama, 1991), so it would not be surprising if conceptualizations or experiences of pride among these individuals were somewhat different from those found in Western cultural contexts. Thus, the finding that, in fact, Chinese and Korean individuals experience and conceive of the same two pride facets as do Americans provides support for the universality of both facets.

What is the difference between these two facets of pride? Studies on their personality correlates have demonstrated that they diverge in a number of ways. At both the trait and state levels, authentic pride is positively related to the socially desirable and generally adaptive Big Five traits of Extraversion, Agreeableness, Conscientiousness, Emotional Stability, and Openness to Experience, whereas hubristic pride is consistently negatively related to the two prosocial traits of Agreeableness and Conscientiousness (Tracy & Robins, 2007c). These distinct personality profiles have also been replicated in a Chinese sample (Shi et al., 2013). Authentic pride is also positively related to both explicit and implicit self-esteem, whereas hubristic pride is negatively related to implicit and explicit self-esteem, yet positively related to narcissism and shame-proneness (Tracy, Cheng, Robins, & Trzesniewski, 2009), consistent with a theoretical distinctions between the two prides as correspondent to the distinction between genuine self-esteem and narcissism (Tracy, Cheng, Martens, & Robins, 2011).

The facets also differ in their links to a range of social behaviors and mental health outcomes; essentially, each facet of pride seems to underlie a different way of engaging with the social world and approaching one's goals. Individuals high in dispositional authentic pride tend to be low in depression, trait anxiety, social phobia, aggression, hostility, and rejection sensitivity; and high in life satisfaction, relationship satisfaction, dyadic adjustment, and social support, and they typically are securely attached to their relationship partners. In contrast, individuals high in dispositional hubristic pride are more likely to experience chronic anxiety and engage in aggression, hostility, and a range of other antisocial misbehaviors (e.g., drug use, petty crimes), and to report lower dyadic adjustment and social support (Orth, Robins, & Soto, 2008; Tracy et al., 2009). Given these highly divergent personality profiles, it is not surprising that the pride facets are located in different quadrants on the Interpersonal Circumplex (i.e., the independent dimensions of agency and communion; Kiesler, 1983). Although both facets are linked to agency, individuals high in communion are prone to authentic pride only; hubristic pride shows a negative relationship with communal traits (Cheng, Tracy, & Henrich, 2010). This distinction plays out in goal striving as well; both facets are positively related to an approach orientation, evidenced by high scores on measures of the behavioral activation system and low scores on the behavioral inhibition system (Carver, Sinclair, & Johnson, 2010). However, individuals high in dispositional authentic pride seem to vigorously engage in their major life goals and are able to put failures in perspective, whereas individuals high in dispositional hubristic pride tend to set unrealistically high goals for fame and success, and to interpret any positive event as indicative of their own greatness (Carver et al., 2010).

Consistent with these distinct approaches to interpreting one's achievements, several studies suggest that the two pride facets are elicited by distinct cognitive appraisals. Pride occurs when individuals appraise a positive event as relevant to their identity, and their goals for their identity, and as internally caused (i.e., due to the self; Ellsworth & Smith, 1988; Lewis, 2000; Roseman, 1991; Tracy & Robins, 2004a; Weiner, 1985); the finding that success elicits pride has now been replicated across American and Japanese samples (Imada & Ellsworth, 2011). Yet studies suggest that authentic and hubristic pride are further distinguished by subsequent attributions: Authentic pride may result from attributions to internal but unstable, specific, and controllable causes, such as effort (e.g., "I won because I practiced"), whereas hubristic pride is more likely to occur from attributions to internal but stable, global, and uncontrollable causes, such as ability (e.g., "I won because I'm great") (Tracy & Robins, 2007c). One study supporting these links found that individuals instructed to attribute a hypothetical success to hard work (unstable, specific attribution) expected to feel authentic pride in response, whereas those instructed to attribute the same success to stable, global ability expected to feel greater hubristic pride. Another study found that individuals who tend to make internal but unstable and controllable attributions for a wide range of events also tend to be dispositionally prone to authentic pride, whereas those who make internal but stable and uncontrollable attributions are more prone to hubristic pride. Finally, a third study examined participants' descriptions of actual pride events and, using content analysis, found that those who reported greater authentic pride in response to these events tended to attribute them to unstable causes, whereas those who reported greater hubristic pride tended to attribute events to stable abilities, and not to their specific behaviors (Tracy & Robins, 2007c).

Recent work in China produced findings that largely replicate these patterns. Based on content coding of Chinese participants' pride descriptions, those who experienced hubristic pride tended to attribute their successes to internal and stable abilities, but *not* to unstable behaviors. Together, these findings suggest that the effort–ability attribution distinction may be a key factor in determining whether an individual experiences authentic or hubristic pride in response to a given success. However, other factors, such as personality and social comparisons, are likely to play a role in this distinction as well, and future research is needed to address this issue further (see also Tracy & Robins, in press, for more on the question of whether these attributions distinguish between the two pride facets). In this vein, a recent set of studies examining judgments of authentic and hubristic pride in others found that although perceptions of a proud target's attributions influenced judgments of the target's authentic or hubristic pride, perceptions about the target's arrogance were also important (Tracy & Prehn, 2012). Arrogance was inferred both from the kinds of attributions targets made (i.e., attributions to ability were perceived as more arrogant than attributions to effort) and the way in which the targets made them (i.e., whether he or she was perceived to be bragging about the success). This suggests that, at least in determining which facet of pride *others* are experiencing, perceived arrogance and modesty may be as important as presumed cognitive appraisal elicitors.

The Pride Nonverbal Expression

One of the most prominent "gold-standard" criteria used to determine whether a particular emotion is likely to be evolved (or "basic") is whether it has a distinct, cross-culturally recognized nonverbal expression (e.g., Ekman & Cordaro, 2011; Tracy & Randles, 2011). Although pride was not included in the pantheon of emotions originally thought to meet this criterion, based on seminal cross-cultural studies by Ekman, Izard, and their colleagues (e.g., Ekman, Sorenson, & Friesen, 1969; Ekman et al., 1987; Izard, 1971), a number of studies in recent years have provided strong evidence for a cross-cultural, reliably recognized pride expression (see Figure 17.2; also see Tracy & Robins, 2007a, for a review). The prototypical pride expression includes the body (i.e., expanded posture, head tilted slightly back, arms akimbo with hands on hips or raised above the head with hands in fists) as well as the face (i.e., small smile) (Tracy & Robins, 2004b, 2007b), and is reliably recognized and distinguished from similar

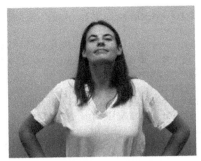

Expression A

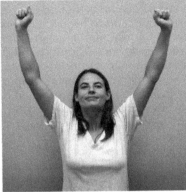

Expression B

FIGURE 17.2. The prototypical pride expression. Both expressions (A and B) are reliably and cross-culturally recognized as pride and spontaneously displayed in response to success.

emotions (e.g., happiness, excitement) by individuals across cultures. Accurate pride recognition has been found even among individuals living in highly isolated, largely preliterate, traditional small-scale societies from two different populations (Burkina Faso and Fiji), who had almost no exposure to Western cultural knowledge (Tracy & Robins, 2008b; Tracy, Shariff, Zhao, & Henrich, 2013). Pride-recognition rates in educated U.S. samples typically range from around 80–90%, comparable to the recognition rates found for more established basic emotions (e.g., anger, sadness). Like those emotions, pride can be recognized quickly and efficiently from a single snapshot image (Tracy & Robins, 2008a).

Importantly, the recognizable pride expression is also spontaneously *displayed* in pride-eliciting situations by successful children as young as 3 years old (Belsky & Domitrovich, 1997; Lewis, Alessandri, & Sullivan, 1992; Stipek, Recchia, & McClintic, 1992), high school students who have performed well on a class exam (Weisfeld & Beresford, 1982), and medal-winning adult Olympic athletes from a wide range of cultures, as well as congenitally blind athletes across cultures, who could not have learned to display pride through visual modeling (Tracy & Matsumoto, 2008). These findings suggest that the pride expression is likely to be a universal and innate behavioral response to success. It is unlikely that the expression (1) would be recognized so consistently and robustly, (2) by individuals who could not have learned it through cross-cultural transmission (i.e., films, television, magazines), or (3) be reliably and spontaneously displayed in pride-eliciting situations by individuals who have never seen others display it, if it were not an innate human universal.

Interestingly, a number of authors have noted that the pride expression differs from other highly recognizable emotion expressions, in that accurate recognition of pride requires bodily and head components, as well as facial muscle movements (Tracy & Robins, 2004b). This distinction, which also characterizes the shame expression (Izard, 1971; Keltner, 1995; Tracy, Robins, & Schriber, 2009), may be indicative of the unique early evolutionary origins of these two self-conscious emotion expressions; they may be homologous with nonhuman dominance and submission displays, which involve similar bodily and head movements (see Tracy & Randles, 2011, for a review). However, several researchers who recently probed this distinction found that pride can be recognized at fairly high levels of accuracy from the face and head alone (i.e., without expanded posture) if shown as a dynamic display (i.e., via video) (Nelson & Russell, 2011). This suggests that though static images of pride require expanded posture for accurate recognition, the observation of a head tilting back or up removes this need, and, therefore, in everyday interpersonal interactions pride displays probably can be reliably recognized even when bodily movements (beyond the head) are not visible.

Studies of vocal displays of emotion have also sought to identify a distinct pride expression, but with somewhat mixed results. While one set of studies failed to find a recognizable vocal burst associated with pride (Simon-Thomas, Keltner, Sauter, Sinicropi-Yao, & Abramson, 2009), another found that vocal bursts of achievement were fairly reliably identified as "achievement." Achievement recognition rates were slightly lower than those typically found for visual pride displays (i.e., $M = 80\%$) but higher than those for vocal bursts intended to convey contentment, relief, and pleasure (Sauter & Scott, 2007). In general, research on vocal expressions of emotion is still somewhat in its infancy, and further work is needed to determine whether pride can be reliably conveyed through this medium.

A broader question for pride expression research, which arises in the face of evidence for two distinct pride facets, is whether each facet is associated with a distinct nonverbal expression. Several studies have addressed this issue by testing whether participants reliably identify different variants of the pride expression (e.g., with arms raised above the head vs. arms akimbo) as either authentic or hubristic pride. Thus far, all recognizable variants of the expression that have been tested have been found to be identified as authentic and hubristic pride at relatively equal rates (Tracy & Robins, 2007a). This suggests that the same expression conveys both facets, and, based on studies mentioned earlier, observers use contextual information (e.g., an expresser's apparent arrogance) to determine which facet he or she is experiencing (Tracy & Prehn, 2012).

Development of Pride

A number of studies have assessed the display, recognition, and understanding of pride in children, resulting in an emerging portrait of the emotion's early developmental trajectory. Like all self-conscious emotions, pride is first experienced later in the course of development than more basic emotions such as fear and joy—at around 3 years of age (e.g., Campos, Barrett, Lamb, Goldsmith, & Stenberg, 1983; Lewis et al., 1992; Stipek et al., 1992). This finding is based on studies that present young children with a challenging task and compare their behavioral and verbal responses after successful completion versus failure, or after successful completion in easy versus difficult conditions. Behavioral components of the pride expression and verbal indicators of pride tend to be shown by children who have reached 2.5 to 3 years of age, but not by younger children, and not in shame-inducing (i.e., failure) situations or easy success conditions.

The capacity to understand pride emerges somewhat later than its (assumed) experience. The earliest emerging form of understanding is the ability to recognize the pride nonverbal expression, which first appears when children reach age 4 (Tracy, Robins, & Lagattuta, 2005)—the same age at which they begin to show accurate recognition of most other expressions, such as surprise. In contrast, the ability to understand the situations and contexts in which pride is elicited seems to develop considerably later. Several studies have found that 7-year-olds have difficulty understanding that pride should be attributed to individuals whose success is due to internal (e.g., effort–ability) but not external (e.g., luck) factors (e.g., Graham & Weiner, 1986; Harris, Olthof, Terwogt, & Hardman, 1987; Thompson, 1989). However, by age 9 or 10, children can make the appropriate attributional distinctions, and grant pride only to individuals who are the cause of their own success (Kornilaki & Chloverakis, 2004; Thompson, 1989).

This developmental trajectory is consistent with the assumption that certain cognitive capacities are prerequisites for the experience of self-conscious emotions: self-awareness, stable self-representations, comparisons between one's own behavior and external standards, and internal attributions (Lagattuta & Thompson, 2007; Lewis, 2000; Tracy & Robins, 2004a). By the age of 3, children demonstrate early-emerging components of self-awareness (i.e., mirror self-recognition, self-referencing, imitation; Hart & Karmel, 1996) and begin to display prideful behavioral responses to success, but cannot yet identify pride in others. The development of a full understanding of the situations and attributions that elicit pride and distinguish it from happiness seems to coincide with the achievement of a global sense of self and self-esteem (Harter, 1983). Future studies are needed to tease apart the likely bidirectional causal links between these shifting pride experiences and children's maturing sense of self.

While no studies have addressed the question of whether and when young children experience and distinguish between the two distinct facets of pride, one study used a cross-sectional approach to delineate a portrait of normative developmental shifts in authentic and hubristic pride across the lifespan (Orth, Robins, & Soto, 2010). These researchers found that authentic pride increased fairly continuously from adolescence to old age, in a trend that paralleled overall well-being. In contrast, hubristic pride peaked in adolescence and young adulthood, declined throughout adulthood, until about age 65, and was stable in old age. These findings suggest that pride follows the maturity principle of personality development (e.g., Roberts, Wood, & Caspi, 2008), wherein maturing social roles are thought to facilitate the experience and expression of socially and intrapsychically adaptive emotions and traits.

Neuroscience of Pride

Neurobiological research on pride remains fairly limited, but several researchers have begun to examine the brain structures and neurochemicals that may be involved in pride experiences. In the single functional magnetic resonance imaging (fMRI) study on pride experiences of which we are aware (Takahashi et al., 2008), greater activation was found in the posterior superior temporal sulcus and left temporal lobe—two brain regions thought to be involved in theory of mind—when participants imagined themselves in pride-eliciting scenarios, compared to when they imagined themselves in neutral scenarios. Although theory of mind may be an important cognitive prerequisite for pride (self-evaluations require the understanding that others can evaluate the self), these researchers had expected to find greater medial prefrontal cortex (mPFC) activation, given previous findings of mPFC activity during negative self-conscious emotional experiences, as well as research linking the mPFC to self-referential thought (e.g., Fossati et al., 2003; Kircher et al., 2002; Takahashi et al., 2004). The failure to find mPFC activity in imagined pride experiences raises a number of questions, but these findings need to be replicated, ideally in studies that compare activation during pride to other positive emotional states, to control for shared variance in positivity or reward.

Other studies have examined the physiological correlates of pride and identified an apparently distinct pattern of cardiac activity. One study found that positive feedback on a laboratory task (assumed to induce pride) led to moderate increases in skin conductance and heart rate, and shifts in heart rate variability indicative of the sympathetic nervous system preparing for controlled action (Fourie et al., 2011). However, another study that compared cardiac arousal levels following pride, anger, and shame inductions found lower arousal for pride compared to that for the negative emotions (Herrald & Tomaka, 2002). Together, these findings may suggest that pride promotes moderate rather than large physiological changes, which help prepare the body for action.

In related work, posing a key component of the pride nonverbal expression—expanded posture—has been shown to promote increases in the hormone testosterone (Carney, Cuddy, & Yap, 2010). This finding may indicate direct links between holding the nonverbal display of pride and its physiological response, or that posing pride led participants to experience pride, which in turn promoted a corresponding hormonal response, consistent with the facial feedback hypothesis (Tomkins, 1962). This theory has been supported by studies showing that individuals who pose certain facial expressions of emotions demonstrate physiological changes corresponding to those emotions (Rosenberg & Ekman, 1994). In the case of pride, an association with testosterone is consistent with long-standing theoretical accounts of pride as the affective mechanism underlying status increases, and with prior research indicating an association between testosterone and dominance (Carré, McCormick, & Hariri, 2011; Mazur, 1983; Mehta & Josephs, 2010; see Tracy et al., 2010, for a review).

These few neurobiological findings are promising and support the suggestion that pride, like other basic emotions, is a bio-logical and fully embodied psychological experience. However, additional research in this area is needed, including experimental studies to uncover the specific neural underpinnings of pride experiences and pride recognition, and direct tests of whether pride experiences are in fact associated with increases in testosterone. Given arguments that distinct neurocircuitry is a prerequisite for categorizing a given phenomenological state as a discrete emotion (Ekman & Cordaro, 2011; Levenson, 2011; Panksepp & Watt, 2011), such future studies may be some of the most important next steps in addressing questions about pride as a distinct positive emotion.

Evolutionary Function of Pride

The findings we just reviewed suggest that pride meets at least one of the central criteria to be considered a "functional universal" (i.e., a psychological entity that evolved to serve a particular adaptive function; Norenzayan & Heine, 2005): Its cross-culturally recognized nonverbal expression is displayed by individuals across cultures in the same contexts and situations. Furthermore, the evidence that pride experiences and pride recognition emerge early in development, and that pride experiences may have distinct neural and physiological correlates, is also consistent with this account. From this perspective, pride is best considered a product of evolutionary processes and thus may be an adaptation for coping with challenges presented by the situations in which it occurs—success, or other opportunities for status enhancement. Several theorists have argued that pride evolved to help individuals transform culturally valued achievements into higher social status, an outcome with clear adaptive benefits (e.g., resource acquisition, mate retention, well-being; e.g., Adler, Epel, Castellazzo, & Ickovics, 2000; Ellis, 1995; von Rueden, Gurven, & Kaplan, 2011).

Based on extant research, there are several ways in which pride may promote status increases. First, a growing body of evidence suggests that the pride nonverbal display functions to signal an individual's deservedness of high status. Behaviors consistent with the pride expression have been observed in the dominance displays of a number of nonhuman animals; these displays are shown when animals seek to exert status or intimidate an opponent. For example, after defeating a rival or prior to an agonistic encounter, high-ranking chimpanzees show "inflated" or "bluff" displays that include behaviors such as arms raised and body expanded—two components of the human pride expression (de Waal, 1989; Martens, Tracy, Cheng, Parr, & Price, 2010). Second, and more directly supporting the link between human pride expressions and status attainment, one study found that individuals manipulated to experience pride prior to engaging in a group task were subsequently perceived by others in the group and outside observers as behaving in a more "dominant" manner, suggesting that the pride experience promoted interpersonal behaviors that increased perceived dominance (Williams & DeSteno, 2009). Results of other studies suggest that those critical dominant behaviors are likely to have been components of the pride expression: Behaviors such as head tilt upward, erect posture, and arms stretched upward and out from the body have been found to be displayed by preschool children who have won a fight (Strayer & Strayer, 1976), high school students who have performed well on a class exam (Weisfeld & Beresford, 1982), children as young as 3 years old in response to task success (Belsky & Domitrovich, 1997; Lewis et al., 1992; Stipek et al., 1992), and sighted and blind adults across cultures who have won an Olympic Games judo match (Tracy & Matsumoto, 2008)—all achievement-related situations that should promote higher social rank. Studies have also shown that posing these pride expression components—most notably, expanded chest—activates feelings of confidence and a tendency to take action, suggesting that the embodiment of pride displays promotes status-related thoughts and motives, perhaps through the facial feedback mechanism mentioned earlier (Fischer, Fischer, Englich, Aydin, & Frey, 2011; Huang, Galinsky, Guenfeld, & Guillory, 2011).

Perhaps the most direct evidence that pride displays function to *communicate* high status comes from studies that addressed this question using implicit measures directly (Shariff & Tracy, 2009). In this work, participants demonstrated an automatic tendency to perceive pride displays as conveying high status, and pride was more strongly implicitly associated with high status than were low-status emotions (e.g., shame, embarrassment), other high-status emotions (e.g., happiness, anger), and emotions not theoretically relevant to status (e.g., disgust, fear). A subsequent study in this same article demonstrated that the association between pride displays and high status cannot be attributed to specific artifacts of the expression's appearance, such as expanded body size or outstretched arms. Furthermore, other research suggests that the status signal uniquely sent by pride displays is powerful enough to override contradictory status cues in the environment (Shariff, Tracy, & Markusoff, 2012). In this work, observers made automatic high-status inferences about targets displaying pride, even when those targets were paired with contextual information indicating that they merited low status. In each of these studies, participants were presented with two identical targets, each displaying different "context-incongruent" emotion expressions. For example, one target was portrayed as obviously high status (i.e., a skilled and respected soccer team captain), but displayed a shame expression, whereas the other target was portrayed as obviously low status (i.e., the soccer team's unskilled, disrespected waterboy) but displayed pride. When participants were probed for their implicit status associations with each target, the low-status but pride-displaying waterboy was automatically judged as higher status than the high-status but shame-displaying captain, suggesting that pride expressions can outweigh contradictory contextual information in informing status judgments. Furthermore, although pride was compared with shame in these studies, other studies in this line of work included a neutral-display comparison, to demonstrate that effects were largely driven by pride rather than shame.

In all of these studies directly assessing perceptions of pride-displaying targets, the communication of high status has consistently been found to occur implicitly; in a study examining explicit status judgments of pride-displaying targets, similar effects emerged but were considerably weaker (Shariff et al., 2012). The automaticity of the pride status signal is relevant to our evolutionary account of pride displays, because if the expression evolved as a prelinguistic, preconscious form of communication, then its perception likely occurs through low-level cognitive processes that can elicit adaptive behavioral responses without any need for conscious reflection (Bargh & Pietromonaco, 1982). If understanding pride's functional message required conscious deliberation, then the expression would be less effective as a rapid source of information.

That said, the most important evidence for our account of pride displays as an *evolved* status signal is the finding that the automatic tendency to perceive these displays as high-status generalizes across diverse populations. Tracy and colleagues (2013) replicated several of the implicit association studies discussed earlier in a highly isolated, traditional, small-scale society on a remote island in Fiji. Despite having no prior computer experience, participants in these studies completed computer-based Implicit Association Tests (Greenwald, McGhee, & Schwartz, 1998) and demonstrated results largely convergent with those of North American university students. Among both groups, pride displays were strongly implicitly associated with high-status concepts. The Fijian villagers who participated in this research hold a set of cultural practices and norms that largely suppress personal displays of status or pride, so the finding that pride displays were nonetheless perceived as indicating high status among these individuals suggests that pride is a universal status signal.

Two Prides, Two Functions?

One question that arises regarding our account of pride as an adaptation for coping with the challenge of status attainment is why such a functional emotion would have a seemingly dysfunctional, hubristic side? How might an antisocial, hubristic pride have evolved? To answer this question, we have drawn on a theoretical account suggesting that humans evolved to attain status using two distinct strategies, labeled *dominance* and *prestige* (Henrich & Gil-White, 2001). In this view, "dominance" is defined as status attained through force, threat, and intimidation, and it contrasts with "prestige," which is status attained through the display of knowledge, valuable skills, and earned respect. Dominant individuals are thought to wield power by controlling costs and benefits in many domains, including access to resources, mates, and well-being. They incite fear in subordinates by withholding resources, and subordinates submit by complying with demands or providing deference. Prestige, in contrast, likely arose in evolutionary history when humans acquired the ability to obtain cultural knowledge from other group members, making it adaptive to selectively attend and defer to the most knowledgeable or skilled others. Prestigious individuals thus acquire power by virtue of their competence and expertise, and by permitting followers to copy them. Support for this account comes from a recent study examining hierarchy formation in small groups of unacquainted individuals, who interacted during a collaborative task. Group members who were rated by their peers as high in *either* dominance or prestige: (1) were viewed by other group members and outside observers as influential over the group's decisions, (2) exerted greater influence over the group's decision making, and (3) received more visual attention (a proxy of status and influence) from observers (Cheng, Tracy, Foulsham, Kingstone, & Henrich, 2013). These findings suggest that both dominance and prestige are likely to be adaptive, in the sense of promoting social influence.

Linking this account to pride, we have argued that the two facets may have separately evolved as the affective mechanisms that, respectively, underpin the dominance and prestige systems (see Cheng et al., 2010; Shariff, Tracy, Cheng, & Henrich, 2010; Tracy et al., 2010). Specifically, hubristic pride may facilitate the attainment of dominance by motivating individuals to behave in an aggressive and intimidating manner, and providing them with a sense of grandiosity and entitlement that allows them to take power rather than earn it, and to feel little empathy for those who get in the way. Indeed, when individuals experience hubristic pride, they evaluate themselves as superior to others, experience a subjective sense of dominance and superiority, and demonstrate low empathy toward those who are different from them (Ashton-James & Tracy, 2012; Tracy et al., 2009). In contrast, authentic pride may facilitate the attainment of prestige by motivating and reinforcing achievements and other indicators of competence, and providing individuals with the feelings of genuine self-confidence that allow them to comfortably demonstrate both social attractiveness and generosity. In order to retain subordinates' respect, prestigious individuals must avoid succumbing to feelings of power and superiority, and authentic pride may allow these individuals to focus on their achievements while maintaining some sense of humility. The findings reviewed earlier, showing that authentic pride is associated with agreeableness, conscientiousness, voluntary moral action, and empathy toward outgroup members (Ashton-James & Tracy, 2012; Hart & Matsuba, 2007; Tracy et al., 2009; Tracy & Robins, 2007c) are consistent with this account. In addition, several prior lines of work suggest a strong connection between pride and achievement motivation (e.g., Herrald & Tomaka, 2002; Pekrun, Elliot, & Maier, 2009; Williams & DeSteno, 2008). These studies did not assess authentic pride in particular, however, so future studies should seek to replicate these results using narrower measures of each pride facet.

In addition to these supportive lines of work, several studies provide direct evidence for the unique theorized associations between each pride facet and the corresponding status-attaining strategy (Cheng et al., 2010). First, in a study assessing dispositional levels of authentic and hubristic pride and dominance and prestige, individuals prone to experiencing authentic pride were found to rate themselves as highly prestigious, whereas those prone to experiencing hubristic pride rated themselves as more dominant. In a second study, this pattern was replicated using peer ratings of dominance and prestige; varsity athletes rated the extent to which team members used each strategy. Individuals high in authentic pride were viewed as prestigious (but not dominant) by their peers, whereas those high in hubristic pride were viewed as dominant (but not prestigious). Follow-up analyses demonstrated that these effects could not be attributed to shared variance in positive affect; when controlling for authentic and hubristic pride, neither peer-rated prestige nor dominance was significantly related to positive affect. These results suggest that

although individuals high in prestige are generally happy, likable, and agreeable (Cheng et al., 2010), the emotion that accounts for their ability to attain high status is not their general positivity but rather their authentic pride. More broadly, these findings suggest that both facets of pride facilitate status attainment, but they do so through distinct mechanisms.

One implication of this account of authentic pride as the emotional mechanism underlying prestige is its suggestion that the pride expression might serve an additional function, beyond communicating high status: it might signal an opportunity for social learning. Given how widely and reliably recognized the pride expression is, even among young children, it is likely that recognizing pride has adaptive benefits for perceivers as well as expressers. In this view, the tendency to display pride in response to success may have coevolved with a tendency to recognize the pride shown by successful others and make functional inferences on that basis (Martens, Tracy, & Shariff, 2012). Specifically, observers may use others' pride displays to determine quickly and effortlessly which group members are high status and therefore likely to have knowledge or expertise that should be copied (if they are prestigious). If this is the case, the ability to rapidly detect and understand the pride expression would benefit observers by biasing their social learning, such that individuals would selectively copy those displaying pride.[1]

Two recent studies tested this account by examining whether financially motivated observers would choose to copy answers to difficult trivia questions provided by another group member (actually a confederate) if the other individual showed pride (Martens & Tracy, 2013). Across both studies, participants copied the answers of pride-displaying confederates more frequently (approximately 80% of the time) than they copied the answers of confederates displaying neutral, shame, or, importantly, happy expressions. This finding further supports the claim that pride's functionality cannot be attributed to positive affect more generally. It also suggests that, to the extent that pride displays are a reliable signal of knowledge or expertise, they are likely to be functional not only for those who display them and acquire higher status, but also for those who observe and automatically interpret pride in others.

Current Directions in Pride Research

Several emerging lines of research have built on the research we have reviewed, suggesting that pride is a distinct and evolved emotion, to examine how pride influences individuals' relationships with others, social behavior, and even mental health. Below, we review some of these exciting new findings.

Pride and Social Interactions

A small but growing literature suggests that pride can have a major impact on interpersonal interactions and social relationships. One line of research exemplifying this trend found that pride displays influence sexual attraction in gender-specific ways (Tracy & Beall, 2011). In a series of four studies using different methodological approaches, men who displayed pride were found to be most attractive to women, compared to men who displayed neutral, shame, or happy displays (male happy displays were, in fact, particularly unattractive). In contrast, women who displayed pride were perceived by male viewers as unattractive compared to women who displayed happy or shame expressions, and generally less attractive than women who displayed neutral expressions. These findings are consistent with the social status account of pride and evolutionary mating theory suggesting that high-status men are perceived as having high mate value, whereas for women status should be less relevant to mate quality. However, these findings are also consistent with social constructivist accounts suggesting that men should appear high status and women submissive, so more research is needed to tease apart these competing explanations.

In another line of work on pride's impact on relationships, several studies found that pride influences prejudicial attitudes (e.g., Ashton-James & Tracy, 2012). Across four studies, a sharp difference emerged between the two facets of pride, in that participants manipulated to experience authentic pride responded with greater positivity toward outgroup members, whereas those manipulated to experience hubristic pride responded with hostility toward these individuals, and even displayed a propensity to discriminate against them. These effects were mediated by empathic concern for outgroup members, suggesting that authentic pride increases, and hubristic pride decreases, empathy toward those who are different. What is particularly surprising about these studies is that results emerged from both dispositional pride tendencies *and* momentarily manipulated pride states, suggesting that any person can become more or less prejudicial depending on the form of pride he or she happens to be experiencing. Given that pride is most typically experienced by high-status individuals—precisely those who have the power to hire, fire, or discriminate against others—these findings have important implications for pride in real-world settings. In related work, researchers are also beginning to examine the ways in which collective pride (e.g., pride in one's nation or social group) can influence intergroup relationships (e.g., Kavetsos, 2011; Luksyte & Avery, 2010; Reeskens & Wright, 2011). By taking into account the findings reviewed earlier suggesting that pride is an evolved part of human nature that has two distinct facets with markedly divergent outcomes, we expect that these emerging research trends will contribute enormously to our understanding of the emotions that underlie nationalism, patriotism, and intergroup hostility and alliances.

Finally, a third set of studies on pride and relationships found effects of pride on perceptions of similarity to others (Oveis, Horberg, & Keltner, 2010). These studies compared pride and compassion, and found that those who felt pride—at both a dispositional and momentary state level—experienced a sense of greater similarity toward strong social groups (e.g., professional athletes), whereas those who felt compassion experienced a sense of greater similarity toward weaker social groups (e.g., young children, the elderly). These studies did not distinguish between authentic and hubristic pride, so it is unclear whether both facets promote these feelings, but they are consistent with the high-status account of pride, given that feeling similar to strong others may motivate power seeking and achievement striving.

Pride and Psychopathology

Consistent with the findings reviewed earlier suggesting that authentic pride is linked to well-being, recent studies have demonstrated that pride can play an ameliorative role in the trajectory of certain mood disorders, such as depression and bipolar disorder (BD). Pride has been found to negatively predict current manic symptoms and future depressive symptoms among individuals at-risk for BD (Gruber & Johnson, 2009; Gruber et al., 2009). In addition, pride may even be diagnostic of these disorders; highly depressive individuals show blunted reactivity when presented with pride-evoking film clips, despite normal reactivity to happiness-evoking clips (Gruber, Oveis, Keltner, & Johnson, 2011).

In contrast to these findings that suggest pride is associated with mental health, other studies indicate that individuals who experience high levels of pride are at greater risk for developing BD (Gruber & Johnson, 2009), and that pride predicts the development of BD above and beyond other positive emotions (e.g., love, compassion). Given the aforementioned positive relation between hubristic pride and unrealistic life goals (Carver et al., 2010), and the finding from this work that those at risk for BD engage in unrealistic goal setting (Gruber & Johnson, 2009), it seems likely that the form of pride most relevant to BD is hubristic pride. That said, this research would benefit greatly from studies that make an explicit distinction between the pride facets, which likely have important consequences for mental health.

Conclusion

A relatively large body of research on pride has emerged in the past decade; these studies suggest that pride is a fundamental emotion in the biological and evolutionary sense, and in the social and interpersonal sense. It plays a major role in interpersonal and, in all likelihood, intergroup functioning, and, importantly, also shapes each individual's self-concept and self-esteem. Perhaps most important, pride is the single most important emotion underpinning the attainment and maintenance of social status; pride experiences motivate status striving in a variety of ways, and pride displays communicate status-relevant information to others. We hope that the research reviewed in this chapter provides a foundation for future work addressing a range of remaining questions about pride and its antecedents, consequences, and impact on the social world.

Note

1. One issue raised by this account is whether observers benefit from recognizing pride shown by dominant rather than prestigious individuals. Though future research is needed to address this issue, one possibility that is consistent with the extant evidence (Shariff et al., 2012; Shariff & Tracy, 2009; Tracy & Prehn, 2012) is that pride displays provide general information about a target's deservingness of high status, and additional contextual information is needed to determine whether the target is prestigious or dominant and should therefore be copied or feared.

References

Adler, N. E., Epel, E. S., Castellazzo, G., & Ickovics, J. R. (2000). Relationship of subjective and objective social status with psychological and physiological functioning: Preliminary data in healthy, white women. *Health Psychology, 19,* 586–592.

Ashton-James, C. E., & Tracy, J. L. (2012). Pride and prejudice: Feelings about the self influence judgments about others. *Personality and Social Psychology Bulletin, 38,* 466–476.

Bargh, J. A., & Pietromonaco, P. (1982). Automatic information processing and social perception: The influence of trait information presented outside of conscious awareness on impression formation. *Journal of Personality and Social Psychology, 43,* 437–449.

Bartlett, M. Y., & DeSteno, D. (2006). Gratitude and prosocial behavior: Helping when it costs you. *Psychological Science, 17,* 319–325.

Belsky, J., & Domitrovich, C. (1997). Temperament and parenting antecedents of individual difference in three-year-old boys' pride and shame reactions. *Child Development, 68,* 456–466.

Campos, J. J., Barrett, K. C., Lamb, M. E., Goldsmith, H. H., & Stenberg, C. (1983). Socioemotional development. In M. M. Haith & J.

J. Campos (Eds.), *Handbook of child psychology: Infancy and developmental psychobiology* (Vol. 2, pp. 783–915). New York: Wiley.

Carney, D. R., Cuddy, A. J. C., & Yap, A. J. (2010). Power posing: Brief non-verbal displays affect neuroendocrine levels and risk tolerance. *Psychological Science, 21,* 1363–1368.

Carré, J. M., McCormick, C. M., & Hariri, A. R. (2011). The social neuroendocrinology of human aggression. *Psychoneuroendocrinology, 36,* 935–944.

Carver, C. S., Sinclair, S., & Johnson, S. L. (2010). Authentic and hubristic pride: Differential relations to aspects of goal regulation, affect, and self-control. *Journal of Research in Personality, 44,* 698–703.

Cheng, J. T., Tracy, J. L., Foulsham, T., & Kingstone, A., & Henrich, J. (2013). Two ways to the top: Evidence that dominance and prestige are distinct yet viable avenues to social rank and influence. *Journal of Personality and Social Psychology, 104*(1), 103–125.

Cheng, J. T., Tracy, J. L., & Henrich, J. (2010). Pride, personality, and the evolutionary foundations of human social status. *Evolution and Human Behavior, 31,* 334–347.

de Waal, F. (1989). *Peacemaking among primates.* Cambridge, MA: Harvard University Press.

Ekman, P., & Cordaro, D. (2011). What is meant by calling emotions basic? *Emotion Review, 3,* 364–370.

Ekman, P., Friesen, W. V., O'Sullivan, M., Chan, A., Diacoyanni- Tarlatzis, I, Heider, K., et al. (1987). Universals and cultural differences in the judgment of facial expressions of emotion. *Journal of Personality and Social Psychology, 53,* 712–717.

Ekman, P., Sorenson, E. R., & Friesen, W. V. (1969). Pan-cultural elements in facial displays of emotion. *Science, 164,* 86–88.

Ellis, L. (1995). Dominance and reproductive success among nonhuman animals: A cross-species comparison. *Ethology and Sociobiology, 16,* 257–333.

Ellsworth, P. C., & Smith, C. A. (1988). Shades of joy: Patterns of appraisal differentiating pleasant emotions. *Cognition and Emotion, 2,* 301–331.

Fischer, J., Fischer, P., Englich, B., Aydin, N., & Frey, D. (2011). Empower my decisions: The effects of power gestures on confirmatory information processing. *Journal of Experimental Social Psychology, 47,* 1146–1154.

Fossati, P., Hevenor, S. J., Graham, S. J., Grady, C., Keightley, M. L., Craik, F., et al. (2003). In search of the emotional self: An fMRI study using positive and negative emotional words. *American Journal of Psychiatry, 160,* 1938–1945.

Fourie, M. M., Rauch, H. G. L., Morgan, B. E., Ellis, G. F. R., Jordaan, E. R., & Thomas, K. F. G. (2011). Guilt and pride are heartfelt, but not equally so. *Psychophysiology, 48,* 888–999.

Fredrickson, B. L. (1998). What good are positive emotions? *Review of General Psychology, 2,* 300–319.

Graham, S., & Weiner, B. (1986). From an attributional theory of emotion to developmental psychology: A round-trip ticket? *Social Cognition, 4,* 152–179.

Greenwald, A. G., McGhee, D. E., & Schwartz, J. L. K. (1998). Measuring individual differences in implicit cognition: The implicit association test. *Journal of Personality and Social Psychology, 74,* 1464–1480.

Griskevicius, V., Shiota, M. N., & Neufeld, S. L. (2010). Influence of positive emotions on persuasion processing: A functional evolutionary approach. *Emotion, 10,* 190–206.

Gruber, J., Culver, J. L., Johnson, S. L., Nam, J. Y., Keller, K. L., & Ketter, T. A. (2009). Do positive emotions predict symptomatic change in bipolar disorder? *Bipolar Disorders, 11,* 330–336.

Gruber, J., & Johnson, S. L. (2009). Positive emotional traits and ambitious goals among people at risk for mania: The need for specificity. *International Journal of Cognitive Therapy, 2,* 179–190.

Gruber, J., Oveis, C., Keltner, D., & Johnson, S. L. (2011). A discrete emotions approach to positive emotion disturbance in depression. *Cognition and Emotion, 25,* 40–52.

Harris, P. L., Olthof, T., Terwogt, M. M., & Hardman, C. E. (1987). Children's knowledge of the situations that provoke emotion. *International Journal of Behavioral Development, 10,* 319–343.

Hart, D., & Karmel, M. P. (1996). Self-awareness and self-knowledge in humans, apes, and monkeys. In A. E. Russon, K. A. Bard, & S. T. Parker (Eds.), *Reaching into thought: The minds of the great apes* (pp. 325–347). New York: Cambridge University Press.

Hart, D., & Matsuba, M. K. (2007). The development of pride and moral life. In J. L. Tracy, R. W. Robins, & J. P. Tangney (Eds.), *The self-conscious emotions: Theory and research.* (pp. 114–133). New York: Guilford Press.

Harter, S. (1983). Developmental perspective on the self-system. In E. M. Hetherington (Ed.) & P. H. Mussen (Series Ed.), *Handbook of child psychology: Vol 4. Socialization, personality, and social development* (4th ed., pp. 275–385). New York: Wiley.

Heine, S. J., Lehman, D. R., Markus, H. R., & Kitayama, S. (1999). Is there a universal need for positive self-regard? *Psychological Review, 106,* 766–794.

Henrich, J., & Gil-White, F. J. (2001). The evolution of prestige: Freely conferred deference as a mechanism for enhancing the benefits of cultural transmission. *Evolution and Human Behavior, 22,* 165–196.

Herrald, M. M., & Tomaka, J. (2002). Patterns of emotion-specific appraisal, coping, and cardiovascular reactivity during an ongoing emotional episode. *Journal of Personality and Social Psychology, 83,* 434–450.

Huang, L., Galinsky, A. D., Gruenfeld, D. H., & Guillory, L. E. (2011). Powerful postures versus powerful roles: Which is the proximate correlate of thought and behavior? *Psychological Science, 22,* 95–102.

Imada, T., & Ellsworth, P. C. (2011). Proud Americans and lucky Japanese: Cultural differences in appraisal and corresponding emotion. *Emotion, 11,* 329–345.

Izard, C. E. (1971). *The face of emotion.* East Norwalk, CT: Appleton-Century-Crofts.

Kavetsos, G. (2011). National pride: War minus the shooting. *Social Indicators Research, 106,* 173–185.

Keltner, D. (1995). Signs of appeasement: Evidence for the distinct displays of embarrassment, amusement, and shame. *Journal of Personality and Social Psychology, 61,* 441–454.

Keltner, D., Haidt, J., & Shiota, M. N. (2006). Social functionalism and the evolution of emotions. In M. Schaller, J. A. Simpson, & D. T. Kenrick (Eds.), *Evolution and social psychology* (pp. 115–142). Madison, CT: Psychosocial Press.

Kiesler, D. J. (1983). The 1982 Interpersonal Circle: A taxonomy for complementarity in human transactions. *Psychological Review, 90,* 185–214.

Kircher, T. T. J., Brammer, M., Bullmore, E., Simmons, A., Bartels, M., & David, A. S. (2002). The neural correlates of intentional and incidental self processing. *Neuropsychologia, 40,* 683–692.

Kornilaki, E. N., & Chloverakis, G. (2004). The situational antecedents of pride and happiness: Developmental and domain differences. *British Journal of Developmental Psychology, 22,* 605–619.

Lagattuta, K. H., & Thompson, R. A. (2007). The development of self-conscious emotions: Cognitive processes and social influences. In J. L. Tracy, R. W. Robins, & J. P. Tangney (Eds.), *The self-conscious emotions: Theory and research* (pp. 91–113). New York: Guilford Press.

Levenson, R. W. (2011). Basic emotion questions. *Emotion Review, 3,* 379–386.

Lewis, M. (2000). Self-conscious emotions: Embarrassment, pride, shame, and guilt. In M. Lewis & J. M. Haviland-Jones (Eds.), *Handbook of emotions* (2nd ed., pp. 623–636). New York: Guilford Press.

Lewis, M., Alessandri, S. M., & Sullivan, M. W. (1992). Differences in shame and pride as a function of children's gender and task difficulty. *Child Development, 63,* 630–638.

Luksyte, A., & Avery, D. R. (2010). The effects of citizenship dissimilarity and national pride on attitudes towards immigrants: Investigating mediators and moderators of intergroup contact. *International Journal of Intercultural Relations, 34,* 629–641.

Markus, H. R., & Kitayama, S. (1991). Culture and the self: Implications for cognition, emotion, and motivation. *Psychological Review, 98,* 224–253.

Martens, J. P., & Tracy, J. L. (2013). The emotional origins of a social learning bias: Does the pride expression cue copying? *Social Psychological and Personality Science, 4,* 492–499.

Martens, J. P., Tracy, J. L., Cheng, J. T., Parr, L. A., & Price, S. (2010, January). *Do the chimpanzee bluff display and human pride expression share evolutionary origins?* Poster presented at the Society for Personality and Social Psychology Preconference on Evolutionary Psychology, Las Vegas, NV.

Martens, J. P., Tracy, J. L., & Shariff, A. F. (2012). Status signals: Adaptive benefits of displaying and observing the non-verbal expressions of pride and shame. *Cognition and Emotion, 26,* 390–406.

Mazur, A. (1983). Hormones, aggression, and dominance in humans. In B. B. Svare (Ed.), *Hormones and aggressive behavior* (pp. 535–562). New York: Plenum Press.

Mehta, P. H., & Josephs, R. A. (2010). Testosterone and cortisol jointly regulate dominance: Evidence for a dual-hormone hypothesis. *Hormones and Behavior, 58,* 898–906.

Nelson, N. L., & Russell, J. A. (2011). When dynamic, the head and face alone can express pride. *Emotion, 11,* 990–993.

Norenzayan, A., & Heine, S. J. (2005). Psychological universals: What are they and how can we know? *Psychological Bulletin, 131,* 763–784.

Orth, U., Robins, R. W., & Soto, C. J. (2010). Tracking the trajectory of shame, guilt, and pride across the lifespan. *Journal of Personality and Social Psychology, 99,* 1061–1071

Oveis, C., Horberg, E. J., & Keltner, D. (2010). Compassion, pride, and social intuitions of self–other similarity. *Journal of Personality and Social Psychology, 98,* 618–630.

Panksepp, J., & Watt, D. (2011). What is basic about basic emotions?: Lasting lessons from affective neuroscience. *Emotion Review, 3,* 387–396.

Pekrun, R., Elliot, A. J., & Maier, M. A. (2009). Achievement goals and achievement emotions: Testing a model of their joint relations with academic performance. *Journal of Educational Psychology, 101,* 115–135.

Reeskens, T., & Wright, M. (2011). Subjective well-being and national satisfaction: Taking seriously the "proud of what" question. *Psychological Science, 22,* 1460–1462.

Roberts, B. W., Wood, D., & Caspi, A. (2008). The development of personality traits in adulthood. In O. P. John, R. W. Robins, & L. A. Pervin (Eds.), *Handbook of personality: Theory and research* (pp. 375–398). New York: Guilford Press.

Roseman, I. J. (1991). Appraisal determinants of discrete emotions. *Cognition and Emotion, 5,* 161–200.

Rosenberg, E. L., & Ekman, P. (1994). Coherence between expressive and experiential systems in emotion. *Cognition and Emotion, 8,* 201–229.

Sauter, D. A., & Scott, S. K. (2007). More than one kind of happiness: Can we recognize vocal expressions of different positive states? *Motivation and Emotion, 31,* 192–199.

Seligman, M. E. P., & Csikszentmihalyi, M. (2000). Positive psychology: An introduction. *American Psychologist, 55,* 5–14.

Shariff, A. F., & Tracy, J. L. (2009). Knowing who's boss: Implicit perceptions of status from the nonverbal expression of pride. *Emotion, 9,* 631–639.

Shariff, A. F., Tracy, J. L., Cheng, J. T., & Henrich, J. (2010). Further thoughts on the evolution of pride/s two facets: A response to Clark. *Emotion Review, 2,* 399–400.

Shariff, A. F., Tracy, J. L., & Markusoff, J. (2012). (Implicitly) judging a book by its cover: The power of pride and shame expressions in shaping judgments of social status. *Personality and Social Psychology Bulletin, 38*(9), 1178–1193.

Shi, Y., Chung, J., Cheng, J. T., Tracy, J. L., Robins, R. W., Chen, X., et al. (2013). *Cross-cultural evidence for the two-facet structure of pride.* Manuscript under review.

Simon-Thomas, E. R., Keltner, D. J., Sauter, D., Sinicropi-Yao, L., & Abramson, A. (2009). The voice conveys specific emotions: Evidence from vocal burst displays. *Emotion, 9,* 838–846.

Stipek, D., Recchia, S., & McClintic, S. (1992). Self-evaluation in young children. *Monographs of the Society for Research in Child Development, 57,* 100.

Strayer, F. F., & Strayer, J. (1976). An ethological analysis of social agonism and dominance relations among preschool children. *Child Development, 47,* 980–989.

Takahashi, H., Matsuura, M., Koeda, M., Yahata, N., Suhara, T., Kato, M., et al. (2008). Brain activations during judgments of positive self-conscious emotion and positive basic emotion: Pride and joy. *Cerebral Cortex, 18,* 898–903.

Takahashi, H., Yahata, N., Koeda, M., Matsuda, T., Asai, K., & Okubo, Y. (2004). Brain activation associated with evaluative processes of guilt and embarrassment: An fMRI study. *NeuroImage, 23,* 967–974.

Tangney, J. P., & Fisher, K. W. (Eds.). (1995). *Self-conscious emotions: The psychology of shame, guilt, embarrassment, and pride.* New York: Guilford Press.

Tangney, J. P., Wagner, P., & Gramzow, R. (1989). *The Test of Self-Conscious Affect.* Fairfax, VA: George Mason University.

Thompson, R. A. (1989). Causal attributions and children's emotional understanding. In C. Saarni & P. L. Harris (Eds.), *Children's understanding of emotion* (pp. 117–150). New York: Cambridge University Press.

Tomkins, S. S. (1962). *Affect imagery consciousness: The positive affects* (Vol. 1). New York: Springer.

Tracy, J. L., & Beall, A. (2011). Happy guys finish last: The impact of emotional expressions on sexual attraction. *Emotion, 11,* 1379–1387.

Tracy, J. L., Cheng, J. T., Martens, J. P., & Robins, R. W. (2011). The affective core of narcissism: Inflated by pride, deflated by shame. In W. K. Campbell & J. Miller (Eds.), *Handbook of narcissism and narcissistic personality disorder* (pp. 330–343). New York: Wiley.

Tracy, J. L., Cheng, J. T., Robins, R. W., & Trzesniewski, K. H. (2009). Authentic and hubristic pride: The affective core of self-esteem and narcissism. *Self and Identity, 8*, 196–213.

Tracy, J. L., & Matsumoto, D. (2008). The spontaneous display of pride and shame: Evidence for biologically innate nonverbal displays. *Proceedings of the National Academy of Sciences, 105*, 11655–11660.

Tracy, J. L., & Prehn, C. (2012). The use of contextual knowledge to differentiate hubristic and authentic pride from a single non-verbal expression. *Cognition and Emotion, 26*, 14–24.

Tracy, J. L., & Randles, D. (2011). Four models of basic emotions: A review of Ekman and Cordaro, Izard, Levenson, and Panksepp and Watt. *Emotion Review, 3*, 397–405.

Tracy, J. L., & Robins, R. W. (2004a). Putting the self into self-conscious emotions: A theoretical model. *Psychological Inquiry, 15*, 103–125.

Tracy, J. L., & Robins, R. W. (2004b). Show your pride: Evidence for a discrete emotion expression. *Psychological Science, 15*, 194–197.

Tracy, J. L., & Robins, R. W. (2007a). Emerging insights into the nature and function of pride. *Current Directions in Psychological Science, 16*, 147–150.

Tracy, J. L., & Robins, R. W. (2007b). The prototypical pride expression: Development of a nonverbal behavioral coding system. *Emotion, 7*, 789–801.

Tracy, J. L., & Robins, R. W. (2007c). The psychological structure of pride: A tale of two facets. *Journal of Personality and Social Psychology, 92*, 506–525.

Tracy, J. L., & Robins, R. W. (2008a). The automaticity of emotion recognition. *Emotion, 7*, 81–95.

Tracy, J. L., & Robins, R. W. (2008b). The nonverbal expression of pride: Evidence for cross-cultural recognition. *Journal of Personality and Social Psychology, 94*, 516–530.

Tracy, J. L., & Robins, R. W. (in press). Conceptual and empirical strengths of the authentic/hubristic model of pride. *Emotion*.

Tracy, J. L., Robins, R. W., & Lagattuta, K. H. (2005). Can children recognize the pride expression? *Emotion, 5*, 251–257.

Tracy, J. L., Robins, R. W. & Schriber, R. A. (2009). Development of a FACS-verified set of basic and self-conscious emotion expressions. *Emotion, 9*, 554–559.

Tracy, J. L., Shariff, A. F., & Cheng, J. T. (2010). A naturalist's view of pride. *Emotion Review, 2*, 163–177.

Tracy, J. L., Shariff, A. F., Zhao, W., & Henrich, J. (2013). Cross-cultural evidence that the pride expression is a universal automatic status signal. *Journal of Experimental Psychology: General, 142*, 163–180.

von Rueden, C., Gurven, M., & Kaplan, H. (2011). Why do men seek status?: Fitness payoffs to dominance and prestige. *Proceedings of the Royal Society B: Biological Sciences, 278*, 2223–2232.

Weiner, B. (1985). An attributional theory of achievement motivation and emotion. *Psychological Review, 92*, 548–573.

Weisfeld, G. E., & Beresford, J. M. (1982). Erectness of posture as an indicator of dominance or success in humans. *Motivation and Emotion, 6*, 113–131.

Williams, L. A., & DeSteno, D. (2008). Pride and perseverance: The motivational role of pride. *Journal of Personality and Social Psychology, 94*, 1007–1017.

Williams, L., & DeSteno, D. (2009). Pride: Adaptive social emotion or seventh sin? *Psychological Science, 20*, 284–288.

CHAPTER 18

Romantic Love

Lisa M. Diamond

The scientific study of human love has undergone dramatic changes during the past several decades. As recently as 1975, Senator Henry Proxmire took the floor of the Senate to publicly denounce the National Science Foundation's award of a research grant to Ellen Berscheid and Elaine Hatfield for the study of romantic love, arguing that there was no hope that the methods and tools of science could be fruitfully applied to this topic (Hatfield, 2001). Nearly 40 years later, it is clear that nothing could be further from the truth. The explosion of scientific research on romantic love and intimate relationships demonstrates that there are few subjects in which the average American is *more* interested than the science of romantic love. Furthermore, this body of research has reliably shown that the experience of love plays a fundamental role in human health and well-being across the lifespan, fostering the development and maintenance of adaptive psychological, behavioral, and physiological responses to the stresses and strains of everyday life (Repetti, Taylor, & Seeman, 2002; Ryff, Singer, Wing, & Love, 2001). Among the most compelling examples of the critical importance of love is the fact that knowing whether an individual "feels loved" significantly and independently predicts his or her future risk of cardiovascular disease (Seeman & Syme, 1987).

Accordingly, extensive research has attempted to understand the basic nature, dynamics, and underlying biology of romantic love. What exactly *is* love, and how does it develop over the lifespan? What are its neurobiological underpinnings? What explains the links that have been detected between the experience of love and long-term mental and physical health? What are the similarities and differences between romantic love and other forms of love? This chapter provides an overview of contemporary research addressing these questions and identifies several key directions for future research.

Love as an Emotion-Motivation System

Aron and Aron (1991) defined romantic love as "the constellation of behaviors, cognitions, and emotions associated with a desire to enter or maintain a close relationship with a specific other person" (p. 26). Notable in this definition is the *multifactorial* nature of love (involving behaviors, cognitions, and emotions) and the *motivational* force of love (i.e., *desire* to enter or maintain a relationship), and its focus on a *single target*. Among the oldest debates about love is whether this complex experience should be conceptualized as a basic emotion, similar to happiness, fear, and disgust (reviewed by Shaver,

Morgan, & Wu, 1996). Studies assessing lay conceptions of love have found that most individuals consider love to be an emotion, similar in valence and intensity to joy (Fehr & Russell, 1984; Shaver, Schwartz, Kirson, O'Connor, & Parrott, 2001), especially during moments when their experience of love for a specific individual is particularly strong and/or salient (Gonzaga, Keltner, Londahl, & Smith, 2001). Yet numerous emotion theorists and relationship researchers have argued against the notion of love as a basic emotion, noting that it does not consistently meet the full range of criteria that have been posited by different scholars for basic emotions (i.e., that it involve distinctive and cross-culturally intelligible signals; that it have a unique physiological signature; that it have clear-cut neural substrates; and that it be relatively brief, sudden, and unbidden; reviewed by Shaver et al., 1996). Some researchers have adopted a cognitive perspective to love, examining how laypeople organize various features (and types) of love at a conceptual level, as cognitive prototypes that comprise both central and peripheral features (Fehr, 1988, 2006; Fehr & Russell, 1991). Aron and Aron's (1986) self-expansion model posits that love involves the process of increasingly incorporating the love object's perspectives and resources into one's own self-concept, and that the speed of this process (in new love relationships) contributes to the intense feelings of exhilaration and preoccupation of passionate love. Sternberg (1998) argued that experiences of love could be viewed as narratives representing the constellation of expectations and preconceptions that individuals unconsciously draw upon when selecting romantic partners.

Perhaps the most influential current conceptualization of love is that of Aron and colleagues (2005; Aron & Aron, 1991; Xu et al., 2010), who view love as a goal-oriented motivational state that *elicits* strong emotions (and often a mixture of emotions, as noted by Izard, 1991). This overall "emotion-motivation system" (Fisher, 1998) functions to motivate specific behaviors toward the love object, most notably proximity seeking, in service of the evolutionary goal of keeping reproductive partners together to rear their offspring successfully (Fisher, 1998). Similarly, Gonzaga and colleagues (2001) argued that love functions as an emotional "commitment device," motivating individuals to sustain their tie to their current partner *and* to decrease their motivation to seek out alternative partners.

In the end, debating whether love is best conceptualized as an emotion, a motivational state, or some combination of the two appears to be less important than understanding the basic nature, functional dynamics, and health implications of this experience at affective, cognitive, behavioral, and biological levels. Toward this end, we begin by making critical distinctions between different *types* of love and reviewing what is known about each type at multiple levels of analysis.

Passionate versus Companionate Love

Most contemporary scholars of love acknowledge a basic distinction between "passionate" love, which typically characterizes the earliest stages of a new romantic relationship, and "companionate" love, which characterizes longer-term affectional bonds. Passionate love is sometimes denoted "infatuation" or "limerence" and is characterized by heightened preoccupation with the love object, proximity seeking, and high rates of sexual desire and behavior (Hatfield, 1987; Hatfield & Rapson, 2006; Tennov, 1979). In contrast, companionate love is characterized by feelings of calm, security, empathy, mutual comfort seeking, giving of the self for the good of the other, and deep affection (Hatfield, 1987; Hazan & Shaver, 1987).

The most influential early research on passionate love was conducted by Tennov (1979), who interviewed over 1,000 individuals about their experiences of passionate love (or "limerence" in her terminology) and meticulously documented the common features of their experiences, such as intense desires for proximity and physical contact, resistance to separation, feelings of excitement and euphoria when receiving attention and affection from the partner, fascination with the partner's behavior and appearance, extreme sensitivity to the love partner's moods and signs of interest, and intrusive thoughts of the partner. Importantly, Jankowiak and Fischer (1992) found that the very same phenomenological features also characterized descriptions of passionate love collected by anthropologists in hundreds of different cultures, supporting the notion that passionate love represents a universal human capacity. Significant contributions to the study of passionate love have been made by Hatfield and Sprecher (1986), who developed a questionnaire measure (called the Passionate Love Scale) specifically designed to assess the intensity of individuals' passionate love experience (sample items include "I would rather be with X than anybody else"; "Sometimes I can't control my thoughts. They are obsessively on X"; "I have an endless appetite for affection from X").

Passionate love appears to be a time-dependent experience, declining progressively over the first several years of a new relationship (Huesmann, 1980; Sternberg, 1986; Traupmann & Hatfield, 1981; Tucker & Aron, 1993). Yet during the same period, companionate love between partners correspondingly increases (Berscheid & Hatfield, 1969; Sternberg, 1986). Hence, passionate love and companionate love are not simply different *types* of love, experienced for different types of partners, but different *stages* in the development of a single love relationship. For example, Sprecher and Regan (1998) collected relationship descriptions from over 200 couples at various stages of relationship development and found that the longer couples had been together, the fewer "passionate" and the more "companionate" characteristics their relationship contained. Zeifman and Hazan (1997) provided a plausible rationale for the distinction between early-stage passionate love and longer-term companionate love: They noted that the establishment of an enduring, long-term affectional bond between two individuals (the type of bond characterized by companionate love) takes time to develop, and requires extended proximity and close contact between partners. Accordingly, the intense preoccupation, proximity seeking, and euphoria that characterize early-stage passionate love provide a potent motivator to keep new partners together long enough for an enduring affectional bond to develop. Fisher (2004) viewed the transition between passionate and companionate love with respect to the evolutionary goal of reproduction, arguing that passionate love keeps reproductive partners together long enough to rear their resulting offspring past the period of greatest vulnerability (i.e., the first few years of life). However, studies suggest that the decline in passionate love in long-term relationships is not, in fact, a foregone conclusion. Several large-scale surveys have found that a small subset of long-term couples report that they continue to experience intense feelings of romantic passion for one another (Acevedo & Aron, 2009; Tucker & Aron, 1993), and experimental research suggests that the couples most likely to preserve feelings of intense romantic passion are those who pursue novel, arousing activities with one another (Aron, Norman, Aron, McKenna, & Heyman, 2000).

Neurobiological Research on Passionate Love

Perhaps the most intriguing body of new research on the distinct characteristics of passionate love comes from functional neuroimaging (most commonly functional magnetic resonance imaging [fMRI], but also positron emission tomography [PET] and, less often, electroencephalography [EEG]). PET and fMRI techniques measure changes in blood flow and oxygenation in response to the presentation of visual, auditory, or tactile stimuli, under the assumption that these changes correspond to regional neural activity. Responses to experimental stimuli are contrasted with responses to control stimuli in order to identify stimulus-specific patterns of brain activity (i.e., responses to sexually arousing photographs or to a photograph of one's romantic partner). The most relevant data on the neurobiological bases of romantic love comes from studies by Bartels and Zeki (2000), Aron and colleagues (Acevedo, Aron, Fisher, & Brown, 2011; Aron et al., 2005; Xu et al., 2010), and Ortigue, Bianchi-Demicheli, Hamilton, and Grafton (2007). The foundational early work of Bartels and Zeki (2000) focused on early-stage passionate love, and found that when participants viewed pictures of their loved one (vs. viewing pictures of friends that were comparable to the loved one with respect to age, sex, and familiarity), activation was detected in the middle insula, anterior cingulate cortex (ACC), putamen, retrsoplenial cortex, and caudate. In contrast, deactivation was detected in the amygdala. The insula and ACC are typically associated with emotion and attentional states, whereas the retrosplenial cortex is involved in episodic memory recall, imagination, and planning for the future. The putamen and caudate are associated with motivational states and reward, while the amygdala processes fear and experiences of threat.

Aron and colleagues (2005) also focused on early-stage passionate love and found that when participants looked at the face of their partner and thought about pleasurable, non-sexual events involving the partner, activation was detected in the right caudate and the ventral tegmental area (VTA), whereas the amygdala showed deactivation (similar to Bartels and Zeki's [2000] findings). Additionally, they found that individuals who reported more intense experiences of passionate love (as assessed with the aforementioned Passionate Love Scale; Hatfield & Sprecher, 1986) showed correspondingly greater activation in the caudate. These findings are in accord with numerous other studies documenting specific activation of the caudate and the VTA during passionate love (Acevedo et al., 2011; Aron et al., 2005; Bartels & Zeki, 2000; Ortigue et al., 2007; Xu et al., 2010), and support the notion that the intense motivation of passionate love is mediated by central release of dopamine. The brain's fundamental reward circuitry comprises a network of dopaminergic projections to the prefrontal cortex from the midbrain region, through the hypothalamus, and in mammals this network plays a critical role in the rewarding nature of social contact. The caudate nucleus contains the vast majority of the brain's dopamine receptors, and the VTA is the origin of dopamine cells that project to numerous brain regions involved in the brain's reward system, including the prefrontal cortex and the caudal brainstem. The fact that these brain regions have shown consistent activation in neuroimaging studies of passionate love is consistent with the fact that the distinct phenomenology of passionate love—intense motivation and goal-seeking, focused attention on the love object, high levels of energy and positive affect—is known to be associated with central release of dopamine (as well as norepinephrine), as reviewed by Fisher (1998).

Ortigue and colleagues (2007) made a notable contribution to the growing body of evidence for passionate love as a dopaminergically mediated motivational state by comparing romantic passion to other forms of passion. Specifically, they compared brain activation in response to subliminal primes of the love object's name with brain activation in response to "generalized passion" primes (i.e., primes describing activities about which individuals had reported feeling passionate). This allowed for the identification of regions specifically associated with *romantic* passion. Results revealed love-specific activation in the bilateral fusiform regions and bilateral angular gyri, which are involved in the integration of abstract representations, particularly abstract representations of the self, and call upon episodic retrieval processes. Hence, this work builds on the emerging view of romantic love as a dopaminergically mediated motivational state by demonstrating that love also fundamentally involves a self-representational component, consistent with Aron and Aron's (1986) model of love as involving the inclusion of the beloved into one's own self-concept. Finally, research using priming tasks (Bianchi-Demicheli, Grafton, & Ortigue, 2006; Ortigue et al., 2007) has also demonstrated that the dopaminergically mediated motivational state of romantic love has powerful effects on cognition, facilitating performance on lexical decision tasks. This body of work is particularly important for demonstrating that although the experience of love may be localized in specific brain regions, its *effects* on other brain functions can be broad and pervasive due to a "love enhanced" neural associative network (Bianchi-Demicheli et al., 2006).

Passionate Love versus Sexual Desire

Among the oldest and most important questions in the study of passionate love concerns its similarities to and differences from sexual desire (typically defined as "a wish, need, or drive to seek out sexual objects or to engage in sexual activities" [Regan & Berscheid, 1995, p. 346]). Historically, sexual desire was presumed to be a necessary precursor for passionate love (reviewed and critiqued by Diamond, 2003), but current theory and research demonstrate that although passionate love and sexual desire frequently occur in concert, they are nonetheless functionally independent social-behavioral systems with distinct evolutionary functions and distinct neural bases (Diamond, 2003; Fisher, 1998; Hatfield, 1987; Hatfield & Rapson, 1987). Most notably, whereas sexual desire is oriented toward the goal of sexual release, numerous studies suggest that passionate love is motivated by desire for proximity to the target partner and signs of reciprocal liking from the target partner. Although sexual union is often desired as well, it is not the sole focal point. For example, Tennov's (1979) exhaustive interview study of passionate love found that 61% of women and 35% of men reported experiencing passionate love without feeling "any need for sex" (p. 74).

This is further supported by research by Hatfield, Schmitz, Cornelius, and Rapson (1988), who assessed the passionate infatuations of over 200 youth between ages 4 and 18. Respondents were asked to think about an other-gender "boyfriend" or "girlfriend" for whom they had intense feelings and to rate their agreement with statements such as "I am always thinking about X" or "When X hugs me my body feels warm all over." The intensity of respondents' infatuation experiences was then correlated with their degree of pubertal maturation (measured with standardized assessments of physical development). If sexual desire were a necessary "ingredient" for the intensity of passionate love, then one would expect to find that the intensity of romantic passion correlated with the respondents' degree of sexual maturity. Yet this was not the case. Not only did younger children report experiences of passionate infatuation that were as intense as the experiences of older children, but there was no association between their degree of sexual maturity and their experiences of romantic passion.

Additional evidence for the functional independence between sexual desire and passionate love comes from cross-cultural and historical evidence that heterosexual individuals often develop feelings of romantic—but not sexual—passion for their closest same-gender friends (Blackwood, 1985; Brain, 1976; Faderman, 1981; Hansen, 1992; Katz, 1976; Rotundo, 1989; Smith-Rosenberg, 1975; W. L. Williams,

1992). These bonds often inspired their own unique terms, such as *romantic friendships* (Faderman, 1981; Rotundo, 1989), *bond friendships* (Firth, 1967), *mummy–baby friendships* (Gay, 1985), *camaradia* (Reina, 1966), or *smashes* (Sahli, 1979). One 19th-century schoolmistress described smashes as "an extraordinary habit which [the schoolgirls'] have of falling violently in love with each other, and suffering all the pangs of unrequited attachment, desperate jealousy etc. etc., with as much energy as if one of them were a man" (Sahli, 1979, p. 22). W. L. Williams's (1992) ethnographic research on North American Indians documented similarly intense but nonsexual bonds between men, which observers likened to romantic infatuation (Trumbull, 1894), similar to the passionate friendships that Brain (1976) documented between young Bangwa men in the Cameroon, which resembled "more the passion of heterosexual lovers than the calm friendship of equals" (pp. 39–40).

Although contemporary Western culture lacks a defined category for platonic same-gender infatuations, they continue to occur (Diamond, 2000; Rothblum, 1993; Von Sydow, 1995), and although it is common for observers reading such accounts to presume that such intense friendships must involve suppressed same-sex sexual attraction, scholars who study and document such relationships have argued against this view, noting that the presumption of a necessary link between same-gender affectional bonds and same-gender sexual desires reflects cultural and historical biases (see, especially, D'Emilio & Freedman, 1988; Faderman, 1981; Nardi, 1992).

Neurobiological Research Distinguishing Sexual Desire from Passionate Love

Additional evidence for the distinction between passionate love and sexual desire comes from comparisons between the distinctive patterns of brain activation found to be associated with each experience. These comparisons are complicated by the fact that research findings on the specific brain regions activated during sexual desire show more variability than research findings on the regions activated during passionate love, which may be attributable to the fact that studies of sexual desire have used a much broader range of eliciting stimuli (Fonteille & Stoleru, 2011; Maravilla & Yang, 2008; Ortigue, Patel, & Bianchi-Demicheli, 2009; Stoleru & Mouras, 2007). Whereas love studies have used pictures of the romantic partner or primes of the partner's name, studies of sexual desire have used a broad range of sexually explicit stimuli, and the form and intensity of participants' neurological response are likely influenced by multiple features of the stimuli (whether the stimulus is visual, auditory, or tactile; whether still photographs or videos are used; whether stimulus presentation is short or long; etc.).

Despite diversity in stimulus properties and experimental protocols, certain regions do appear to be reliably activated in response to sexual stimuli, such as the hypothalamus, putamen, visual cortical areas and inferotemporal cortex, the orbitofrontal cortex (OFC), ACC, parietal cortex, temporal–parietal junction, insula, ventral striatum, anterior temporal areas, interior frontal and cingulate areas, amygdala, and basal ganglia (for comprehensive examples and reviews, see Ferretti et al., 2005; Fonteille & Stoleru, 2011; Karama et al., 2002; Maravilla & Yang, 2007, 2008; Moulier et al., 2006; Redoute et al., 2000; Walter et al., 2008). Most importantly, studies of sexual arousal or desire have *not* detected the distinctive pattern of predominant caudate and VTA activation that reliably characterizes passionate love, supporting the notion that love and desire are distinct on both experiential and neurobiological levels (Aron, Fisher, & Strong, 2006). Yet there is some involvement of the caudate in sexual desire, along with other regions that have shown activation during passionate love, such as the insula, putamen, and ACC (reviewed in S. Cacioppo, Bianchi-Demicheli, Frum, Pfaus, & Lewis, 2012). The fact that love and desire share a subset of neural substrates provides a potential neurobiological basis for the fact that these experiences often occur in concert and are perceived to be phenomenologically intertwined.

Given that the putamen and the caudate are both associated with motivational states and reward, their joint relevance for both sexual desire and romantic love likely reflects the fact that love and desire both involve strong motivation to seek the love object (albeit for different rewards: proximity in the case of romantic love, and sexual activity in the case of desire). The joint relevance of the ACC for both love and sexual desire is notable given that the specific region of the ACC that was found to be activated in Bartels and Zeki's (2000) study of love-specific brain activation was the rostral (rACC) or perigenual ACC. This is the same region found by Walter and colleagues (2008) to be particularly sensitive to the *emotional valence* of sexual stimuli. This pattern of findings is consistent with the fact that the rACC is generally considered the "affective" component of the ACC (in contrast to the dorsal ACC, which is more relevant for cognition, attention, and motor control, and hence appears more important for physiological arousal). It is also notable that rACC activation has also been found to be related to the personal relevance and self-relatedness of stimuli (Heinzel et al., 2006; Phan, Wager, Taylor, & Liberzon, 2002), which is consistent with its role in romantic love.

Hence, in answer to the question of whether love and desire are distinct or interconnected at the neural level, the most accurate answer may be "It depends." Sexual arousal and desire clearly involve *both* "sex-specific" forms of neurological activity *and* more cognitively and affectively mediated forms of activity, the latter of which show more overlap with patterns of activation detected for romantic love. Hence, certain types of sexual desire might be more independent of romantic love than others (both experientially and neurologically), and certain types of love might be more independent of sexual desire than others. Cacioppo and colleagues (2012) concluded from their comprehensive meta-analysis of research targeting the brain regions involved in love versus desire that love might best be viewed as an experience that grows out of the neural circuitry and sensorimotor experiences of pleasure and desire, but additionally involves brain regions associated with reward expectancy and habit formation. Clearly, understanding the specific nature of the links and distinctions between romantic love and sexual desire is a critical goal for future neurobiological research.

Companionate Love as Attachment

Up until now, our focus has been on the earliest, most intense stage of passionate love. As noted earlier, this stage tends to decline over the first several years of a new relationship as companionate love develops and deepens. The dominant theoretical model used to explain the formation, function, expression, and underlying biology of companionate love is *attachment theory* (Bowlby, 1958, 1982). Bowlby conceptualized attachment as an evolved social-behavioral system that serves the purpose of forming and maintaining enduring bonds between mothers and their offspring. Because mammalian (and particularly primate) offspring require substantial care and feeding after birth, the psychological mechanism of attachment is theorized to have evolved to ensure that infants maintain close proximity to their caregivers at all costs during the first few years of life, thereby dramatically increasing their chances for survival. The attachment system is driven by emotions. When infants are too far from their caregivers, they experience distress and signal the caregiver for attention. Once the caregiver is sufficiently close, the infant feels calmed and can resume species-typical, developmentally appropriate behaviors such as exploration. Over time, the infant comes to associate the presence of the attachment figure with emotional security and distress alleviation. Even when the attachment figure is not consistently effective at alleviating distress, infants typically develop a unique, exclusive, emotionally primary relationship with the attachment figure, such that he or she becomes the preferred target for proximity and security seeking. Hence, attachment represents the form of love experienced by children for their caregivers.

It takes approximately 6–12 months of regular contact for infants to develop a basic, functional attachment to their caregivers, a period of time that has been described as "attachment-in-the-making" (Ainsworth, Blehar, Waters, & Wall, 1978). During this period, the infant displays an increasingly intense fixation on the caregiver. By the end of this period, the infant's relationship with the caregiver (now denoted the "attachment figure") is notably distinct from his or her other social relationships. Although there is no single marker that an attachment bond is in place, its core characteristics involve heightened seeking of proximity and contact with the attachment figure (accompanied by distinct physiological responses to such contact) and intense resistance to separation from the attachment figure (again, accompanied by distinct physiological responses to such separations). These characteristics have been observed not only in humans (Ainsworth et al., 1978; Bowlby, 1973, 1982; Field, 1994) but also across a variety of mammalian species, such as rats (Hofer, 1987, 1994), guinea pigs (Graves & Hennessy, 2000), and nonhuman primates (Berman, Rasmussen, & Suomi, 1994; Hoffman, Mendoza, Hennessy, & Mason, 1995; Suomi, 1999).

How does this relate to adult romantic love? Among the most important "revolutions" in research on intimate relationships over the past 20 years was the notion, advanced by Hazan and Shaver in 1987, that adult romantic relationships are, in essence, adult "versions" of infant–caregiver attachment bonds, governed by the same evolved social-behavioral system and characterized by the same emotional and behavioral dynamics (see also Shaver, Hazan, & Bradshaw, 1988). As with infant–caregiver attachment, the evolutionary function of adult attachment is reproduction. Given the developmental immaturity of human infants, the provision of care by *both* parents in the early years of life greatly increased the chances of survival in the environment in which humans evolved. This introduced the critical evolutionary problem of how to keep reproductive partners together long enough to rear their offspring past the initial, most dangerous stage of development (Mellen, 1982). Hence, the affectional bonding program of infant–caregiver attachment is thought to have been co-opted for this purpose (Panksepp, 1998). Hazan and Shaver (1987) martialed considerable support for the notion that adult romantic relationships are adult attachment bonds, noting that infant–caregiver and adult romantic attachments share the same unique features: heightened proximity seeking, intense resistance to separation, and utilization of the partner as a preferred target for comfort and security seeking (reviewed in Hazan & Zeifman, 1999). Furthermore, Hazan and Zeifman (1994) also observed that these two types of bonds share the same types of distinctive intimate physical contact: nuzzling, kissing, stroking, sustained mutual gazing, and sustained chest-to-chest cuddling.

Even more powerful evidence for the fundamental correspondence between infant–caregiver attachment and adult romantic attachment comes from the emerging body of research on the neurobiological substrates of these systems. Considerable animal research indicates that the intense, distinctive proximity maintenance and separation distress associated with attachment formation (from its passionate onset to its development into a stable, enduring affectional bond) are mediated by an array of interacting neurochemicals that undergird the fundamental reward circuitry of the mammalian brain, such as endogenous opioids, dopamine, corticosterone, oxytocin, and vasopressin (reviewed in Carter, 1998; Panksepp, 1998; Panksepp, Nelson, & Bekkedal, 1997). Perhaps the most important evidence regarding the correspondence between infant–caregiver attachment and adult romantic attachment comes from research on oxytocin, a neuropeptide hormone produced in the hypothalamus that is released into circulation from the posterior pituitary; oxytocin is also released directly into the brain from neurons in the paraventricular nucleus. Brain oxytocin receptors are found throughout the limbic system and in the brainstem, particularly in areas associated with emotion, autonomic control, and reproductive and social behavior. Oxytocin is most well known for stimulating the contractions of labor and facilitating milk let-down in nursing mothers, but it is also involved in multiple processes of mammalian attachment and affiliation over the life course. Oxytocin is released during (and subsequently reinforces) physical contact between social affiliates (Knox & Uvnäs-Moberg, 1998; Martel, Nevison, Rayment, Simpson, & Keverne, 1993; Uvnäs-Moberg, Bruzelius, Alster, & Lundeberg, 1993; Witt, Winslow, & Insel, 1992), and has been shown to influence maternal feeding behavior, maternal–infant bonding, and kin recognition (Carter, 1998; Nelson & Panksepp, 1996; Pedersen, Caldwell, Walker, & Ayers, 1994; Uvnäs-Moberg, 1994). Oxytocin facilitates conditioning (Liberzon,

Trujillo, Akil, & Young, 1997; Ostrowski, 1998) and plays a role in the formation of stable preferences for both places and social partners (Nelson & Panksepp, 1996, 1998; J. R. Williams, Insel, Harbaugh, & Carter, 1994). Most notably, research on monogamous prairie voles has demonstrated that administration of central oxytocin facilitates adult pair-bonding, whereas administration of oxytocin antagonists interferes with it (Cho, DeVries, Williams, & Carter, 1999; Insel & Hulihan, 1995; J. R. Williams et al., 1994). Oxytocin has pronounced antistress effects (Chiodera et al., 1991; Uvnäs-Moberg, 1997), and this has been suggested as an additional mechanism through which it facilitates social bonding. Specifically, Uvnäs-Moberg (1998) and Carter (1998) have argued that attachment formation—from infancy to adulthood—involves three main processes: (1) the triggering of oxytocin release by physical contact and/or sustained proximity to a potential attachment figure; (2) the subsequent, oxytocin-mediated down-regulation of stress reactivity in the hypothalamic–pituitary–adrenal (HPA) axis and the autonomic nervous system; and (3) the development of conditioned associations between the potential attachment figure and these effects.

Neuroimaging Research on Attachment

There has been considerably less neuroimaging work on the companionate, "attachment" stage of love than the early, passionate stage, yet a number of neuroimaging studies have investigated whether companionate love directed toward romantic partners differs from companionate love directed toward other close social partners. For example, one study (Acevedo et al., 2011) compared brain activation in response to viewing a picture of one's spouse versus viewing a picture of a close, long-term friend, a highly familiar acquaintance, and a relatively low-familiar person. When participants viewed the partner compared to the close friend, activation was detected in the VTA, substantia nigra, caudate, putamen, ventral striatum, insula, posterior hippocampus, ACC, angular gyrus (also known as the temporal–parietal junction [TPJ]), and the amygdala, suggesting that the experience of companionate love for romantic partners may be categorically different from companionate love directed toward friends. Further evidence for this conclusion comes from the fact that certain brain regions appear to be particularly sensitive to differences in interpersonal closeness between friends and romantic partners. Acevedo and colleagues asked participants to complete the Inclusion of Other in the Self (IOS) scale with regard to their close friends and their spouse. The IOS represents different degrees of interpersonal closeness via pairs of overlapping circles. At the lowest level of closeness, the two circles (representing oneself and the other person) are completely separate; at the highest level, they overlap almost completely. Among individuals with larger discrepancies between the IOS scores given to partners versus friends (indicating much greater closeness to the partner), greater activation was detected in the right VTA, the right insula, and the left ACC when they viewed their spouse versus the friend. Hence, these regions appear to be particularly sensitive to the unique type of interconnectedness that is characteristic of romantic bonds.

As for romantic love versus familial love, Bartels and Zeki (2004) contrasted brain activation in mothers viewing pictures of their own child versus a child with whom they were well acquainted, and directly compared their findings with results from their previous study on romantic love (Bartels & Zeki, 2000). They found overlapping patterns of activation for maternal love and romantic love in the following regions: the putamen, globus pallidus, caudate nucleus, middle insula, and ACC, consistent with the view that romantic and maternal love have a shared dopaminergic–motivational substrate reflecting their shared basis in the social-behavioral system of attachment (Carter, 1998; Carter & Keverne, 2002). They also detected joint activation in the substantia nigra and globus pallidus, both of which are rich in receptors for oxytocin and vasopressin, which are known to play critical roles in the formation and functioning of attachment bonds formed between parents and children, as well as adult reproductive partners (Carter, 1998; Carter & Keverne, 2002).The regions that were only activated during romantic love included the hippocampus, hypothalamus, and anterior portion of

the VTA. In contrast, they only detected periaqueductal gray matter (PAG) activation during maternal love. The PAG is also rich in oxytocin receptors, and is thought to play a critical role in maternal attachment formation. Notably, PAG activation has also been found to be associated with feelings of unconditional love (Beauregard, Courtemanche, Paquette, & St-Pierre, 2009), and in long-term couples, PAG activation is correlated with the duration of marriage (Acevedo et al., 2011). This suggests a potential role for the PAG in emotionally intense but nonsexual experiences of love.

Overall, the brain imaging data are strongly consistent with the notion that romantic attachments and parent–child attachments, despite their differences, have parallel bases and functions (Shaver et al., 1988), which may be traceable to their shared patterns of brain activation. More importantly, both appear to be highly distinct from close friendships. A promising direction for future research on links and distinctions between love and desire is to evaluate *changes* in patterns of neurological activation elicited by romantic partners over time. Both sexual desire and passionate infatuation are known to decline in long-term relationships, but Acevedo and colleagues (2011) found that some long-term couples report experiencing—and show patterns of brain activation consistent with—the sort of passionate infatuation that is more typical of new couples (i.e., greater activation in the VTA, caudate, putamen, and posterior hippocampus). Future research should examine whether longitudinal changes in couples' subjective experiences of their relationship (i.e., a shift from passionate infatuation to unconditional, companionate devotion) correspond to changes in the constellation of brain regions activated by the partner (i.e., reductions in VTA, and caudate, and putamen activation and increases in PAG activation).

Attachment, Romantic Love, and Health

The research reviewed earlier demonstrates that both passionate and companionate love are fundamentally psychobiological phenomena, involving complex patterns of activation in the brain's dopaminergic reward circuitry. We enter this world as infants, psychobiologically "wired" to fall in love with our caregivers, driven to seek proximity and contact with these figures at all costs, and as adults, we direct the same intense focus on our romantic partners. Notably, research has long shown that infants deprived of love from their caregivers suffer notable deficits in physical and mental well-being (Bowlby, 1951; Rutter, 1972), and a parallel body of research on adults has found that the lack of substantive emotional ties in adulthood—known as emotional loneliness—confers profound risks for compromised cardiovascular, neuroendocrine, and immune system functioning (J. T. Caccioppo et al., 2002; Hawkley, Burleson, Berntson, & Cacioppo, 2003; Hawkley & Cacioppo, 2003, 2010). More specifically, researchers have found that the lack of an enduring, committed romantic relationship is associated with poorer health and lower happiness over the lifespan (Cheung, 1998; Horwitz, McLaughlin, & White, 1998; Kitigawa & Hauser, 1973; Mastekaasa, 1994; Murphy, Glaser, & Grundy, 1997; Ross, 1995; Ryff et al., 2001; Stack, 1998; Stack & Eshleman, 1998). This effect cannot be attributed to low overall social integration given that individuals' *most intimate* relationships appear to promote health and well-being above and beyond generalized social support (Ross, 1995; Ryff et al., 2001). Rather, the key variable appears to be the existence of an enduring, emotionally intimate affectional bond (Ross, 1995). As noted earlier, simply knowing whether an individual "feels loved" significantly predicts his or her future cardiovascular disease risk (Seeman & Syme, 1987).

Extensive research has therefore investigated the processes through which satisfying love relationships may influence health-related processes (Esch & Stefano, 2005; Maggi & Corona, 2011). Many of these studies focus on the social support provided by romantic partners, which can, of course, be provided within many other types of close social ties (Uchino, 2006), and there has been increasing interest in determining whether romantic relationships confer distinct and unique benefits (for a review and critique of this literature, see DePaulo & Morris, 2005). One of the paradoxes that has emerged from this line of

research is that although global perceptions of support availability are reliably linked to health-related outcomes (Collins & Feeney, 2000; Reis, Clark, & Holmes, 2004; Srivastava, McGonigal, Richards, Butler, & Gross, 2006), the process of *actually receiving* concrete, observable acts of support—whether from a romantic partner or other close social partners—does not appear to be beneficial, a finding that has been attributed to the possibility that such clear-cut acts of support inadvertently reinforce the recipient's feelings of stress or weakness, implicitly suggesting that he or she is perceived as incompetent (Bolger & Amarel, 2007; Bolger, Zuckerman, & Kessler, 2000; Gleason, Iida, Shrout, & Bolger, 2008; Shrout, Herman, & Bolger, 2006). This work has been interpreted to suggest that the *emotions* experienced (and regulated) on a day-to-day level within love relationships play a more central role in shaping immediate and long term health-related processes than concrete interpersonal acts. Interactions with romantic partners that amplify positive emotions and attenuate negative emotions appear to have the most direct and measurable consequences for health-related physiological processes, including cardiovascular, neuroendocrine, and immune functioning (Brown, Smith, & Benjamin, 1998; Grewen, Girdler, Amico, & Light, 2005; Holt-Lunstad, Birmingham, & Light, 2008; Kiecolt-Glaser, Malarkey, Chee, & Newton, 1993; Mayne, O'Leary, McCrady, & Contrada, 1997; Miller, Dopp, Myers, Stevens, & Fahey, 1999; Powers, Pietromonaco, Gunlicks, & Sayer, 2006; Smith et al., 2011).

Hence, one way to interpret these data is to suggest that the "secret ingredient" of well-functioning romantic relationships—with regard to health outcomes—is not a particular form of "supportive" behavior but *the positive emotional experience of love itself.* In other words, well-functioning love relationships are healthy because the subjective experience of giving and receiving love on a day-to-day basis has a cascade of beneficial psychological and physical consequences. Numerous lines of evidence provide support for this view. For example, there is substantial evidence that the chronic emotional states elicited within social relationships—both romantic and otherwise—represent a primary pathway through which social relationships "get under our skin" (Kiecolt-Glaser, McGuire, Robles, & Glaser, 2002; Repetti et al., 2002; Ryff et al., 2001; Seeman, 2001) to shape long-term health-related physiological functioning. Although the bulk of research on this topic has focused on negative emotions (reviewed in Kiecolt-Glaser et al., 2002; Richman et al., 2005), an increasing body of research suggests that the experience of positive emotions enhances multiple health-related processes. For example, inductions of positive affective states are associated with corresponding increases in natural killer (NK) cell activity (Berk, Felten, Tan, Bittman, & Westengard, 2001; Takahashi et al., 2001), and lymphocyte proliferative response (Futterman, Kemeny, Shapiro, & Fahey, 1994), and individuals who report a chronic disposition to experience happiness and joy show less vulnerability to cold infections (Cohen, Doyle, Turner, Alper, & Skoner, 2003; Doyle, Gentile, & Cohen, 2006; Marsland, Cohen, Rabin, & Manuck, 2006). These processes may account for the links that have been established between chronic positive emotionality and longevity (Danner, Snowdon, & Friesen, 2001; Moskowitz, 2003).

Hence, given that the experience of love within a well-functioning relationship is typically associated with strong positive emotions (notably, Fredrickson [1998] considers love to be one of the four primary types of positive emotion—along with joy, interest, and contentment—that foster well-being by increasing individuals' physical, cognitive, and social resources), such chronic positive emotions may represent a key pathway through which love promotes health. This is supported by the fact that the dopaminergic brain reward system that mediates the rewarding aspects of social affiliation, passionate love, and attachment formation is also associated with immune functioning, specifically, NK cell activity (Wenner, Kawamura, Ishikawa, & Matsuda, 2000; Wrona & Trojniar, 2003, 2005). Increases in peripheral dopamine have been shown to correlate with the experience of positive emotions, and with corresponding increases in NK cell activity (Mizuno, Oda, Takeda, Mizuno, & Moriya, 2003). One study found that individuals watching a positive film or the image of a favorite person showed increases in serum dopamine concentra-

tion and NK cell activity (Matsunaga et al., 2008). Such findings provide further evidence that the experience of love, by fostering activation of the dopaminergic brain reward and corresponding experiences of positive emotions, facilitates robust immune system functioning and hence long-term health.

Oxytocin release may provide another pathway through which love may enhance physical health. As reviewed earlier, oxytocin is critically involved in social bonding, and several researchers have suggested that oxytocin may partially account for the health benefits of well-functioning love relationships (Carter, 1998; Knox & Uvnäs-Moberg, 1998; McCarthy & Altemus, 1997; Uvnäs-Moberg, 2004). The potential health benefits of oxytocin are supported by findings that indicate oxytocin release is associated with positive emotional experience (Turner, Altemus, Enos, Cooper, & McGuinness, 1999); that oxytocin release is enhanced by warm physical touch between romantic partners (Holt-Lunstad et al., 2008); that individuals who receive more frequent physical affection from their romantic partners show higher levels of oxytocin (Light, Grewen, & Amico, 2005); that higher oxytocin levels are associated with lower cardiovascular reactivity to stress (Grewen & Light, 2011), lower blood pressure (Knox & Uvnäs-Moberg, 1998; Light et al., 2005; Uvnäs-Moberg, 2004) and faster healing of experimentally induced wounds (Gouin et al., 2010); that exogenous administration of oxytocin enhances the ability of social support to buffer individuals from cortisol reactivity to stress (Heinrichs, Baumgartner, Kirschbaum, & Ehlert, 2003) and has been associated with reduced cortisol reactivity to marital conflict (Ditzen et al., 2009). Hence, love relationships that foster sustained oxytocin release through the provision of consistent affection and positive emotion may yield a range of health benefits over the lifespan, most notably by reducing both blood pressure and cardiovascular and neuroendocrine responses to stress.

Conclusion

Research on the experience of love at behavioral, psychological, and biological levels, and love's implications for mental and physical functioning over the lifespan, remains one of the most exciting areas of interdisciplinary research in psychology. Directly contrary to early assumptions that there was little about the "mystery" of love and of romantic relationships that could be rendered intelligible by the conventional methods of social-scientific inquiry, the past several decades of research have made incredible strides in revealing the underlying neurobiology of love, its evolved underpinnings with respect to our mammalian heritage, its profound implications for health and well-being, and the mechanisms underlying such links. This line of research has much in common with the parallel lines of inquiry over the past several decades into the fundamental importance of positive emotions for human health and happiness. Regardless of whether one considers love to be a basic emotion or merely a context for the experience and distillation of positive emotions, love's fundamental importance to human nature is without question, and critical discoveries lie ahead with regard to the development of a thoroughgoing, lifespan understanding of the multiple interacting biobehavioral processes that account for its lasting effects on human health and well-being.

References

Acevedo, B. P., & Aron, A. (2009). Does a long-term relationship kill romantic love? *Review of General Psychology, 13,* 59–65.

Acevedo, B. P., Aron, A., Fisher, H. E., & Brown, L. L. (2011). Neural correlates of long-term intense romantic love. *Social Cognitive and Affective Neuroscience, 7,* 145–159.

Ainsworth, M. D. S., Blehar, M. C., Waters, E., & Wall, S. (1978). *Patterns of attachment: A psychological study of the Strange Situation.* Hillsdale, NJ: Erlbaum.

Aron, A., Fisher, H., Mashek, D. J., Strong, G., Li, H., & Brown, L. L. (2005). Reward, motivation, and emotion systems associated with early-stage intense romantic love. *Journal of Neurophysiology, 94,* 327–337.

Aron, A., Fisher, H., & Strong, G. (2006). Romantic love. In A. Vangelisti & D. Perlman (Eds.), *Cambridge handbook of personal relationships* (pp. 595–614). New York: Cambridge University Press.

Aron, A., Norman, C. C., Aron, E. N., McKenna, C., & Heyman, R. E. (2000). Couples' shared participation in novel and arousing activities and experienced relationship quality. *Journal of Personality and Social Psychology, 78,* 273–284.

Aron, A. P., & Aron, E. N. (1986). *Love as the expansion of self: Understanding attraction and satisfaction.* New York: Hemisphere.

Aron, A. P., & Aron, E. N. (1991). Love and sexuality. In K. McKinney & S. Sprecher (Eds.), *Sexuality in close relationships* (pp. 25–48). Hillsdale, NJ: Erlbaum.

Bartels, A., & Zeki, S. (2000). The neural basis of romantic love. *NeuroReport, 11,* 3829–3834.

Bartels, A., & Zeki, S. (2004). The neural correlates of maternal and romantic love. *NeuroImage, 21,* 1155–1166.

Beauregard, M., Courtemanche, J., Paquette, V., & St-Pierre, E. L. (2009). The neural basis of unconditional love. *Psychiatry Research: Neuroimaging, 172,* 93–98.

Berk, L. S., Felten, D. L., Tan, S. A., Bittman, B. B., & Westengard, J. (2001). Modulation of neuroimmune parameters during the eustress of humor-associated mirthful laughter. *Alternative Therapies in Health and Medicine, 7,* 62–72, 74–76.

Berman, C. M., Rasmussen, K. L. R., & Suomi, S. J. (1994). Responses of free-ranging rhesus monkeys to a natural form of maternal separation: I. Parallels with mother–infant separation in captivity. *Child Development, 65,* 1028–1041.

Berscheid, E., & Hatfield, E. H. (1969). *Interpersonal attraction.* New York: Addison-Wesley.

Bianchi-Demicheli, F., Grafton, S. T., & Ortigue, S. (2006). The power of love on the human brain. *Social Neuroscience, 1,* 90–103.

Blackwood, E. (1985). Breaking the mirror: The construction of lesbianism and the anthropological discourse on homosexuality. *Journal of Homosexuality, 11,* 1–17.

Bolger, N., & Amarel, D. (2007). Effects of social support visibility on adjustment to stress: Experimental evidence. *Journal of Personality and Social Psychology, 92,* 458–475.

Bolger, N., Zuckerman, A., & Kessler, R. C. (2000). Invisible support and adjustment to stress. *Journal of Personality and Social Psychology, 79,* 953–961.

Bowlby, J. (1951). *Maternal care and mental health.* Geneva: World Health Organization.

Bowlby, J. (1958). The nature of the child's tie to his mother. *International Journal of Psychoanalysis, 39,* 350–373.

Bowlby, J. (1973). *Attachment and loss: Vol. 2. Separation: Anxiety and anger.* New York: Basic Books.

Bowlby, J. (1982). *Attachment and loss: Vol. 1. Attachment* (2nd ed.). New York: Basic Books.

Brain, R. (1976). *Friends and lovers.* New York: Basic Books.

Brown, P. C., Smith, T. W., & Benjamin, L. S. (1998). Perceptions of spouse dominance predict blood pressure reactivity during marital interactions. *Annals of Behavioral Medicine, 20,* 286–293.

Cacioppo, J. T., Hawkley, L. C., Crawford, E., Ernst, J. M., Burleson, M. H., Kowalewski, R. B., et al. (2002). Loneliness and health: Potential mechanisms. *Psychosomatic Medicine, 64,* 407–417.

Cacioppo, S., Bianchi-Demicheli, F., Frum, C., Pfaus, J. G., & Lewis, J. W. (2012). The common neural bases between sexual desire and love: A multilevel kernel density fMRI analysis. *Journal of Sexual Medicine, 9,* 1048–1054.

Carter, C. S. (1998). Neuroendocrine perspectives on social attachment and love. *Psychoneuroendocrinology, 23,* 779–818.

Carter, C. S., & Keverne, E. B. (2002). The neurobiology of social affiliation and pair bonding. In J. Pfaff, A. P. Arnold, A. E. Etgen, & S. E. Fahrbach (Eds.), *Hormones, brain and behavior* (Vol. 1, pp. 299–377). New York: Academic Press.

Cheung, Y. B. (1998). Accidents, assaults, and marital status. *Social Science and Medicine, 47,* 1325–1329.

Chiodera, P., Salvarani, C., Bacchi-Modena, A., Spallanzani, R., Cigarini, C., Alboni, A., et al. (1991). Relationship between plasma profiles of oxytocin and adrenocorticotrophic hormone during suckling or breast stimulation in women. *Hormone Research, 35,* 119–123.

Cho, M. M., DeVries, A. C., Williams, J. R., & Carter, C. S. (1999). The effects of oxytocin and vasopressin on partner preferences in male and female prairie voles (*Microtus ochrogaster*). *Behavioral Neuroscience, 113,* 1071–1079.

Cohen, S., Doyle, W. J., Turner, R. B., Alper, C. M., & Skoner, D. P. (2003). Emotional style and susceptibility to the common cold. *Psychosomatic Medicine, 65,* 652–657.

Collins, N. L., & Feeney, B. C. (2000). A safe haven: An attachment theory perspective on support seeking and caregiving in intimate relationships. *Journal of Personality and Social Psychology, 78,* 1053–1073.

Danner, D. D., Snowdon, D. A., & Friesen, W. V. (2001). Positive emotions in early life and longevity: Findings from the nun study. *Journal of Personality and Social Psychology, 80,* 804–813.

D'Emilio, J., & Freedman, E. B. (1988). *Intimate matters: A history of sexuality in America.* New York: Harper & Row.

DePaulo, B. M., & Morris, W. L. (2005). Singles in society and in science. *Psychological Inquiry, 16,* 57–83.

Diamond, L. M. (2000). Passionate friendships among adolescent sexual-minority women. *Journal of Research on Adolescence, 10,* 191–209.

Diamond, L. M. (2003). What does sexual orientation orient?: A biobehavioral model distinguishing romantic love and sexual desire. *Psychological Review, 110,* 173–192.

Ditzen, B., Schaer, M., Gabriel, B., Bodenmann, G., Ehlert, U., & Heinrichs, M. (2009). Intranasal oxytocin increases positive communication and reduces cortisol levels during couple conflict. *Biological Psychiatry, 65,* 728–731.

Doyle, W. J., Gentile, D. A., & Cohen, S. (2006). Emotional style, nasal cytokines, and illness expression after experimental rhinovirus exposure. *Brain, Behavior, and Immunity, 20,* 175–181.

Esch, T., & Stefano, G. B. (2005). Love promotes health. *Neuroendocrinology Letters, 26,* 264–267.

Faderman, L. (1981). *Surpassing the love of men.* New York: Morrow.

Fehr, B. (1988). Prototype analysis of the concepts of love and commitment. *Journal of Personality and Social Psychology, 55,* 557–579.

Fehr, B. (2006). A prototype approach to studying love. In R. J. Sternberg & K. Weis (Eds.), *The new psychology of love* (pp. 225–246). New Haven, CT: Yale University Press.

Fehr, B., & Russell, J. A. (1984). Concept of emotion viewed from a prototype perspective. *Journal of Experimental Psychology: General, 113,* 464–486.

Fehr, B., & Russell, J. A. (1991). The concept of love viewed from a prototype perspective. *Journal of Personality and Social Psychology, 60,* 425–438.

Ferretti, A., Caulo, M., Del Gratta, C., Di Matteo, R., Merla, A., Montorsi, F., et al. (2005). Dynamics of male sexual arousal: Distinct components of brain activation revealed by fMRI. *NeuroImage, 26,* 1086–1096.

Field, T. (1994). The effects of mother's physical and emotional unavailability on emotion regulation. In N. Fox (Ed.), The development of emotion regulation: Biological and behavioral considerations. *Monographs of the Society for Research in Child Development, 59,* (2–3, Serial No. 240), 208–227.

Firth, R. W. (1967). *Tikopia ritual and belief.* Boston: Allen & Unwin.

Fisher, H. E. (1998). Lust, attraction, and attachment in mammalian reproduction. *Human Nature, 9,* 23–52.

Fisher, H. E. (2004). *Why we love: The nature and chemistry of romantic love.* New York: Holt.

Fonteille, V., & Stoleru, S. (2011). The cerebral correlates of sexual desire: Functional neuroimaging approach. *Sexologies, 20*(3), 142–148.

Fredrickson, B. L. (1998). What good are positive emotions? *Review of General Psychology, 2,* 300–319.

Futterman, A. D., Kemeny, M. E., Shapiro, D., & Fahey, J. L. (1994). Immunological and physiological changes associated with induced positive and negative mood. *Psychosomatic Medicine, 56,* 499–511.

Gay, J. (1985). "Mummies and babies" and friends and lovers in Lesotho [Special issue]. *Journal of Homosexuality, 11,* 97–116.

Gleason, M. E. J., Iida, M., Shrout, P. E., & Bolger, N. (2008). Receiving support as a mixed blessing: Evidence for dual effects of support on psychological outcomes. *Journal of Personality and Social Psychology, 94,* 824–838.

Gonzaga, G. C., Keltner, D., Londahl, E. A., & Smith, M. D. (2001). Love and the commitment problem in romantic relations and friendship. *Journal of Personality and Social Psychology, 81,* 247–262.

Gouin, J.-P., Carter, C. S., Pournajafi-Nazarloo, H., Glaser, R., Malarkey, W. B., Loving, T. J., et al. (2010). Marital behavior, oxytocin, vasopressin, and wound healing. *Psychoneuroendocrinology, 35,* 1082–1090.

Graves, F. C., & Hennessy, M. B. (2000). Comparison of the effects of the mother and an unfamiliar adult female on cortisol and behavioral responses of pre and postweaning guinea pigs. *Developmental Psychobiology, 36,* 91–100.

Grewen, K. M., Girdler, S. S., Amico, J., & Light, K. C. (2005). Effects of partner support on resting oxytocin, cortisol, norepinephrine, and blood pressure before and after warm partner contact. *Psychosomatic Medicine, 67,* 531–538.

Grewen, K. M., & Light, K. C. (2011). Plasma oxytocin is related to lower cardiovascular and sympathetic reactivity to stress. *Biological Psychology, 87,* 340–349.

Hansen, K. V. (1992). "Our eyes behold each other": Masculinity and intimate friendship in antebellum New England. In P. Nardi (Ed.), *Men's friendships* (pp. 35–58). Newbury Park, CA: Sage.

Hatfield, E. (1987). Passionate and companionate love. In R. J. Sternberg & M. L. Barnes (Eds.), *The psychology of love* (pp. 191–217). New Haven, CT: Yale University Press.

Hatfield, E. (2001). Elaine Hatfield. In A. N. O'Connell (Ed.), *Models of achievement: Reflections of eminent women in psychology* (Vol. 3, pp. 136–147). New York: Columbia University Press.

Hatfield, E., & Rapson, R. L. (1987). Passionate love/sexual desire: Can the same paradigm explain both? *Archives of Sexual Behavior, 16,* 259–277.

Hatfield, E., & Rapson, R. L. (2006). Passionate love, sexual desire, and mate selection: Cross-cultural and historical perspectives. In P. Noller & J. A. Feeney (Eds.), *Close relationships: Functions, forms and processes* (pp. 227–243). Hove, UK: Psychology Press/Taylor & Francis.

Hatfield, E., Schmitz, E., Cornelius, J., & Rapson, R. L. (1988). Passionate love: How early does it begin? *Journal of Psychology and Human Sexuality, 1,* 35–52.

Hatfield, E., & Sprecher, S. (1986). Measuring passionate love in intimate relationships. *Journal of Adolescence, 9,* 383–410.

Hawkley, L. C., Burleson, M. H., Berntson, G. G., & Cacioppo, J. T. (2003). Loneliness in everyday life: Cardiovascular activity, psychosocial context, and health behaviors. *Journal of Personality and Social Psychology, 85,* 105–120.

Hawkley, L. C., & Cacioppo, J. T. (2003). Loneliness and pathways to disease. *Brain, Behavior, and Immunity, 17,* S98–S105.

Hawkley, L. C., & Cacioppo, J. T. (2010). Loneliness matters: A theoretical and empirical review of consequences and mechanisms. *Annals of Behavioral Medicine, 40,* 218–227.

Hazan, C., & Shaver, P. R. (1987). Romantic love conceptualized as an attachment process. *Journal of Personality and Social Psychology, 52,* 511–524.

Hazan, C., & Zeifman, D. (1994). Sex and the psychological tether. In D. Perlman & K. Bartholomew (Eds.), *Advances in personal rela-*

tionships: A research annual (Vol. 5, pp. 151–177). London: Jessica Kingsley.

Hazan, C., & Zeifman, D. (1999). Pair-bonds as attachments: Evaluating the evidence. In J. Cassidy & P. R. Shaver (Eds.), Handbook of attachment: Theory, research, and clinical applications (pp. 336–354). New York: Guilford Press.

Heinrichs, M., Baumgartner, T., Kirschbaum, C., & Ehlert, U. (2003). Social support and oxytocin interact to suppress cortisol and subjective responses to psychosocial stress. Biological Psychiatry, 54, 1389–1398.

Heinzel, A., Walter, M., Schneider, F., Rotte, M., Matthiae, C., Tempelmann, C., et al. (2006). Self-related processing in the sexual domain: Parametric event-related fMRI study reveals neural activity in ventral cortical midline structures. Social Neuroscience, 1, 41–51.

Hofer, M. (1994). Hidden regulators in attachment, separation, and loss. Monographs of the Society for Research in Child Development, 59, (2–3, Serial No. 240), 192–207.

Hofer, M. A. (1987). Early social relationships: A psychobiologist's view. Child Development, 58, 633–647.

Hoffman, K. A., Mendoza, S. P., Hennessy, M. B., & Mason, W. A. (1995). Responses of infant titi monkeys, Callicebus moloch, to removal of one or both parents: Evidence for paternal attachment. Developmental Psychobiology, 28, 399–407.

Holt-Lunstad, J., Birmingham, W. A., & Light, K. C. (2008). Influence of a "warm touch" support enhancement intervention among married couples on ambulatory blood pressure, oxytocin, alpha amylase, and cortisol. Psychosomatic Medicine, 70, 976–985.

Horwitz, A. V., McLaughlin, J., & White, H. R. (1998). How the negative and positive aspects of partner relationships affect the mental health of young married people. Journal of Health and Social Behavior, 39, 124–136.

Huesmann, L. R. (1980). Toward a predictive model of romantic behavior. In K. Pope (Ed.), On love and loving (pp. 152–171). San Francisco: Jossey-Bass.

Insel, T. R., & Hulihan, T. J. (1995). A gender-specific mechanism for pair bonding: Oxytocin and partner preference formation in monogamous voles. Behavioral Neuroscience, 109, 782–789.

Izard, C. E. (1991). The psychology of emotions. New York: Plenum Press.

Jankowiak, W. R., & Fischer, E. F. (1992). A cross-cultural perspective on romantic love. Ethnology, 31, 149–155.

Karama, S., Lecours, A. R., Leroux, J.-M., Bourgouin, P., Beaudoin, G., Joubert, S., et al. (2002). Areas of brain activation in males and females during viewing of erotic film excerpts. Human Brain Mapping, 16, 1–13.

Katz, J. (1976). Gay American history. New York: Crowell.

Kiecolt-Glaser, J. K., Malarkey, W. B., Chee, M., & Newton, T. (1993). Negative behavior during marital conflict is associated with immunological down-regulation. Psychosomatic Medicine, 55, 395–409.

Kiecolt-Glaser, J. K., McGuire, L., Robles, T. F., & Glaser, R. (2002). Emotions, morbidity, and mortality: New perspectives from psychoneuroimmunology. Annual Review of Psychology, 53, 83–107.

Kitigawa, E. M., & Hauser, P. M. (1973). Differential mortality in the United States: A study in socio-economic epidemiology. Cambridge, MA: Harvard University Press.

Knox, S. S., & Uvnäs-Moberg, K. (1998). Social isolation and cardiovascular disease: An atherosclerotic pathway? Psychoneuroendocrinology, 23, 877–890.

Liberzon, I., Trujillo, K. A., Akil, H., & Young, E. A. (1997). Motivational properties of oxytocin in the conditioned place preference paradigm. Neuropsychopharmacology, 17, 353–359.

Light, K. C., Grewen, K. M., & Amico, J. A. (2005). More frequent partner hugs and higher oxytocin levels are linked to lower blood pressure and heart rate in premenopausal women. Biological Psychology, 69, 5–21.

Maggi, M., & Corona, G. (2011). Love protects lover's life. Journal of Sexual Medicine, 8, 931–935.

Maravilla, K. R., & Yang, C. C. (2007). Sex and the brain: The role of fMRI for assessment of sexual function and response. International Journal of Impotence Research, 19, 25–29.

Maravilla, K. R., & Yang, C. C. (2008). Magnetic resonance imaging and the female sexual response: Overview of techniques, results, and future directions. Journal of Sexual Medicine, 5, 1559–1571.

Marsland, A. L., Cohen, S., Rabin, B. S., & Manuck, S. B. (2006). Trait positive affect and antibody response to hepatitis B vaccination. Brain, Behavior, and Immunity, 20, 261–269.

Martel, F. L., Nevison, C. M., Rayment, F. D., Simpson, M. J. A., & Keverne, E. B. (1993).

Opioid receptor blockade reduces maternal affect and social grooming in rhesus monkeys. *Psychoneuroendocrinology, 18*, 307–321.

Mastekaasa, A. (1994). Marital-status, distress, and well-being: An international comparison. *Journal of Comparative Family Studies, 25*, 183–205.

Matsunaga, M., Isowa, T., Kimura, K., Miyakoshi, M., Kanayama, N., Murakami, H., et al. (2008). Associations among central nervous, endocrine, and immune activities when positive emotions are elicited by looking at a favorite person. *Brain, Behavior, and Immunity, 22*, 408–417.

Mayne, T. J., O'Leary, A., McCrady, B., & Contrada, R. (1997). The differential effects of acute marital distress on emotional, physiological and immune functions in maritally distressed men and women. *Psychology and Health, 12*, 277–288.

McCarthy, M. M., & Altemus, M. (1997). Central nervous system actions of oxytocin and modulation of behavior in humans. *Molecular Medicine Today, 3*, 269–275.

Mellen, S. L. W. (1982). *The evolution of love*: San Francisco: Freeman.

Miller, G. E., Dopp, J. M., Myers, H. F., Stevens, S. Y., & Fahey, J. L. (1999). Psychosocial predictors of natural killer cell mobilization during marital conflict. *Health Psychology, 18*, 262–271.

Mizuno, T., Oda, S., Takeda, H., Mizuno, M., & Moriya, K. (2003). Immunological, hormonal, and psychological effects of comfortable self-paced running as compared to bed-resting relaxation in untrained healthy men. *Medicine and Science in Sport and Exercise, 35*(5, Suppl.), S379.

Moskowitz, J. (2003). Positive affect predicts lower risk of AIDS mortality. *Psychosomatic Medicine, 65*, 620–626.

Moulier, V., Mouras, H., Pelegrini-Isaac, M., Glutron, D., Rouxel, R., & Grandjean, B. (2006). Neuroanatomical correlates of penile erection evoked by photographic stimuli in human males. *NeuroImage, 33*, 689–699.

Murphy, M., Glaser, K., & Grundy, E. (1997). Marital status and long-term illness in Great Britain. *Journal of Marriage and the Family, 59*, 156–164.

Nardi, P. M. (1992). "Seamless souls": An introduction to men's friendships. In P. Nardi (Ed.), *Men's friendships* (pp. 1–14). Newbury Park, CA: Sage.

Nelson, E. E., & Panksepp, J. (1996). Oxytocin mediates acquisition of maternally associated odor preferences in preweanling rat pups. *Behavioral Neuroscience, 110*, 583–592.

Nelson, E. E., & Panksepp, J. (1998). Brain substrates of infant–mother attachment: Contributions of opioids, oxytocin, and norepinephrine. *Neuroscience and Biobehavioral Reviews, 22*, 437–452.

Ortigue, S., Bianchi-Demicheli, F., Hamilton, A. F., & Grafton, S. T. (2007). The neural basis of love as a subliminal prime: An event-related functional magnetic resonance imaging study. *Journal of Cognitive Neuroscience, 19*, 1218–1230.

Ortigue, S., Patel, N., & Bianchi-Demicheli, F. (2009). New electroencephalogram (EEG) neuroimaging methods of analyzing brain activity applicable to the study of human sexual response. *Journal of Sexual Medicine, 6*, 1830–1845.

Ostrowski, N. L. (1998). Oxytocin receptor mRNA expression in rat brain: Implications for behavioral integration and reproductive success. *Psychoneuroendocrinology, 23*, 989–1004.

Panksepp, J. (1998). *Affective neuroscience: The foundations of human and animal emotions*. New York: Cambridge University Press.

Panksepp, J., Nelson, E., & Bekkedal, M. (1997). Brain systems for the mediation of social separation-distress and social-reward: Evolutionary antecedents and neuropeptide intermediaries. *Annals of the New York Academy of Sciences, 807*, 78–100.

Pedersen, C. A., Caldwell, J. D., Walker, C., & Ayers, G. (1994). Oxytocin activates the postpartum onset of rat maternal behavior in the ventral tegmental and medial preoptic areas. *Behavioral Neuroscience, 108*, 1163–1171.

Phan, K. L., Wager, T., Taylor, S. F., & Liberzon, I. (2002). Functional neuroanatomy of emotion: A meta-analysis of emotion activation studies in PET and fMRI. *NeuroImage, 16*, 331–348.

Powers, S. I., Pietromonaco, P. R., Gunlicks, M., & Sayer, A. (2006). Dating couples' attachment styles and patterns of cortisol reactivity and recovery in response to a relationship conflict. *Journal of Personality and Social Psychology, 90*, 613–628.

Redoute, J. R. M., Stolery, S., Gregoire, M.-C., Costes, N., Cinotti, L., Lavenne, F., et al. (2000). Brain processing of visual sexual stimuli in human males. *Human Brain Mapping, 11*, 162–177.

Regan, P. C., & Berscheid, E. (1995). Gender differences in beliefs about the causes of male and female sexual desire. *Personal Relationships, 2,* 345–358.

Reina, R. (1966). *The law of the saints: A Pokoman pueblo and its community culture.* Indianapolis, IN: Bobbs-Merrill.

Reis, H. T., Clark, M. S., & Holmes, J. G. (2004). Perceived partner responsiveness as an organizing construct in the study of intimacy and closeness. In D. J. Mashek & A. P. Aron (Eds.), *Handbook of closeness and intimacy* (pp. 201–225). Mahwah, NJ: Erlbaum.

Repetti, R. L., Taylor, S. E., & Seeman, T. E. (2002). Risky families: Family social environments and the mental and physical health of offspring. *Psychological Bulletin, 128,* 330–366.

Richman, L. S., Kubzansky, L., Maselko, J., Kawachi, I., Choo, P., & Bauer, M. (2005). Positive emotion and health: Going beyond the negative. *Health Psychology, 24,* 422–429.

Ross, C. E. (1995). Reconceptualizing marital-status as a continuum of social attachment. *Journal of Marriage and the Family, 57,* 129–140.

Rothblum, E. D. (1993). Early memories, current realities. In E. D. Rothblum & K. A. Brehony (Eds.), *Boston marriages* (pp. 14–18). Amherst: University of Massachusetts Press.

Rotundo, E. A. (1989). Romantic friendships: Male intimacy and middle-class youth in the northern United States, 1800–1900. *Journal of Social History, 23,* 1–25.

Rutter, M. (1972). *Maternal deprivation reassessed.* Harmondsworth, UK: Penguin.

Ryff, C. D., Singer, B. H., Wing, E., & Love, G. D. (2001). Elective affinities and uninvited agonies: Mapping emotion with significant others onto health. In C. D. Ryff & B. H. Singer (Eds.), *Emotions, social relationships, and health* (pp. 133–174). New York: Oxford University Press.

Sahli, N. (1979). Smashing: Women's relationships before the fall. *Chrysalis, 8,* 17–27.

Seeman, T. E. (2001). How do others get under our skin?: Social relationships and health. In C. D. Ryff & B. H. Singer (Eds.), *Emotion, social relationships, and health* (pp. 189–209). New York: Oxford University Press.

Seeman, T. E., & Syme, S. L. (1987). Social networks and coronary artery disease: A comparison of the structure and function of social relations as predictors of disease. *Psychosomatic Medicine, 49,* 341–354.

Shaver, P. R., Hazan, C., & Bradshaw, D. (1988). Love as attachment: The integration of three behavioral systems. In J. Sternberg & M. L. Barnes (Eds.), *The psychology of love* (pp. 193–219). New Haven, CT: Yale University Press.

Shaver, P. R., Morgan, H. J., & Wu, S. (1996). Is love a "basic" emotion. *Personal Relationships, 3,* 81–96.

Shaver, P. R., Schwartz, J., Kirson, D., O'Connor, C., & Parrott, W. G. (2001). Emotion knowledge: Further exploration of a prototype approach. In W. G. Parrott (Ed.), *Emotions in social psychology: Essential readings* (pp. 26–56). New York: Psychology Press.

Shrout, P. E., Herman, C. M., & Bolger, N. (2006). The costs and benefits of practical and emotional support on adjustment: A daily diary study of couples experiencing acute stress. *Personal Relationships, 13,* 115–134.

Smith-Rosenberg, C. (1975). The female world of love and ritual: Relations between women in nineteenth century America. *Signs, 1,* 1–29.

Smith, T. W., Cribbet, M. R., Nealey-Moore, J. B., Uchino, B. N., Williams, P. G., MacKenzie, J. J., et al. (2011). Matters of the variable heart: Respiratory sinus arrhythmia response to marital interaction and associations with marital quality. *Journal of Personality and Social Psychology, 100*(1), 103–119.

Sprecher, S., & Regan, P. C. (1998). Passionate and companionate love in courting and young married couples. *Sociological Inquiry, 68,* 163–185.

Srivastava, S., McGonigal, K. M., Richards, J. M., Butler, E. A., & Gross, J. J. (2006). Optimism in close relationships: How seeing things in a positive light makes them so. *Journal of Personality and Social Psychology, 91,* 143–153.

Stack, S. (1998). Marriage, family and loneliness: A cross-national study. *Sociological Perspectives, 41,* 415–432.

Stack, S., & Eshleman, J. R. (1998). Marital status and happiness: A 17-nation study. *Journal of Marriage and the Family, 60,* 527–536.

Sternberg, R. J. (1986). A triangular theory of love. *Psychological Review, 93,* 119–135.

Sternberg, R. J. (1998). *Love is a story: A new theory of relationships.* New York: Oxford University Press.

Stoleru, S., & Mouras, H. (2007). Brain functional imaging studies of sexual desire and arousal in human males. In E. Janssen (Ed.), *The psychophysiology of sex* (pp. 3–34). Bloomington: Indiana University Press.

Suomi, S. J. (1999). Attachment in rhesus monkeys. In J. Cassidy & P. R. Shaver (Eds.), *Handbook of attachment: Theory, research, and clinical applications* (pp. 181–197). New York: Guilford Press.

Takahashi, K., Iwase, M., Yamashita, K., Tatsumoto, Y., Ue, H., Kuratsune, H., et al. (2001). The elevation of natural killer cell activity induced by laughter in a crossover designed study. *International Journal of Molecular Medicine, 8,* 645–650.

Tennov, D. (1979). *Love and limerence: The experience of being in love.* New York: Stein & Day.

Traupmann, J., & Hatfield, E. (1981). Love and its effect on mental and physical health. In R. W. Fogel, E. Hatfield, S. B. Keisler, & E. Shanas (Eds.), *Aging: Stability and change in the family* (pp. 253–274). New York: Academic Press.

Trumbull, H. C. (1894). *Friendship the master passion.* Philadelphia: Wattles.

Tucker, P., & Aron, A. (1993). Passionate love and marital satisfaction at key transition points in the family life cycle. *Journal of Social and Clinical Psychology, 12,* 135–147.

Turner, R. A., Altemus, M., Enos, T., Cooper, B., & McGuinness, T. (1999). Preliminary research on plasma oxytocin in normal cycling women: Investigating emotion and interpersonal distress. *Psychiatry, 62,* 97–113.

Uchino, B. N. (2006). Social support and health: A review of physiological processes, potentially underlying links to disease outcomes. *Journal of Behavioral Medicine, 29,* 377–387.

Uvnäs-Moberg, K. (1994). Oxytocin and behaviour. *Annals of Medicine, 26,* 315–317.

Uvnäs-Moberg, K. (1997). Physiological and endocrine effects of social contact. *Annals of the New York Academy of Science, 807,* 146–163.

Uvnäs-Moberg, K. (1998). Oxytocin may mediate the benefits of positive social interaction and emotions. *Psychoneuroendocrinology, 23,* 819–835.

Uvnäs-Moberg, K. (2004). *The oxytocin factor: Tapping the hormone of calm, love, and healing* (R. W. Francis, Trans.). Cambridge, MA: Da Capo Press.

Uvnäs-Moberg, K., Bruzelius, G., Alster, P., & Lundeberg, T. (1993). The antinociceptive effect of non-noxious sensory stimulation is mediated partly through oxytocinergic mechanisms. *Acta Physiologica Scandinavica, 149,* 199–204.

Von Sydow, K. (1995). Unconventional sexual relationships: Data about German women ages 50 to 91 years. *Archives of Sexual Behavior, 24,* 271–290.

Walter, M., Bermpohl, F., Mouras, H., Schiltz, K., Tempelmann, C., Rotte, M., et al. (2008). Distinguishing specific sexual and general emotional effects in fMRI–subcortical and cortical arousal during erotic picture viewing. *NeuroImage, 40,* 1482–1494.

Wenner, M., Kawamura, N., Ishikawa, T., & Matsuda, Y. (2000). Reward linked to increased natural killer cell activity in rats. *Neuroimmunomodulation, 7,* 1–5.

Williams, J. R., Insel, T. R., Harbaugh, C. R., & Carter, C. S. (1994). Oxytocin administered centrally facilitates formation of a partner preference in female prairie voles (*Microtus ochrogaster*). *Journal of Neuroendocrinology, 6,* 247–250.

Williams, W. L. (1992). The relationship between male–male friendship and male–female marriage. In P. Nardi (Ed.), *Men's friendships* (pp. 187–200). Newbury Park, CA: Sage.

Witt, D. M., Winslow, J. T., & Insel, T. R. (1992). Enhanced social interactions in rats following chronic, centrally infused oxytocin. *Pharmacology, Biochemistry and Behavior, 43,* 855–861.

Wrona, D., & Trojniar, W. (2003). Chronic electrical stimulation of the lateral hypothalamus increases natural killer cell cytotoxicity in rats. *Journal of Neuroimmunology, 141,* 20–29.

Wrona, D., & Trojniar, W. (2005). Suppression of natural killer cell cytotoxicity following chronic electrical stimulation of the ventromedial hypothalamic nucleus in rats. *Journal of Neuroimmunology, 163,* 40–52.

Xu, X., Aron, A., Brown, L., Cao, G., Feng, T., & Weng, X. (2010). Reward and motivation systems: A brain mapping study of early-stage intense romantic love in Chinese participants. *Human Brain Mapping, 32,* 249–257.

Zeifman, D., & Hazan, C. (1997). A process model of adult attachment formation. In S. Duck (Ed.), *Handbook of personal relationships* (2nd ed., pp. 179–195). Chichester, UK: Wiley.

CHAPTER 19

■ ■ ■ ■ ■ ■ ■ ■ ■

Compassion

Jennifer E. Stellar
Dacher Keltner

Compassion features in the ancient philosophical musings of Aristotle and Confucius and is a central component of the Bible and Buddhist writings. Compassion provides the emotional underpinnings to one of the most sacred moral values: *care for the weak, do not harm others* (Haidt & Joseph, 2004; Horberg, Oveis, & Keltner, 2011). Along with other prosocial emotions such as gratitude, love, and forgiveness, compassion is crucial for sustaining harmonious group living because it promotes cooperation, caretaking, and social connection with others (Goetz, Keltner, & Simon-Thomas, 2010).

Although compassion is elicited by negatively valenced stimuli—occurrences and signals of harm and suffering—it is in many ways a positive emotion and a fitting topic for this handbook. Compassion is associated with feelings of warmth, tenderness, kindness, and caring, that encourage social connection (Campos et al., 2009). When participants were asked to categorize emotions by valence, compassion was consistently grouped with other positive emotions (Shaver, Schwartz, Kirson, & O'Connor, 1987). Like other positive emotions, compassion also yields benefits for the mind and body (Fredrickson, 2001). For instance, individuals who report experiencing more dispositional compassion are buffered from

the physiological costs of participating in stressful tasks when there are even minimal signs of social support (Cosley, McCoy, Saslow, & Epel, 2010), and caregivers who experience more compassion report lower levels of stress (Monin, Martire, Schulz, & Clark, 2009). Cultivating compassion has become the focus of a burgeoning interest in meditation (Fredrickson, Cohn, Coffey, Pek, & Finkel, 2008) and novel research is even assessing how focusing compassion inward, termed *self-compassion*, may be a better predictor of self-worth than traditional constructs such as self-esteem (Neff & Vonk, 2009). These findings support the claim that compassion is inherently a positive interpersonal emotion, despite its negative triggers.

We argue that compassion is a discrete emotion, distinct from other emotions such as sadness, distress, or love, but part of a family of other-focused affective responses, including empathy, sympathy, and pity. We begin this chapter by defining compassion, its antecedents and appraisals, and its behavioral consequences. We then highlight the evolutionary functions of compassion that suggest why this emotion is found universally in human cultures and can be observed in our closest primate relatives. We next consider how novel methods of measuring emotion expression are uncovering recognizable and potentially universal signals of compassion (Hertenstein, Keltner, App, Bulleit, & Jaskolka, 2006; Simon-Thomas, Keltner, Sauter, Sinicropi-Yao, & Abramson, 2009) and outline the rapidly emerging physiological profile of this emotion (e.g., Eisenberg et al., 1989). Last, we examine the current state of research in compassion and discuss potential future lines of inquiry.

Defining Compassion

Compassion is defined as feeling sorrow or concern for the suffering of another person, coupled with the desire to alleviate that suffering (Eisenberg & Miller, 1987; Lazarus, 1991). This definition situates compassion in the realm of emotions as a feeling or affective response rather than a mere attitude toward suffering (Sprecher & Fehr, 2005). Compassion has specific antecedents, appraisals, and behavioral consequences. It is elicited by the emotional or physical suffering of another person. Laboratory studies have used narratives, pictures, and film clips about individuals with illnesses (Batson, Sager, Garst, & Kang, 1997; Stellar, Manzo, Kraus, & Keltner, 2012), disabled children (Eisenberg, Fabes, et al., 1988), painful responses to shocks (Batson O'Quin, Fultz, Vanderplas, & Isen, 1983), and starvation and poverty (Oveis, Horberg, & Keltner, 2010) to evoke compassion.

Suffering is the core antecedent of compassion, but suffering does not always lead to a compassionate response. Three basic appraisals determine whether compassion, as opposed to other emotions, is elicited. First, to generate compassion, the suffering of an individual needs to be relevant to the self or the goals of the individual perceiving the suffering. This claim is supported by higher levels of compassion, which are reported for kin (Burnstein, Crandall, & Kitayama, 1994) and emotionally close others, such as friends (Korchmaros & Kenny, 2001). Even temporary manipulations that generate perceived similarity can make another's suffering feel more self-relevant. Using a minimal manipulation of similarity, tapping fingers with a partner in synchrony versus asynchrony, Valdesolo and DeSteno (2011) demonstrated that participants who were made to feel similar reported greater compassion when witnessing their partner being victimized by unfair behavior and engaged in more helping behavior. If the suffering of an individual is not relevant to the self, then it is likely to elicit other affective states or little emotion at all. In certain cases, when someone's suffering actually *supports* the goal or values of the self, that suffering may lead to the experience of *schadenfraude*—taking pleasure in another's suffering (Ortony, Clore, & Collins, 1988).

A second critical appraisal centers on the sufferer's deservingness of compassion. Compassion can quickly turn to anger when an individual is perceived to be responsible for the event that caused the suffering (Nussbaum, 1996). Participants who learned an individual had no control over his illness or disease (e.g., contracting AIDS through a blood transfusion) reported greater compassion and less anger for him than participants who learned the individual had contracted the illness or disease through some fault of his own (e.g., AIDS through unprotected sexual contact) (Weiner, Perry, & Magnusson, 1988). A meta-analysis of over 60 studies revealed that the degree of perceived controllability correlated positively with anger and negatively with compassion, and that compassion (but not anger) predicted subsequent prosocial behavior (Rudolph, Roesch, Greitemeyer, & Weiner, 2004). In addition, perceptions of flawed moral character may also lead to appraisals that the sufferer is not worthy of compassion, and accordingly, is unworthy of altruistic behavior and cooperation. Concerns about deservingness, whether founded in perceived responsibility or moral character, are vital to the elicitation of compassion.

Third, appraisals of the ability to cope with the suffering of another person determine the likelihood of the experience of compassion. Responding to someone in need incurs many kinds of costs—the direction of resources to others, potential exploitation, and so on. If an individual perceives these costs to be manageable, whether they be material (e.g., money) or emotional, compassion will be elicited. In support of this claim, a sense of self-efficacy promotes greater compassion in response to suffering. If these costs exceed the capabilities of the observer, then experiences of distress rather than compassion are likely (Hoffman, 1981). One prediction is that individuals who encounter the suffering of large numbers of people (e.g., starvation in Sudan) are more likely to respond with sadness, distress, or even apathy as a result of their inability to cope with suffering of such a large magnitude.

With someone's emotional or physical pain as the core antecedent of compassion, its behavioral consequences center on ameliorating such suffering. Compassion promotes altruistic behavior in an effort to help, care for, or soothe the individual who is suffering (Batson, Fultz, & Schoenrade, 1987). Batson, Duncan, Ackerman, Buckley, and Birch (1981) demonstrated that when levels of compassion were high in response to a confederate being painfully shocked, participants were more likely to offer to take her place, even when escape from the situation was made easy by the experimenter. In addition, the behaviors of compassion are accompanied by cognitions that encourage and reinforce these behaviors, such as a sense of similarity or closeness with the sufferer (Oveis et al., 2010).

Compassion as a Discrete Emotion

Despite the fact that compassion has unique antecedents, appraisals, and behavioral consequences, it has not traditionally been considered part of the taxonomy of basic emotions (e.g., Smith & Ellsworth, 1985). Compassion has often been described as a variation of love mixed with sadness (Shaver et al., 1987; Sprecher & Fehr, 2005; Underwood, 2002) or vicarious distress (Ekman, 2003). However, inspired by several recent studies, we argue that compassion has different antecedents, appraisals, and behavioral consequences than sadness, distress, or love. Studies also suggest that the expressions of these emotions have different patterns in the face and body than compassion (e.g., Eisenberg et al., 1989), a point that we return to later in the chapter.

Although individuals report feeling sadness when they witness others suffer, there are important distinctions between the two emotions. Sadness is a negative emotion based on an appraisal of personal loss and is experienced in response to negative events with clear consequences for the self, such as the loss of a loved one or the dissolution

of an important relationship (Ortony et al., 1988; Shaver et al., 1987). It is associated with behaviors such as withdrawal from social engagement with others (Lazarus, 1991), which clearly distinguishes it from compassion. Sadness may represent a form of emotion contagion rather than a complimentary response to suffering.

Vicarious distress is a natural response to the suffering of another person, but instead of overlapping with compassion, distress can interfere with its experience (Batson et al., 1987). Distress differs from compassion in its focus. Whereas distress and sadness move one's attention inward to the concerns and needs of the self, compassion drives one's attention outward to the person who is suffering. Eisenberg and colleagues (1989) found that self-reports of compassion by children shown a video of another child confronting the death of his parents predicted greater helping behavior, but that self-reports of distress predicted lower levels of helping. Although distress and compassion can share the same antecedent of suffering, their distinct appraisals promote very different behavioral patterns.

Factor analysis can provide insight into the distinctions and relationships among compassion, sadness, and vicarious distress. In studies in which a participant was exposed to someone suffering, factor analysis of the endorsement of a variety of emotion words revealed that compassion-related words loaded onto a different factor than sadness- or distress-related words (Batson et al., 1987; Fultz, Schaller, & Cialdini, 1988). In a separate study, when grouped into positive and negative emotions categories, compassion was considered a positive emotion, whereas sadness and distress were classified as negative emotions. In addition, sadness and distress create motivations to avoid and withdraw, whereas compassion promotes approach and caretaking (Goetz et al., 2010).

Compassion has also been conceived of as a subtype of love (Sprecher & Fehr, 2005; Underwood, 2002). Although fewer empirical studies have teased apart these two emotions, some initial researchers argue that they have different antecedents. While both love and compassion may promote a desire for closeness, love centers on an appreciation of the positive attributes of another, which is often elicited by sharing positive events together (Shaver et al., 1987). In contrast, compassion is based on the experience of suffering. More empirical research will be important to distinguish compassion from love. Studies that measure the expression of sadness, distress, love, and compassion also have further distinguished between these emotions (e.g., Eisenberg et al., 1989), a point that we return to later in the chapter.

More recently, compassion has been conceptualized as part of an emotion family that also contains empathy, sympathy, and pity (Batson et al., 1981; Campos et al., 2009; Goetz et al., 2010). These compassion-related states have similar antecedents, behavioral consequences, signals, and physiological experience (Keltner & Lerner, 2010). Although we argue that empathy, sympathy, and pity are part of an emotion family, we now briefly discuss the distinctions between them. *Empathy* or *empathic concern*, like compassion, is considered to be a state wherein an individual's attention is focused outward on another rather than inward, and it is considered to include feelings such as sympathy, compassion, and tenderness (Batson et al., 1991). As the research on empathy matures, the definition of *empathy* is no longer restricted to feeling negative affect in response to another's suffering, but can be experienced in response to a wide variety of negative and even positive emotions (Rameson, Morelli, & Lieberman, 2012; Royzman & Rozin, 2006). Whereas empathy is characterized as the sharing of another's emotions and perspective, compassion is a complementary emotional response to another's suffering (Lazarus 1991). Sympathy is the most similar to compassion and overlaps in the feeling of sorrow or concern for another person (Batson et al., 1987; Eisenberg et al., 1994). Colloquially, *compassion* and *sympathy* are used interchangeably, and research very rarely distinguishes between the two. *Pity* differs from compassion in that it incorporates hierarchical appraisals of the sufferer's inferiority that can reduce a sense of similarity to the sufferer (Ben Ze'ev, 2000; Fiske, Cuddy, Glick, & Xu, 2002). Interestingly, their valence is one of the few distinctions among sympathy, pity, and compassion. Individuals place sympathy and pity in the same broad emotion category with compassion. However, when categorized by valence, sympathy and pity are categorized as negative, sadness-related emotions, unlike compassion, which is considered to be positive (Shaver et al., 1987). Future work may further define differences among empathy, sympathy, pity, and compassion; however, these compassion-related states are a family of emotions bound by their similarity.

Evolutionary Roots of Compassion

When taking a functional approach to compassion it is helpful to imagine our society without this emotion. Like other basic emotions, compassion serves critical functions and prioritizes particular behaviors. When these behaviors increase the likelihood of survival or the passing on of genetic information, the emotions that motivate these behaviors are selected for by evolution. Darwin recognized the importance of compassion-related emotions, claiming they would be maintained and even encouraged through natural selection processes (Darwin, 1871/2004).

Two arguments have been made by evolutionary theorists for why compassion would be encouraged through different selection processes. First, compassion promotes caretaking behaviors critical to enabling offspring to reach the age of reproduction (Keltner & Haidt, 2001; Trivers, 1971). Adaptations that would encourage caretaking in response to cues of distress in infants would be necessary for infant survival, especially in species where offspring are characterized by an extended period of vulnerability (Berry & McArthur, 1986; Hrdy, 1999). Consistent with this argument, stronger compassion responses are reported for vulnerable targets, such as children and the disabled (Keltner, Horberg, & Oveis, 2006; Zahn-Waxler, Friedman, & Cummings, 1983), individuals who are closely related (Cialdini, Brown, Lewis, Luce, & Neuberg, 1997; Eisenberg & Miller, 1987), and those who are seen as similar to the self (Batson et al., 1981; Oveis et al., 2010). The link between caretaking and compassion is evident even in the literature on attachment styles. Mikulincer and Shaver (2005) found that compassion was more readily felt by individuals with secure attachment styles, as well as those who were induced to feel securely attached.

A second argument posits that compassion evolved to promote cooperation among nonkin (Frank, 1988; Trivers, 1971). Compassion for strangers, this position argues, promotes helping behavior and perpetuates the formation and maintenance of long-term relationships rooted in the benefits of direct reciprocity (Sober & Wilson, 1998; Trivers, 1971). Compassion, along with a suite of other emotions, such as gratitude and anger, may be important for initiating and monitoring valuable reciprocal relationships (Nesse, 1990). In keeping with this argument, individuals who report high levels of dispositional compassion also report more trusting, cooperative, and positive relationships with others (Zhou et al., 2002). It is plausible that compassion may have initially developed to promote caretaking for kin and was later extended to nonkin as a result of the benefits it afforded through increased cooperation (see Goetz et al., 2010).

If compassion evolved universally in humans to promote caretaking and cooperation, it should be detected in a variety of human cultures and be found in closely-related species that share similar societal characteristics. Compassion has been observed by anthropologists and psychologists in both preindustrialized and industrialized cultures (e.g., Eibl-Eibesfeldt, 1989; Eisenberg, Zhou, & Koller, 2001; Konner, 2003). Compassionate behavior has also been recorded among higher-order primate species, and there is mounting evidence that it existed in early hominid societies. A variety of cases of compassionate acts oriented toward harm reduction and caregiving in chimpanzees has been systematically observed (de Waal, 2007; Goodall, 1990; Warneken & Tomasello, 2006). Chimpanzees have assumed costly behaviors such as jumping into water without being able to swim in order to save an unrelated, crying infant (Goodall, 1990) or embracing an unrelated female who has just participated in a painful conflict (de Waal, 2007). In addition, recent analyses of archeological remains of early hominids suggest that compassion was a robust emotion early in our species' history. Examinations of skeletons reveal that children with extreme cases of congenital diseases—which should have led

to death in infancy—received care from others for years, and that elderly individuals lived long after serious levels of deterioration (Hublin, 2009). These lines of evidence suggest that compassion is universal and part of our evolutionary history.

Signal and Measurement of Compassion

Given the likely role of compassion in caregiving interactions and mutual cooperation, evolutionary theorists would argue that its display and recognition in another would be critical (Frank, 1988; Hertenstein et al., 2006). Empirical attempts to document a universal facial signal of compassion have had mixed results. As measures of emotion expand beyond the face, emotion researchers are discovering that compassion is among a host of positive emotions expressed in multiple modalities, along with facial muscle movements.

Facial expressions of compassion can be distinguished from similar emotions such as distress, sadness, or love (Goetz et al., 2010). Expressions of compassion are defined by a furrowing in the center of the brow and relaxation of the lower face with the mouth sometimes open or in a frown (Eisenberg et al., 1989). This display of compassion can be compared to expressions of distress, which include a lowering and pulling forward of the eyebrows and nervous mouth movements, such as tensing of the mouth or biting of the lip (Eisenberg et al., 1989). Sadness shares a similar facial configuration to compassion, most notably in the furrowing of the eyebrows, but sadness has a different bodily posture, which we will discuss shortly (Ekman, Friesen, & Hager, 2002a, 2002b). Love is characterized by Duchenne smiles, and does not include furrowed eyebrows or lip presses (Gonzaga, Keltner, Londahl, & Smith, 2001; Gonzaga, Turner, Keltner, Campos, & Altemus, 2006).

When facial configurations of compassion were recorded as static images, independent of context, two separate studies—one in the United States, the other in India—failed to find high levels of accuracy in recognition of the display (Haidt & Keltner, 1999; Keltner & Buswell, 1996). Compassion images were correctly identified 33–43% of the time (chance guessing between 6 and 12%), but were often confused with sadness, which was used to label slides of expressions portraying compassion 36% of the time. These accuracy rates were lower than those for other emotions, which ranged from the high 50s to the 80s. In a relatively recent study, accuracy rates in identifying compassion from photographs were lower when participants were given the option to respond freely rather than select from a list of emotion choices (Widen, Christy, Hewett, & Russell, 2011).

Positive emotions such as compassion are often expressed when individuals are in close proximity and may utilize other modes of expression, such as body movements, touch, or vocalizations. A remarkable study on emotion encoding assessed whether participants preferred to rely on different modes of communication for different emotions (App, McIntosh, Reed, & Hertenstein, 2011). App and colleagues (2011) discovered that for disgust and anger, the face was the preferred method for discerning emotions, but for love and sympathy, touch was the preferred method. Importantly, accuracy rates for recognizing these emotions were much higher when participants were allowed to use the preferred channel for that emotion.

Touch is a critical component of the expression of compassion and has been demonstrated, especially in times of distress, to reduce levels of cortisol in the body (Francis & Meaney, 1999) and activate brain areas associated with reward (Rolls, 2000) that are critical in recovery from suffering (Keltner & Buswell, 1996). Compassion is readily recognized through touch (Hertenstein et al., 2006). In a paradigm used in both the United States and Spain, a toucher touched a touchee on the forearm in an attempt to communicate different emotions. Participants who were touched within this paradigm reliably identified compassion 48–57% of the time when it was embedded in a forced-choice paradigm (where accuracy rates for random selection of an answer would be around 8%). The communication of compassion was characterized by patting and stroking of the touchee's arm with moderate intensity and for an average duration of 7.6 seconds, which is longer than that for other emotions, such as anger. Furthermore, it appears that the tactile signal of compassion is so robust that feeling the actual touch

is not required; observers who watched the videos of past participants using touch to communicate emotions were also able to identify compassion's expression reliably.

In addition to touch, studies have noted the role of body posture and voice in communicating compassion. Compassion includes an orientation of the head and body forward and a forward lean, which suggest connection and engagement with the sufferer (Eisenberg, Schaller, et al., 1988; Eisenberg et al., 1989). When this stance is contrasted with the posture of sadness, which includes a hunched and withdrawn posture (Coulson, 2004; Shaver et al., 1987) and eye gaze aversion (Adams & Kleck, 2005), it becomes clear that compassion and sadness are signaled in different ways.

Compassion is also communicated through the voice. When participants were presented with half-second, nonword vocal bursts that attempted to communicate different emotions, compassion was identified 24% of the time in a forced-choice paradigm among 12 other positive emotions (again, accuracy rates for random answering would be around 8%; Simon-Thomas et al., 2009). Accurate and reliable measurement of the expression of compassion requires a more global coding system that includes facial expression, movements and orientation of the head and body, touch, and vocalizations, or that at least allows participants to recognize emotions using their preferred channel.

Compassion and the Autonomic Nervous System

Witnessing the suffering of another person is associated with changes in the peripheral autonomic nervous system that not only are useful tools in the measurement of compassion but also elucidate how this emotion mobilizes the body for action. What is known about the basic correlates of autonomic processes lays the groundwork for predictions about the relationship of compassion to changes in heart rate. For instance, heart rate tends to decelerate in association with an outward focus of attention (Cacioppo & Sandman, 1978), which is a core aspect of compassion in response to suffering. For example, Eisenberg and colleagues (1991) have indeed documented that compassion at the subjective and expressive levels tends to covary with heart rate deceleration, which in turn predicts downstream helping behavior. Participants induced to feel compassion show decreases in heart rate from neutral state inductions, and the magnitude of the physiological response distinguished between those who reported more or less compassion (Stellar et al., 2013).

Changes in heart rate associated with compassion differentiate the autonomic profile of compassion from that of distress. When individuals respond with distress to someone's suffering, heart rate tends to accelerate (Eisenberg et al., 1991). Distress appears to activate the sympathetic, fight-or-flight system, and signals autonomic arousal. In support of this claim, skin conductance—a pure measure of sympathetic activity that is traditionally associated with general arousal and stress (Dawson, Schell, & Filion, 2000)—has reliably been associated with distress but not compassion (Eisenberg et al., 1991).

More recent work suggests that the parasympathetic system, particularly the vagus nerve, may have an important association with compassion. The autonomic nervous system has two branches, the parasympathetic and sympathetic, which in most cases act antagonistically with one another (Brownley, Hurwitz, & Schneiderman, 2000). Whereas the sympathetic system prepares the body for defensive or offensive behaviors, the parasympathetic system has been implicated in recovery from stress, as well as in processes that take place during restful, calm states (Mezzacappa, Kelsey, Katkin, & Sloan, 2001). The vagus nerve, a critical component of the parasympathetic system, is thought to enable the individual to focus on another and to approach and soothe (Porges, 2003). The vagus nerve is the 10th cranial nerve and projects from the nucleus ambiguus and dorsal motor nucleus, innervating muscles involved in communication (e.g., facial muscles and those that coordinate head movements), as well as organs such as the heart and stomach. It is most often measured through the noninvasive index of respiratory sinus arrhythmia (RSA) (Brownley et al., 2000). The vagus nerve has been linked to facial and vocal displays, attention, nodding of the head when listening, and motor behaviors such as tactile contact, which are all involved in compassion. Some researchers have theorized that the portion of the vagus nerve that is unique to mammals may have evolved to encourage social engagement in humans and feelings of connection to others (Beauchaine, 2001; Kok & Fredrickson, 2010; Porges 2003). In support of this claim, RSA is often inversely related to heart rate and is higher during sustained attention, which both occur during compassion (Suess, Porges, & Plude, 1994). As further support, individuals shown compassion-inducing stimuli, compared to neutral video clips, exhibit higher RSA (Stellar & Keltner, 2013). In children, higher vagal tone predicted greater levels of self-reported compassion when watching a video about another child's response to a stranger lurking outside his house (Fabes, Eisenberg, & Eisenbud, 1993). Further evidence for the link between vagal tone and compassion comes from clinical samples. Children with autism, who show some of the most significant deficits in the capacity to experience compassion and social connection with others, have low vagal activity (Ming, Julu, Brimacombe, Connor, & Daniels, 2005). Individuals who show high risk for mania, which is characterized by the extreme experience of positive emotion and a heightened sense of connection with others, exhibit extremely high levels of vagal activity (Gruber, Johnson, Oveis, & Keltner, 2008). If emotions are associated with changes in the body in preparation for certain action patterns, it is provocative to ask how heart rate deceleration and increased vagal activity serve to promote compassion-related behavior. While emotions such as anger move blood to the periphery in order to engage in aggression (Levenson, 2003), changes in the body associated with compassion and social engagement may calm the body to prepare it to engage soothingly and in a caring manner with those who are suffering.

Compassion and the Central Nervous System

The emerging field of neuroscience has identified a network of areas thought to be associated with empathy and compassion (see Simon-Thomas et al., 2011). Recent work has investigated how the desire to approach and care for someone who is suffering, a core component of compassion, activates unique areas associated with caregiving, such as the periaqueductal gray (PAG) (Simon-Thomas et al., 2011). The PAG is an older area of the brain that is associated with the monitoring of pain, as well as caregiving behavior (Heinricher, Tavares, Leith, & Lumb, 2009; Lovick & Adamec, 2009). For instance, the PAG shows greater activation when mothers are shown pictures of infants exhibiting attachment-soliciting behaviors such as smiling or crying (Bartels & Zeki, 2004; Nitschke et al., 2004; Noriuchi, Kikuchi, & Senoo, 2008; Swain, 2010). The PAG plays a critical role during the experience of compassion. It shows greater activation when participants viewed images of sad faces with instructions to view them with a compassionate attitude (Kim et al., 2009), heard compassion-inducing narratives (Immordino-Yang, McColl, Damasio, & Damasio, 2009) and watched compassion-inducing slides (Simon-Thomas et al., 2011). Activation of the PAG during compassionate responding supports a deep link between compassion and caretaking.

Current and Future Directions in Compassion Research

The scientific study of positive emotion, once an afterthought in the emotion revolution, has made great advances. The young science of positive emotion has elucidated important distinctions between different positive emotions and their place in thought and action. However, there are still several unanswered questions in the study of compassion. These include broad questions as to the boundary conditions, how individual differences shape compassion, and the role of emotion regulation in compassion.

Defining the boundary conditions of compassion is critical for understanding why it may be attenuated in some situations and exaggerated in others. For example, in their classic "From Jerusalem to Jericho" study, Darley and Batson (1973) found that creating a context with time pressure reduced participants' compassionate responses to those in need. More is needed to understand the various contextual forces that shape the compassion experience. Certain environments that prioritize a focus on the self should be particularly likely to diminish the experience of compassion. We argue that even small primes (e.g., making money or wealth salient) would have large effects on the experience of compassion. In addition, environments that are competitive and stressful would likely reduce compassion by shifting one's focus almost exclusively to the self. According to a report by the American Psychological Association (2010), the impact of stressful environments on compassionate responding will be an important line of inquiry as perceptions of daily stress levels continue to rise. It is of critical importance to understand whether our current society facilitates environments that are damaging to the experience of compassion.

In addition to contextual information, the qualities of both the observer and the sufferer are certain to moderate compassionate responding. In terms of observer qualities, dispositional measures of compassion suggest that certain individuals experience this emotion more than others (Shiota, Keltner, & John, 2006). Cultural identities may also attenuate or intensify the experience of compassion for observers. For instance, lower social class individuals experience greater compassion in response to the suffering of others than their upper-class counterparts (Stellar et al., 2012). These differences in compassion are posited to be responsible for greater levels of prosocial behavior among individuals of lower socioeconomic status (Piff, Kraus, Côté, Cheng, & Keltner, 2010). Studies examining power mirror results of studies of social class; people with high power display a more attenuated compassion response than do people with low power (van Kleef et al., 2008).

Compassion is inherently a social emotion, and little is known about how individual differences in the sufferer influence compassionate responses in others. Compassion is not felt equally for everyone. Evolutionary accounts would predict reduced compassion for those who, because of selfish qualities, may not reciprocate altruistic behavior (Trivers, 1971). Moral judgments about individuals' dishonesty or lack of trustworthiness may act in similar ways to attentuate compassion in response to their suffering. Future work should examine whether individuals who hold opposing moral values (e.g., abortion or capital punishment) would also elicit less compassion. Drawing distinctions between ingroup and outgroup membership has a variety of interpersonal consequences that suggest reduced compassion for outgroup members and increased compassion for ingroup members (Chiao & Mathur, 2010). Future work should examine whether reduced compassion for racial or ethnic outgroups is part of the larger set of psychological effects evoked by different group membership.

And finally, the experience of compassion can be regulated like any other emotion. One argument holds that emotion regulation while witnessing another person suffer should reduce negative affect and personal distress, thus allowing for more compassion. Down-regulation of distress may be critical for achieving a compassionate response. As mentioned earlier in this chapter, appraisals centered on the ability to cope with the suffering of another individual are critical in promoting compassion instead of distress. Studies that reduce coping skills via cognitive load or depletion of emotional capacities may promote a more negative affective response, leading to greater distress rather than compassion. One study provides suggestive results related to this line of reasoning, demonstrating a positive relationship between trait emotion regulation strategies and self-reported compassion (Eisenberg et al., 1994), but these results do not indicate how regulation strategies interact with emotional responses to suffering to predict compassionate responding in the moment.

At the same time, one can readily imagine instances in which emotion regulation might reduce compassionate responding. Recent research has documented that when regulation strategies such as reappraisal were engaged while watching compassion-inducing images and information, compassion diminishes (Cameron & Payne, 2011). The relationship between emotion regulation and compassion may also depend on the particular type of regulation strategy being used. There are many different styles of emotion regulation, and two of the most commonly studied forms, expressive suppression and cognitive reappraisal (Gross & John, 2003), may have diverging influences on compassion.

Conclusion

Recent research has documented that compassion, an approach-oriented, positively valenced emotion, is different from related emotions such as sadness, distress, and love. Compassion is part of a family of prosocial emotions, including empathy, sympathy, and pity, that motivate helping and soothing behaviors in response to suffering. Compassion is universally signaled through touch and vocalizations and a physiological profile of this emotion is emerging. These multiple methods of measurement will allow more accurate assessment of this vital interpersonal emotion in laboratory settings. Future work aimed at understanding the social contexts, individual differences, appraisals, and regulation strategies that attenuate or amplify compassion are important avenues of future research, with deep societal implications. Compassion propels us to form connections, bonding us to others when they suffer and need help the most. Morality and altruism captivated the minds of scientists even before Darwin and Aristotle, yet little attention has been given to its emotional underpinnings.

References

Adams, R. B., & Kleck, R. E. (2005). Effects of direct and averted gaze on the perception of facially communicated emotion. *Emotion, 5,* 3–11.

American Psychological Association. (2010). *Stress in America findings.* Washington, DC: Author.

App, B., McIntosh, D. N., Reed, C. L., & Hertenstein, M. J. (2011). Nonverbal channel use in communication of emotion: How may depend on why. *Emotion, 11,* 603–617.

Bartels, A., & Zeki, S. (2004). The neural correlates of maternal and romantic love. *NeuroImage, 21*(3), 1155–1166.

Batson, C. D., Duncan, B. D., Ackerman, P., Buckley, T., & Birch, K. (1981). Is empathic emotion a source of altruistic motivation? *Journal of personality and Social Psychology, 40*(2), 290–302.

Batson, C. D., Fultz, J., & Schoenrade, P. A. (1987). Distress and empathy: Two qualitatively distinct vicarious emotions with different motivational consequences. *Journal of Personality, 55,* 19–39.

Batson, C. D., O'Quin, K., Fultz, J., Vanderplas, M., & Isen, A. M. (1983). Influence of self-reported distress and empathy on egoistic versus altruistic motivation to help. *Journal of Personality and Social Psychology, 45,* 706–718.

Batson, C. D., Sager, K., Garst, E., & Kang, M. (1997). Is empathy-induced helping due to self–other merging? *Journal of Personality and Social Psychology, 73,* 495–509.

Beauchaine, T. (2001). Vagal tone, development, and Gray's motivational theory: Toward an integrated model of autonomic nervous system functioning in psychopathology. *Development and psychopathology, 13,* 183–214.

Ben Ze'ev, A. (2000). *The subtlety of emotions.* Cambridge, MA: MIT Press.

Berry, D. S., & McArthur, L. Z. (1986). Perceiving character in faces: The impact of age-related craniofacial changes on social perception. *Psychological Bulletin, 100,* 3–18.

Brownley, K. A., Hurwitz, B. E., & Schneiderman, N. (2000). Cardiovascular psychophysiology. In J. T. Cacioppo, L. G. Tassinary, & G. G. Bernston (Eds.), *Handbook of psychophysiology.* (pp. 224–264). Cambridge, UK: Cambridge University Press.

Burnstein, E., Crandall, C., & Kitayama, S. (1994). Some neo-Darwinian decision rules for altruism: Weighing cues for inclusive fitness as a function of the biological importance of the decision. *Journal of Personality and Social Psychology, 67,* 773–789.

Cacioppo, J. X., & Sandman, C. A. (1978). Physiological differentiation of sensory and cognitive tasks as a function of warning, processing demands, and reported unpleasantness. *Biological Psychology, 6,* 181–192.

Cameron, C. D., & Payne, B. K. (2011). Escaping affect: How motivated emotion regulation creates insensitivity to mass suffering. *Journal of Personality and Social Psychology, 100,* 1–15.

Campos, B., Shiota, M. N., Keltner, D., Gonzaga, G., Goetz, J. L., & Shin, M. (2009). *Amusement, awe, contentment, happiness, love, pride, and sympathy: An empirical exploration of positive emotions in language, internal experience, and facial expression.* Unpublished manuscript, Department of Psychology, University of California, Berkeley.

Chiao, J. Y., & Mathur, V. A. (2010). Intergroup empathy: How does race affect empathic neural responses? *Current Biology, 20,* R478–R480.

Cialdini, R. B., Brown, S. L., Lewis, B. P., Luce, C., & Neuberg, S. L. (1997). Reinterpreting the empathy–altruism relationship: When one into one equals oneness. *Journal of Personality and Social Psychology, 73*(3), 481–494.

Cosley, B. J., McCoy, S. K., Saslow, L. R., & Epel, E. S. (2010). Is compassion for others stress buffering?: Consequences of compassion and social support for physiological reactivity to stress. *Journal of Experimental Social Psychology, 46,* 816–823.

Coulson, M. (2004). Attributing emotion to static body postures: Recognition accuracy, confusions, and viewpoint dependence. *Journal of Nonverbal Behavior, 28,* 117–139.

Darley, J. M., & Batson, C. D. (1973). "From Jerusalem to Jericho": A study of situational and dispositional variables in helping behavior. *Journal of Personality and Social Psychology, 27,* 100–108.

Darwin, C. (2004). *The descent of man, and selection in relation to sex.* London: Penguin Books. (Original work published 1871)

Dawson, M. E., Schell, A. M., & Filion, D. L. (2000). The electrodermal system. In J. T. Cacioppo, L. G. Tassinary, & G. G. Bernston (Eds.), *Handbook of psychophysiology* (pp. 200–223). Cambridge, UK: Cambridge University Press.

de Waal, F. B. (2007). With a little help from a friend. *PLoS Biology, 5,* e190.

Eibl-Eibesfeldt, I. (1989). *Human ethology.* New York: de Gruyter.

Eisenberg, N., Fabes, R. A., Bustamante, D., Mathy, R. M., Miller, P. A., & Lindholm, E. (1988). Differentiation of vicariously induced emotional reactions in children. *Developmental Psychology, 24,* 237–246.

Eisenberg, N., Fabes, R. A., Miller, P. A., Fultz, J., Shell, R., Mathy, R. M., et al. (1989). Relation of sympathy and personal distress to prosocial behavior: A multimethod study. *Journal of Personality and Social Psychology, 57,* 55–66.

Eisenberg, N., Fabes, R. A., Murphy, B., Karbon, M., Maszk, P., Smith, M., et al. (1994). The relations of emotionality and regulation to dispositional and situational empathy-related responding. *Journal of Personality and Social Psychology, 66,* 776–797.

Eisenberg, N., Fabes, R. A., Schaller, M., Miller, P., Carlo, G., Poulin, R., et al. (1991). Personality and socialization correlates of vicarious emotional responding. *Journal of Personality and Social Psychology, 61,* 459–470.

Eisenberg, N., & Miller, P. A. (1987). The relation of empathy to prosocial and related behaviors. *Psychological Bulletin, 101,* 91–119.

Eisenberg, N., Schaller, M., Fabes, R. A., Bustamante, D., Mathy, R. M., Shell, R., et al. (1988). Differentiation of personal distress and sympathy in children and adults. *Developmental Psychology, 24,* 766–775.

Eisenberg, N., Zhou, Q., & Koller, S. (2001). Brazilian adolescents' prosocial moral judgment and behavior: Relations to sympathy, perspective taking, gender-role orientation, and demographic characteristics. *Child Development, 72*(2), 518–534.

Ekman, P. (2003). *Emotions revealed: Recognizing faces and feelings to improve communication and emotional life.* New York: Holt.

Ekman, P., Friesen, W. V., & Hager, J. C. (2002a). *Facial Action Coding System: The investigator's guide.* Salt Lake City, UT: Research Nexus.

Ekman, P., Friesen, W. V., & Hager, J. C. (2002b). *Facial Action Coding System: The manual.* Salt Lake City, UT: Research Nexus.

Fabes, R. A., Eisenberg, N., & Eisenbud, L. (1993). Behavioral and physiological correlates of children's reactions to others in distress. *Developmental Psychology, 29*(4), 655–663.

Fiske, S. T., Cuddy, A. J. C., Glick, P., & Xu, J. (2002). A model of (often mixed) stereotype content: Competence and warmth respectively follow from perceived status and competition. *Journal of Personality and Social Psychology, 82,* 878–902.

Francis, D., & Meaney, M. J. (1999). Maternal care and the development of stress responses. *Development, 9,* 128–134.

Frank, R. H. (1988). *Passions within reason: The strategic role of the emotions.* New York: Norton.

Fredrickson, B. L. (2001). The role of positive emotions in positive psychology: The broaden-and-build theory of positive emotions. *American Psychologist, 56,* 218–226.

Fredrickson, B. L., Cohn, M. A., Coffey, K. A., Pek, J., & Finkel, S. M. (2008). Open hearts build lives: Positive emotions, induced through loving-kindness meditation, build consequential personal resources. *Journal of Personality and Social Psychology, 95,* 1045–1062.

Fultz, J., Schaller, M., & Cialdini, R. B. (1988). Empathy, sadness, and distress: Three related but distinct vicarious affective responses to another's suffering. *Personality and Social Psychology Bulletin, 14,* 312–325.

Goetz, J. L., Keltner, D., & Simon-Thomas, E. (2010). Compassion: An evolutionary analysis and empirical review. *Psychological Bulletin, 136,* 351–374.

Gonzaga, G. C., Keltner, D., Londahl, E. A., & Smith, M. D. (2001). Love and the commitment problem in romantic relationships and friendship. *Journal of Personality and Social Psychology, 81,* 247–262.

Gonzaga, G. C., Turner, R. A., Keltner, D., Campos, B. C., & Altemus, M. (2006). Romantic love and sexual desire in close bonds. *Emotion, 6,* 163–179.

Goodall, J. (1990). *Through a window: My thirty years with the chimpanzees of Fombe.* Boston: Houghton Mifflin.

Gross, J. J., & John, O. P. (2003). Individual differences in two emotion regulation processes: Implications for affect, relationships, and well-being. *Journal of Personality and Social Psychology, 85,* 348–362.

Gruber, J., Johnson, S. L., Oveis, C., & Keltner, D. (2008). Risk for mania and positive emotional responding: Too much of a good thing? *Emotion, 8*(1), 23–33.

Haidt, J., & Joseph, C. (2004). Intuitive ethics: How innately prepared intuitions generate culturally variable virtues [Special issue]. *Daedalus, 133,* 55–66.

Haidt, J., & Keltner, D. (1999). Culture and facial expression: Open-ended methods find more expression and a gradient of recognition. *Cognition and Emotion, 13,* 225–266.

Heinricher, M. M., Tavares, I., Leith, J. L., Lumb, B. M. (2009). Descending control of nociception: specificity, recruitment and plasticity. *Brain Research Review, 60*(1), 214–225.

Hertenstein, M. J., Keltner, D., App, B., Bulleit, B. A., & Jaskolka, A. R. (2006). Touch communicates distinct emotions. *Emotion, 6,* 528–533.

Hoffman, M. L. (1981). Is altruism part of human nature? *Journal of Personality and Social Psychology, 40,* 121–137.

Horberg, E. J., Oveis, C., & Keltner, D. (2011). Emotions as moral amplifiers: An appraisal tendency approach to the influences of distinct emotions upon moral judgment. *Emotion Review, 3,* 237–242.

Hrdy, S. H. (1999). *Mother Nature: A history of mothers, infants, and natural selection.* New York: Pantheon.

Hublin, J. J. (2009). The prehistory of compassion. *Proceedings of the National Academy of Sciences, 106,* 6429–6430.

Immordino-Yang, M. H., McColl, A., Damasio, H., & Damasio, A. (2009). Neural correlates of admiration and compassion. *Proceedings of the National Academy of Sciences USA, 106,* 8021–8026.

Keltner, D., & Buswell, B. N. (1996). Evidence for the distinctness of embarrassment, shame, and guilt: A study of recalled antecedents and facial expressions of emotion. *Cognition and Emotion, 10,* 155–172.

Keltner, D., & Haidt, J. (2001). Social functions of emotions. In T. J. Mayne & G. A. Bonanno (Eds.), *Emotions: Current issues and future directions* (pp. 192–213). New York: Guilford Press.

Keltner, D., Horberg, E. J., & Oveis, C. (2006). Emotions as moral intuitions. In J. P. Forgas (Ed.), *Affect in thinking and social behavior* (pp. 161–175). New York: Psychology Press.

Keltner, D., & Lerner, J. S. (2010). Emotion. In S. Fiske & D. Gilbert (Eds.), *The handbook of social psychology* (5th ed., pp. 312–347). Hoboken, NJ: Wiley.

Kim, J. W., Kim, S. E., Kim, J. J., Jeong, B., Park, C. H., Son, A. R., et al. (2009). Compassionate attitude towards others' suffering activates the mesolimbic neural system. *Neuropsychologia, 47,* 2073–2081.

Kok, B. E., & Fredrickson, B. L. (2010). Upward spirals of the heart: Autonomic flexibility, as indexed by vagal tone, reciprocally and prospectively predicts positive emotions and social connectedness. *Biological Psychology, 85,* 432–436.

Konner, M. (2003). *The tangled wing: Biological constraints on the human spirit.* New York: Holt.

Korchmaros, J. D., & Kenny, D. A. (2001). Emotional closeness as a mediator of the effect of genetic relatedness on altruism. *Psychological Science, 12,* 262–265.

Lazarus, R. S. (1991). *Emotion and adaptation.* Oxford, UK: Oxford University Press.

Levenson, R. W. (2003). Autonomic specificity and emotion. In R. J. Davidson & K. R. Scherer (Eds.), *Handbook of affective sciences* (pp. 212–224). New York: Oxford University Press.

Lovick, T. A., & Adamec, R. (2009). The periaqueductal gray (PAG). *Neural Plasticity, 2009,* 360907.

Mezzacappa, E. S., Kelsey, R. M., Katkin, E. S., & Sloan, R. P. (2001). Vagal rebound and recovery from psychological stress. *Psychosomatic Medicine, 63,* 650–657.

Mikulincer, M., & Shaver, P. R. (2005). Attachment security, compassion and altruism. *Current Directions in Psychological Science, 14,* 34–38.

Ming, X., Julu, P. O., Brimacombe, M., Connor, S., & Daniels, M. L. (2005). Reduced cardiac parasympathetic activity in children with autism. *Brain and Development, 27,* 509–516.

Monin, J. K., Martire, L. M., Schulz, R., & Clark, M. S. (2009). Willingness to express emotions to caregiving spouses. *Emotion, 9,* 101–106.

Neff, K. D., & Vonk, R. (2009). Self-compassion versus global self-esteem: Two different ways of relating to oneself. *Journal of Personality, 77,* 23–50.

Nesse, R. M. (1990). Evolutionary explanations of emotions. *Human Nature, 1,* 261–289.

Nitschke, J. B., Nelson, E. E., Rusch, B. D., Fox, A. S., Oakes, T. R., & Davidson, R. J. (2004). Orbitofrontal cortex tracks positive mood in mothers viewing pictures of their newborn infants. *NeuroImage, 21,* 583–592.

Noriuchi, M., Kikuchi, Y., Senoo, A. (2008). The functional neuroanatomy of maternal love: Mother's response to infant's attachment behaviors. *Biological Psychiatry, 63,* 415–423.

Nussbaum, M. C. (1996). Compassion: The basic social emotion. *Social Philosophy and Policy, 13,* 27–58.

Ortony, A., Clore, G. L., & Collins, A. (1988). *The cognitive structure of emotions.* New York: Cambridge University Press.

Oveis, C., Horberg, E. J., & Keltner, D. (2010). Compassion, pride, and social intuitions of self–other similarity. *Journal of Personality and Social Psychology, 98,* 618–630.

Piff, P. K., Kraus, M. W., Côté, S., Cheng, B. H., & Keltner, D. (2010). Having less, giving more: the influence of social class on prosocial behavior. *Journal of Personality and Social Psychology, 99*(5), 771–784.

Porges, S. W. (2003). The polyvagal theory: Phylogenetic contributions to social behavior. *Physiology and Behavior. 79,* 503–513.

Rameson, L. T., Morelli, S. A., & Lieberman, M. D. (2012). The neural correlates of empathy: experience, automaticity, and prosocial behavior. *Journal of Cognitive Neuroscience, 24*(1), 235–245.

Rolls, E. T. (2000). The orbitofrontal cortex and reward. *Cerebral Cortex, 10,* 284–294.

Royzman, E. B., & Rozin, P. (2006). Limits of symhedonia: The differential role of prior emotional attachment in sympathy and sympathetic joy. *Emotion, 6,* 82–93.

Rudolph, U., Roesch, S. C., Greitemeyer, T., & Weiner, B. (2004). A meta-analytic review of help giving and aggression from an attributional perspective: Contributions to a general theory of motivation. *Cognition and Emotion, 18,* 815–848.

Shaver, P. R., Schwartz, J., Kirson, D., & O'Connor, C. (1987). Emotion knowledge: Further exploration of a prototype approach. *Journal of Personality and Social Psychology, 52,* 1061–1086.

Shiota, M. N., Keltner, D., & John, O. P. (2006). Positive emotion dispositions differentially associated with Big Five personality and attachment style. *Journal of Positive Psychology, 1,* 61–71.

Simon-Thomas, E. R., Godzik, J., Castle, E., Antonenko, O., Ponz, A., Kogan, A., et al. (2011). An fMRI study of caring vs self-focus during induced compassion and pride. *Social Cognitive and Affective Neuroscience, 1,* 635–648.

Simon-Thomas, E. R., Keltner, D. J., Sauter, D., Sinicropi-Yao, L., & Abramson, A. (2009). The voice conveys specific emotions: Evidence from vocal burst displays. *Emotion, 9,* 838–846.

Smith, C. A., & Ellsworth, P. C. (1985). Patterns of cognitive appraisal in emotion. *Journal of Personality and Social Psychology, 48,* 813–838.

Sober, E., & Wilson, D. S. (1998). *Unto others: The evolution and psychology of unselfish behavior.* Cambridge, MA: Harvard University Press.

Sprecher, S., & Fehr, B. (2005). Compassionate love for close others and humanity. *Journal of Social and Personal Relationships, 22,* 629–651.

Stellar, J. E., & Keltner, D. (2013). *Vagal reactivity and compassionate responses to the suffering of others.* Manuscript submitted for publication.

Stellar, J. E., Manzo, V. M., Kraus, M. W., & Keltner, D. (2012). Class and compassion:

Socioeconomic factors predict responses to suffering. *Emotion, 12,* 449–459.

Suess, P. A., Porges, S. W., & Plude, D. J. (1994). Cardiac vagal tone and sustained attention in school-age children. *Psychophysiology, 31,* 17–22.

Swain, J. E. (2010). The human parental brain: In vivo neuroimaging. *Progress in Neuro-Psychopharmacology and Biological Psychiatry, 35,* 1242–1254.

Trivers, R. L. (1971). The evolution of reciprocal altruism. *Quarterly Review of Biology, 46,* 35–57.

Underwood, L. G. (2002). The human experience of compassionate love: Conceptual mapping and data from selected studies. In S. G. Post, L. G. Underwood, J. P. Schloss, & W. B. Hurlbut (Eds.), *Altruism and altruistic love: Science, philosophy, and religion in dialogue* (pp. 72–88). New York: Oxford University Press.

Valdesolo, P., & DeSteno, D. (2011). Synchrony and the social tuning of compassion. *Emotion, 11,* 262–266.

van Kleef, G. A., Oveis, C., van der Löwe, I., LuoKogan, A., Goetz, J., & Keltner, D. (2008). Power, distress, and compassion: Turning a blind eye to the suffering of others. *Psychological Science, 19,* 1315–1322.

Warneken, F., & Tomasello, M. (2006). Altruistic helping in human infants and young chimpanzees. *Science, 311,* 1301–1303.

Weiner, B., Perry, R. P., & Magnusson, J. (1988). An attributional analysis of reactions to stigmas. *Journal of Personality and Social Psychology, 55,* 738–748.

Widen, S. C., Christy, A. M., Hewett, K., & Russell, J. A. (2011). Do proposed facial expressions of contempt, shame, embarrassment, and compassion communicate the predicted emotion? *Cognition and Emotion, 25,* 898–906.

Zahn-Waxler, C., Friedman, S. L., & Cummings, E. M. (1983). Children's emotions and behaviors in response to infants' cries. *Child Development, 54,* 1522–1528.

Zhou, Q., Eisenberg, N., Losoya, S. H., Fabes, R. A., Reiser, M., Guthrie, I. K., et al. (2002). The relations of parental warmth and positive expressiveness to children's empathy-related responding and social functioning: A longitudinal study. *Child Development, 73,* 893–915.

CHAPTER 20

■ ■ ■ ■ ■ ■ ■ ■

Gratitude

Anthony H. Ahrens
Courtney N. Forbes

A joyful and pleasant thing it is to be thankful.
—*Book of Common Prayer* (1892)

Can a day go by without the experience of gratitude, whether in response to the cashier who sells the morning coffee, the roommate or romantic partner who completes household chores, the colleague who helps with difficult tasks, or the experience of beauty in nature? Gratitude has been called "foundational to well-being and mental health throughout the lifespan" (Emmons & Mishra, 2011, p. 249).

Research on the psychology of gratitude has only recently become common, but it has been growing. A search of the database PsycINFO for the subject heading *gratitude* yielded just four articles in 2004 and three in 2005, but 35 in 2010 and 27 in 2011. The rate of publication on gratitude has become sufficient that there have been multiple excellent recent reviews of it (e.g., Emmons & Mishra, 2011; Watkins, Van Gelder, & Frias, 2009; Wood, Froh, & Geraghty, 2010). Given the promise of initial research on gratitude, the Greater Good Science Center, funded by the John Templeton Foundation, has launched a nearly $6 million

program to support research on gratitude (Lattin, 2012). In just the last few years, more and more psychologists have shown interest in learning how gratitude contributes to human well-being and social life.

This growing interest in gratitude has yielded several interrelated lines of research. In this review, we emphasize four such lines. First we examine the "grateful disposition," which is correlated with a variety of measures of physical and mental health. Next we turn to interventions designed to increase gratitude. These have shown promise for improving well-being. Third, we discuss gratitude in the context of interpersonal relationships. Might gratitude facilitate the building and maintenance of good relationships? Finally, we focus on insights that might be drawn from considering people's reports of gratitude as arising from a set of related emotions rather than from a single emotion. Our chapter emphasizes recent research, especially that conducted since the extensive review by Wood and colleagues (2010).

Gratitude as a Disposition

Gratefulness is the key to a happy life that we hold in our hands because if we are not grateful, then no matter how much we have we will not be happy—because we will always want to have something else or something more.

—Brother David Steindl-Rast
(in Lesowitz & Sammons, 2009)

If gratitude is indeed the key to a happy life, then it is not surprising that one of the important developments in gratitude research has been the description of the "grateful disposition," and the demonstration that this disposition is related to well-being. In a foundational paper, McCullough, Emmons, and Tsang (2002) defined it as "a generalized tendency to recognize and respond with grateful emotion to the roles of other people's benevolences in the positive experiences and outcomes that one obtains" (p. 112). Dispositionally grateful people are particularly likely to feel and express thankfulness for benefits received from others, and this tendency is consistent across varied situations.

Research has confirmed that grateful people may indeed hold the keys to a happy life. McCullough and his colleagues (2002) found a link between the grateful disposition and several qualities, such as being low in Neuroticism and high in Agreeableness and Extraversion. They also developed an individual-differences measure for the disposition toward gratitude, the Gratitude Questionnaire (GQ-6), in which participants indicate the degree to which they endorse statements such as "I have much in life to be thankful for." When researchers controlled for the Big Five traits, higher dispositional gratitude was still related to less envy and feelings of depression, and to greater life satisfaction and happiness. Considerable subsequent work has confirmed the association of dispositional gratitude, using both the GQ-6 and other related measures, with well-being, construed broadly (see Wood et al., 2010, for a review).

Recent work has extended the range of psychological health variables to which the grateful disposition is related. For instance, one study (Breen, Kashdan, Lenser, & Fincham, 2010) examined whether undergraduate students' dispositional tendencies toward gratitude and forgiveness could be used to predict other person-level variables reliably. High levels of gratitude and forgiveness were negatively associated with neuroticism, anger, loneliness, and depressive symptoms, and positively associated with acceptance and self-compassion. Participants' self-ratings of dispositional gratitude and forgiveness were also correlated with others' reports of participants' well-being. Highly grateful and forgiving people were less unhappy and more accepting, both in their own eyes and in the eyes of others.

The link between gratitude, health, and happiness appears to be consistent across diverse populations, from adolescents to older adults. For instance, in a sample of youth ages 10–19, high scores on the GQ-6 correlated with positive affect and life satisfaction (Froh, Fan, et al., 2011). In the same sample, dispositionally grateful adolescents ages 12–19 reported less negative affect. Similarly, in a recent study of high school students (Froh, Emmons, Card, Bono, & Wilson, 2011), those who reported high trait-level gratitude did better in school, were more satisfied with their lives, felt more connected to those around them, and reported fewer depressive symptoms than their less grateful peers. And, among 16- to 18-year-olds, those whose life satisfaction rankings were in the top one-third among their peers reported more gratitude than those in the middle and lower one-thirds (Proctor, Linley, & Maltby, 2010). Overall, highly grateful adolescents appear to flourish.

Trait-level gratitude is also associated with well-being in older groups. In a sample of Christian adults ages 60–89 (Scheidle, 2011), participants' grateful dispositions, as measured by both the GQ-6 and the Gratitude, Resentment, and Appreciation Test (GRAT; Watkins, Woodward, Stone, & Kolts, 2003), predicted positive affect, life satisfaction, and healthy attitudes toward aging, indicating that older adults who are disposed toward high levels of gratitude may also be more content with their lives. The grateful disposition appears to predict increased happiness, adjustment, and psychological well-being across the lifespan.

Although the majority of research to date has examined the correlates of dispositional gratitude among Westerners, preliminary cross-cultural work suggests that the GQ-6 may also have predictive value in East Asian populations (Chen & Kee, 2008). For instance, dispositional gratitude was positively associated with life satisfaction among adolescent athletes in Taiwan, and high scores on the GQ-6 were negatively related to athlete burnout. And in a sample of Taiwanese undergraduates (Chen, Chen, Kee, & Tsai, 2009), dispositional gratitude was linked to several positive traits, including optimism, happiness, and agreeableness. Additional research is needed to build on these early findings on the cross-cultural similarities and differences in the grateful disposition.

While the bulk of initial research on the grateful disposition has used cross-sectional designs (but see Wood, Maltby, Gillett, Linley, & Joseph, 2008, for an exception), some more recent work has examined the ability of dispositional gratitude to predict well-being later on. Froh, Bono, and Emmons (2010), for instance, measured changes in gratitude, prosocial behavior, life satisfaction, and social engagement in middle school students over a 6-month period. Participants who reported high levels of gratitude at the beginning of the study experienced more social integration (that is, a stronger sense of purpose and belongingness), as well as a greater desire to give back to their communities, at the 6-month follow-up, even when the researchers controlled for demographics and initial social integration. More grateful students also reported more prosocial behavior (e.g., offering to help other classmates with schoolwork) and greater life satisfaction at 3 months. High life satisfaction, in turn, predicted greater social integration at the conclusion of the study.

A recent series of studies has demonstrated that the grateful disposition predicts not only the presence of social integration, but also the relative absence of negative symptoms (Lambert, Fincham, & Stillman, 2012). Undergraduate students high in trait gratitude experienced fewer depressive symptoms than their less grateful peers at a 6- and 12-week follow-up, with researchers controlling for initial depressive symptoms. "Positive reframing," that is, a tendency to reframe challenging circumstances in a positive light, was identified as a mediator. A third study identified positive emotion as yet another mediator of the relationship

between gratitude and depressive symptoms. Similarly, another recent study (Li, Zhang, Li, Li, & Ye, 2012) found that Chinese adolescents who scored higher on a measure of dispositional gratitude were less likely to report that they had considered or attempted suicide, even when researchers controlled for participants' age, gender, and family socioeconomic status. Furthermore, this relationship was mediated by participants' self-esteem.

A disposition toward gratefulness is clearly linked with numerous positive attributes and attitudes. Growing evidence indicates that this relationship extends across age and culture. Furthermore, several studies have now shown that trait gratitude predicts subsequent well-being, though there are still relatively few studies on this topic. Despite this progress, much remains to be done to understand the relation of dispositional gratitude to well-being. For instance, little is known about the mediators of the relation of gratitude to well-being. (See Emmons & Mishra, 2011, for a particularly extensive list of candidates.) Our suggestions for future research draw from two traditions in individual-differences research: emotion regulation and social-cognitive approaches to individual differences.

Emotion regulation involves five families of strategies: situation selection, situation modification, attentional deployment, cognitive change, and response modulation (Gross & Thompson, 2007). People place themselves in different situations, adjust those situations, shift their attention within situations, change what they think about situations, and control how they respond to the situations. Might individual differences in the use of these strategies (John & Gross, 2007) be used to understand the disposition to gratitude? Perhaps the grateful disposition reflects the experience of a greater frequency of instances of gratitude, and this frequency might reflect the disposition to engage in different strategies to regulate emotion.

Consider situation selection. People sometimes place themselves in situations in which they are more likely to experience desired emotions (Harmon-Jones, Harmon-Jones, Amodio, & Gable, 2011). Might individual differences in the grateful disposition be due in part to differences in the frequency of being in situations that make a particular person grateful? We know of no data bearing on this point. If there are such differences, then one way to increase the grateful disposition might be to help people identify and place themselves in the sorts of contexts that make them, in particular, grateful.

Alternatively, might individual differences in gratitude reflect individual differences in reappraisal of an event? For instance, gratitude has been linked to resilience in the face of crisis (Fredrickson, 2004; Fredrickson, Tugade, Waugh, & Larkin, 2003). Similarly, benefit finding is linked with growth after trauma (Helgeson, Reynolds, & Tomich, 2006). Perhaps the grateful disposition involves, in part, finding benefits in the aftermath of a traumatic experience. Indeed, in a cross-sectional study of undergraduates with a history of trauma (Vernon, 2012), those who had reported having experienced more gratitude and appreciation for life in the hours and days immediately following the traumatic event reported fewer symptoms of posttraumatic stress disorder at the time of the study, even when the researcher controlled for respondents' gender and trauma history. Perhaps those who experienced more gratitude in the immediate aftermath of a trauma were more focused on the benefits of the experience than on its negative aspects, though the retrospective nature of this recollection calls for particular caution.

Consideration of cognitive changes raises an interesting question about the relation of dispositional gratitude to depression. Gratitude is typically construed as involving attribution of one's good experiences to the actions of others, an external cause (e.g., McCullough et al., 2002; Roberts, 2004). Gratitude might be increased, then, by helping people attribute their positive experiences to the actions of other people (but see Lefcourt, Martin, & Ware, 1984, for a study in which externality was not related to gratitude). However, the disposition to attribute good experiences to external causes has been linked to depression (Sweeney, Anderson, & Bailey, 1986). Learned helplessness suggests that attributing good outcomes to external sources will lead people to conclude that their own actions do not matter, that is, that they are helpless, which leads to depression (Seligman, 1975) or reduction in their self-esteem (Abramson, Metalsky, & Alloy, 1989; Abramson, Seligman, & Teasdale, 1978). Thus, external attributions are linked to well-being in the gratitude literature, but to depression and reduced self-esteem in the helplessness literature. What circumstances and personality variables moderate whether the disposition to attribute positive outcomes to others leads to gratitude versus depression?

Research on the grateful disposition has largely utilized a trait approach to individual differences, suggesting cross-situational consistency in gratitude. In contrast, social-cognitive theory suggests that coherence in personality often reflects individual differences in reactions to particular situations (Cervone, 2004; Mischel & Shoda, 1999). For instance, two people might be equally grateful on average, yet one could consistently be more grateful than the other in one sort of situation (e.g., with close friends), and less grateful in a different sort of situation (e.g., when contemplating nature). Trait-level gratitude might suggest that these two people are equally grateful and miss an important individual difference. Measurement of gratitude, then, might focus on development of idiographic measures of personality designed to predict intraindividual variability in gratitude (Caldwell, Cervone, & Rubin, 2008).

Gratitude Interventions

The hardest arithmetic to master is that which enables us to count our blessings.

—ERIC HOFFER (1973)

Given the association of dispositional gratitude with well-being and the growing evidence that it can predict various positive outcomes, the question arises as to how to increase gratitude. Indeed, a second foundational paper in gratitude research described a set of three such experiments on counting blessings (Emmons & McCullough, 2003). In two of the studies, participants were undergraduates; in the third, adults with neuromuscular disease. Those assigned to list recent occurrences for which they felt grateful experienced higher well-being at the conclusion of the study than did those recording daily hassles and, in some cases, other control groups.

Research by several laboratories on a variety of interventions has followed. Wood and colleagues (2010) reviewed a dozen studies of gratitude interventions involving clinically relevant outcomes, including seven "gratitude list" studies similar to those reported in the original Emmons and McCullough (2003) paper, as well as other studies of grateful contemplation and behavioral expressions of gratitude. These studies targeted a variety of populations, including schoolchildren (Froh, Sefick, & Emmons, 2008) and a community sample with body image impairments (Geraghty, Wood, & Hyland, 2010). In reviewing this work, Wood and his colleagues concluded:

The 12 studies clearly suggest that interventions to increase gratitude are effective in improving well-being. As such, they have been widely promoted as being the most successful positive psychology intervention, and one that should be used widely, perhaps even on a national scale.... Such conclusions, however, seem premature. (p. 898)

The authors note several reasons why these conclusions might be premature, even though initial studies have been promising (if mixed; see Koo, Algoe, Wilson, & Gilbert, 2008). One of the most important reasons is that while gratitude interventions have been compared to hassles and neutral control conditions, they have rarely been compared to controls that would cause expectancy effects similar to those evoked by gratitude exercises. The positive outcomes observed in these experiments may be influenced more by participants' expectations than by the specific effects of any gratitude manipulation. Another reason is that many of the gratitude intervention studies did not examine whether the observed effects were mediated by increases in gratitude (but see Emmons & McCullough, 2003, for exceptions). It is possible, then, that some of the effects of "gratitude" exercises could be due to other mediators, such as relief or contentment. Nonetheless, gratitude exercises are promising. How might they be improved?

When gratitude exercises are done over and over, might they become boring? How can gratitude exercises be made fresh, so as to avoid adaptation (Sheldon & Lyubomirsky, 2012)? Some evidence suggests

that spacing out the exercises might help to prevent adaptation (Lyubomirsky, Sheldon, & Schkade, 2005). Perhaps another way to prevent adaptation is to have those doing the exercises consider "counterfactuals," or what might have been. If people think about how things could have been different, then they might be made to see their actual experiences as more surprising, and surprise might temper adaptation. Indeed, in a pair of studies, participants described why an event for which they said they were grateful was surprising (Koo et al., 2008). In comparison to other groups, including those writing about why the event was not surprising, participants who wrote about the surprising nature of the event reported higher positive affect.

One significant counterfactual is imagining that we are no longer alive. In one relatively recent study, undergraduates were asked to imagine vividly their own death in an apartment fire, then to reflect on their family members' reactions to the event and how they [the undergraduates] would expect to feel about their lives up to that point (Frias, Watkins, Webber, & Froh, 2011). Participants in this death reflection condition experienced a greater increase in gratitude than those in a traditional mortality salience condition (who were asked to describe their thoughts, feelings, and emotions regarding their own death), and those in a control condition, who reflected on their own and their family members' reactions to the events of a typical day. Drawing on anecdotal reports of increased gratitude following life-threatening experiences, the authors suggest that vividly imagining a potential death scene might prompt a heightened sense of gratefulness and appreciation for life itself, a benefit that often is otherwise taken for granted.

Perhaps empathy might also make gratitude-evoking events more vivid and surprising. Conversely, a lack of empathy might make it more difficult to imagine the cost to others when they provide the benefit that might cause gratitude. Indeed, gratitude is related to empathic concern (DeWall, Lambert, Pond, Kashdan, & Fincham, 2012; McCullough, Tsang, & Emmons, 2004). Gratitude interventions, then, might benefit from attention to research on increasing empathy because interventions designed to induce empathy may increase gratitude as well.

One method by which empathy has been increased is training in "mindfulness," that is, nonjudgmental attention to the present moment (Block-Lerner, Adair, Plumb, Rhatigan, & Orsillo, 2007; Shapiro, Brown, Thoresen, & Plante, 2011). If mindfulness increases empathy, then perhaps providing those who are least empathic with mindfulness training might make it easier for them to understand the costs that their benefactors have borne, and so lead them to greater gratitude. Indeed, in one study, those who were higher in trait mindfulness reported more subsequent gratitude in a daily diary task (Ahrens, Breetz, & Forbes, 2011).

McIntosh and Ahrens (2012) compared a single-session, standard gratitude list task to a gratitude task that involved mindfulness instructions and to a neutral control condition. The mindful gratitude list condition included, for instance, instructions for participants to refrain from judgment and to bring their minds back gently to the task if they found their attention wandering. Among those high in empathy, both gratitude list tasks boosted positive affect and reduced negative affect compared to the neutral control condition; the tasks did not differ from one another in terms of these effects. However, among those low in empathy, just listing things for which they were grateful did not influence affect, whereas the mindfulness list did. Future work should continue to refine gratitude interventions and to delineate which types of people may benefit most from practicing gratitude. (See also Emmons & Mishra, 2011, for more suggestions on future gratitude interventions.)

Recent studies have explored an expanded range of outcomes of gratitude interventions. For instance, brief gratitude inductions have been shown to reduce moral hypocrisy (Batson, Thompson, Seuferling, Whitney, & Strongman, 1999) among undergraduates (Tong & Yang, 2011), as well as death anxiety in older individuals (Lau & Cheng, 2011). This study on death anxiety is also one of the few to examine the benefits of "counting one's blessings" in non-Western cultures. In another such study, Chinese schoolteachers wrote down three good things that happened to them each week over an 8-week period, and reflected on those benefits at the end of each week using a traditional Confucian self-questioning method (Chan, 2010). After the intervention, participants experienced significant increases in gratitude, life satisfaction, and positive affect. Interestingly, those who scored lower on the GQ-6 benefited most from the gratitude list task, suggesting that individuals who are less grateful to begin with may stand to gain more from gratitude interventions. However, since this study lacked a nonintervention control group, particular care should be taken in drawing causal inferences.

In summary, early work on gratitude interventions suggests that making a conscious effort to attend to and record the things for which one is thankful may have positive effects on well-being. However, much of the work on gratitude interventions to date has used limited control groups and/or failed to examine the mediating effects of gratitude. Additionally, little research has examined the moderators of gratitude interventions. People differ in their preferences for positive psychology exercises, so gratitude research might benefit by tailoring the intervention to the individual (Schueller, 2010).

Gratitude interventions might be enhanced by consideration of what causes gratitude. For instance, emotional experience depends on people's beliefs and emotions about emotions, that is, "meta-emotion" (Gottman, Katz, & Hooven, 1996; Harmon-Jones et al., 2011; Mitmansgruber, Beck, Hofer, & Schussler, 2009; Salovey, Mayer, Golman, Turvey, & Palfai, 1995). People differ in which emotions they find most desirable (Tsai, 2007). If gratitude is more desired, it seems likely it would more often be up-regulated. Indeed, those who prefer to count their blessings adhere more to the exercise and benefit more from it (Schueller, 2010). In contrast, are others more afraid of emotion (Williams, Chambless, & Ahrens, 1997), and so less likely to expand the positive experience of giftedness? How might gratitude exercises be tailored to those who are less comfortable with positive emotions or with the associates of gratitude? Perhaps they might be particularly likely to benefit from gratitude exercises that include training in acceptance, such as mindfulness (Baer & Lykins, 2011; Klainin-Yobas, Cho, & Creedy, 2012). Indeed, in one study, brief mindfulness training increased positive emotion experienced via a subsequent film clip (Erisman & Roemer, 2010). By accepting their emotional experiences, people may be more likely to remain with them and see their benefits. In the last section of this chapter, we examine other ways in which consideration of the causes of gratitude might enhance gratitude interventions.

Gratitude interventions might also benefit from attention to the goal of the intervention. What aspect of well-being is being targeted? Consider the distinction between happiness as pleasure and happiness as meaning (Peterson, Park, & Seligman, 2005). Perhaps counting blessings helps in part by increasing the degree to which people savor their experiences and, thereby experience pleasure. To experience pleasure at gratitude for something likely involves close attention to and appreciation of that thing. Indeed, counting one's blessings is related to savoring (Beaumont, 2011). Perhaps, then, gratitude interventions geared to promoting pleasure might benefit from emphasis on what helps people to savor that for which they are grateful.

Alternatively, perhaps gratitude can help to enhance meaning (Lambert, Graham, Fincham, & Stillman, 2009). Gratitude increases positive feelings, and feeling good does seem to increase meaning (King, 2012). The practice of gratitude might also be an instance of mindfulness practice, enhancing meaning by drawing a connection between ourselves and something beyond (Baumeister & Vohs, 2005; Hicks & King, 2007). In one study, students whose stress management training was supplemented with gratitude journaling subsequently found their classwork more meaningful and engaging than did those who only engaged in stress management (Flinchbaugh, Moore, Chang, & May, 2012). If gratitude exercises target the development of meaning, then they might be paired with other practices that enhance meaning. They might also be paired with exercises emphasizing other transcendent emotions, such as elevation (Haidt, 2003) and awe (Shiota, Keltner, & Mossman, 2007), which connect people to something beyond themselves.

We have focused on intrapersonal well-being. Gratitude might also enhance interpersonal relationships. Indeed, we review in the next section some recently developed interventions that involve relational components of gratitude.

Relational Aspects of Gratitude

Gratitude is the most exquisite form of courtesy.
—JACQUES MARITAIN (1975)

Gratitude involves not only a subjective feeling but also an action tendency, one often oriented toward others. After receiving help from a friend or coworker, we would be remiss if we did not express appreciation to them and ask how we can return the favor. We teach children to write thank-you notes upon receiving presents, and encourage them to buy gifts for coaches and teachers to thank them for their hard work. And we often see authors, musicians, and performers going to a great deal of effort to show appreciation to those who have helped them along the way. Indeed, expressions of gratitude are woven into the social fabric of our lives.

As such, a third major line of gratitude research has examined interpersonal aspects of gratitude, such as the benefits of expressing thankfulness to those around us. In one early study, participants were given a week to write and deliver a letter expressing gratitude to someone they felt they had never properly thanked (Seligman, Steen, Park, & Peterson, 2005). Compared to a control condition in which participants recalled early childhood memories for that week, the "gratitude visit" increased participants' happiness and decreased their depression symptoms over the next month. The experience of feeling grateful to others and the act of expressing that gratitude may have important consequences for our interpersonal relationships.

Several additional variations on this "gratitude letter" paradigm have produced positive results. In one recent experiment, participants were asked to write letters of gratitude to three separate recipients over a 3-week period (Toepfer, Cichy, & Peters, 2011). After 3 weeks, those who wrote gratitude letters reported increases in happiness and life satisfaction compared to both the control group, who did not write letters, and to their pretest levels. Participants in the letter-writing group also experienced fewer depression symptoms, both over time and compared to nonwriters. In another study, among children and young adults who completed the exercise, those who initially scored the lowest on a premanipulation measure of positive emotion experienced the greatest boost in well-being after writing and delivering a gratitude letter (Froh, Kashdan, Ozimkowski, & Miller, 2009). That the least happy children experienced the most benefits from the exercise seems similar to the result that the least grateful benefited most in one previously mentioned gratitude list study (Chan, 2010).

The effects of the gratitude visit have also been tested among culturally diverse groups. In one study (Boehm, Lyubomirsky, & Sheldon, 2011), Anglo American and Asian American participants wrote letters of gratitude once a week for 6 weeks. At the conclusion of the study, Anglo Americans experienced a significantly greater boost in life satisfaction than did Asian Americans, perhaps because the latter group tends to focus more on communal goals than on increasing individual happiness. This preliminary evidence suggests that the ability of gratitude expression exercises to improve well-being may be somewhat limited by culture.

Since the gratitude visit exercise is a fairly recent development, it may be too early to draw conclusions about its effectiveness. However, existing research suggests that this is a promising intervention. Over the past several years, researchers have demonstrated that writing and (sometimes) delivering a letter of gratitude to someone the writer has never properly thanked have positive psychological effects among diverse populations, including cardiovascular patients (Huffman et al., 2011), schoolchildren (see McCabe, Bray, Kehle, Theodore, & Gelbar 2011, for a review), and undergraduate students (Watkins et al., 2003). The exercise is also inexpensive and time-limited, and likely has social benefits. In the future, additional research may confirm that this is a useful exercise in both clinical and community populations.

What is the function of gratitude in interpersonal relationships? Perhaps it serves to build relationships. Algoe and colleagues (Algoe, 2012; Algoe, Haidt, & Gable, 2008) propose that gratitude serves to "find,

remind, and bind"; that is, gratitude serves to help people find new relationship partners or remind them of known partners, and to bind together those who give and the recipients of those gifts. Initial research supports this view.

One recent experiment (Lambert et al., 2013) examined the effect of repeatedly sharing experiences for which one is grateful with a close friend or romantic partner. Participants who kept a daily journal of gratitude-inducing events and shared those experiences with a partner twice a week for 4 weeks experienced greater positive affect, happiness, and life satisfaction over the course of the study than did those who simply thought about grateful experiences. This preliminary data indicate that the simple act of discussing things for which we are thankful with those around us may promote well-being (see also Gable, Reis, Impett, & Asher, 2004).

Perhaps gratitude builds communal relationships (Algoe, 2012; Clark & Mills, 1993). Gratitude draws attention to "the opportunity to solidify a connection with someone who would be a high-quality dyadic relationship partner, that is, someone who will be there through thick and thin, both providing support and enriching one's life" (Algoe, 2012, p. 9). Indeed, in one longitudinal study (Algoe, Gable, & Maisel, 2010), members of cohabitating couples kept a daily diary of thoughtful things they had done for a partner, their partner's thoughtful behaviors toward them, and their emotional responses to those actions over a 2-week period. Predictably, participants who reported that their partners had acted more thoughtfully toward them experienced more gratitude. One partner's self-reports of his or her own thoughtful behaviors also predicted the other partner's gratitude. When participants experienced more gratitude to a partner, they were more likely to feel that their relationship was stronger on the following day. Consistent with this, in a 2-week study of couples who on average had been married for 21 years, each partner's feelings of gratitude on a given day significantly predicted his or her own relationship satisfaction, as well as his or her spouse's feelings about the relationship (Gordon, Arnette, & Smith, 2011). Interestingly, one partner's expression of gratitude on a particular day only predicted his or her own subsequent relationship satisfaction, not his or her partner's satisfaction.

These relationship-building effects of gratitude apply to nonromantic relationships as well. In one study, undergraduates were asked to increase expressions of gratitude to a close friend over a 3-week period (Lambert, Clark, Durtschi, Fincham, & Graham, 2010). At the end of the study, those in the gratitude expression condition perceived more communal strength—that is, the degree to which partners feel responsible for each other's needs—in their friendship with the target person than did control participants. Lambert and Fincham (2011) also demonstrated that students who increased expressions of gratitude to a friend viewed the friend more positively and felt more comfortable voicing concerns about the relationship.

One way that gratitude may promote healthy relationships is through encouraging relationship maintenance behaviors, or prosocial actions taken by a partner to maintain a relationship even at a cost to him- or herself (e.g., completing one's household chores, or doing a special favor for a partner who has had a stressful day). Perceptions of responsiveness of the giver to one's needs should enhance such behaviors (Algoe, 2012). In a longitudinal study of newlywed couples, Partner A's perception of Partner B's responsiveness at time 1 predicted Partner A's gratitude 1 year later (Kubacka, Finkenauer, Rusbult, & Keijsers, 2011). Each partner's gratitude also predicted his or her relationship maintenance behaviors over time. Seeing that the relationship partner has been responsive to one's needs should prompt the perception that the partner cares and is therefore a potential high-quality relationship partner (Reis, Clark, & Holmes, 2004). Indeed, those who have been thanked are more likely to initiate and maintain prosocial behaviors in the future, and these effects may be mediated by changes in social worth (Grant & Gino, 2010).

Gratitude may also benefit close social relationships by protecting against destructive interpersonal tendencies. Several recent studies (e.g., DeWall et al., 2012) have supported the hypothesis that grateful people may be less likely to act in ways that threaten the well-being of others, since gratitude so often involves action tendencies toward prosocial behavior. In one experiment, people who, prior to receiving negative feedback on an essay, had written about things for which they were grateful were less likely than control participants to deliver a blast of noise to the person who gave the negative feedback. Empathy may mediate this relationship. Grateful people tend to feel more empathy toward others, which may in turn limit their tendencies toward aggressive behavior.

The expression of gratitude, not just its experience, seems important for building relationships. Therefore, an individual's willingness to communicate gratitude to others might influence the effects of gratitude expression. In two studies of Taiwanese undergraduates (Chen, Chen, & Tsai, 2012), the positive relationship between gratitude and happiness was not as strong for participants who were uncomfortable expressing emotions. And among women with breast cancer, for those high in willingness to express emotion, gratitude predicted increased social support 3 months later (Algoe & Stanton, 2012). In contrast, gratitude did not predict increased social support over time for those more ambivalent about expressing emotion. These findings suggest that individuals must be willing to express gratitude in order to experience its full benefits.

Overall, recent work supports the idea that gratitude strengthens social relationships by providing opportunities to grow closer to friends and romantic partners through reciprocal positive interactions. This research suggests that gratitude's influence extends far beyond isolated expressions of thanks for favors given; instead, all of those singular instances may add up over time in ways that shape our long-term social relationships. Indeed, the studies reviewed earlier indicate that the experience and expression of gratitude are beneficial to children (Froh et al., 2009), adolescents (Froh, Emmons, Card, et al., 2011), college students (Watkins et al., 2003), and older adults (Scheidle, 2011), in part through their effects on their interpersonal functioning. Abundant research has demonstrated the importance of interpersonal relationships to psychological functioning across the lifespan (Ainsworth, 1985; Carstensen,

1993). It is likely that gratitude contributes to well-being by strengthening the close relationships that accompany individuals from childhood to old age.

In our daily lives, we express gratitude not only to significant others but also to many people with whom we interact for only brief periods of time. In fact, the action tendency to return a favor for which one feels grateful may be stronger among strangers than among friends (Clark, 1984). In a recent study of gratitude and economic exchange (DeSteno, Bartlett, Baumann, Williams, & Dickens, 2010), participants' level of gratitude toward a confederate who had recently helped them with a tedious experimental task predicted the extent of their cooperation with the confederate in a resource allocation game. Gratitude appears to reduce selfishness and encourage behaviors aimed at cooperation and relationship maintenance in both friends and strangers.

In addition to encouraging one-to-one reciprocations of helpful gestures, gratitude may also inspire us to direct positive acts toward people in our social network, creating a self-perpetuating chain of prosocial behavior. Termed "upstream reciprocity" or the "pay it forward effect" (McCullough, Kimeldorf, & Cohen, 2008; Nowak & Roch, 2007), this phenomenon may play a role in building strong communities and organizations. After recalling a time when they had received a kindness, people were inclined to help not only the person who had given the kindness but also those who were close to them and, to a lesser degree, strangers or persons who had been unkind to them (Exline, Lisan, & Lisan, 2012). Among Taiwanese students working in groups during a semester-long business class, more grateful people helped their teammates more often over the course of the semester (Chang, Lin, & Chen, 2012). These students were also more likely to initiate and propagate chain reactions of helping behaviors. Gratitude may indeed strengthen social bonds by encouraging individuals to pass on prosocial behaviors.

The effects of gratitude expression have been demonstrated in several interesting contexts. In one study, registered voters who were randomly selected to receive a post card thanking them for voting in a previous election were more likely to vote in an upcoming election than voters who simply received a reminder encouraging them to vote (Panagopoulos, 2011). And, in another study (Cho & Fast, 2012), individuals who were assigned a "supervisory" role in a laboratory task were less likely to put down a "subordinate" after receiving negative feedback on a test if they had received a grateful note from the subordinate; this effect was mediated by the extent to which the participant felt valued by the subordinate. Receiving an expression of gratitude makes people more likely to behave in ways that contribute to the well-being of others or of the community.

Overall, recent work confirms the conventional wisdom that it is a good thing to say "thanks." Expressing one's gratitude to another person—whether verbally, in written form, once, several times, or every day—is beneficial for the person doing the expressing, the target of the appreciation, and the quality of the relationship between the two individuals. However, much work remains to be done with regard to the interpersonal effects of gratitude expression.

For instance, what increases the desire of grateful people to give not just to their benefactors, but to others, paying it forward? In one study, the receipt of a non-normative kindness, such as one from someone in a more distant relationship, made it more likely that people would want to give to strangers or to those who had been unkind to them (Exline et al., 2012). What else affects this phenomenon? Would gratitude lead to more help for strangers and enemies among those who believe that friends and strangers are all part of a common humanity? Would being from a culture that values independence limit this response of generosity?

Several other aspects of work on gratitude and relationships might also be fertile ground for future research. Some of the experiments noted earlier did not measure gratitude as a mediator, so one task for future researchers will be to determine whether an increase in gratefulness is truly responsible for the observed effects. Furthermore, aside from the work on emotional ambivalence and gratitude expression discussed earlier (Algoe & Stanton, 2012; Chen et al., 2012), little attention has been given to the moderators of gratitude interventions in interpersonal relationships. One relatively recent study (Sergeant & Mongrain, 2011) has suggested that people who are more self-critical may respond more favorably to gratitude exercises, and that those who are more needy, less so, perhaps even showing negative effects in response to the exercises. Might gratitude lead those who are needy to worry about rejection? In the next section, we turn to the possibility that people's reports of "gratitude" reflect different experiences. This might help to identify mediators and moderators of gratitude effects.

Varieties of Gratitude

No metaphysician ever felt the deficiency of language so much as the grateful.
—CHARLES CALEB COLTON (in Douglas, 1917)

When different people report that they are grateful, are they referring to the same emotion? Some recent research suggests that they are not. Lambert, Graham, and Fincham (2009) identified two different meanings of gratitude: *benefit-triggered* and *generalized*. Others (e.g., Steindl-Rast, 2004) have also suggested that there are varieties of gratitude. William James (1890/1983) wrote that "the first steps in most of the sciences are purely classificatory. Where facts fall easily into rich and intricate series (as plants and animals and chemical compounds do), the mere sight of the series fills the mind with a satisfaction *sui generis*" (p. 1342, original emphasis). Indeed, research on cancer, for instance, proceeds in part by identifying different subtypes (Shah et al., 2012). This very book is possible in large part because of advances in distinguishing between different positive emotions (e.g., Ellsworth & Smith, 1988; Fredrickson, 2001). Might distinguishing different sorts of gratitude prove fruitful as a next step in the science of gratitude?

To understand the possibility that reports of gratitude might be reports of different emotional experiences, it is useful to draw on appraisal theories of emotion (Arnold, 1960; Ellsworth & Scherer, 2003; Schorr, 2001). Appraisal theories suggest that emotions involve an assessment of an object, along with the subjective experience and action tendencies that arise from this assessment. For instance, fear might involve the judgment that something is a threat with which

one cannot cope. This judgment might lead to the desire to run, and the subjective experience that one is afraid. Particular emotions are identified by not only the label (e.g., "fear"), but also the appraisals leading to them and the action tendencies arising from them. If there are varieties of gratitude, these should arise from different appraisals and prompt different action tendencies.

Appraisal theories have often been used in the attempt to understand gratitude (e.g., Lazarus & Lazarus, 1994; Ortony, Clore, & Collins, 1988; Smith, 1991; Weiner, Russell, & Lerman, 1979). Perhaps the most common formulation of the appraisals involved in gratitude is a variation on the idea that it arises when a person "construes himself or herself (the beneficiary) as the recipient of some good (the benefice) from a giver (the benefactor)" (Roberts, 2004, p. 61). Roberts indicates that this good need not be seen as the person's legal or moral due; rather, the recipient must see the benefit as having been freely given. Furthermore, several studies have demonstrated that appraisals related to both benefactors and goods received do influence the experience of gratitude. For instance, when helpers are perceived as more selfish, their assistance evokes less gratitude (Tsang, 2006). More subtle motivations on the part of the helper can also affect gratitude (Weinstein, DeHaan, & Ryan, 2010). In three studies, participants were asked to imagine themselves in hypothetical situations that involved receiving help from another person. Helpers with more autonomous motivations, that is, those arising from the person's values and interests, evoked more gratitude than did those with more controlled motivations, those arising from internal or external pressure, mediated in part by perceived closeness to the helper.

Similarly, the appraised magnitude of a gift should influence the amount of gratitude resulting from it, with more gratitude arising from a greater gift. Australian postgraduates who perceived that their supervisors' helpful acts had a more powerful effect on their PhD life reported more grateful affect in response to that help (Unsworth, Turner, Williams, & Piccin-Houle, 2010). (Happily, only six of the 189 students could not think of an act by their supervisors that made them feel grateful!) The appraisal of gift magnitude appears to depend on the distribution of help one has received. Participants in one study imagined receiving help from 11 friends (Wood, Brown, & Maltby, 2011). The overall help was the same in each condition. But for some participants, most helpers clustered toward the top end of the distribution of help, with a few helping little, whereas for others, most clustered toward the bottom of the distribution, with a few helping a great deal. Even with the amount of overall help held constant, participants reported more gratitude when help was clustered toward the top of the range of help than toward the bottom. The authors suggest one reason for ingratitude might be mistaken recollection of the distribution of help. Many people helping a fair amount might increase the memory of generosity, whereas many helping only a little might hinder it.

While appraisals clearly influence the experience of gratitude, laypeople seem to use the word *gratitude* in several different ways (Lambert, Graham, & Fincham, 2009). The gratitude one feels upon receiving a birthday gift from a friend is different, for instance, from the deep appreciation children may feel for the parents (or other adults) who raised them, although similar words might be used to express both feelings. Does this varied use of the word *gratitude* reflect the use of different appraisals? If distinct appraisals can lead people to report the subjective experience of "gratitude," then the dispositions related to, methods to increase, and relational aspects of these different "gratitudes" might to some degree be distinct.

Perhaps people's use of the word *gratitude* to describe different subjective states arises because gratitude is closely related to other emotions with similar appraisals (e.g., Algoe & Haidt, 2009). We began this chapter with the quotation, "A joyful and pleasant thing it is to be thankful." But according to Samuel Johnson, "there are minds so impatient of inferiority that their gratitude is a species of revenge, and they return benefits, not because recompense is a pleasure, but because obligation is a pain" (cited in Bate & Strauss, 1969, p. 96). Sometimes people's reports of "gratitude" refer to the appraisals, subjective experience, and action tendencies of "indebtedness," such as that described by Dr. Johnson.

Indebtedness increases (and gratitude decreases) with the perception that others expect more in return for a gift (Algoe & Stanton, 2012; Watkins, Scheer, Ovnicek, & Kolts, 2006). Given this, those more attuned to thinking of exchange (e.g., those with more interdependent self-construals) should be more prone to experience indebtedness than those less attuned to exchange (e.g., those with more independent self-construals). Indeed, in a series of five studies, Asian participants were less willing to accept small gifts from casual acquaintances than were North Americans, due in part to the feelings of indebtedness (Shen, Wan, & Wyer, 2011). This cultural difference did not extend to gifts given in close relationships, in which both groups would likely feel interdependent.

Indebtedness can be increased by self-focus (Mathews & Green, 2010). In one study, trait public self-consciousness was positively associated with indebtedness. In a second, self-focus was manipulated by the presence of a mirror. Those made to be more self-focused also reported more indebtedness in response to a recently received favor that they were asked to recall. In this study, though, self-consciousness did not affect gratitude.

While the word *gratitude* might also be used to label the subjective state of indebtedness, some have distinguished different forms of gratitude as a positive emotion (e.g., Shelton, 2004). Steindl-Rast (2004) distinguishes between personal and transpersonal gratitude. He frames personal gratitude in terms of being "thankful to" and transpersonal gratitude in terms of being "grateful for." One might be thankful *to* a stranger for giving directions, for example, but grateful *for* humanity's goodness in general. Steindl-Rast argues further that "[the] construal of gratitude in terms of beneficiary, benefice, and benefactor . . . produces many valuable insights regarding thankfulness but is ill-equipped to deal with gratefulness" (p. 287).

Lambert, Graham, and Fincham (2009) make a distinction similar to that of Steindl-Rast (2004), that between benefit-triggered and generalized gratitude. "Benefit-triggered gratitude" refers to being "grateful to" a benefactor for the experience of transfer of a benefit, the sort of gratitude emphasized by the beneficiary–benefice–benefactor view of gratitude. "Generalized gratitude" is more about being "grateful for" all the good things in life. One way of uniting the sorts of gratitude described by Steindl-Rast and Lambert, Graham, and Fincham (2009) is that each (personal and transpersonal, benefit-triggered and generalized gratitude) involves an appraisal that something is good and undeserved. But they differ in whether there is an emphasis on the idea that this undeserved goodness is caused by another. Both Steindl-Rast and Lambert, Graham, and Fincham distinguish being "grateful to," with a focus on the benefactor, and "grateful for," with a focus on undeserved goodness. Perhaps it would be helpful to construe being "grateful to" and "grateful for" as distinct emotions.

An analogy might be drawn to the distinction between shame and guilt. People often do not distinguish between the two, yet the two can be distinguished. Tangney and Salovey (2010; see also Lewis, 1971) suggest that the distinction between shame and guilt is a matter of focus: "When people feel shame, their focus is on the self ('I did that horrible thing'), whereas when people feel guilt, their focus is on a behavior ('I *did* that horrible *thing*')" (Tangney & Salovey, 2010, p. 248, original emphasis). By analogy, the two types of gratitude might be distinguished by whether the focus is on agency (grateful to) or on the benefit (grateful for).

A series of studies indicates that people do appear to report both benefit-triggered gratitude and generalized gratitude (Lambert, Graham, & Fincham, 2009). When asked to explain gratitude to others, some participants' descriptions appeared to reflect benefit-triggered gratitude, while others' descriptions reflected generalized gratitude. Given scenarios representing the two forms of gratitude, participants reported feeling gratitude in response to both, but reported more gratitude in response to the generalized gratitude scenario. In another study, participants read one scenario evoking benefit-triggered gratitude (a neighbor fixing one's computer) and a second designed to evoke generalized gratitude (feeling grateful for the beauty of nature and for family). Though participants thought both scenarios were representative of gratitude, a substantial minority (27%) chose the latter scenario as more representative of gratitude. Finally, when asked to think of a time when they felt grateful, over 40% of participants in each

of two studies reported an instance involving generalized gratitude, suggesting that appreciating an object or event without a clear benefactor falls within many people's concept of "gratitude."

In a study reporting a similar distinction, participants wrote daily about positive events (Ahrens & McIntosh, 2012). Half were asked to record events in which something good was caused by others, to evoke benefit-triggered gratitude. The other half were asked to record daily events in which something good was caused by neither themselves nor others, to trigger generalized gratitude. Prior to starting the daily diaries, participants completed the GQ-6, the short form of the GRAT, and a new vignette-based measure of individual differences in gratitude. One subscale of this measure was designed to assess Benefit-Triggered Gratitude (BTG-V). Participants imagined themselves in situations in which an explicit other caused a benefit for them, such as helping them to succeed in a class in which they were struggling. The other subscale was designed to assess Generalized Gratitude (GG-V). Participants imagined themselves in situations in which they experienced goodness with no explicit benefactor, such as being at the beach on a sunny day.

Consistent with previous results concerning hypothetical situations (Lambert, Graham, & Fincham, 2009), participants writing about daily events with no explicit benefactor still reported gratitude. Interestingly, reported gratitude had different associates in the two conditions. The daily relation of gratitude to happiness was stronger when there was no benefactor than when there was one, whereas the daily relation of gratitude to obligation was stronger when there was a benefactor than when there was none. Finally, the GG-V predicted additional variance in daily diary gratitude, above and beyond the GQ-6 and the GRAT, but the GQ-6 and GRAT did not predict unique variance in daily diary gratitude. This work supports that of Lambert, Graham, and Fincham (2009) and the suggestion by Steindl-Rast (2004) that people reporting gratitude sometimes are referring to at least two distinct positive states.

Reports of the subjective experience of "gratitude" may reflect multiple at least somewhat distinct emotions. These include indebtedness, arising from feeling an unpleasant burden in response to a gift, benefit-triggered gratitude, or being "grateful to," and generalized gratitude, or being "grateful for." We now discuss the implications of people's varied usage of the term *gratitude*. These implications extend across all three other topics we have discussed: the grateful disposition, gratitude interventions, and relational aspects of gratitude.

Appraisal theories emphasize that emotions involve not only the judgments that give rise to emotional experience but also the action tendencies arising from the experience (Frijda, 1986). If there are distinct sets of appraisals that sometimes lead people to report the experience of gratitude, one focused on the benefactor ("gratitude to"), and another on the undeserved goodness one has received ("gratitude for"), what distinct action tendencies might these emotions prompt? Steindl-Rast (2004, p. 286) argues that personal gratitude, or "gratitude to," "expresses itself in thanks given to the giver by the receiver of the gift." In contrast, Steindl-Rast suggests, transpersonal gratitude involves "the full response of a person to gratuitous belonging" (p. 286). If the emphasis is on the fact of undeserved goodness rather than the cause of the undeserved goodness, the action tendency may be less likely to involve the cause, that is, the benefactor. Steindl-Rast suggests that the action tendency arising from transpersonal gratitude is celebration. Shelton (2004) argues that "gratitude's intrinsic function allows one to approach the world by *embracing it, nourishing it, and transforming it*" (p. 274, original emphasis). Perhaps with transpersonal gratitude, or Lambert and colleagues' (2009) generalized gratitude, or "gratitude for," the action tendency is celebration with and giving to any and all, rather than just return to the benefactor. Future research should examine the possibility that gratitude variously experienced will, indeed, prompt different actions, in particular actions directed at different targets, such as paying it forward.

If different appraisals give rise to different reports of gratitude, then different factors should moderate the effects of gratitude interventions. Consider the exercise of counting one's blessings. Might those most inclined to focus on the debts they incur from gifts be more prone to indebtedness and, consequently, experience less of a boost in well-being from the exercise? Might they benefit most from exercises focused on the gift rather than the giver? That is, might it be easier for those prone to focus on debt to experience generalized gratitude, "gratitude for," than benefit-triggered gratitude, "gratitude to"? Does empathy affect appraisals of giver more than it does of gift? If so, will empathy affect more the results of gratitude exercises focused on the giver, such as the gratitude letter, than on the gift?

In recent years, narcissism has been on the rise in the United States (Twenge, Konrath, Foster, Campbell, & Bushman, 2008). Might gratitude exercises serve as an antidote to this trend? While some have suggested that narcissism is inversely related to gratitude (e.g., Emmons & Shelton, 2002), little research has examined this topic. Would gratitude exercises focused more on being "grateful for" rather than "grateful to" (which might imply that one is not self-sufficient) be more easily accepted by those high in narcissism?

Consideration of the different appraisals giving rise to reports of "gratitude" suggests the importance of refining measurement of gratitude. Initial dispositional gratitude measures have been important in demonstrating that gratitude is related to other variables of interest. More refined measurement techniques should make it easier to study the effects of gratitude. For instance, in addition to examining participants' subjective experience (feeling gratitude), measures might ask about their appraisals and action tendencies, so as to differentiate "gratitude" that reflects indebtedness, "gratitude to," and generalized gratitude, "gratitude for" (Smith & Kirby, 2012). The report of being "grateful," with an appraisal focused on the benefactor and the action tendency of giving back to that benefactor, may illuminate a different state than a similar report of being "grateful," with an appraisal focused on the good one has received and a desire to celebrate.

Summary and Conclusion

Gratitude research is still young, and as a result much work has yet to be done. However, even with the remaining mysteries, recent research on gratitude has illuminated a number of phenomena. The grateful disposition is associated with well-being, broadly construed. Several methods have been developed for increasing gratitude, and for using gratitude to increase well-being. While further work on these interventions is important, initial findings are promising. Gratitude has been tied to healthy interpersonal relationships between friends, romantic partners, and even strangers. And studies on the varieties of gratitude described by laypersons' language have contributed to a deeper understanding of gratitude as an interpersonal and transpersonal emotion (Steindl-Rast, 2004). We are grateful to the scholars who have built the burgeoning gratitude literature, and grateful for the literature itself. In light of what has been given, we anticipate that research on gratitude will continue to grow as it has in recent years.

Acknowledgments

The authors thank Kate Gunthert, Leslie Kirby, and Kate Stewart for their helpful comments on earlier drafts of this chapter.

References

Abramson, L. Y., Metalsky, G. I., & Alloy, L. B. (1989). Hopelessness depression: A theory-based subtype of depression. *Psychological Review, 96,* 358–372.

Abramson, L. Y., Seligman, M. E. P., & Teasdale, J. D. (1978). Learned helplessness in humans: Critique and reformulation. *Journal of Abnormal Psychology, 87,* 49–74.

Ahrens, A. H., Breetz, A. A., & Forbes, C. N. (2011, May). *Facets of mindfulness as predictors of gratitude: A daily diary study.* Poster session presented at the annual meeting of the Association for Psychological Science, Washington, DC.

Ahrens, A. H., & McIntosh, E. (2012). *A daily diary comparison of benefit-triggered and generalized gratitude.* Unpublished manuscript, Department of Psychology, American University, Washington, DC.

Ainsworth, M. D. (1985). Attachment across the life span. *Bulletin of the New York Academy of Medicine, 61*(9), 792–812.

Algoe, S. B. (2012). Find, remind, and bind: The functions of gratitude in everyday relationships. *Social and Personality Psychology Compass, 6,* 455–469.

Algoe, S. B., Gable, S. L., & Maisel, N. C. (2010). It's the little things: Everyday gratitude as a booster shot for romantic relationships. *Personal Relationships, 17,* 217–233.

Algoe, S. B., & Haidt, J. (2009). Witnessing excellence in action: The "other-praising" emotions of elevation, gratitude, and admiration. *Journal of Positive Psychology, 4,* 105–127.

Algoe, S. B., Haidt, J., & Gable, S. L. (2008). Beyond reciprocity: Gratitude and relationships in everyday life. *Emotion, 8,* 425–429.

Algoe, S. B., & Stanton, A. L. (2012). Gratitude when it is needed most: Social functions of gratitude in women with metastatic breast cancer. *Emotion, 12,* 163–168.

Arnold, M. B. (1960). *Emotion and personality: Vol. 1. Psychological aspects.* New York: Columbia University Press.

Baer, R. A., & Lykins, E. L. B. (2011). Mindfulness and positive psychological functioning. In K. M. Sheldon, T. B. Kashdan, & M. F. Steger (Eds.), *Designing positive psychology: Taking stock and moving forward* (pp. 335–348). Oxford, UK: Oxford University Press.

Bate, W. J., & Strauss, A. B. (Eds.). (1969). *Works of Samuel Johnson, Yale edition* (Vol. 4). New Haven, CT: Yale University Press.

Batson, C. D., Thompson, E. R., Seuferling, G., Whitney, H., & Strongman, J. A. (1999). Moral hypocrisy: Appearing moral to oneself without being so. *Journal of Personality and Social Psychology, 77,* 525–537.

Baumeister, R. F., & Vohs, K. D. (2005). The pursuit of meaningfulness in life. In C. R. Snyder & S. J. Lopez (Eds.), *Handbook of positive psychology* (pp. 608–618). Oxford, UK: Oxford University Press.

Beaumont, S. L. (2011). Identity styles and wisdom during emerging adulthood: Relationships with mindfulness and savoring. *Identity: An International Journal of Theory and Research, 11,* 155–180.

Block-Lerner, J., Adair, C., Plumb, J. C., Rhatigan, D. L., & Orsillo, S. M. (2007). The case for mindfulness-based approaches to the cultivation of empathy: Does nonjudgmental, present-moment awareness increase capacity for perspective-taking and empathic concern? *Journal of Marital and Family Therapy, 33,* 501–516.

Boehm, J. K., Lyubomirsky, S., & Sheldon, K.

M. (2011). A longitudinal experimental study comparing the effectiveness of happiness-enhancing strategies in Anglo Americans and Asian Americans. *Cognition and Emotion, 25*, 1263–1272.

Book of Common Prayer. (1892). A form of prayer and thanksgiving to almighty God. Retrieved from *http://justus.anglican.org/resources/bcp/1892Standard/harvest&family.pdf.*

Breen, W. E., Kashdan, T. B., Lenser, M. L., & Fincham, F. D. (2010). Gratitude and forgiveness: Convergence and divergence on self-report and informant ratings. *Personality and Individual Differences, 49*, 932–937.

Caldwell, T. L., Cervone, D., & Rubin, L. H. (2008). Explaining intra-individual variability in social behavior through idiographic assessment: The case of humor. *Journal of Research in Personality, 42*, 1229–1242.

Carstensen, L. L. (1993). Motivation for social contact across the life span: A theory of socioemotional selectivity. In J. E. Jacobs (Ed.), *Nebraska Symposium on Motivation 1992* (pp. 209–254). Lincoln: University of Nebraska Press.

Cervone, D. (2004). The architecture of personality. *Psychological Review, 111*, 183–204.

Chan, D. W. (2010). Gratitude, gratitude intervention and subjective well-being among Chinese school teachers in Hong Kong. *Educational Psychology: An International Journal of Experimental Educational Psychology, 30*, 139–153.

Chang, Y. P., Lin, Y. C., & Chen, L. H. (2012). Pay it forward: Gratitude in social networks. *Journal of Happiness Studies, 13*(5), 761–781.

Chen, L. H., Chen, M.-Y., Kee, Y. H., & Tsai, Y.-M. (2009). Validation of the Gratitude Questionnaire (GQ) in Taiwanese undergraduate students. *Journal of Happiness Studies, 10*, 655–664.

Chen, L. H., Chen, M. Y., & Tsai, Y. M. (2012). Does gratitude always work?: Ambivalence over emotional expression inhibits the beneficial effect of gratitude on well-being. *International Journal of Psychology, 47*(5), 381–392.

Chen, L. H., & Kee, Y. H. (2008). Gratitude and adolescent athletes' well-being. *Social Indicators Research, 89*, 361–373.

Cho, Y., & Fast, N. J. (2012). Power, defensive denigration, and the assuaging effect of gratitude expression. *Journal of Experimental Social Psychology, 48*, 778–782.

Clark, M. S. (1984). Record keeping in two types of relationships. *Journal of Personality and Social Psychology, 47*, 549–557.

Clark, M. S., & Mills, J. (1993). The difference between communal and exchange relationships: What it is and is not. *Personality and Social Psychology Bulletin, 19*, 684–691.

DeSteno, D., Bartlett, M. Y., Baumann, J., Williams, L. A., & Dickens, L. (2010). Gratitude as moral sentiment: Emotion-guided cooperation in economic exchange. *Emotion, 10*, 289–293.

DeWall, C. N., Lambert, N. M., Pond, R. S., Kashdan, T. B., & Fincham, F. D. (2012). A grateful heart is a nonviolent heart: Cross-sectional, experience sampling, longitudinal, and experimental evidence. *Social Psychological and Personality Science, 3*, 232–240.

Douglas, C. N. (Ed.). (1917). *Forty thousand quotations: Prose and poetical choice extracts on history, science, philosophy, religion, literature, etc.: Selected from the standard authors of ancient and modern times.* New York: Halcyon House.

Ellsworth, P. C., & Scherer, K. R. (2003). Appraisal processes in emotion. In R. J. Davidson, K. R. Scherer, & H. H. Goldsmith (Eds.), *Handbook of affective sciences* (pp. 572–595). New York: Oxford University Press.

Ellsworth, P. C., & Smith, C. A. (1988). Shades of joy: Patterns of appraisal differentiating pleasant emotions. *Cognition and Emotion, 2*, 301–331.

Emmons, R. A., & McCullough, M. E. (2003). Counting blessings versus burdens: An experimental investigation of gratitude and subjective well-being in daily life. *Journal of Personality and Social Psychology, 84*, 377–389.

Emmons, R. A., & Mishra, A. (2011). Why gratitude enhances well-being: What we know, what we need to know. In K. M. Sheldon, T. B. Kashdan, & M. F. Steger (Eds.), *Designing positive psychology: Taking stock and moving forward* (pp. 248–262). New York: Oxford University Press.

Emmons, R. A., & Shelton, C. M. (2002). Gratitude. In C. R. Synder & S. J. Lopez (Eds.), *Handbook of positive psychology* (pp. 459–471). New York: Oxford University Press.

Erisman, S. M., & Roemer, L. (2010). A preliminary investigation of the effects of experimentally induced mindfulness on emotional responding to film clips. *Emotion, 10*, 72–82.

Exline, J. J., Lisan, A. M., & Lisan, E. R. (2012). Reflecting on acts of kindness toward the self: Emotions, generosity, and the role of social norms. *Journal of Positive Psychology, 7,* 45–56.

Flinchbaugh, C. L., Moore, E. W. G., Chang, Y. K., & May, D. R. (2012). Student well-being interventions: The effects of stress management techniques and gratitude journaling in the management education classroom. *Journal of Management Education, 36,* 191–219.

Fredrickson, B. L. (2001). The role of positive emotions in positive psychology: The broaden-and-build theory of positive emotions. *American Psychologist, 56,* 218–226.

Fredrickson, B. L. (2004). Gratitude, like other positive emotions, broadens and builds. In R. A. Emmons & M. E. McCullough (Eds.), *The psychology of gratitude* (pp. 145–166). New York: Oxford University Press.

Fredrickson, B. L., Tugade, M. M., Waugh, C. E., & Larkin, G. R. (2003). What good are positive emotions in crises?: A prospective study of resilience and emotions following the terrorist attacks on the United States on September 11th, 2001. *Journal of Personality and Social Psychology, 84,* 365–376.

Frias, A., Watkins, P. C., Webber, A. C., & Froh, J. J. (2011). Death and gratitude: Death reflection enhances gratitude. *Journal of Positive Psychology, 6,* 154–162.

Frijda, N. H. (1986). *The emotions.* Cambridge, UK: Cambridge University Press.

Froh, J. J., Bono, G., & Emmons, R. A. (2010). Being grateful is beyond good manners: Gratitude and motivation to contribute to society among early adolescents. *Motivation and Emotion, 34,* 144–157.

Froh, J. J., Emmons, R. A., Card, N. A., Bono, G., & Wilson, J. A. (2011). Gratitude and the reduced costs of materialism in adolescents. *Journal of Happiness Studies, 12,* 289–302.

Froh, J. J., Fan, J., Emmons, R. A., Bono, G., Huebner, E. S., & Watkins, P. (2011). Measuring gratitude in youth: Assessing the psychometric properties of adult gratitude scales in children and adolescents. *Psychological Assessment, 23,* 311–324.

Froh, J. J., Kashdan, T. B., Ozimkowski, K. M., & Miller, N. (2009). Who benefits the most from a gratitude intervention in children and adolescents?: Examining positive affect as a moderator. *Journal of Positive Psychology, 4,* 408–422.

Froh, J. J., Sefick, W. J., & Emmons, R. A. (2008). Counting blessings in early adolescents: An experimental study of gratitude and

subjective well-being. *Journal of School Psychology, 46,* 213–233.

Gable, S. L., Reis, H. T., Impett, E. A., & Asher, E. R. (2004). What do you do when things go right?: The intrapersonal and interpersonal benefits of sharing positive events. *Journal of Personality and Social Psychology, 87,* 228–245.

Geraghty, A. W. A., Wood, A. M., & Hyland, M. E. (2010). Attrition from self-directed interventions: Investigating the relationship between psychological predictors, intervention content and dropout from a body dissatisfaction intervention. *Social Science and Medicine, 71,* 30–37.

Gordon, C. L., Arnette, R. A. M., & Smith, R. E. (2011). Have you thanked your spouse today?: Felt and expressed gratitude among married couples. *Personality and Individual Differences, 50,* 339–343.

Gottman, J. M., Katz, L. F., & Hooven, C. (1996). Parental meta-emotion philosophy and the emotional life of families: Theoretical models and preliminary data. *Journal of Family Psychology, 10,* 243–268.

Grant, A. M., & Gino, F. (2010). A little thanks goes a long way: Explaining why gratitude expressions motivate prosocial behavior. *Journal of Personality and Social Psychology, 98,* 946–955.

Gross, J. J., & Thompson, R. A. (2007). Emotion regulation: Conceptual foundations. In J. J. Gross (Ed.), *Handbook of emotion regulation* (pp. 3–24). New York: Guilford Press.

Haidt, J. (2003). Elevation and the positive psychology of morality. In C. L. M. Keyes & J. Haidt (Eds.), *Flourishing: Positive psychology and the life well-lived* (pp. 275–289). Washington DC: American Psychological Association.

Harmon-Jones, E., Harmon-Jones, C., Amodio, D. M., & Gable, P. A. (2011). Attitudes toward emotions. *Journal of Personality and Social Psychology, 101,* 1332–1350.

Helgeson, V. S., Reynolds, K. A., & Tomich, P. L. (2006). A meta-analytic review of benefit finding and growth. *Journal of Consulting and Clinical Psychology, 74,* 797–816.

Hicks, J. A., & King, L. A. (2007). Meaning in life and seeing the big picture: Positive affect and global focus. *Cognition and Emotion, 21,* 1577–1584.

Hoffer, E. (1973). *Reflections on the human condition.* New York: Harper & Row.

Huffman, J. C., Mastromauro, C. A., Boehm, J. K., Seabrook, R., Fricchione, G. L., Denninger, J. W., et al. (2011). Development of a positive psychology intervention for patients with acute cardiovascular disease. *Heart International, 6*, 47–54.

James, W. (1983). *Principles of psychology.* Cambridge, MA: Harvard University Press. (Original work published 1890)

John, O. P., & Gross, J. J. (2007). Individual differences in emotion regulation. In J. J. Gross (Ed.), *Handbook of emotion regulation* (pp. 351–372). New York: Guilford Press.

King, L. A. (2012). Meaning: Ubiquitous and effortless. In P. S. Shaver & M. Mikulincer (Eds.), *Meaning, mortality, and choice: The social psychology of existential concerns* (pp. 129–144). Washington, DC: American Psychological Association.

Klainin-Yobas, P., Cho, M. A. A., & Creedy, D. (2012). Efficacy of mindfulness-based interventions on depressive symptoms among people with mental disorders: A meta-analysis. *International Journal of Nursing Studies, 49*, 109–121.

Koo, M., Algoe, S. B., Wilson, T. D., & Gilbert, D. T. (2008). It's a wonderful life: Mentally subtracting positive events improves people's affective states, contrary to their affective forecasts. *Journal of Personality and Social Psychology, 95*, 1217–1224.

Kubacka, K. E., Finkenauer, C., Rusbult, C. E., & Keisjers, L. (2011). Maintaining close relationships: Gratitude as a motivator and detector of maintenance behavior. *Personality and Social Psychology Bulletin, 37*, 1362–1375.

Lambert, N. M., Clark, M. S., Durtschi, J., Fincham, F. D., & Graham, S. M. (2010). Benefits of expressing gratitude: Expressing gratitude to a partner changes one's view of the relationship. *Psychological Science, 21*, 574–580.

Lambert, N. M., & Fincham, F. D. (2011). Expressing gratitude to a partner leads to more relationship maintenance behavior. *Emotion, 11*, 52–60.

Lambert, N. M., Fincham, F. D., & Stillman, T. F. (2012). Gratitude and depressive symptoms: The role of positive reframing and positive emotion. *Cognition and Emotion, 26*, 615–633.

Lambert, N. M., Graham, S. M., & Fincham, F. D. (2009). A prototype analysis of gratitude: Varieties of gratitude experiences. *Personality and Social Psychology Bulletin, 35*, 1193–1207.

Lambert, N. M., Graham, S. M., Fincham, F. D., & Stillman, T. F. (2009). A changed perspective: How gratitude can affect sense of coherence through positive reframing. *Journal of Positive Psychology, 4*, 461–470.

Lambert, N. M., Gwinn, A. M., Baumeister, R. F., Strachman, A., Washburn, I. J., Gable, S. L., et al. (2013). A boost of positive affect: The perks of sharing positive experiences. *Journal of Social and Personal Relationships, 30*, 24–43.

Lattin, D. (2012, June 18). Gratitude movement leader to speak in S.F. *San Francisco Chronicle.* Retrieved from *www.sfgate.com/cgi-bin/article.cgi?f=/c/a/2012/06/17/ddsp1oujst. dtl&type=science.*

Lau, R. W. L., & Cheng. S. T. (2011). Gratitude lessens death anxiety. *European Journal of Ageing, 8*, 169–175.

Lazarus, R. S., & Lazarus, B. N. (1994). *Passion and reason: Making sense of our emotions.* New York: Oxford University Press.

Lefcourt, H. M., Martin, R. A., & Ware, E. E. (1984). Locus of control, causal attributions, and affects in achievement-related contexts. *Canadian Journal of Behavioral Science, 16*, 57–64.

Lesowitz, N., & Sammons, M. B. (2009). *Living life as a thank you: The transformative power of daily gratitude.* Berkeley, CA: Viva Editions.

Lewis, H. B. (1971). Shame and guilt in neurosis. *Psychoanalytic Review, 58*, 419–438.

Li, D., Zhang, W., Li, X., Li, N., & Ye, B. (2012). Gratitude and suicide ideation and suicide attempts among Chinese Adolescents: Direct, mediated, and moderated effects. *Journal of Adolescence, 35*, 55–66.

Lyubomirsky, S., Sheldon, K. M., & Schkade, D. (2005). Pursuing happiness: The architecture of sustainable change. *Review of General Psychology, 9*, 111–131.

Maritain, J. (1975). *Reflections on America.* New York: Gordian Press.

Mathews, M. A., & Green, J. D. (2010). Looking at me, appreciating you: Self-focused attention distinguishes between gratitude and indebtedness. *Cognition and Emotion, 24*, 710–718.

McCabe, K., Bray, M. A., Kehle, T. J., Theodore, L. A., & Gelbar, N. W. (2011). Promoting happiness and life satisfaction in school children. *Canadian Journal of School Psychology, 26*, 177–192.

McCullough, M. E., Emmons, R. A., & Tsang, J. A. (2002). The grateful disposition: A conceptual and empirical topography. *Journal of Personality and Social Psychology, 82*, 112–127.

McCullough, M. E., Kimeldorf, M. B., & Cohen, A. D. (2008). An adaptation for altruism?: The social causes, social effects, and social evolution of gratitude. *Current Directions in Psychological Science, 17,* 281–285.

McCullough, M. E., Tsang, J. A., & Emmons, R. A. (2004). Gratitude in intermediate affective terrain: Links of grateful moods to individual differences and daily emotional experience. *Journal of Personality and Social Psychology, 86,* 295–309.

McIntosh, E., & Ahrens, A. H. (2012). *The roles of empathy and mindfulness in gratitude induction.* Unpublished manuscript, Department of Psychology, American University, Washington, DC.

Mischel, W., & Shoda, Y. (1999). Integrating dispositions and processing dynamics within a unified theory of personality: The cognitive-affective personality system. In L. A. Pervin & O. P. John (Eds.), *Handbook of personality: Theory and research* (2nd ed., pp. 197–218). New York: Guilford Press.

Mitmansgruber, H., Beck, T. N., Hofer, S., & Schussler, G. (2009). When you don't like what you feel: Experiential avoidance, mindfulness and meta-emotion in emotion regulation. *Personality and Individual Differences, 46,* 448–453.

Nowak, M., & Roch, S. (2007). Upstream reciprocity and the evolution of gratitude. *Proceedings of the Royal Society of London B, 274,* 605–609.

Ortony, A., Clore, G. L., & Collins, A. (1988). *The cognitive structure of emotions.* New York: Cambridge University Press.

Panagopoulos, C. (2011). Thank you for voting: Gratitude expression and voter mobilization. *Journal of Politics, 73,* 707–717.

Peterson, C., Park, N., & Seligman, M. E. P. (2005). Orientations to happiness and life satisfaction: The full life versus the empty life. *Journal of Happiness Studies, 6,* 25–41.

Proctor, C., Linley, P. A., & Maltby, J. (2010). Very happy youths: Benefits of very high life satisfaction among adolescents. *Social Indicators Research, 98,* 519–532.

Reis, H. T., Clark, M. S., & Holmes, J. G. (2004). Perceived partner responsiveness as an organizing construct in the study of intimacy and closeness. In D. J. Mashek & A. Aron (Eds.), *Handbook of closeness and intimacy* (pp. 201–226). Mahwah, NJ: Erlbaum.

Roberts, R. C. (2004). The blessing of gratitude: A conceptual analysis. In R. A. Emmons & M. E. McCullough (Eds.), *The psychology of gratitude* (pp. 58–80). New York: Oxford University Press.

Salovey, P., Mayer, J. D., Golman, S. L., Turvey, C., & Palfai, T. P. (1995). Emotional attention, clarity, and repair: Exploring emotional intelligence using the trait meta-mood scale. In J. W. Pennebaker (Ed.), *Emotion, disclosure, and health* (pp. 125–154). Washington, DC: American Psychological Association.

Scheidle, L. E. (2011). Forgiveness and gratitude as predictors of elderly subjective well-being. Retrieved from ProQuest Dissertations and Theses (UMI 3415859) at *http://search.proquest.com/docview/750172966.*

Schorr, A. (2001). Appraisal: The evolution of an idea. In K. R. Scherer, A. Schorr, & T. Johnstone (Eds.), *Appraisal processes in emotion: Theory, methods, research* (pp. 20–34). New York: Oxford University Press.

Schueller, S. M. (2010). Preferences for positive psychology exercises. *Journal of Positive Psychology, 5,* 192–203.

Sergeant, S., & Mongrain, M. (2011). Are positive psychology exercises helpful for people with depressive personality styles? *Journal of Positive Psychology, 6,* 260–272.

Seligman, M. E. P. (1975). *Helplessness: On depression, development, and death.* San Francisco: Freeman.

Seligman, M. E. P., Steen, T. A., Park, N., & Peterson, C. (2005). Positive psychology progress: Empirical validation of interventions. *American Psychologist, 60,* 410–421.

Shah, S. P., Roth, A., Goya, R., Oloumi, A., Ha, G., Zhao, Y., et al. (2012). The clonal and mutational evolution spectrum of primary triple-negative breast cancers. *Nature, 486,* 395–399.

Shapiro, S. L., Brown, K. W., Thoresen, C., & Plante, T. G. (2011). The moderation of mindfulness-based stress reduction effects by trait mindfulness: Results from a randomized controlled trial. *Journal of Clinical Psychology, 67,* 267–277.

Sheldon, K. M., & Lyubomirsky, S. (2012). The challenge of staying happier: Testing the Happiness Adaptation Prevention model. *Personality and Social Psychology Bulletin, 38,* 670–680.

Shelton, C. M. (2004). Gratitude: Considerations from a moral perspective. In R. A. Emmons & M. E. McCullough (Eds.), *The psychology of gratitude* (pp. 257–281). New York: Oxford University Press.

Shen, H., Wan, F., & Wyer, R. S. (2011). Cross-cultural differences in the refusal to accept a small gift: The differential influence of reciprocity norms on Asians and North Americans. *Journal of Personality and Social Psychology, 100,* 271–281.

Shiota, M. N., Keltner, D., & Mossman, A. (2007). The nature of awe: Elicitors, appraisals, and effects on self-concept. *Cognition and Emotion, 21,* 944–963.

Smith, C. A. (1991). The self, appraisal, and coping. In C. R. Snyder & D. R. Forsyth (Eds.), *Handbook of social and clinical psychology* (pp. 116–137). New York: Pergamon.

Smith, C. A., & Kirby, L. D. (2012, January). *The motivational functions of emotion: Action tendencies, emotivational goals, and enacted behaviors.* Paper presented at the 13th Annual Meeting of the Society of Personality and Social Psychology, San Diego, CA.

Steindl-Rast, D. (2004). Gratitude as thankfulness and gratefulness. In R. A. Emmons & M. E. McCullough (Eds.), *The psychology of gratitude* (pp. 282–290). New York: Oxford University Press.

Sweeney, P. D., Anderson, K., & Bailey, S. (1986). Attributional style in depression: A meta-analytic review. *Journal of Personality and Social Psychology, 50,* 974–991.

Tangney, J. P., & Salovey, P. (2010). Emotions of the imperiled ego: Shame, guilt, jealousy, and envy. In J. E. Maddux & J. P. Tangney (Eds.), *Social psychological foundations of clinical psychology* (pp. 245–271). New York: Guilford Press.

Toepfer, S. M., Cichy, K., & Peters, P. (2011). Letters of gratitude: Further evidence for author benefits. *Journal of Happiness Studies, 13,* 187–201.

Tong, E. M. W., & Yang, Z. (2011). Moral hypocrisy: Of proud and grateful people. *Social Psychological and Personality Science, 2,* 159–165.

Tsai, J. L. (2007). Ideal affect: Cultural causes and behavioral consequences. *Perspectives on Psychological Science, 2,* 242–259.

Tsang, J. A. (2006). The effects of helper intention on gratitude and indebtedness. *Motivation and Emotion, 30,* 198–204.

Twenge, J. M., Konrath, S., Foster, J. D., Campbell, W. K., & Bushman, B. J. (2008). Egos inflating over time: A cross-temporal meta-analysis of the Narcissistic Personality Inventory. *Journal of Personality, 76,* 875–901.

Unsworth, K. L., Turner, N., Williams, H. M., & Piccin-Houle, S. (2010). Giving thanks: The relational context of gratitude in postgraduate supervision. *Studies in Higher Education, 35,* 871–888.

Vernon, L. L. (2012). Relationships among proactive coping, posttrauma gratitude, and psychopathology in a traumatized college sample. *Journal of Aggression, Maltreatment and Trauma, 21,* 114–130.

Watkins, P., Scheer, J., Ovnicek, M., & Kolts, R. (2006). The debt of gratitude: Dissociating gratitude and indebtedness. *Cognition and Emotion, 20,* 217–241.

Watkins, P. C., Van Gelder, M., & Frias, A. (2009). Furthering the science of gratitude. In C. R. Snyder & S. J. Lopez (Eds.), *Oxford handbook of positive psychology* (pp. 437–445). New York: Oxford University Press.

Watkins, P. C., Woodward, K., Stone, T., & Kolts, R. L. (2003). Gratitude and happiness: Development of a measure of gratitude, and relationships with subjective well-being. *Social Behavior and Personality: An International Journal, 31,* 431–451.

Weiner, B., Russell, D., & Lerman, D. (1979). The cognition-emotion process in achievement related contexts. *Journal of Personality and Social Psychology, 37,* 1211–1220.

Weinstein, N., DeHaan, C. R., & Ryan, R. M. (2010). Attributing autonomous versus introjected motivation to helpers and the recipient experience: Effects on gratitude, attitudes, and well-being. *Motivation and Emotion, 34,* 418–431.

Williams, K. E., Chambless, D. L., & Ahrens, A. H. (1997). Are emotions frightening?: An extension of the fear of fear construct. *Behaviour Research and Therapy, 35,* 239–248.

Wood, A. M., Brown, G. D., & Maltby, J. (2011). Thanks, but I'm used to better: A relative rank model of gratitude. *Emotion, 11,* 175–180.

Wood, A. M., Froh, J. J., & Geraghty, A. W. A. (2010). Gratitude and well-being: A review and theoretical integration. *Clinical Psychology Review, 7,* 890–905.

Wood, A. M., Maltby, J., Gillett, R., Linley, P. A., & Joseph, S. (2008). The role of gratitude in the development of social support, stress, and depression: Two longitudinal studies. *Journal of Research in Personality, 42,* 854–871.

CHAPTER 21

Transcending the Self

Awe, Elevation, and Inspiration

Michelle N. Shiota
Todd M. Thrash
Alexander F. Danvers
John T. Dombrowski

As described by Western science, emotion is fundamentally about the self. While major theories of emotion differ in many important regards, most agree that emotions reflect an "assessment of one's own current state" (Russell, 2003, p. 149) and/or evaluation of the significance of events for one's goals and well-being (e.g., Lazarus, 1991; Scherer, 2009). Positive emotions are no exception. Theories of positive emotion and analyses of its neural substrates often emphasize key roles in identifying goal-conducive situations and promoting approach/appetitive states that support acquisition of material and social rewards (e.g., Burgdorf & Panksepp, 2006; Carver & White, 1994; Knutson & Cooper, 2005; Watson, Wiese, Vaidya, & Tellegen, 1999). Even the social emotions of pride in our accomplishments, love for attachment figures, and gratitude toward those who have helped us are arguably self-focused, reflecting on our own actions or what others do for us (Haidt & Morris, 2009).

Emotions also tend to turn attention inward. Negative emotions lead to an increase in self-focused attention, as measured by use of first-person pronouns in sentence-completion tasks (e.g., Salovey, 1992; Salovey & Rodin, 1985; Wood, Saltzberg, & Goldsamt, 1990). Positive emotions have this effect as well, provided that participants are not anticipating a subsequent task that might elicit performance concerns (e.g., Abele, Silvia, & Zöller-Utz, 2005; Silvia & Abele, 2002). Positive emotion is thought to increase reliance on internal knowledge structures and dominant modes of cognition, another way in which the mind can turn inward rather than out to the environment (e.g., Bless, Bohner, Schwarz, & Strack, 1990; Bodenhausen, Kramer, & Süsser, 1994; Fiedler, 2001; Forgas, 1998; although see Fredrickson, 2001, for a different perspective).

The emotions (awe, elevation) and emotional state (inspiration) addressed in this chapter are thought to do the opposite, turning our minds outward rather than inward, encouraging us to transcend the self and its expectations. While they differ from each other in important ways, awe, elevation, and inspiration all involve challenging our expectations about what is and what can be. They pull attention outside the self toward something to be understood and appreciated—a feature of the natural world, the actions of another human being, a practical or creative problem to be solved. Moreover, they draw attention to that which is greater than the self, inviting us to transcend our day-to-day agendas and limits. In this chapter we discuss each of these three constructs, offering a detailed theoretical description, as well as reviewing the available empirical evidence. We then discuss broader issues raised by awe, elevation, and inspiration, offering suggestions for future research on these relatively understudied states.

Awe

Albert Einstein once said, "One cannot help but be in awe when contemplating the mysteries of eternity, of life, of the marvelous structure of reality. It is enough if one tries merely to comprehend a little of the mystery every day. The important thing is not to stop questioning; never lose a holy curiosity" (statement to William Miller, as quoted in Einstein's obituary in *Life* magazine, May 2, 1955). Like other great thinkers, Einstein highlights the transcendence of one's current understanding as a core feature of awe in this comment, and also points the way to important functions that awe might serve.

Theoretical Definition

Drawing extensively on literature in philosophy, sociology, and religious studies, as well as psychology, Keltner and Haidt (2003) proposed a theoretical definition of "awe." Their analysis identifies two themes characterizing stimuli that are likely to elicit the experience of awe: perceived vastness and need for accommodation. "Vastness" means that the stimulus strongly challenges the perceiver's accustomed frame of reference. While this may be a matter of sheer physical size (e.g., the Grand Canyon or the Eiffel Tower), a stimulus can also be vast in terms of explanatory power (e.g., a theory of physics), social import (e.g., a person or historical event that affects millions of people), sensory detail (e.g., a complex musical

or visual piece), conceptual breadth (e.g., a work of art or literature that ties together a rich range of ideas, breaking new conceptual ground), or volume of unexpected information (e.g., the drop of pond water that contains an elaborate world of its own). Because such stimuli are not easily accounted for by one's current understanding of the world, they require "cognitive accommodation"—updating one's worldview in order to include and make sense of the new experience.

Consideration of awe as a possible "basic" emotion—a functionally discrete emotion category thought to be a product of our evolutionary heritage (see Shiota, Chapter 3, this volume)—was long prevented by inability to identify a plausible adaptive function. However, Keltner and Haidt (2003) proposed two ways in which awe might enhance fitness. The first of these is suggested by Einstein's comment, quoted earlier. At the individual level of analysis, the cognitive and behavioral effects of awe should promote greater encoding of new information from the environment, or cognitive accommodation. All animals require knowledge about their environment in order to survive. We humans may be unique in the extent of our ability to gather new information from our surroundings, however, and to store that information in the form of internal mental representations or "schemas" (Piaget, 1973). Schemas are efficient and protective, allowing us to apply old knowledge to new situations and mentally "test out" possible plans of action without actually performing those actions and facing their consequences. However, when old schemas cannot make sense of a new stimulus or experience, a new one must be formed.

If the definition of awe offered earlier is correct, awe should reduce reliance on existing schemas, heuristics, and other current knowledge structures in processing new stimuli, and instead facilitate the intake of new information and formation of new schemas. Notably, this is the opposite of previously observed effects of positive emotions, which typically have been found to promote *greater* reliance on prior schemas and other mental shortcuts in approaching the environment (e.g., Bless et al., 1990; Bodenhausen et al., 1994; Fiedler, 2001; Forgas, 1998). As we see below, this aspect of Keltner and

Haidt's (2003) theory has been highly useful in generating empirical research.

At the group level of analysis, feelings of awe toward powerful leaders may help stabilize social hierarchies by encouraging submissive and cooperative behavior among subordinates. As a species, humans are "ultrasocial," performing many tasks that are crucial for survival and reproductive fitness (food acquisition and production, protection against attack by predators and out-groups, creating shelter, raising offspring) in large groups of loosely related individuals (Campbell, 1983). Large groups require leadership to be effective, but conflict over leadership can be costly for both the group and the individuals in it. Drawing from philosophical and sociological accounts, Keltner and Haidt (2003) suggest that one function of awe is to provide a nonviolent mechanism for allocating power, in which potential or actual leaders use awe-inspiring displays to elicit buy-in from their communities. While this proposal has not, to date, been translated into much psychological research, it is consistent with observations in sociology and cultural anthropology (e.g., Durkheim, 1887/1972; Weber, 1978/2002).

Empirical Research

Like the other constructs addressed in this chapter, awe has received far less empirical attention than positive emotions such as joy/enthusiasm, contentment, amusement, love and pride. Nonetheless, the research currently available for review supports the theoretical portrait offered earlier.

Antecedents

English speakers report that awe is elicited by the kinds of stimuli suggested by Keltner and Haidt's (2003) analysis, and by the construct definition proposed earlier. In one study a sample of undergraduates was invited to describe a recent event in which they felt awe, without further suggestion about type of experience (Shiota, Keltner, & Mossman, 2007). The most commonly reported elicitors were panoramic nature views, extraordinary works of art or music encountered for the first time, and one's own or another's remarkable accomplishment. Notably, all of the eliciting events were described in positive terms, and all emphasized some aspect of vastness in the experience. Even descriptions of potentially negative or primarily social events (e.g., death of a grandparent, a friend's marriage) focused on the magnitude of the life transition in question and the impossibility of knowing what would follow, rather than personal loss or social pleasure. Descriptions of participants' own accomplishments as awe elicitors emphasized amazement bordering on disbelief, rather than pride. These descriptions are highly consistent with the conceptual definition of awe suggested by Keltner and Haidt (2003).

Subjective Experience and Individual Differences

The subjective experience of awe is also consistent with the notion of self-transcendence. Compared with those asked to relive a personal pride-inducing accomplishment, those asked to relive an awe-inspiring natural scene report significantly greater feelings of awe, love, rapture, and contentment, as well as feeling that the self is small or insignificant, sensing the presence of something greater than the self, being unaware of normal day-to-day concerns, feeling connected with the surrounding world, and wanting to prolong the experience as long as possible (Shiota et al., 2007). Awe experiences were *not* rated as challenging or tiring (in fact, they were rated significantly less so than accomplishments), suggesting that the kind of cognitive activity involved in awe does not require effortful, controlled processing. Correlations of dispositional awe-proneness with Extraversion ($r = .34$), Openness to Experience ($r = .49$), and Need for Cognitive Closure ($r = -.39$) also link awe to a tendency to push one's own experiential and intellectual boundaries (Shiota, Keltner, & John, 2006; Shiota et al., 2007).

Physiological and Expressive Aspects

Physiological and expressive aspects of awe have not been widely studied. The one study that explicitly compared autonomic nervous system responding in awe versus other positive emotions and a neutral state found that awe led to a pronounced and unique increase in cardiac preejection period, indicating withdrawal of sympathetic nervous system influence on the heart via beta$_1$-adrenergic receptors (Shiota, Neufeld, Yeung, Moser, & Perea, 2011; see Figure 21.1). This effect is consistent with prior studies demonstrating heart rate reduction during the intake of information (Bradley, 2009). In this study awe was also associated with an increase in respiration rate and decrease in respiratory sinus arrhythmia.

Feelings of goosebumps or "goosetingles" are also commonly associated with the experience of awe (e.g., Maruskin, Thrash, & Elliot, 2012; Schurtz et al., 2012). Although, to our knowledge, this effect has yet to be examined via objective measures of physiological responding, the subjective sense of goosetingles in awe likely reflects contraction of piloerector muscles, making body hair stand on end and literally producing goosebumps. Piloerection is caused by activation of alpha$_1$-adrenergic receptors on these muscles via the sympathetic nervous system—a different mechanism from that driving the cardiac effect described earlier. If future, laboratory-based evidence confirms a consistent role of piloerection in awe, this would suggest a novel and complex autonomic profile. Much further research is needed to document the physiological aspects of awe, and to assess whether these aspects play a role in mediating effects of awe on cognitive outcomes.

A recent study also documented a prototype facial/postural expression associated with awe. Participants were asked to recall a personal experience with awe (as well as several other positive emotions), then to freely pose the way they would express awe to others. Posed expressions commonly included raised inner (but not outer) eyebrows, raised eyelids, loosely opened mouth with parted lips, and slight postural leaning forward (Campos, Shiota, Keltner, Gonzaga, & Goetz, 2013; see Figure 21.1). The absence of an outer brow raise distinguished this expression from the prototypical surprise expression (e.g., Ekman et al., 1987), although both may facilitate intake of visual information. The absence of a smile (Duchenne or otherwise) is striking in comparison with expressions of most other positive emotions and may emphasize the primarily cognitive rather than affiliative nature of awe.

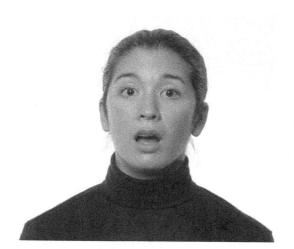
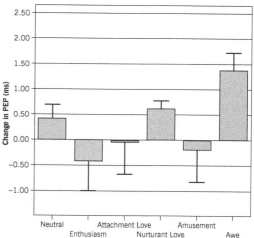

FIGURE 21.1. Prototype facial expression and baseline-to-trial change in cardiac preejection period associated with awe. Prototype facial expression is based on data from Campos, Shiota, Keltner, Gonzaga, and Goetz (2013). Graph of change in cardiac preejection period is reprinted with permission from Shiota, Neufeld, Yeung, Moser, and Perea (2011). Copyright 2011 by the American Psychological Association. Reprinted by permission.

Implications for Cognition, Perception, and Self-Concept

So far, the bulk of empirical research on awe has emphasized this emotion's effects on cognition, perception, and self-concept. Although this research is still very young, some studies already support the proposal that awe inhibits reliance on previously held schemas, mental heuristics/shortcuts, and other internal knowledge structures in processing new information. For example, one set of studies found that participants who had just completed an awe-induction task were less influenced than those in a neutral condition by persuasive messages containing several weak arguments (Griskevicius, Shiota, & Neufeld, 2010). Previously, other positive emotions had been found to *increase* one's susceptibility to weak but prolific persuasive messages relative to a neutral control, indicating reliance on a simple "more is better" heuristic. Griskevicius and colleagues (2010) replicated this original finding with anticipatory enthusiasm, amusement, contentment, and love for attachment figures, but awe showed the opposite effect. Preliminary studies are also finding that awe, relative to other positive emotions, leads to reduced reliance on stereotypes in rating the personalities of people in fictional profiles (Yee & Shiota, 2013), as well as a more conservative bias in deciding whether or not specific details were present in a lengthy audio story about a common event—going out to dinner at a romantic restaurant (Danvers & Shiota, 2013).

Much further research is needed to examine the implications of awe for activation and use of internal knowledge structures, such as mental schemas, and to establish the specific mechanisms and boundary conditions of these effects. In developing this research, it is important to note that demonstrating reduced reliance on prior knowledge structures does not necessarily demonstrate *increased* effective intake of information from the environment; these processes are dissociable and must be demonstrated using different measures.

Studies of schema/heuristic activation emphasize the "need for accommodation" aspect of awe. Other studies of cognitive outcomes have emphasized the "vastness" aspect of the awe experience. Experimentally elicited awe has been found to alter the self-concept in a way consistent with this proposed aspect, increasing the number of "universals" such as "I am a human" and "I am a living being" offered by participants as self-descriptors in the Twenty Statements Test (Shiota et al., 2006), and increasing feelings of oneness with others "in general," as well as with personal friends (Van Cappellen & Saroglou, 2012). Other studies have found that viewing awe-inspiring videos on nature and childbirth led to an increase in spirituality, defined as a "tendency to orient oneself toward a larger transcendent reality" (Saroglou, Buxant, & Tilquin, 2008, p. 169). This effect was not observed after participants viewed a comic video, and the effect did not extend to formal religiosity. Instead, awe appeared to have a distinctive effect on participants' sense of themselves as part of a vast, greater, and meaningful reality.

Most recently, new studies have examined the implications of awe for our perception of time, and the downstream effects of low time pressure for prosocial behavior and well-being (Rudd, Vohs, & Aaker, 2012). Across three studies, experimentally elicited awe was found to increase the perception of available time and reduce feelings of impatience. These changes mediated effects of awe on self-reported willingness to volunteer time to help others, preference for experiences rather than material objects, and life satisfaction. In interpreting these effects, Rudd and colleagues (2012) suggest that, as a consequence of need for accommodation, the experience of awe focuses our attention on the present moment, effectively stretching it out. Further research efforts examining the effects of awe on attention per se are suggested by this analysis, and mediation studies would be a helpful addition to this new line of research.

When asked to offer examples of things that elicit awe, laypeople and great thinkers alike tend to point to the natural world, or to physical creations that, though conceived and built by humans, give a sense of transcending human capacity. Awe may also have an amoral quality, in that vastness and need for accommodation may characterize great horrors as well as great beauty. We now turn to a second self-transcending positive emotion, elevation, which places greater emphasis on social elicitors and the exemplification of moral values.

Elevation

When witnessing an exemplary moral act performed by another person, we may experience a powerful emotional response. Haidt (2000) has identified this response as the emotion *elevation*, "a warm, uplifting feeling that people experience when they see unexpected acts of human goodness, kindness, and compassion" (pp. 1–2). Keltner and Haidt (2003) propose that elevation shares with awe the feature of need for accommodation, but that elevation need not involve the perceptions of vastness or power that characterize awe. Elevation is most commonly elicited by others' actions exemplifying virtues such as charity, gratitude, courage, and loyalty (Haidt, 2000; Landis et al., 2009).

Theoretical Definition

Theoretical analyses of elevation emphasize its role as a "moral emotion," guiding our judgments of others' morality and our own subsequent moral decision making in ways that bypass and may even precede logical moral reasoning (Haidt, 2001, 2003; Horberg, Oveis, & Keltner, 2011). In this sense, elevation may be the opposite of disgust, a negative emotion that frames the social world in terms of a contrast between degradation and moral purity, much as physical disgust emphasizes the contrast between disease or filth and cleanliness (Haidt, 2000, 2001; Rozin, Haidt, & McCauley, 2000).

This aspect of elevation points to a possible adaptive function. Elevation inspires us to help others, but it also helps those who experience it. As members of an ultrasocial species humans feel a need to belong, and we derive great adaptive benefit from cooperating with group members in interdependent relationships (Baumeister & Leary, 1995; Campbell, 1983). Emotions—especially positive emotions—can help support the process of forming and maintaining strong, healthy relationships of this kind (Shiota, Campos, Keltner, & Hertenstein, 2004). At the individual level of analysis, elevation helps us to identify exemplary cooperators and good trade partners by triggering affection for those who display altruism (Haidt, 2000). People who prioritize other people's interests are good relationship partners, and elevation may help point our attention toward these individuals (Frank, 1988). At the group level, elevation can help support community norms of helping. When one member of a group helps, other members are likely to see—and respond by helping yet other group members. Haidt (2000) likens this elevation-driven upward spiral of helping within the group to the upward spiral of individual positive emotion and well-being in Fredrickson's (2001) broaden-and-build model (see Tugade, Devlin, & Fredrickson, Chapter 2, this volume).

Empirical Research

Although elevation was only recently proposed as a distinct positive emotion construct, research has identified several of its characteristics and effects. Elevation is most commonly elicited by "seeing someone else give help or aid to a person who was poor or sick, or stranded in a difficult situation" (Haidt, 2000, p. 2), but it may be evoked by actions exemplifying other moral values, particularly those emphasizing social connection (Haidt, 2000; Landis et al., 2009).

Individual Differences

The tendency to experience elevation may be a stable personality trait. Landis and colleagues (2009) examined the relationship of self-reported disposition to experience elevation with various personality traits, spirituality, and self-reported altruism in a sample of 188 undergraduates (Costa & McCrae, 1992; Piedmont, 2004; Rushton, Chrisjohn, & Fekken, 1981). While supporting the notion of individual differences in elevation-proneness, the research identified two distinct factors in this trait. Items loading heavily on "Elevation-Factor I" emphasized connectedness to others, whereas those loading on "Elevation-Factor II" emphasized physiological reactions experienced while witnessing acts of helping.

Importantly, these two factors were linked to somewhat different aspects of personality. Factor I (connectedness) predicted self-reported altruism, whereas Factor II (physiological reactions) did not. Instead, Factor II better predicted self-reported spiritual transcendence and Openness to Experience. Recent research using a modified version of the Elevation Scale suggests the possibility of a third factor emphasizing an affective component, which captures feeling like a better, more open person (Vianello, Galliani, & Haidt, 2010).

Physiological Aspects

Elevation has been associated with subjective physical sensations, such as feelings of warmth in the chest, as well as some objective physiological changes (Haidt, 2000; Silvers & Haidt, 2008). Thomas Jefferson once suggested that reading about virtue can elicit "dilation of the breast" (cited in Haidt, 2003, p. 275), but participants experiencing elevation in empirical studies also describe a feeling of warmth in the chest (Haidt, 2000; Schnall, Roper, & Fessler, 2010). The physiological mechanisms underlying this sensation have not yet been established and merit new research. Videos that inspire elevation have been found to produce a decrease in vagal parasympathetic influence on the heart (Silvers & Haidt, 2008), but it is not clear whether this would account for the subjective sensations of warmth described earlier. More research is needed to establish whether elevation has a distinctive physiological profile across a range of autonomic nervous system mechanisms.

Elevation may increase circulating levels of the hormone oxytocin, which is known to support lactation, as well as pair-bonding, in humans and a number of other mammals (Insel & Hulihan, 1995; Silvers & Haidt, 2008). In an indirect test of the hypothesis that elevation promotes oxytocin release, Silvers and Haidt (2008) asked nursing mothers and their babies to watch video clips inducing either elevation or amusement. Mothers watching the elevation video were more likely to nurse, leak milk into a nursing pad, and hug their children—all actions linked to oxytocin in prior research. Although replication with direct measurement of oxytocin and comparison of elevation to a neutral control condition are both needed before strong conclusions are warranted, these results suggest one possible hormonal mechanism underlying physiological aspects of elevation.

Implications for Prosocial Behavior and Cooperation

The best-documented effect of elevation is its ability to inspire one's own prosocial behavior. Witnessing an altruistic act increases motivation to perform prosocial and affiliative actions, and views on humanity as a whole may improve (Haidt, 2000). In one set of experiments, participants watched either an elevation-inducing video clip, showing professional musicians expressing gratitude toward the teachers who had mentored them, or a neutral emotion video (Schnall et al., 2010). Those who saw the elevation video were more likely to volunteer to help with a subsequent, unpaid study. In a second study, participants viewed an elevation-inducing, neutral, or funny video clip and were then asked to help the experimenter by completing boring math problems for as long as they were willing, ostensibly for the purpose of establishing norms for the task. Participants in the elevation condition helped for significantly longer than those in either the humor or neutral conditions (41 minutes compared to 24 and 20 minutes). Importantly, helping time was strongly predicted by self-reported aspects of subjective elevation, such as wanting to help others and feeling optimistic about humanity, but not by overall positive affect. In addition to this laboratory-based, experimental research, a study of college students on a service trip found that those who reported more intense and frequent experiences of elevation during the trip performed more trip-related volunteer activities after returning (Cox, 2010).

Elevation elicited by a leader can affect followers' ethical inclinations, with downstream implications for cooperative behavior in and commitment to the workplace (Vianello et al., 2010). In one study, workers at an Italian company read scenarios about a fictitious leader. When the leader was described as interpersonally fair, workers reported higher intentions to perform

"Organizational Citizenship Behaviors" reflecting altruism, courtesy, and compliance at work, as well as greater affective commitment to their organization. In a study of nurses in a public hospital, the current supervisors' fairness and tendency to self-sacrifice predicted elevation in the nurses under their management, which in turn predicted greater commitment and organizational citizenship intentions (mediation analyses demonstrated a significant effect). A similar effect was reported with a sample of preschool teachers.

Awe and elevation have typically been described by psychologists as possible "basic" or "discrete" emotions—complex packages of cognitive, physiological, expressive, and behavioral responses to particular kinds of eliciting situations, thought to serve fairly specific adaptive functions in the context of those situations. The next construct we discuss, inspiration, has not been conceptualized in this way. However, the experience of inspiration is rich with positive affect, and it is interesting to consider how inspiration might intersect with the experience of self-transcending positive emotions.

Inspiration

Although the intellectual history of inspiration is deep and broad, scientific research on inspiration began just in the last decade. According to the *Oxford English Dictionary*, inspiration can be defined as "a breathing in or infusion of some idea, purpose, etc. into the mind; the suggestion, awakening, or creation of some feeling or impulse, especially of an exalted kind" (Simpson & Weiner, 1989, p. 1036). Inspiration is not an emotion, although instances of inspiration are certainly emotion-laden (Thrash & Elliot, 2003, 2004). Whereas emotions are typically defined in terms of specific kinds of eliciting situations, such as "loss of a loved one" (sadness) or "observing acts of human goodness" (elevation), inspiration can be elicited by a wide variety of highly valued objects or events. Emotions are also thought to activate specific motivational goals. Inspiration involves an important motivational component, but the actual goal depends on the thing that elicited inspiration rather than

being inherent in the inspiration construct itself. Rather than an emotion, one may conceptualize inspiration as a psychological *state* that varies in intensity over time and across individuals. In this sense, inspiration may be present as an element in a variety of self-transcending positive emotions, including elevation, admiration, and awe. Moreover, it is helpful to think of inspiration as an *episode* including multiple processes that unfold across time.

Theoretical Definition

Thrash and Elliot (2003) proposed that three core characteristics are necessary and collectively sufficient to define the subjective state of inspiration in a way that distinguishes it from other constructs: transcendence, evocation, and approach motivation. "Transcendence" refers to gaining an awareness of possibilities that are better than the current state of affairs. "Evocation" refers to the passive manner by which inspiration occurs; one does not feel directly responsible for becoming inspired, and ascribes responsibility for inspiration to something beyond one's own will. Finally, inspiration involves an intensified "approach motivation" that compels one to transmit, express, or actualize one's new idea or vision.

Thrash and Elliot (2004) further proposed that an episode of inspiration can be decomposed into two conceptually and empirically distinct processes: being inspired *by* and being inspired *to*. Being inspired *by* refers to being moved by the perceived intrinsic value of an eliciting object, whether that object is a work of art, a creative idea, a role model, or other exemplar. Being inspired *to* refers to the motivation to transmit or extend the valued qualities exemplified in that object. These processes are linked differentially to the core characteristics of inspiration, such that being inspired *by* involves transcendence and evocation, and being inspired *to* involves approach motivation. This framing suggests a temporal sequence for the core characteristics of inspiration that has been helpful in guiding empirical research. Transcendence and evocation are intertwined as two aspects of the same process. As Thrash and Elliot put it, one cannot actively awaken oneself to better possibilities through an act of will any more than one can awaken oneself from sleep; transcendence requires evocation. However, the inspired *by* process responsible for transcendence and evocation is separable from the inspired *to* motivational process to which it gives rise. While it is important to differentiate these two processes, disinterested *appreciation* of the evocative object (i.e., being inspired *by*) often sparks a nondisinterested *motivation* to transmit the qualities exemplified in that object (i.e., being inspired *to*). If such a desire is sparked, then a full episode of inspiration is present.

The proposed link between the inspired *by* and *to* processes highlights the function inspiration may serve. Specifically, inspiration is posited to mediate transmission of a perceived intrinsic value, exemplified by the inspiration-evoking stimulus, into future acts and/or creations (Thrash, Maruskin, Cassidy, Fryer, & Ryan, 2010). For instance, parents who are particularly selfless and caring (antecedent stimulus) are likely to be inspiring (mediator) to their children, who may in turn strive to be more selfless and caring themselves (future consequence). This mediation process may take any of several forms, depending on the nature of the evoking object—one may seek to *embody* a role model's virtue (as in the previous example), to *record* the content of a spiritual revelation, or to *actualize* a creative idea.

Whereas prior theorists have generally emphasized differences among *domains* of inspiration (e.g., creative, spiritual), distinguishing among these *forms* of transmission may do a better job of carving nature at its joints. For instance, the domain of "creative inspiration" is too heterogeneous to be regarded as a type of inspiration—being inspired to record a verse of poetry that comes to mind spontaneously is quite different from being inspired to embody some characteristic of a particular poet, such as Edgar Allen Poe. Likewise, the domain of "spiritual inspiration" is heterogeneous—a prophet's inspiration to record the content of a revelation as scripture is quite different from a reader's inspiration to be more Christ-like. Organizing these instances of inspiration by form of transmission rather than content domain, one sees important similarities between *recording* poetry and scripture (e.g., spontaneous insight, fol-lowed by vigorous writing), and between *embodying* the virtues of Poe and Christ (e.g., admiration of a role model, followed by motivation to pursue a future self modeled after the role model).

Empirical Research

The theoretical model described earlier links diverse instances of inspiration, which may be superficially quite different, to a process that is fundamentally similar. Regardless of content domain and form of transmission, one is moved by an intrinsically valued stimulus object, then compelled to transmit its inspiring qualities to a new object. Empirical research has tested a number of these propositions regarding the construct of inspiration, as well as implications of inspiration for a variety of important outcomes.

Subjective Experience

Research on the subjective experience of inspiration has supported the construct validity of the theoretical model described earlier. In a study by Thrash and Elliot (2004), participants were asked to write about an occasion when they were inspired. Compared with control experiences, inspiration experiences were found to involve elevated levels of variables representing the proposed core characteristics of transcendence (e.g., spirituality), evocation (e.g., passive self), and approach motivation (e.g., activated positive affect [PA]). In subsequent studies, Thrash and Elliot contrasted inspiration with another appetitive state: activated PA. As expected, inspiration involved a comparable level of approach motivation but higher levels of transcendence and evocation. Thrash (2007) further differentiated inspiration and activated PA by documenting different distributions of these states across days of the week. Whereas activated PA was relatively stable across days of the week, inspiration declined on weekends. This divergence was most pronounced on Fridays, which apparently are more conducive to fun and leisure than to embodying virtue or channeling one's Muse.

The distinction between inspired *by* and *to* processes has also received empirical support (Thrash & Elliot, 2004). In a confirmatory factor analysis of state inspiration items, being inspired *by* and being inspired *to* converged as indicators of a general inspiration construct, while still having the hypothesized distinct associations with indicators of transcendence, evocation, and approach motivation. Specifically, being inspired *by* was uniquely positively related to transcendence and evocation, whereas being inspired *to* was uniquely negatively related to transcendence and evocation, and uniquely positively related to approach motivation.

Antecedents

Research on the antecedents of inspiration has identified situations and states that function as proximal antecedents, as well as personality traits that function as distal antecedents. In some studies, proximal antecedents have been operationalized in terms of specific sources of intrinsic value in specific eliciting objects (e.g., extraordinary competence in role models; Thrash, Elliot, Maruskin, & Cassidy, 2010); in other studies, proximal antecedents have been operationalized in terms of more general insight or "illumination" experiences that are posited to accompany any of a variety of elicitor objects.

Thrash and Elliot (2004) proposed that the antecedents of inspiration are quite different than those of other appetitive states (e.g., activated PA) because inspiration begins with the nonmotivational process of being inspired *by*. They found that the tendency to become inspired in daily life was predicted proximally by the experience of illumination (but not by reward salience) and distally by openness-related traits (but not by approach temperament). The tendency to experience activated PA in daily life showed the opposite pattern; it was predicted proximally by reward salience and distally by approach temperament. Although approach temperament did not predispose individuals to become inspired more often, it did predict inspiration intensity and motivation strength during episodes of inspiration. In summary, consistent with the *by–to* distinction, openness-related traits predispose individuals to the kinds of illumination experiences that precede inspiration; once the individual is inspired by something, the approach temperament system is recruited to support motivation and action.

Thrash, Maruskin, and colleagues (2010) reported similar findings in the context of the creative process. In a cross-lagged analysis of data from a 5-week panel study, they found that creative insight early in the study preceded appraisals of inspiration at later time points during the writing process. Trait openness to aesthetics predicted creativity of individuals' initial ideas, and in turn the tendency to feel inspired. Behavioral activation system (BAS) scale scores, an indicator of approach temperament, did not predict the creativity of initial ideas; rather, it amplified the effect of the creativity of this idea on inspiration. Across both these lines of research, openness-related traits predisposed individuals to the proximal elicitors of inspiration; thereafter, approach temperament facilitated inspired motivation.

Individual Differences

Thrash and Elliot (2003) developed and validated an 8-item trait questionnaire, the Inspiration Scale. This measure comprises four stem statements (e.g., "I feel inspired"), each of which is rated in terms of both frequency and intensity using 7-point Likert scales. The frequency and intensity subscales tend to be highly correlated and may be combined into an overall index of inspiration, but they may also be used individually to measure inspired *by* versus *to* processes as needed (Thrash & Elliot, 2004). Instructions may be adapted for assessment of inspiration over specified time periods, such as the prior week (Thrash, Maruskin, et al., 2010) or half-day (Thrash, Elliot, et al., 2010), or to assess inspiration in specific domains, such as stages of the creative process (Thrash, Maruskin, et al., 2010).

The Inspiration Scale has strong psychometric properties, demonstrating the expected frequency-versus-intensity two-factor structure suggested by the inspired *by* versus *to* distinction. Inspiration is also factorially distinct from activated PA, the strongest known correlate of inspiration. The Frequency and Intensity subscales, as well as the overall Inspiration Index, are internally consistent, with Cronbach alphas above .90. Scores on the two subscales predict inspiration frequency and intensity, respectively, as assessed using daily diary methods. Two-month test–retest reliabilities are high, $r = .77$, for both subscales. Finally, the Inspiration Scale has invariant measurement properties (e.g., factor structure, loadings, and intercepts) across time (2 months) and across populations (university alumni, patent holders).

Trait inspiration, as assessed by the Inspiration Scale, converges meaningfully with a variety of individual difference variables. Regarding Big Five traits, Thrash and Elliot (2003) theorized that Openness to Experience should promote the process of being inspired *by*, whereas Extraversion, an indicator of approach temperament (Elliot & Thrash, 2002), should promote the process of being inspired *to*. As expected, Openness to Experience and Extraversion have consistently emerged as significant and robust predictors of trait inspiration (Thrash & Elliot, 2003; Thrash, Elliot, et al., 2010; Milyavskaya, Ianakieva, Foxen-Craft, Colantuoni, & Koestner, 2012). In contrast, Neuroticism, an indicator of avoidance temperament (Elliot & Thrash, 2002), has consistently failed to predict inspiration. Conscientiousness and Agreeableness have shown weak and sporadic relations to inspiration.

Those higher in trait inspiration are also higher in intrinsic motivation, BAS strength, absorption, work-mastery motivation, activated PA, optimism, perceived competence, self-esteem, and self-determination (Thrash & Elliot, 2003). Students higher in trait inspiration are more likely than those lower in trait inspiration to pursue majors in the humanities, and they pursue more majors simultaneously (Thrash & Elliot, 2003). These studies provide further support for the theoretical model of inspiration described earlier, with particular emphasis on the inspired *by* versus *to* processes.

Implications for Creativity, Productivity, and Well-Being

The transmission function of inspiration implies a variety of desirable consequences. Here we review evidence that inspiration leads to enhanced creativity, work efficiency and productivity, and well-being.

Findings from a number of studies support a relation between inspiration and creativity. Thrash and Elliot (2003) found that trait inspiration is positively related to a trait measure of creativity; moreover, inspira-

tion has a cross-lagged effect on subsequent self-reported creativity. Thrash and Elliot also found that frequency of felt inspiration among U.S. patent holders was related to the number of patents held, an objective indicator of creative output. In addition, patent holders were found to experience inspiration more frequently and intensely than individuals from a matched comparison sample.

In three studies by Thrash, Maruskin, and colleagues (2010), felt inspiration during the writing process was found to predict expert ratings of the creativity of the completed written products. These findings held regardless of the type of writing (scientific writing, poetry, mystery stories), research context (naturalistic, laboratory), and level of analysis (e.g., across persons, across written pages). Moreover, the findings were robust when a variety of covariates were controlled, including aptitude (e.g., Scholastic Aptitude Test [SAT] verbal scores), traits (e.g., openness), states (e.g., PA), behaviors (e.g., deletion), and other aspects of writing quality (e.g., technical merit).

We have noted that the creativity of a writer's initial idea is an antecedent of felt inspiration, and that the creativity of the completed product is a consequence, a pattern that is consistent with the posited transmission function. Thrash, Maruskin, and colleagues (2010) tested this transmission model directly in two studies. As expected, inspiration was found to mediate the relation between the creativity of the seminal idea and the creativity of the completed product. Other covariates of inspiration (effort, awe, activated PA) did not mediate transmission of creativity, suggesting that the transmission function is unique to inspiration.

Thrash, Maruskin, and colleagues (2010) also proposed that inspired action is likely to be efficient and productive because the inspiring object provides a concrete exemplar to serve as a guide. For instance, inspired writing is expected to proceed fluidly because it is guided by a compelling idea; uninspired writing proceeds without such guidance, resulting in a more labored process. Thrash, Maruskin, and colleagues used a screen capture technique to test this proposal—"efficiency" was defined as the proportion of typed words that were retained in the completed product, and "productivity" was defined as the number of words in the final product, after they adjusted for writing time. As predicted, inspiration while writing positively predicted both efficiency and productivity. It is noteworthy that this efficiency and productivity did not come at the cost of writing quality; indeed, inspiration predicted greater creativity in this same study.

Finally, Thrash, Elliot, and colleagues (2010) proposed that inspiration should promote psychological well-being. Two variables known to promote well-being were expected independently to mediate this effect: gratitude and purpose in life. Being inspired *by* was posited to promote a sense of gratitude toward the source of inspiration, and being inspired *to* was posited to instill a sense of direction and purpose. In one study, viewing a Michael Jordan highlight film was found to increase activated PA, and this effect was explained by inspiration. In two cross-lagged longitudinal studies, trait inspiration was found to lead to increases in a variety of positive well-being variables, such as activated PA, life satisfaction, vitality, and self-actualization. These findings held when a variety of covariates (e.g., the Big 5 traits, social desirability biases, and initial levels of well-being) were controlled. In a diary study, morning inspiration was found to predict evening levels of well-being variables. These effects were mediated partially by gratitude and partially by purpose. Milyavskaya and colleagues (2012) recently reported that trait inspiration predicts greater progress toward personal goals, and they proposed that goal progress may serve as an additional mediator of the relation between inspiration and well-being.

Conclusions and Future Directions

Psychological research on positive emotion was long delayed, compared with that on negative emotions such as fear, sadness, anger, and disgust, by difficulty identifying plausible adaptive functions that could provide a foundation for clear construct definition and hypothesis generation. While this has certainly changed in the new millennium, much research on positive emotion has solved the "function" problem by emphasizing its role in the immediate pursuit, acquisition, and consumption of material rewards.

Empirical research on positive emotion is still young enough that findings on this kind of positive emotion are sometimes generalized to all positive affect. One such finding was emphasized at the beginning of the chapter—the tendency for positive emotion to turn our focus inward toward the self, its assumptions and its needs. One of our key aims in this chapter was to describe three positive emotion/emotional constructs whose theoretical definitions predict sharp divergence from the characteristics of positive emotion in the context of short-term rewards. Awe, elevation, and inspiration all direct attention firmly outside the self, away from one's mundane expectations and immediate needs. These three constructs do not exhaust the list of self-transcending emotional states. Compassion, amusement, and admiration, among others, may also focus attention away from the self (Haidt & Morris, 2009). What is distinctive about awe, elevation, and inspiration is the element of "breaking set" in terms of beliefs about what is possible, focusing attention not only outside the self but also on that which is greater than the self and beyond its perceived boundaries.

Moving beyond reward acquisition and personal need fulfillment as the basis for positive emotion need not undercut the potential for talking about these states in terms of adaptive function. In fact, proposed functionality was a key basis for hypotheses in each of the lines of research described here. Once we acknowledge that adaptiveness reflects "total lifetime fitness consequences" (Cosmides & Tooby, 2000, p. 96), as well as immediate consequences for survival, we open to door to emotional mechanisms that treat knowledge about the world, the well-being of other people, and the transmission of key social values as important fitness-relevant resources. Indeed, the broaden-and-build model emphasizes this aspect of the function of positive emotion—impact on *enduring* personal resources, not just short-term rewards (e.g., Fredrickson, 2001).

One more substantial challenge to framing these states in evolutionary terms lies in the very feature that binds them together. The notion of "breaking set" implies that a mental set is present in the first place, and that it can be broken based on new experience. This requires a number of cognitive processes—schema formation, exemplar identification, abstract thinking, and so forth—that may be uniquely human. This feature presents something of a dilemma for theories of awe and elevation, which have been posited as emotional responses that (presumably) draw upon mechanisms with roots deep in our evolutionary past. To truly understand these states, it would help to know their origin, as well as their current form. To address this dilemma, theorists may need to consider these states as exaptations of more evolutionarily ancient processes. Such an approach could provide further guidance for hypotheses regarding overlap with other positive emotional states, some of which are already more widely studied.

As is clear from this overview, empirical research on self-transcending positive emotion is still very new, and has been limited to the efforts of a small number of laboratories. Potential future directions are many. Most research so far has been on social and cognitive implications of these states, but many gaps remain to be filled. Research on awe has emphasized a limited number of high-level cognitive processes (e.g., stereotyping, persuasion, and time perception), but these presumably entrain lower-level sensory and cognitive mechanisms that have not yet been explored. Research on elevation has emphasized effects on social intentions and behaviors, but further research on the psychological mechanisms mediating these effects is needed. Research on inspiration has emphasized the products of inspiration, consistent with the "transmission" model of this state's function. However, there is much to learn about the process by which one becomes "inspired *by*" in the first place, and whether inspirational things have common elements or are idiosyncratic. Across all three of these states, research has often addressed one of these constructs at a time, rather than comparing them with other positive emotion constructs, or examining how they relate to each other. Beyond social and cognitive outcomes, there is very little objective research on the physiological or expressive aspects of these states, or on their central neural substrates.

These gaps in the current research are pointed out as opportunities rather than limitations. The self-transcending positive emotions, and emotional states such as inspiration, offer tremendous potential to enrich our understanding of the human condition. Emotions are often thought of as the bestial, selfish, irrational side of human nature. What if emotions also support the best human nature has to offer? Much work has yet to be done before we can answer this question.

Acknowledgments

Contribution by Michelle N. Shiota and Alexander F. Danvers to the writing of this chapter was supported by a grant from the John Templeton Foundation. The opinions expressed in this chapter are those of the authors, and do not necessarily reflect the views of the John Templeton Foundation.

References

Abele, A. E., Silvia, P. J., & Zöller-Utz, I. (2005). Flexible effects of positive mood on self-focused attention. *Cognition and Emotion, 19*, 623–631.

Baumeister, R. F., & Leary, M. R. (1995). The need to belong: Desire for interpersonal attachments as a fundamental human motivation. *Psychological Bulletin, 117*, 497–529.

Bless, H., Bohner, G., Schwarz, N., & Strack, F. (1990). Mood and persuasion: A cognitive response analysis. *Personality and Social Psychology Bulletin, 16*, 331–345.

Bodenhausen, G. V., Kramer, G. P., & Süsser, K. (1994). Happiness and stereotypic thinking in social judgment. *Journal of Personality and Social Psychology, 66*, 621–632.

Bradley, M. M. (2009). Natural selective attention: Orienting and emotion. *Psychophysiology, 46*(1), 1–11.

Burgdorf, J., & Panksepp, J. (2006). The neurobiology of positive emotions. *Neuroscience and Biobehavioral Reviews, 30*, 173–187.

Campbell, D. T. (1983). The two distinct routes beyond kin selection to ultrasociality: Implications for the humanities and social sciences. In D. Bridgeman (Ed.), *The nature of prosocial development: Theories and strategies* (pp. 11–39). New York: Academic Press.

Campos, B., Shiota, M. N., Keltner, D., Gonzaga, G. C., & Goetz, J. (2013). What is shared, what is different?: Core relational themes and expressive displays of eight positive emotions. *Cognition and Emotion, 27*(1), 37–52.

Carver, C. S., & White, T. L. (1994). Behavioral inhibition, behavioral activation, and affective responses to impending reward and punishment: The BIS/BAS scales. *Journal of Personality and Social Psychology, 67,* 319–333.

Cosmides, L., & Tooby, J. (2000). Evolutionary psychology and the emotions. In M. Lewis & J. M. Haviland-Jones (Eds.), *Handbook of emotions* (2nd ed., pp. 91–115). New York: Guilford Press.

Costa, P. T., Jr., & McCrae, R. R. (1992). *The NEO PI-R professional manual.* Odessa, FL: Psychological Assessment Resources.

Cox, K. S. (2010). Elevation predicts domain-specific volunteerism 3 months later. *Journal of Positive Psychology, 5,* 333–341.

Danvers, A. F., & Shiota, M. N. (2013, January). *Positive emotions and recognition of details from a "going out to dinner" story.* Poster presented at the annual meeting of the Society for Personality and Social Psychology, New Orleans, LA.

Durkheim, E. (1887). Review of Guyau: L'irreÂligion de l'avenir. In *Revue Philosophique, 23,* 1887. Reprinted in A. Giddens (Ed.), *Emile Durkheim, selected writings (1972).* Cambridge, UK: Cambridge University Press.

Ekman, P., Friesen, W. V., O'Sullivan, M., Chan, A., Diacoyanni-Tarlatzis, I., Heider, K., et al. (1987). Universals and cultural differences in the judgments of facial expressions of emotion. *Journal of Personality and Social Psychology, 51,* 712–717.

Elliot, A. J., & Thrash, T. M. (2002). Approach–avoidance motivation in personality: Approach and avoidance temperaments and goals. *Journal of Personality and Social Psychology, 82,* 804–818.

Fiedler, K. (2001). Affective states trigger processes of assimilation and accommodation. In L. L. Martin & G. L. Clore (Eds.), *Theories of mood and cognition: A user's guidebook* (pp. 85–98). Mahwah, NJ: Erlbaum.

Forgas, J. P. (1998). On being happy and mistaken: Mood effects on the fundamental attribution error. *Journal of Personality and Social Psychology, 75,* 318–331.

Frank, R. (1988). *Passions within reason: The strategic role of the emotions.* New York: Norton.

Fredrickson, B. L. (2001). The role of positive emotions in positive psychology: The broaden-and-build theory of positive emotions. *American Psychologist, 56,* 218–226.

Griskevicius, V., Shiota, M. N., & Neufeld, S. L. (2010). Influence of different positive emotions on persuasion processing: A functional evolutionary approach. *Emotion, 10,* 190–206.

Haidt, J. (2000). The positive emotion of elevation. *Prevention and Treatment, 3,* 1–5.

Haidt, J. (2001). The emotional dog and its rational tail: A social intuitionist approach to moral judgment. *Psychological Review, 108,* 814–834.

Haidt, J. (2003). Elevation and the positive psychology of morality. In C. L. Keyes & J. Haidt (Eds.), *Flourishing: Positive psychology and the life well-lived* (pp. 275–289). Washington, DC: American Psychological Association.

Haidt, J., & Morris, J. P. (2009). Finding the self in self-transcendent emotions. *Proceedings of the National Academy of Sciences, 106,* 7687–7688.

Horberg, E. J., Oveis, C., & Keltner, D. (2011). Emotions as moral amplifiers: An appraisal tendency approach to the influences of distinct emotions upon moral judgment. *Emotion Review, 3,* 237–244.

Insel, T. R., & Hulihan, T. J. (1995). A gender-specific mechanism for pair bonding: Oxytocin and partner preference formation in monogamous voles. *Behavioral Neuroscience, 109,* 782–789.

Keltner, D., & Haidt, J. (2003). Approaching awe, a moral, spiritual, and aesthetic emotion. *Cognition and Emotion, 17,* 297–314.

Knutson, B., & Cooper, J. C. (2005). Functional magnetic resonance imaging of reward prediction. *Current Opinion in Neurology, 18,* 411–417.

Landis, S. K., Sherman, M. F., Piedmont, R. L., Kirkhart, M. W., Rapp, E. M., & Bike, D. H. (2009). The relation between elevation and self-reported prosocial behavior: Incremental validity over the five-factor model of personality. *Journal of Positive Psychology, 4,* 71–84.

Lazarus, R. S. (1991). Goal congruent (positive) and problematic emotions. In *Emotion and adaptation* (pp. 264–296). New York: Oxford University Press.

Maruskin, L. A., Thrash, T. M., & Elliot, A. J. (2012). The chills as a psychological construct: Content universe, factor structure, affective composition, elicitors, trait antecedents, and consequences. *Journal of Personality and Social Psychology, 103,* 135–157.

Milyavskaya, M., Ianakieva, I., Foxen-Craft, E.,

Colantuoni, A., Koestner, R. (2012). Inspired to get there: The effects of trait and goal inspiration on goal progress. *Personality and Individual Differences, 52,* 56–60.

Piaget, J. (1973). *The child and reality* (A. Rosin, Trans.). New York: Grossman.

Piedmont, R. L. (2004). *Assessment of spirituality and religious sentiments: Manual.* Baltimore: Author.

Rozin, P., Haidt, J., & McCauley, C. R. (2000). Disgust. In M. Lewis & J. M. Haviland-Jones (Ed.), *Handbook of emotions* (2nd ed., pp. 637–653). New York: Guilford Press.

Rudd, M., Vohs, K. D., & Aaker, J. (2012). Awe expands people's perception of time, alters decision making, and enhances well-being. *Psychological Science, 23*(10), 1130–1136.

Rushton, J. P., Chrisjohn, R. D., & Fekken, G. C. (1981). The altruistic personality and the Self-Report Altruism Scale. *Personality and Individual Differences, 2,* 293–302.

Russell, J. A. (2003). Core affect and the psychological construction of emotion. *Psychological Review, 110,* 145–172.

Salovey, P. (1992). Mood-induced self-focused attention. *Journal of Personality and Social Psychology, 62,* 699–707.

Salovey, P., & Rodin, J. (1985). Cognitions about the self: Connecting feeling states and social behavior. In P. Shaver (Ed.), *Self, situations and social behavior* (pp. 143–166). Beverly Hills, CA: Sage.

Saroglou, V., Buxant, C., & Tilquin, J. (2008). Positive emotions as leading to religion and spirituality. *Journal of Positive Psychology, 3,* 165–173.

Scherer, K. R. (2009). The dynamic architecture of emotion: Evidence for the component process model. *Cognition and Emotion, 23,* 1307–1351.

Schnall, S., Roper, J., & Fessler, D. M. T. (2010). Elevation leads to altruistic behavior. *Psychological Science, 21,* 315–320.

Schurtz, D. R., Blincoe, S., Smith, R. H., Powell, C. A. J., Combs, D. J. Y., & Kim, S. H. (2012). Exploring the social aspects of goose bumps and their role in awe and envy. *Motivation and Emotion, 36,* 205–217.

Shiota, M. N., Campos, B., Keltner, D., & Hertenstein, M. J. (2004). Positive emotion and the regulation of interpersonal relationships. In P. Philippot & R. S. Feldman (Eds.), *The regulation of emotion* (pp. 127–155). Mahwah, NJ: Erlbaum.

Shiota, M. N., Keltner, D., & John, O. P. (2006). Positive emotion dispositions differentially associated with Big Five personality and attachment style. *Journal of Positive Psychology, 1,* 61–71.

Shiota, M. N., Keltner, D., & Mossman, A. (2007). The nature of awe: Elicitors, appraisals, and effects on self-concept. *Cognition and Emotion, 21,* 944–963.

Shiota, M. N., Neufeld, S. L., Yeung, W. H., Moser, S. E., & Perea, E. F. (2011). Feeling good: Autonomic nervous system responding in five positive emotions. *Emotion, 11,* 1368–1378.

Silvers, J. A., & Haidt, J. (2008). Moral elevation can induce nursing. *Emotion, 8,* 291–295.

Silvia, P. J., & Abele, A. E. (2002). Can positive affect induce self-focused attention?: Methodological and measurement issues. *Cognition and Emotion, 16,* 845–853.

Simpson, J. A., & Weiner, S. C. (Eds.). (1989). *Oxford English dictionary* (2nd ed., Vol. 7). Oxford, UK: Clarendon Press.

Thrash, T. M. (2007). Differentiation of the distributions of inspiration and positive affect across days of the week: An application of logistic multilevel modeling. In A. D. Ong & M. Van Dulmen (Eds.), *Oxford handbook of methods in positive psychology* (pp. 515–529). New York: Oxford University Press.

Thrash, T. M., & Elliot, A. J. (2003). Inspiration as a psychological construct. *Journal of Personality and Social Psychology, 84,* 871–889.

Thrash, T. M., & Elliot, A. J. (2004). Inspiration: Core characteristics, component processes, antecedents, and function. *Journal of Personality and Social Psychology, 87,* 957–973.

Thrash, T. M., Elliot, A. J., Maruskin, L. A., & Cassidy, S. E. (2010). Inspiration and the promotion of well-being: Tests of causality and mediation. *Journal of Personality and Social Psychology, 98,* 488–506.

Thrash, T. M., Maruskin, L. A., Cassidy, S. E., Fryer, J. W., & Ryan, R. M. (2010). Mediating between the muse and the masses: Inspiration and the actualization of creative ideas. *Journal of Personality and Social Psychology, 98,* 469–487.

Van Cappellen, P., & Saroglou, V. (2012). Awe activates religious and spiritual feelings and behavioral intentions. *Psychology of Religion and Spirituality, 4*(3), 223–236.

Vianello, M., Galliani, E. M., & Haidt, J.

(2010). Elevation at work: The effects of leaders' moral excellence. *Journal of Positive Psychology, 5,* 390–411.

Watson, D., Wiese, D., Vaidya, J., & Tellegen, A. (1999). The two general activation systems of affect: Structural findings, evolutionary considerations, and psychobiological evidence. *Journal of Personality and Social Psychology, 76,* 820–838.

Weber, M. (2002). Economy and society: An outline of interpretive sociology. In N. W. Biggart (Ed.), *Readings in economic sociology* (pp.24–37). Malden, MA: Wiley-Blackwell. (Original work published 1978)

Wood, J. V., Saltzberg, J. A., & Goldsamt, L. A. (1990). Does affect induce self-focused attention? *Journal of Personality and Social Psychology, 58,* 899–908.

Yee, C. I., & Shiota, M. N. (2013, January). *Beyond expectations: Effects of awe on stereotype-based personality ratings.* Poster presented at the annual meeting of the Society for Personality and Social Psychology, New Orleans, LA.

CHAPTER 22

The Challenge of Challenge

Pursuing Determination as an Emotion

Leslie D. Kirby
Jannay Morrow
Jennifer Yih

What Is Challenge?

You have been spending a fair bit of time trying to solve a difficult problem that is part of an important project on which you have been working. So far you have been unable to solve the problem, but you believe that a solution is possible and you know that if you keep at it, you will be able to solve the problem and make the project a success.

Challenge arises when people are engaged in striving toward an as yet unobtained goal. It is an emotion with which every athlete, every employee, every student is familiar. The example we just cited (taken from Kirby, Tugade, Morrow, Ahrens, & Smith, Chapter 14, this volume, p. 251) describes the subjective feelings that accompany challenge, illustrates the kinds of circumstances that give rise to challenge, and shows how challenge promotes engagement and persistence in the face of potential obstacles. These properties suggest that challenge is a motivationally important emotion, yet it has received relatively little attention as such in the literature. In this chapter, we detail the antecedents of

challenge, apply the componential approach to support the view of challenge as an emotion, discuss the connections between state and trait challenge, and explore applications of challenge research. The body of evidence presents a strong case for classifying challenge as an emotion.

Psychologists have investigated challenge from several theoretical vantage points (e.g., emotion, trait, and motivation perspectives) and levels of analysis; however, relative to other emotions, challenge has heretofore been largely neglected. This trend may reflect a number of factors including the motivation literature's focus on "challenge" primarily in a stress context, as the situational hindrance to be overcome rather than as the resulting psychological state that motivates one's efforts to overcome those situated challenges. In emotions research, the preference historically has been to focus on a few core/basic emotions, of which few have been positive until recently. Challenge research suffered even more than research on other positive emotions because of the absence of evidence showing its association with a discrete facial expression. In addition, the valence of the most studied emotions has been either clearly positive (e.g., happiness) or clearly negative (sadness, fear, disgust, etc.). As we discuss, the valence of challenge is more complicated than that for many other emotions.

Gross and Barrett (2011) echo the frequently expressed sentiment that nearly everything in affective science is up for debate. They note two exceptions: widespread agreement that emotions are central to models of human behavior, and that emotions comprise subjective experience, physiological responses, and expressive behavior (which we interpret as including action tendencies, enacted behaviors, and nonverbal expressions of emotion; e.g., Frijda, 1986; Smith & Lazarus, 1990). This agreement has led many researchers to define emotions by their component parts. This "componential approach" provides a clear set of inquiry points for research, despite continued disagreements about formal definitions of emotion (Cornelius, 2000). The body of empirical evidence indicates that "challenge" readily satisfies all of these conditions.

In terms of eliciting conditions, challenge has a consistent appraisal pattern that is distinct from those eliciting other emotions (Smith & Kirby, 2009b), including positive ones (Ellsworth & Smith, 1988), specifically involving appraisals of low congruence (indicating a goal obstacle) combined with high coping potential (indicating the obstacle can be effectively overcome). Challenge entails distinct expressive displays including furrowed brows (Smith, 1989) and closed lips or frowning (Harmon-Jones, Schmeichel, Mennitt, & Harmon-Jones, 2011) associated with effort. Challenge also produces a distinct pattern of physiological arousal involving low total peripheral resistance combined with high cardiac output (Blascovich, 2008), also often reflected in systolic blood pressure (Wright & Kirby, 2001). People readily describe their subjective experiences of challenge (Frijda, Kuipers, & ter Schure, 1989; Smith & Ellsworth, 1985), which they characterize as feeling confident, determined, excited, and motivated (Abuhamdeh & Csikszentmihalyi, 2012; Carver & Scheier, 1994; Smith & Kirby, 2009b). Action tendencies associated with challenge involve an approach orientation, attentional focus, and willingness to expend effort (Fri-

jda et al., 1989). This fits with proposals that challenge functions to mobilize an individual to overcome situational demands and to sustain effort to improve his or her situation or skills (Lazarus & Folkman, 1984). In terms of applications, ample research on emotion, stress, and coping demonstrates that feeling challenged is associated with active coping, better physical health, and greater well-being (Carver & Scheier, 1994; Folkman & Moskowitz, 2007; Schwarzer & Knoll, 2003). Challenge also predicts higher levels of persistence, satisfaction, and performance in achievement settings (Gardner & Fletcher, 2009; Pekrun & Stephens, 2010), and appears to have a beneficial impact on interpersonal relationships (Feinberg & Aiello, 2010; Fitzell & Pakenham, 2010), and across the lifespan (Hunter, Boyle, & Warden, 2004; Ong, 2010).

A Note on Lexicon

In English, the word *challenge* is problematic for a number of reasons. First, as both a noun and a verb, it represents both the obstacle to be overcome and the act of overcoming itself. Colloquially, *challenged* has recently been used to describe someone who is handicapped or limited in some way (i.e., "mentally challenged," "developmentally challenged"). For emotion theorists, people's association with the word *challenge* appears to have shifted. Based on data collected in our laboratories, participants seem to perceive challenge as the obstacle itself, and to describe the feeling of challenge as more like the feelings of frustration that result from perceiving the obstacle, rather than describing the feelings theoretically meant to be encompassed by the term, which includes the effort and engagement associated with actively striving to overcome those obstacles. In this chapter we primarily use the word *challenge* to conform with the majority of existing literature. Because the term seems to be moving off the mark of what has been intended theoretically and to avoid confusion going forward, we suggest that *determination* would be a better descriptor of this emotional state, and the better choice in self-report measures. The Felt Emotional Experience List (FEEL) assesses this state with the adjective cluster "determined, persistent, motivated" (Kirby, Yih, Lagotte,

& Smith, 2013); the Positive and Negative Affect Schedule (PANAS) also assesses this state as "determined" (Tellegen, Watson, & Clark, 1988).

The Antecedent Appraisal Structure of Challenge

Appraisal theory hypothesizes that appraisals both "cause and constitute emotional experience" (Silvia, 2006, p. 55). That is, appraisals produce the emotional reaction by eliciting and organizing the components of the emotion around the adaptational implications of the appraisals; however, in addition, the appraisals themselves continue on and contribute to the subjective feeling state (Lazarus, 1999). Different emotions should not only be elicited by distinctive appraisal profiles, but they should also be associated with distinctive subjective feeling states and motivational properties that influence subsequent behavior in distinctive ways (e.g., Roseman & Smith, 2001).

Appraisal Components

Within the componential approach to emotion, various dimensions of appraisal combine to elicit each particular emotion. Key appraisal dimensions for challenge include motivational relevance, motivational congruence, problem-focused coping potential, and future expectancy (Smith, 1991; Smith & Kirby, 2009b; Smith & Lazarus, 1990). *Motivational relevance* is an evaluation of the degree to which a situation is applicable to an individual's concerns and goals. In many ways, the evaluation of importance is an intensity gauge, and maps roughly onto the "arousal" dimension commonly discussed in two-dimensional models of emotion (e.g., Russell, 1980). *Motivational congruence* is the degree to which the current situation is consistent with an individual's concerns and goals. In other models (Roseman, 2001), this dimension is deconstructed into two components, situational state (what you have or do not have) and motivational state (what you want or do not want)—if the two match, the situation is congruent; if not, it is incongruent. *Problem-focused coping potential* is an evaluation of one's ability to act on a situation to bring it into congruence with one's

goals. *Future expectancy* is an evaluation of potential changes that could (for any reason) make a situation more or less congruent. The outcome of the appraisal process elicits a specific, distinct emotional state.

Challenge is a positive emotion that fits a unique emotional profile, in that it shares appraisal properties with both positive and negative emotions. Challenge serves the unique adaptive function of motivating active coping in a person to reach or sustain a goal, and it is associated with the "core themes" of effortful optimism and the potential for success (Smith, 1991). These themes are exactly defined by the appraisal components for challenge. In other words, evaluations of motivational relevance, motivational incongruence, high problem-focused coping potential, and positive future expectations combine to form effortful optimism and the potential for success. The appraisal dimensions of challenge come together such that the experience of the emotion motivates active coping behavior that prepares an individual to persevere through adversity. Thus, challenge is a strong motivator of task engagement or persistence.

The Paradox of Challenge

This unique appraisal structure creates a "paradox of challenge," since challenge is a positive emotion that is elicited by appraisals of motivational *incongruence*, rather than the appraisals of motivational *congruence* that typically precede positive emotions. This paradoxical quality separates challenge from other positive emotions such as happiness, interest, or pride, as well as negative emotions such as anger, sadness, or fear. In general, negative emotions are about self-protection and harm avoidance—the possibility or actuality that one's situation contains things one does not want (Lazarus, 1991). In Roseman's (2001) terms, something that you do not want (motivational state) is (or might well be) present in the situation (situational state). In contrast, positive emotions, including challenge, are about opportunities (potential benefits) and realized benefits (Smith & Kirby, 2011). That is, they are about the presence, or potential presence (situational state), of wanted things (motivational state) in the situation. Thus, the motivational incongruence in challenge is different from that associated with most negative emotions. Rather than something unwanted being present in the situation, in challenge, something wanted is not yet present in the situation. In addition, the overall motivational congruence of the situation may be greater than that for most negative emotions because there is a belief that one will be able to attain what is desired, even though the desire is not yet realized. So rather than feeling frustrated, threatened, or overwhelmed by motivational incongruence, in challenge, the individual perceives opportunity—the goal is attainable, if enough work is put in.

Although the broaden-and-build theory of positive emotions (Fredrickson, 2001) would suggest that challenge should broaden thought–action repertoires in a similar manner as other positive emotions, recent data suggest that challenge appears to do just the opposite; in other words, like typical negative emotions, challenge may narrow rather than broaden attention (Matthews & Campbell, 2009; Smith & Kirby, 2009b). A closer look at the appraisal dimensions of challenge, combined with a motivational examination of the broaden-and-build model, may shed light on this anomaly. As described earlier, challenge is elicited by appraisals of motivational relevance and motivational incongruence, making it similar to negative emotions. However, evaluations of high problem-focused coping potential associated with challenge distinguish it from these other negative, stress-related emotions because these evaluations give challenge a positive flavor in that they indicate that, with effort, it is possible to attain one's goals. It may be that prototypical positive emotions can broaden one's attentional scope because one's circumstances and goals are in alignment—the individual has gotten what he or she wants, one way or the other,

and nothing needs to be done right now. As a result, one has the luxury of expanding one's mind in the classic broaden-and-build sense. But in challenge, the discrepancy between one's goals and one's circumstances demands attention. The high coping potential helps provide motivation to get one to do the work to bring things into alignment. Thus, the combination of incongruence plus high coping potential signifies an *opportunity* for a positive outcome, but the focus is still on that discrepancy and the need to deal with it to realize that opportunity. This is similar to the way in which prototypical negative emotions focus attention on the motivational discrepancies that are at the core of the potential threats and harms signaled by the negative feeling.

Research on the Appraisal Structure of Challenge

Empirical evidence supports the theorized appraisal dimensions of challenge. Ellsworth and Smith (1988) demonstrated that challenge can be distinguished from other positive emotions such as happiness, hope, and interest on the basis of appraisals of perceived goal obstacles and a desire to expend effort (presumably aimed at overcoming the goal obstacles). Moreover, aggregating across numerous previous studies, we examined data across over 1,500 undergraduate students at multiple universities (Kirby, 2006). Table 22.1 shows correlations between the predicted appraisal dimensions and the experience of challenge. As expected, motivational relevance and problem-focused coping potential were both positively correlated with challenge. However, the results for motivational congruence were not as predicted. We expected challenge to be negatively correlated with motivational congruence. It seems likely that because partici-

TABLE 22.1. Correlations between Appraisal Dimensions of Challenge and the Experience of Challenge

	Correlation	Beta-weight	p-value
Motivational relevance	.09	.08	= .001
Motivational congruence	.32	.24	< .001
Problem-focused coping potential	.30	.19	< .001

Note. Multiple $R = .37$; $N = 1,530$.

pants believe they can ultimately get what they want, they report the *overall situation* as being consistent with their goals. Compared to the item we used ("When you were in this situation, how consistent was what was happening with what you wanted to happen?"), perhaps separate assessments of motivational and situational state (cf. Roseman, 2001) would have yielded a clearer indication of the challenge-eliciting situation involving an as-yet-unfulfilled goal.

Historical Roots of Challenge

Darwin (1872) dealt with determination as an emotion, primarily focusing on cross-species evidence for a determined face. According to Darwin, determination was reflected by a "firmly closed mouth," which he tied very closely and explicitly to effort and a "frowning brow," which he tied to encountering obstacles. Although he discussed emotions generally, Darwin focused primarily on expressions rather than experience of emotions, including determination. Alexander Bain, considered by many to be one of the first psychologists and emotion theorists (e.g., Hergenhahn, 2009), wrote detailed accounts of emotions and distinguished them from other psychological constructs. Bain's writings (1859, 1876) on the emotion "pursuit" contain perhaps some of earliest explanations of challenge. Bain (1859) described the emotion of pursuit as positive feelings that come from working toward an end, and differentiated the pleasure experienced during pursuit from both the pleasure inherent in the end itself and the satisfaction derived from success. Some of the factors Bain saw as necessary for making pursuit pleasurable also appear in the appraisal model of challenge, and others of his observations represent intriguing hypotheses for future investigation. For example, the desired outcome must be important to the individual, implying appraisals of motivational relevance, in line with contemporary theory—it "should not be too trivial or insignificant, it must not be overpowering or excessive" (Bain, 1876, p. 221). However, he continues by noting that if the person has an "enormous stake" in the outcome, working toward the outcome can be filled "with unrelieved misery," which may place a boundary condition on

how motivationally relevant a situation can be and still be challenging rather than fear-evoking or resignation-inducing, in line with current theorizing about appraisals of coping potential. Bain specified that one must have the suitable skills for the situation, and that the demands and effort required must fit with the person's resources; however, going beyond this, he also explained that optimal levels of anticipation and uncertainty engender delight and excitement, whereas too much uncertainty brings about dread and despair (Bain, 1859, 1876).

The Componential Approach to Challenge

Challenge consists of the sensibility that although difficulties stand in the way of gain, they can be overcome with verve, persistence, and self-confidence.
                              —LAZARUS (1999, p. 33)

Recalling the Gross and Barrett (2011) criteria, we begin by analyzing challenge in terms of the componential approach to emotions, focusing on the emotion being generated by appraisals, and including subjective feeling state, physiological arousal, and the associated expressions (action tendencies, enacted behaviors, and nonverbal expressions; see Figure 22.1). Figure 22.2 shows these components mapped onto specific outcomes associated with challenge. The idea is that the appraisals of high relevance, low congruence, and high problem-focused coping potential combine to produce the emotion *challenge*, which has three component parts. The appraisals themselves become the subjective feeling state, in this case, a feeling of effortful optimism. The action tendency

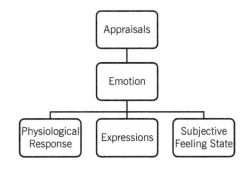

FIGURE 22.1. Components of an emotional response.

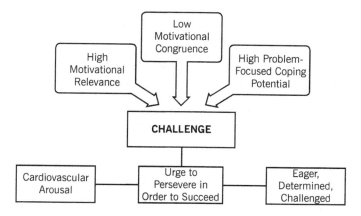

FIGURE 22.2. Componential approach to challenge.

is to put forth the effort needed to bring the situation in line with one's goals, which will lead to task engagement (and expressions of determination). The physiological arousal is geared toward making the effort possible.

Subjective Feeling State

A number of studies have described feelings of challenge in terms of other positive emotional and motivational states. *Challenge* has been described as a positive, energized state in which feelings of confidence, control, motivation, and eagerness prevail (Folkman & Lazarus, 1985; Folkman & Moskowitz, 2007; Matthews, Warm, Reinerman, Langheim, & Saxby, 2010; Skinner & Brewer, 2002). During intrinsic goal pursuit, challenge is perceived as pleasurable (fun, excitement, and interest), even after researchers control for skills level and performance outcomes (Abuhamdeh & Csikszentmihalyi, 2012), which complements the appraisal data discussed previously (Kirby, 2006). In a study of emotional experiences during college exams, challenge loaded with other positive emotions (e.g., happiness, hope, pride, interest) on a single factor, and when coping potential was high, feelings of pleasantness, engagement, and ability to control emotions were also high (Schmidt, Tinti, Levine, & Testa, 2010). When challenged, people find it easy to immerse themselves and stay engaged in what they are doing. Matthews and colleagues (2010) view challenge appraisals and emotions as closely related to task engagement, and engagement is accompanied by

energetic arousal, hedonic tone, motivation, curiosity, confidence, and control.

Challenge is not purely positive, though, since it is directed at goal pursuit rather than celebration of something already attained. For example, during challenge, people may experience dejection, anxiety, anger, or other negative feelings (Matthews et al., 2010; Skinner & Brewer, 2002). One of the strengths of challenge, however, may be its power to transform the meaning of negative experiences. This may be because challenge is infused with agency and optimism. That is, when feeling challenge, people feel confident in their coping ability, so positive outcomes seem likely, negative emotions are seen as facilitating goal attainment, and stressful situations are viewed less in threatening terms, or even as holding opportunities for growth and self-enhancement (Folkman & Moskowitz, 2007; Skinner & Brewer, 2002; Williams, Cumming, & Balanos, 2010). Furthermore, through down-regulation, challenge may dampen the duration and intensity of negative feelings (Tugade & Fredrickson, 2004).

A number of appraisal-based studies move beyond these general findings to differentiate challenge from other emotions. A series of studies by Blascovich and colleagues (e.g., Blascovich, 2008) examined threat and challenge using a biopsychosocial (BPS) model of motivation. Although there are some issues with the conceptualization and interpretation in the BPS model (see Wright & Kirby, 2003), challenged individuals consistently perceive the possibility of gains and losses in a potentially stressful situation, and tend to strive for those gains, whereas threatened individuals tend to perceive only the losses. In a study explicitly comparing hope and challenge (Kirby, Smith, & Garden, 2012), hope involved more nonhuman agency (implying a faith in divine intervention to remove goal obstacles), whereas challenge involved greater self-accountability (implying a need to rely on the self to remove the goal obstacle). The experience of challenge also involved elevated problem-focused coping potential and a need for action.

As a whole, these studies argue for a consistent subjective feeling state associated with challenge that involves a positive, energized feeling stemming from the believed ability to overcome actual and potential obstacles to achieve one's goals.

Physiological Arousal

Many researchers have tried (and largely failed) to find specific physiological patterns associated with discrete emotional states (e.g., Larsen, Bernston, Poehlmann, Ito, & Cacioppo, 2008); however, some theorists argue that, conceptually, it makes more sense for the physiological activation to support the action tendency of the emotion rather than the subjective feeling component (Smith & Scott, 1997). In other words, physiological activation is organized around what the individual is about to do rather than how the individual feels. This would explain why there is so much overlap in terms of physiological arousal across emotional states. So, for example, anger, fear, and excitement are all associated with increased heart rate, skin conductance and respiration. (e.g., Marwitz & Stemmler, 1998; Smith, 1989).

Effort is the action tendency believed to be associated with challenge. So the specific physiological arousal expected to be associated with challenge should reflect effort. Obrist (1981) described what he referred to as an active coping proposition, specifically that sympathetic nervous system (SNS) effects on the heart are proportional to task engagement (effort). Since systolic blood pressure (SBP) is the "purest" measure of sympathetic activation in the cardiovascular (CV) system, it is the most likely CV measure to reflect effort. And, in fact, across a variety of laboratory-based problem-solving tasks requiring engagement, SBP does indeed reflect effort (Gendolla & Krüsken, 2001; Wright & Kirby, 2001). Data on the aforementioned BPS model suggest consistent CV findings for people who perceive motivated performance tasks to be a challenge as opposed to a threat, with challenged individuals exhibiting a pattern of increased cardiac output coupled with low total peripheral resistance (Blascovich, 2008). This type of pattern means the heart is beating faster and/or stronger, pumping more blood, and the vasculature is relaxed. This means blood flows optimally throughout the body, efficiently enervating the muscles and effectively preparing the body for action.

Expressive Behaviors

Action Tendencies

In a study of 288 students on two campuses, participants recalled a past experience associated with a particular emotion (i.e., awe, challenge, contentment, gratitude, happiness, hope, interest, pride), and answered questions on felt action tendencies and expressive behaviors (Kirby, Tugade, et al., 2013). Relative to these other emotions, participants in the challenge condition reported a greater tendency toward motivational urges to stay focused, to persevere, to take on another challenge, and to worry; these participants reported the lowest motivational urge to savor the moment. Other studies indicate action tendencies of self-agency (Frijda et al., 1989), as well as effort–task focus and active coping (Matthews et al., 2010). All of these felt action tendencies are theoretically consistent with the appraisal structure and physiological arousal of challenge, with a focus on removing obstacles and achieving a goal, and further evidence for challenge as a distinct emotion.

Enacted Behaviors

In a series of studies examining relational models of appraisal (Smith & Kirby, 2009a), feelings of challenge were associated with greater success on a math problem-solving task, as well as greater persistence, measured by more time spent working on the problems (Smith & Kirby, 2009b). In another series of experiments comparing the effects of challenge and pride on task engagement, challenge was a better motivator of task engagement, as indexed by perseverance in a math problem-solving task (Yih, Christian, Kirby, & Smith, 2013). Interestingly, in the Kirby, Yih, and colleagues (2013) study described earlier, participants in the challenge condition experienced three significant discrepancies between their action tendencies and their enacted behaviors (differences between what they wanted to do, and what they actually did). Challenge participants reported a desire to celebrate, reward themselves, and relax but did not report actually doing those things. This corresponds with the appraisal data reported earlier, indicating a confidence about how the situation will resolve and a desire to be at that point or resolution, combined with a knowledge that the situation is not yet resolved and there is still work to be done to get to that point. Finally, a recent review of studies using different tasks designed to overload the attention system showed that people who appraised the attention-demanding tasks as challenging and controllable experienced greater task engagement (i.e., energetic arousal, task interest, success motivation and concentration), used more task-focused coping and less avoidant coping when dealing with the taxing demands of the tasks, and also performed better on the tasks (Matthews et al., 2010). This indicates that challenge promotes sustained effort and attention, which in turn influences performance. Again, all of these findings are theoretically consistent with the proposed model of challenge as an emotion.

Nonverbal Expressions

Contemporary appraisal theorists do not endorse the notion of fixed categorical displays for each emotion; rather they expect to see dynamic displays that reflect, moment-to-moment, what the person is doing, or trying to do (Scherer, 2001). Thus, we would expect expressive variations depending on where people are in their goal pursuit. If individuals are temporarily stumped, or at times when they are working very hard, then the brow likely furrows and the lips compress; if they become confused, then the brow may rise in uncertainty; and when they are approaching a solution, zygomatic hints of smiling may emerge.

Data on facial, vocal, and bodily expressions of challenge bear out this theoretical expectation of a dynamic expression. In studies explicitly examining the association of facial expressions and appraisals, corrugator supercilii activity (eyebrow frown) was more pronounced the more participants focused on anticipated effort and obstacle imagery relative to a goal (Smith, 1989; Smith & Scott, 1997). This eyebrow frowning was more directly related to focusing on obstacles to goals than to effort. In these studies, cheek elevation occurred while participants focused on the situation in general, suggesting the overall pleasantness of the challenge situation, which is consistent with the appraisal data presented in Table 22.1. Similarly, during task immersion and flow states, zygomatic activity is apparent during challenge experiences, but sometimes corrugator activity appears as well (de Manzano, Theorell, Harmat, & Ullén, 2010; Nacke, Stellmach, & Lindley, 2011). These patterns may reflect online changes in task demands, attention, or coping expectancies, as well as changes in the ratio of positive versus negative emotions.

During challenge, the eyes settle quickly and remain focused longer, and eye movements tend to be task relevant (Moore, Vine, Wilson, & Freeman, 2012). Challenge expressions also involve pressed lips (Harmon-Jones et al., 2011), which may reflect appraisals of confidence, positive expectations, and effort (Darwin, 1872; Kaiser & Wehrle, 2001). However, because of changing demands or obstacles, challenge may co-occur with uncertainty or novelty appraisals, which produce raised eyebrows and upper eyelids (Kaiser & Wehrle, 2001; Smith & Scott, 1997). During some challenge experiences, goal obstruction and situational demands may sometimes produce appraisals associated with anger (Kaiser & Wehrle, 2001), which fit with recent work on similarities between facial expressions of determination and anger (Harmon-Jones et al., 2011).

These studies suggest that the nonverbal expressions accompanying challenge are distinguishable from those of other emotions, and that a *challenge expression* reflects anticipated or actual effort to remove goal obstacles, and telegraphs engagement and confidence.

Connections between State and Trait Challenge

Like many psychological phenomena, challenge exists on a continuum ranging from momentary feelings (state challenge), to a more stable and consistent way of approaching a variety of experiences and situations (trait challenge). Generally speaking, *emotional traits* are enduring tendencies to experience particular emotional responses (e.g., Kuppens & Tong, 2010). Much of the research on trait challenge to date has focused on challenge appraisal styles and challenge as a facet of other traits (e.g., resilience, grit, optimism). Our main purpose in this section is to elucidate the properties of trait-level challenge, and to examine the likely consequences of being a person who experiences challenge across a fairly broad range of potentially relevant situations relatively easily, strongly, and frequently.

Emotional Thresholds

Emotional traits, including challenge, organize, guide and modulate an individual's response to emotionally relevant circumstances by affecting appraisals, attention, motivation, and construals of situations and people. One important aspect of this is that they establish the threshold for eliciting particular emotional states, moods, and expressive behaviors (e.g., Davidson, 2004; Rosenberg, 1998), and determine the tonic level of activation, magnitude of response, latency to peak response, and recovery time of particular emotions (e.g., Gross, Sutton, & Ketelaar, 1998).

Individuals who are relatively high in trait challenge have a lower threshold for challenge elicitation (Lazarus, 1991): They are more likely to experience challenge and challenge-congruent emotions than challenge-incongruent ones. Furthermore, if emotional traits and states share the same underlying features and consequences (Gross et al., 1998), individuals high in trait challenge would experience feelings of challenge—along with relevant appraisals, motivational tendencies, and behaviors—more often, for longer periods, more intensely, and in more kinds of situations than would individuals who are low in trait challenge.

Appraisal Styles

A challenge appraisal style involves the dispositional tendency to perceive a variety of well-being-relevant experiences as holding potential for mastery, gain, or growth (e.g., Folkman & Moskowitz, 2007). The goal of an appraisal style is to predict how a particular individual will appraise and therefore respond emotionally to a particular context (Smith & Kirby, 2013). In this case, challenge appraisal styles should specify particular circumstances under which individuals are likely to appraise high coping potential in an important and (currently) incongruent situation.

A number of consistent findings with regard to dispositional appraisals have emerged, which is striking given the considerable variation in how challenge appraisal styles have been measured. Challenge appraisal styles predict greater well-being and decreased symptoms of mental illness, including anxiety, depression, and somatization (Maltby & Day, 2003; Roesch & Rowley, 2005). In the face of demands and obstacles, people with challenge appraisal styles tend to use task-focused coping, preventive/proactive coping, and positive reinterpretation/benefit finding rather than avoidant coping (Gardner & Fletcher, 2009; Peacock & Wong, 1990). They also are able to focus their attention and thoughts on the task at hand: Challenge appraisal styles are positively correlated with task-directed behaviors and cognitions, including attentional deployment, task engagement, effort, and task-relevant cognitions (Hemenover & Dienstbier, 1996; Matthews & Campbell, 2009). Dispositional challenge appraisals tend to predict situation-specific challenge appraisals and emotions (Lengua, Long, & Meltzoff, 2006; Skinner & Brewer, 2002; Smith & Kirby, 2013), which lends further credence to our arguments that challenge can be positioned on a continuum that extends from feeling state to emotional trait.

Evidence suggests that challenge appraisal styles influence the thresholds concerning perceptions of stress, coping potential, and goal attainment. People with challenge appraisal styles perceive negative life events as less stressful (Roesch & Rowley, 2005) or even view them in positive light (Anshel, Robertson, & Caputi, 1997; Skinner &

Brewer, 2002). Challenge appraisal styles may promote feelings of control and influence perceptions of coping resources and skills (Peacock & Wong, 1990). Skinner and Brewer (2002) found that individuals with challenge appraisal styles tend to perceive state appraisals and emotions, regardless of valence, as being beneficial and motivating. Challenge appraisal style was the strongest predictor of confident coping expectancies in their studies; however, compared to trait appraisals, state challenge appraisals were the more proximate predictor of positive emotions and exam performance, which is theoretically consistent with appraisal style models (Smith & Kirby, 2013).

Challenge-Related Traits

Overall, research on appraisal styles provides support for the idea that challenge appraisal styles influence the threshold for triggering state-level challenge. Research on other challenge-related traits suggests that a number of other traits serve similar functions. Rather than providing an extensive discussion of this research, we highlight the central findings to shed light on the experience of challenge as an emotion.

Resilience

Trait resilience reflects the capacity to calibrate behavior in response to situational demands and opportunities (Letzring, Block, & Funder, 2005). Tugade (2011) argues that resilience derives from the capacity to capitalize on positive emotions, and defines *resilience* as flexibility coupled with "the ability to bounce back from negative emotional experiences" (Tugade, Fredrickson, & Barrett, 2004, p. 1168). Positive emotions and resilience build on each other to promote health (Tugade, 2011). The effectiveness of positive emotions in "undoing" the physiological and psychological effects of negative emotions and threat states (e.g., Fredrickson, 2001; Tugade et al., 2004) supports these points. The down-regulation of negative emotions via positive emotions may become more automatic with time or practice, thereby helping to build resilience. Challenge itself can be used to cope with negative feelings. People who are high in trait resilience tend to view impending

stressors as challenges; thus, they experience challenge-related emotions, which down-regulate negative emotion (Tugade & Fredrickson, 2004). The findings of Ong Bergeman, Bisconti, and Wallace (2006) suggest that resilient individuals rebound from daily stress experiences because of the positive emotions they experience. Moreover, people recognize the effectiveness of challenge in coping with negative emotions. Following an emotion induction, participants indicted that they would be most likely to use challenge (compared to interest, pride, or contentment/serenity) to reduce anxiety and anger, and to use happiness and contentment to cope with sadness (Kirby, Tugade, et al., 2013). Resilience research illuminates the relevance of challenge for coping with negative emotions and rebounding after negative events.

Grit

Grit has been defined as "perseverance and passion for long term goals" (Duckworth, Peterson, Matthews, & Kelly, 2007, p. 1087). Studies demonstrate that across a variety of performance situations, the grittier an individual is, the more successful he or she will likely be over time (Duckworth, Kirby, Tsukayama, Berstein, & Ericsson, 2010; Maddi, Matthews, Kelly, Villarreal, & White, 2012). It appears that state-level challenge might be the mechanism for grit. Duckworth and colleagues (2007, p. 1088) explain that "the gritty individual approaches achievement as a marathon; his or her advantage is stamina. Whereas disappointment or boredom signals to others that it is time to change trajectory and cut losses, the gritty individual stays the course." From this, one can infer that the gritty individual stays the course precisely *because* he or she is experiencing high levels of challenge, among perhaps other positive emotions.

A recent study examining the relationship among grit, trait challenge, the Big Five personality traits, and coping behaviors (Morrow & Tugade, 2011) found that challenge and grit were both negatively correlated with Neuroticism and positively correlated with Conscientiousness. Challenge, but not grit, was positively correlated with Extraversion and Openness to Experience. Moreover, challenge explained unique variance in threat appraisal after controlling for grit, with lower levels of challenge predicting threat appraisal styles. When participants reported how they would feel and cope after imagining themselves experiencing specific negative events, trait challenge was a more consistent predictor of experiencing positive emotions and a stronger predictor of finding benefits in potentially threatening situations. These patterns of associations suggest that challenge may foster cognitive and behavioral flexibility and openness that aid in problem solving and coping that may not be as closely related to grit. Trait challenge may give rise to appraisals, positive coping, and positive emotions that help promote long-term grittiness.

Optimism

Trait optimism represents a broad behavioral tendency to be confident and persistent in the face of adversity (Carver, Schier, & Segerstrom, 2010). Optimists tend to expect positive outcomes and subsequently experience more positive emotions compared to pessimists (Carver et al., 2010), which may help to explain the role of optimism in promoting well-being and physical health. Essentially, optimism lowers the threshold for appraisals of problem-focused coping potential and is in this way another pathway to state challenge.

Optimism and challenge share two important commonalities: (1) associations with active coping behavior and (2) positive expectancies for the future (Carver et al., 2010). Both optimism and challenge have been correlated with higher engagement in adaptive coping behaviors, such as approach rather than avoidance coping (Scheier, Carver, & Bridges, 2001; Smith, 1991). As we have discussed, the appraisal of high problem-focused coping potential is a key appraisal dimension of challenge, and importantly, trait optimism has been demonstrated to predict problem-focused coping with controllable stressors (Carver et al., 2010). Therefore, it may be the case that optimists are predisposed to experience challenge because optimists are confident and persistent in their attempts to change stressful situations. In other words, optimism seems to embody the characteristics that may be described as the antecedents of the appraisal dimensions of challenge.

Applications of Challenge Research

One of the strengths of challenge research is its applicability to a variety of benefits related to success and quality of life. Simply put, challenge leads to outcomes that people desire in both personal and professional domains. Although much of the applied research on challenge deals with trait-level challenge, we would argue that state-level experiences are driving many of these beneficial outcomes and, as always, understanding the link between state and trait challenge is crucial. We begin with the stress and coping literature, linking challenge to positive health outcomes, then discuss the role challenge plays in success in achievement situations, and finally examine the growth and social reward produced by challenge in interpersonal relationships.

Health and Well-Being

Numerous studies link feeling challenged to enhanced physical health, as well as mental well-being. Finding meaning or even benefits in highly stressful circumstances (loss of a loved one, dealing with chronic/terminal illnesses, etc.) is linked to better outcomes, including better physical health, illness resistance, and survival rates (Folkman & Moskowitz, 2007). In a study of teachers, Schwarzer and Knoll (2003) found that proactive coping (which combines a view of demanding situations as challenges to be met, taking action to meet ones goal, and having high coping potential) predicted lower burnout and a greater sense of accomplishment. Challenge experiences may lead to meaning in a number of ways, including promotion of problem-focused coping and positive reappraisal (e.g., Folkman & Moskowitz, 2007).

Ample evidence suggests that the challenge aspect of hardiness (Ong, 2010) explains unique variance in indices of well-being, adjustment, and health (e.g., occupational stress, family conflict, posttraumatic stress disorder, emotional exhaustion, depression, mental health, physical health indices, and personal accomplishment; for a recent meta-analysis see Eschleman, Bowling, & Alarcon, 2010). For example, a study of Type A personality, hardiness, and physiological reactivity found that hardiness moderated the effects Type A personality on blood pressure reactivity during a difficult task, and the effects of hardiness on reactivity were largely a result of the effects of challenge (Contrada, 1989).

These findings also hold up across the lifespan. In a study of fifth graders, challenge appraisals predicted better psychological adjustment, as measured by lower levels of internalizing problems, and these appraisals moderated the effects of negative events on internalizing problems (Lengua & Long, 2002). Building on the undoing effects of positive emotions and challenge appraisals, Ong's (2010) model of successful aging focuses on how positive emotion mediates the stress-buffering effects of trait hardiness/resilience on emotional well-being and physical health.

Achievement

Challenge has implications in a wide variety of achievement situations because of its impact on coping, health, and productivity. Challenge allows for engagement at work, which is an antidote for burnout-related physical and mental exhaustion (Folkman & Moskowitz, 2007). Challenge is also related to daily creativity and proactive behavior at work, which may be attributed to the connections among challenge, creativity, and flow (Ohly & Fritz, 2009). O'Connor, Arnold, and Maurizio (2010) demonstrated that those who appraised an upcoming negotiation as a challenge had more accurate perceptions of priorities, used more aggressive tactics, and therefore reached higher quality deals compared to those who appraised the same negotiation as a threat. Challenge-related appraisals are associated with higher levels of job-related well-being and satisfaction (Cavanaugh, Boswell, Roehling, & Boudreau, 2000; Gardner & Fletcher, 2009), which may result from the stress-buffering effects of challenge appraisals. In this sense, potential stressors (e.g., role ambiguity, conflict, and workload) can be perceived as both challenges and hindrances (Webster, Beehr, & Love, 2011). To the extent that these potential stressors are judged to be related to favorable outcomes, they are appraised as challenges, which is a central idea borrowed from the transactional theory of stress (Lazarus & Folk-

man, 1984). In fact, when task demands are manipulated or objectively measured, challenge appraisals predict perceptions of decreased workload, demand, or difficulty (Feinberg & Aiello, 2010; Matthews et al., 2010). In applied settings, challenge appraisals predict positive emotions and proactive coping when workplaces hassles, negative events, and workload are high. Optimism is quite likely related to how these attributes are appraised, with optimism serving as a dispositional antecedent to challenge, leading to increased feelings of mastery and agency. Future research would benefit by incorporating constructs such as resilience, grit, and optimism into applied settings to observe their relations to challenge.

The findings from occupational settings fit well with the research on academic achievement, which we have touched on throughout our discussion. This research has focused on challenge in applied settings (e.g., Skinner & Brewer, 2002) as well as on achievement-relevant tasks and situations (Blascovich, 2008; Hemenover & Dienstbier, 1996; Smith & Kirby, 2009b). Across studies and achievement domains, more proximate challenge indices (states/emotions) tend to be the strongest predictors of coping, performance, and satisfaction (Matthews et al., 2010; Pekrun & Stephens, 2010; Webster et al., 2011). At the same time, these studies also indicate that mastery goals, achievement-relevant traits, and appraisal styles provide additional information that adds to our understanding of the role of challenge in achievement settings, furthering the idea that continued exploration of the relationship between state and trait challenge is crucial to understanding motivated performance in such settings.

Sports psychology researchers have begun to hone in on the study of challenge due to the link between challenge and outcomes in sporting situations. Jones, Meijen, McCarthy, and Sheffield (2009) proposed a model theorizing that achievement goals, perceptions of control, and self-efficacy are the key factors that contribute to appraisals of either challenge or threat during athletic competition, which is similar to research on relational models of appraisal predicting circumstances under which people will be likely to appraise an event in a particular way (Smith & Kirby, 2009a, 2009b). In a study of novice golfers, those experiencing challenge putted better than those experiencing threat; in addition, the body movements and swing of the challenged novices were more like those of expert golfers (Moore et al., 2012). Imagery studies inducing appraisals in competitive athletes have shown that both challenge and threat cause increases in anxiety, but this increased anxiety is perceived as facilitative during challenge and debilitative during threat, since threat may produce worry and other cognitions that interfere with concentration (Cumming, Olphin, & Law, 2007; Williams et al., 2010).

Whether perceptions of anxiety as beneficial consistently translate into better athletic performance may depend on other factors, including skill and attention (Moore et al., 2012). Yet perceptions of challenge and its effects on performance do seem to correspond. In one induction study, when asked to choose whether challenge, neutral, or threat appraisal states would be most beneficial to their performance, 70% of the sample identified challenge as the most helpful, 30% selected neutrality, and no one chose threat (Williams et al., 2010). The selection of neutrality by 30% of participants may suggest the role of individual differences, not only in perceptions of challenge, but in perceptions of emotions experienced during challenge states, including anxiety. Finally, in a study of dancers (Quested et al., 2011) threat, but not challenge appraisals, predicted anxiety and mediated the effects of need satisfaction (autonomy, competence, and relatedness) on cognitive anxiety. However, challenge, but not threat, mediated the relationship between need satisfaction and cortisol levels following a performance. The link to cortisol suggests the importance of examining the long-term effects of challenge on performance, health, and well-being.

Interpersonal Relationships

A number of studies has also explored applications of challenge in the interpersonal domain. For example, research on caregivers suggests that challenge may be a unique predictor of psychological adjustment. Fitzell and Pakenham (2010) found that compared to stress appraisals, challenge appraisals were the strongest predictor of adjustment outcomes. Challenge also explained unique variance in life satisfaction. Mackay and Pak-enham (2011) found that the positive effects of challenge appraisals were not explained by optimism, and that challenge, not optimism, predicted benefit finding when caring for a loved one dealing with mental illness.

Challenge appraisals may also be useful in dealing with interpersonal conflict or discord. For instance, 9- to 14-year-old bullying victims who experienced the bullying as a challenge were more likely to seek social support and report the bullying; threat appraisals were not a significant predictor of coping with bullying (Hunter et al., 2004). A number of studies show the relationship between challenge appraisals and secure attachment styles, and suggest the importance of challenge appraisals in coping effectively with interpersonal transgressions, loss, and conflict (e.g., Shaver & Mikulincer, 2008).

Feinberg and Aiello (2010) demonstrated that challenge promotes social facilitation, which implies that challenge promotes mastery goals and decreases evaluation apprehension. This may be due to the confidence associated with challenge. The social facilitation findings have interesting implications for studies of possible effects of challenge on teamwork. Some of the BPS findings add to the interpersonal effects, demonstrating that a challenge response is facilitated by social support, even if the social support comes from a pet (Blascovich, 2008). It would be interesting to examine directionality with these findings to see whether, for example, induced challenge appraisals lead to reduced stereotype threat or stigma response.

The beneficial effects of challenge in the interpersonal domain may arise from improved emotion regulation, problem solving, and sustained effort. Or these benefits may arise because challenge mitigates the debilitating effects of threat and rejection. Research in this area also importantly focuses on social achievements rather than the traditional performance-based outcomes associated with mastery.

In general, investigations of applications of challenge would benefit from considering the role of coping potential and discrete positive emotions rather than focusing so extensively on threat "versus" challenge, as if they are independent, polar opposites, and the full spectrum of possibilities for motivated performance. The emotional experience of challenge may be more powerful/effective under certain circumstances, so collapsing across motivational states in this manner is not only overly simplistic but it may also result in a loss of information (e.g., Carver & Scheier, 1994; Smith & Kirby, 2011), particularly in light of data suggesting that challenge and threat can coexist (Lengua & Long, 2002; Skinner & Brewer, 2002).

Lessons learned from research on stress and coping and trait-level challenge suggest the importance of the experience of emotion for longer-term outcomes. State-level challenge may well explain the effects of personality traits in outcomes research, either through mediation or moderation, depending on the trait, and help us better understand the threshold argument.

Conclusions

Challenge/determination is a legitimate, unique, and positive emotion. It differs from most other positive emotions in that it is associated with current goal incongruence. Challenge serves a vital and basic motivational function (task engagement and perseverance leading to success and personal growth) that does not seem to be covered by any other emotions. Although current research is somewhat scarce, as reviewed in the chapter, all indications are that when considered at the state level, indeed, challenge fits a unique emotional profile, and that it motivates task engagement and mastery as proposed. Importantly, this is reinforced by the study of challenge at the trait or dispositional level, where as an appraisal style, as well as other related dispositional constructs, challenge clearly plays a positive role in longer-term adaptation to stress—showing clear and consistent associations with outcomes such as health, success, job satisfaction, and social rewards. Given this, it is vital to place challenge, both as a state and as a trait, under our research lens more often, so that we might better understand it, its properties, and its consequences.

Acknowledgments

We would like to thank Craig A. Smith, Debra Zeifman, Randy R. Cornelius, and Elisabeth Sandberg for their extremely helpful (and speedy) feedback on this chapter.

References

Abuhamdeh, S., & Csikszentmihalyi, M. (2012). The importance of challenge for the enjoyment of intrinsically motivated, goal-directed activities. *Personality and Social Psychology Bulletin, 38,* 317–330.

Anshel, M. H., Robertson, M., & Caputi, P. (1997). Sources of acute stress and their appraisals and reappraisals among Australian police as a function of previous experience. *Journal of Occupational and Organizational Psychology, 70,* 337–357.

Bain, A. (1859). *The emotions and the will.* London: John W. Parker & Son/West Strand.

Bain, A. (1876). *The emotions and the will* (3rd ed.). New York: Appleton.

Blascovich, J. (2008). Challenge, threat, and health. In J. Y. Shah & W. L. Gardner (Eds.), *Handbook of motivation science* (pp. 481–493). New York: Guilford Press.

Carver, C. S., & Scheier, M. F. (1994). Situational coping and coping dispositions in a stressful transaction. *Journal of Personality and Social Psychology, 66,* 184–184.

Carver, C. S., Scheier, M. F., & Segerstrom, S. C. (2010). Optimism. *Clinical Psychology Review, 30,* 879–889.

Cavanaugh, M. A., Boswell, W. R., Roehling, M. V., & Boudreau, J. W. (2000). An empirical examination of self-reported work stress among US managers. *Journal of Applied Psychology, 85,* 65–74.

Contrada, R. J. (1989). Type A behavior, personality hardiness, and cardiovascular responses to stress. *Journal of Personality and Social Psychology, 57*(5), 895–903.

Cornelius, R. R. (2000). Theoretical approaches to emotion. In R. Cowie, E. Douglas-Cowie, & M. Schöder (Eds.), *Speech and emotion: A conceptual framework for research* (pp. 3–10). Belfast: Textflow.

Cumming, J., Olphin, T., & Law, M. (2007). Self-reported psychological states and physiological responses to different types of motivational general imagery. *Journal of Sport and Exercise Psychology, 29,* 629–644.

Darwin, C. (1872). *The expression of emotions in man and animals.* New York: Philosophical Library.

Davidson, R. J. (2004). Affective style: Causes

and consequences. In R. Davidson (Ed.), *Essays in social neuroscience* (pp. 77–91). Cambridge, MA: MIT Press.

de Manzano, Ö., Theorell, T., Harmat, L., & Ullén, F. (2010). The psychophysiology of flow during piano playing. *Emotion, 10*, 301–311.

Duckworth, A. L., Peterson, C., Matthews, M. D., & Kelly, D. R. (2007). Grit: Perseverance and passion for long-term goals. *Journal of Personality and Social Psychology, 92*, 1087–1101.

Duckworth, A. L., Kirby, T., Tsukayama, E., Berstein, H., & Ericsson, K. (2010). Deliberate practice spells success: Why grittier competitors triumph at the National Spelling Bee. *Social Psychological and Personality Science, 2*, 174–181.

Ellsworth, P. C., & Smith, C. A. (1988). Shades of joy: Patterns of appraisal differentiating pleasant emotions. *Cognition and Emotion, 2*, 301–331.

Eschleman, K. J., Bowling, N. A., & Alarcon, G. M. (2010). A meta-analytic examination of hardiness. *International Journal of Stress Management, 17*, 277–307.

Feinberg, J. M., & Aiello, J. R. (2010). The effect of challenge and threat appraisals under evaluative presence. *Journal of Applied Social Psychology, 40*, 2071–2104.

Fitzell, A., & Pakenham, K. I. (2010). Application of a stress and coping model to positive and negative adjustment outcomes in colorectal cancer caregiving. *Psycho-Oncology, 19*, 1171–1178.

Folkman, S., & Lazarus, R. S. (1985). If it changes it must be a process: Study of emotion and coping during three stages of a college examination. *Journal of Personality and Social Psychology, 48*, 150–170.

Folkman, S., & Moskowitz, J. T. (2007). Positive affect and meaning-focused coping during significant psychological stress. In M. Hewstone, H. Schut, J. de Wit, K. Van Den, & M. Stroebe (Eds.), *The scope of social psychology: Theory and applications* (pp. 193–208). East Sussex, UK: Psychology Press.

Fredrickson, B. L. (2001). The role of positive emotions in positive psychology: The broaden-and-build theory of positive emotions. *American Psychologist, 56*, 218–226.

Frijda, N. H. (1986). *The emotions.* New York: Cambridge University Press.

Frijda, N. H., Kuipers, P., & ter Schure, E. (1989). Relations among emotion, appraisal, and emotional action readiness. *Journal of Personality and Social Psychology, 57*, 212–228.

Gardner, D., & Fletcher, R. (2009). Demands, appraisal, coping and outcomes: Positive and negative aspects of occupational stress in veterinarians. *International Journal of Organizational Analysis, 17*, 268–284.

Gendolla, G. H., & Krüsken, J. (2001). The joint impact of mood state and task difficulty on cardiovascular and electrodermal reactivity in active coping. *Psychophysiology, 38*, 548–556.

Gross, J. J., & Barrett, L. F. (2011). Emotion generation and emotion regulation: One or two depends on your point of view. *Emotion Review, 3*, 8–16.

Gross, J. J., Sutton, S. K., & Ketelaar, T. V. (1998). Relations between affect and personality: Support for the affect-level and affective-reactivity views. *Personality and Social Psychology Bulletin, 24*, 279–288.

Harmon-Jones, C., Schmeichel, B. J., Mennitt, E., & Harmon-Jones, E. (2011). The expression of determination: Similarities between anger and approach-related positive affect. *Journal of Personality and Social Psychology, 100*, 172–181.

Hemenover, S. H., & Dienstbier, R. A. (1996). The effects of an appraisal manipulation: Affect, intrusive cognitions, and performance for two cognitive tasks. *Motivation and Emotion, 20*, 319–340.

Hergenhahn, B. R. (2009). *An introduction to the history of psychology.* Belmont, CA: Wadsworth, Cengage Learning.

Hunter, S. C., Boyle, J. M., & Warden, D. (2004). Help seeking amongst child and adolescent victims of peer-aggression and bullying: The influence of school-stage, gender, victimisation, appraisal, and emotion. *British Journal of Educational Psychology, 74*, 375–390.

Jones, M., Meijen, C., McCarthy, P. J., & Sheffield, D. (2009). A theory of challenge and threat states in athletes. *International Review of Sport and Exercise Psychology, 2*, 161–180.

Kaiser, S., & Wehrle, T. (2001). Facial expressions as indicators of appraisal processes. In K. R. Scherer, A. Schorr, & T. Johnstone (Eds.), *Appraisal processes in emotion: Theory, methods, research* (pp. 285–300). New York: Oxford University Press.

Kirby, L. D. (2006, November). *The challenge of challenge: The emotional basis of task engagement.* Presented at the 28th Annual Meeting of the Society for Southeastern Social Psychologists, Knoxville, TN.

Kirby, L. D., Smith, C. A., & Garden, R. (2012, January). *Not all positive emotions look the same: Differentiating hope and challenge.* Presented at the 13th Annual Meeting of the Society of Personality and Social Psychology, San Diego, CA.

Kirby, L. D., Tugade, M., Morrow, J. & Smith, C.A. (2013). *The motivational functions of positive emotions: Action tendencies and enacted behaviors.* Manuscript submitted for publication.

Kirby, L. D., Yih, J., Lagotte, A., & Smith, C. A. (2013). *The felt emotional experience list (FEEL): A development and validation study.* Manuscript submitted for publication.

Kuppens, P., & Tong, E. M. (2010). An appraisal account of individual differences in emotional experience. *Social and Personality Psychology Compass, 4,* 1138–1150.

Larsen, J. T., Berntson, G. G., Poehlmann, K. M., Ito, T. A., & Cacioppo, J. T. (2008). The psychophysiology of emotion. In M. D. Lewis, J. M. Haviland-Jones, & L. F. Barrett (Eds.), *Handbook of emotions* (pp. 180–195). New York: Guilford Press.

Lazarus, R. S. (1991). Cognition and motivation in emotion. *American Psychologist, 46,* 352–367.

Lazarus, R. S. (1999). *Stress and emotion: A new synthesis.* New York: Springer.

Lazarus, R. S., & Folkman, S. (1984). *Stress, appraisal, and coping.* New York: Springer.

Lengua, L. J., & Long, A. C. (2002). The role of emotionality and self-regulation in the appraisal–coping process: Tests of direct and moderating effects. *Journal of Applied Developmental Psychology, 23,* 471–493.

Lengua, L. J., Long, A. C., & Meltzoff, A. N. (2006). Pre-attack stress-load, appraisals, and coping in children's responses to the 9/11 terrorist attacks. *Journal of Child Psychology and Psychiatry, 47,* 1219–1227.

Letzring, T. D., Block, J., & Funder, D. C. (2005). Ego-control and ego-resiliency: Generalization of self-report scales based on personality descriptions from acquaintances, clinicians, and the self. *Journal of Research in Personality, 39,* 395–422.

Mackay, C., & Pakenham, K. I. (2011). Identification of stress and coping risk and protective factors associated with changes in adjustment to caring for an adult with mental illness. *Journal of Clinical Psychology, 67,* 1064–1079.

Maddi, S., Matthews, M., Kelly, R., Villarreal, B. & White, M. (2012). The role of hardiness and grit in predicting performance and retention of USMA cadets. *Military Psychology, 24,* 19–28.

Maltby, J., & Day, L. (2003). Religious orientation, religious coping and appraisals of stress: Assessing primary appraisal factors in the relationship between religiosity and psychological well-being. *Personality and Individual Differences, 34,* 1209–1224.

Marwitz, M., & Stemmler, G. (1998). On the status of individual response specificity. *Psychophysiology, 35,* 1–15.

Matthews, G., & Campbell, S. E. (2009). Sustained performance under overload: Personality and individual differences in stress and coping. *Theoretical Issues in Ergonomics Science, 10,* 417–442.

Matthews, G., Warm, J. S., Reinerman, L. E., Langheim, L. K., & Saxby, D. J. (2010). Task engagement, attention, and executive control. In A. Gruzka, G. Matthews, & B. Szymura (Eds.), *Handbook of individual differences in cognition* (pp. 205–230). New York: Springer.

Moore, L. J., Vine, S. J., Wilson, M. R., & Freeman, P. (2012). The effect of challenge and threat states on performance: An examination of potential mechanisms. *Psychophysiology, 49,* 1417–1425.

Morrow, J. & Tugade, M. M. (2011, January). *Explorations of dispositional challenge: Distinctions between challenge and interest.* Paper presented at the 12th Annual Meeting of the Society for Personality and Social Psychology, San Antonio, TX.

Nacke, L. E., Stellmach, S., & Lindley, C. A. (2011). Electroencephalographic assessment of player experience: A pilot study in affective ludology. *Simulation and Gaming, 42,* 632–655.

Obrist, P. A. (1981). *Cardiovascular psychophysiology: A perspective.* New York: Plenum Press.

O'Connor, K. M., Arnold, J. A., & Maurizio, A. M. (2010). The prospect of negotiating: Stress, cognitive appraisal, and performance. *Journal of Experimental Social Psychology, 46,* 729–735.

Ohly, S., & Fritz, C. (2009). Work characteristics, challenge appraisal, creativity, and proactive behavior: A multi-level study. *Journal of Organizational Behavior, 31,* 543–565.

Ong, A. D. (2010). Pathways linking positive emotion and health in later life. *Current Directions in Psychological Science, 19(6),* 358–362.

Ong, A. D., Bergeman, C. S., Bisconti, T. L., & Wallace, K. A. (2006). Psychological resilience, positive emotions, and successful adaptation to stress in later life. *Journal of Personality and Social Psychology, 91,* 730–749.

Peacock, E. J., & Wong, P. T. P. (1990). The Stress Appraisal Measure (SAM): A multidimensional approach to cognitive appraisal. *Stress Medicine, 6,* 227–236.

Pekrun, R., & Stephens, E. J. (2010). Achievement emotions: A control-value approach. *Social and Personality Psychology Compass, 4,* 238–255.

Quested, E., Bosch, J., Burns, V. E., Cumming, J., Ntoumanis, N., & Duda, J. L. (2011). Basic psychological need satisfaction, stress-related appraisals, and dancers' cortisol and anxiety responses. *Journal of Sport and Exercise Psychology, 2011,* 828–846.

Roesch, S. C., & Rowley, A. A. (2005). Evaluating and developing a multidimensional, dispositional measure of appraisal. *Journal of Personality Assessment, 85,* 188–196.

Roseman, I. J. (2001). A model of appraisal in the emotion system: Integrating theory, research, and applications. In K. R. Scherer, A. Schorr, & T. Johnstone (Eds.), *Appraisal processes in emotion: Theory, methods, research* (pp. 68–91). New York: Oxford University Press.

Roseman, I. J., & Smith, C. A. (2001). Appraisal theory: Overview, assumptions, varieties, controversies. In K. R. Scherer, A. Schorr, & T. Johnstone (Eds.), *Appraisal processes in emotion: Theory, methods, research* (pp. 68–91). New York: Oxford University Press.

Rosenberg, E. L. (1998). Levels of analysis and the organization of affect. *Review of General Psychology, 2,* 247–270.

Russell, J. A. (1980). A circumplex model of affect. *Journal of Personality and Social Psychology, 39,* 1161–1178.

Scheier, M. F., Carver, C. S., & Bridges, M. W. (2001). Optimism, pessimism, and psychological well-being. In E. C. Chang (Ed.), *Optimism and pessimism: Implications for theory, research, and practice* (pp. 189–216). Washinton, DC: American Psychological Association.

Scherer, K. R. (2001). Appraisal considered as a process of multilevel sequential checking. In K. R. Scherer, A. Schorr, & T. Johnstone (Eds.), *Appraisal processes in emotion: Theory, methods, research* (pp. 92–120). New York: Oxford University Press.

Schmidt, S., Tinti, C., Levine, L. J. & Testa, S. (2010). Appraisals, emotions and emotion reg-

ulation: An integrative approach. *Motivation and Emotion, 34,* 63–72.

Schwarzer, R., & Knoll, N. (2003). Positive coping: Mastering demands and searching for meaning. In S. J. Lopez & C. R. Snyder (Eds.), *Handbook of positive psychological assessment* (pp. 393–409). Washington, DC: American Psychological Association.

Shaver, P. R., & Mikulincer, M. (2008). Adult attachment and cognitive and affective reactions to positive and negative events. *Social and Personality Psychology Compass, 2,* 1844–1865.

Silvia, P. J. (2006). *Exploring the psychology of interest.* New York: Oxford University Press.

Skinner, N., & Brewer, N. (2002). The dynamics of threat and challenge appraisals prior to stressful achievement events. *Journal of Personality and Social Psychology, 83,* 678–692.

Smith, C. A. (1989). Dimensions of appraisal and physiological response in emotion. *Journal of Personality and Social Psychology, 56,* 339–353.

Smith, C. A. (1991). The self, appraisal, and coping. In C. R. Snyder & D. R. Forsyth (Eds.), *Handbook of social and clinical psychology: The health perspective* (pp. 116–137). Needham Heights, MA: Allyn & Bacon.

Smith, C. A., & Ellsworth, P. C. (1985). Attitudes and social cognition. *Journal of Personality and Social Psychology, 48,* 813–838.

Smith, C. A., & Kirby, L. D. (2009a). Putting appraisal in context: Toward a relational model of appraisal and emotion. *Cognition and Emotion, 23,* 1352–1372.

Smith, C. A., & Kirby, L. D. (2009b). Relational antecedents of appraised problem-focused coping potential and its associated emotions. *Cognition and Emotion, 23,* 481–503.

Smith, C. A., & Kirby, L. D. (2011). The role of appraisal and emotion in coping and adaptation. In R. J. Contrada & A. Baum (Eds.), *Handbook of stress science: Biology, psychology, and health* (pp. 195–208). New York: Springer.

Smith, C. A. & Kirby, L.D. (2013). *From state to trait and back: Introducing a multidimensional measure of appraisal style.* Manuscript submitted for publication.

Smith, C. A., & Lazarus, R. S. (1990). Emotion and adaptation. In L. A. Pervin (Ed.), *Handbook of personality: Theory and research* (pp. 609–637). New York: Guilford Press.

Smith, C. A., & Scott, H. S. (1997). A componential approach to the meaning of facial expressions. In J. A. Russell & J. M. Fernández-Dols (Eds.), *The psychology of facial expression* (pp. 229–254). New York: Cambridge University Press.

Tellegen, A., Watson, D., & Clark, L. A. (1988). Development and validation of brief measures of positive and negative affect: The PANAS scales. *Journal of Personality and Social Psychology, 54*, 1063–1070.

Tugade, M. M. (2011). Positive emotion and coping: Examining dual-process models of resilience. In S. Folkman (Ed.), *The Oxford handbook of stress, health, and coping* (pp. 186–199). New York: Oxford University Press.

Tugade, M. M., & Fredrickson, B. L. (2004). Resilient individuals use positive emotions to bounce back from negative emotional experiences. *Journal of Personality and Social Psychology, 86*, 320–333.

Tugade, M. M., Fredrickson, B. L., & Barrett, L. F. (2004). Psychological resilience and positive emotional granularity: Examining the benefits of positive emotions on coping and health [Special issue]. *Journal of Personality, 72*, 1161–1190.

Webster, J. R., Beehr, T. A., & Love, K. (2011). Extending the challenge-hindrance model of occupational stress: The role of appraisal. *Journal of Vocational Behavior, 79*, 505–516.

Williams, S. E., Cumming, J., & Balanos, G. M. (2010). The use of imagery to manipulate challenge and threat appraisal states in athletes. *Journal of Sport and Exercise Psychology, 32*, 339–358.

Wright, R. A., & Kirby, L. D. (2001). Effort determination of cardiovascular response: An integrative analysis with applications in social psychology. In M. Zanna (Ed.), *Advances in experimental social psychology* (Vol. 33, pp. 255–307). San Diego, CA: Academic Press.

Wright, R. A., & Kirby, L. D. (2003). Cardiovascular correlates of challenge and threat appraisals: A critical examination of the biopsychosocial analysis. *Personality and Social Psychological Review, 7*, 216–233.

Yih, J., Christian, F. L., Kirby, L. D., & Smith, C. A. (2013). *The effects of challenge and pride on perseverance*. Paper presented at the 14th Annual Meeting of the Society for Personality and Social Psychology, New Orleans, LA.

CHAPTER 23

Hope Theory

Jennifer S. Cheavens
Lorie A. Ritschel

Hope, a construct that is both easily recognizable and difficult to define, may therefore be associated with more questions than answers. Scholars have debated whether hope is a process or an outcome; they have discussed whether hope is an emotion or cognition. Additionally, questions have been raised about whether hope enhances the life of the individual by opening the mind to new possibilities or whether it is a fool's errand that puts the individual at risk of ignoring realistic information in the environment. In Greek mythology, hope was all that remained in Pandora's jar after she unknowingly let loose all the evils of mankind into the world; the myth does not clarify whether hope was one of evils intended to plague the world by creating a false sense of security and optimism or whether it was construed as a mitigating force against the evils of the world.

Although long part of philosophical and religious discussions, the construct of hope was not featured strongly in the scientific literature until the latter part of the 20th century. In 1959, Karl Menninger's presidential address to the American Psychiatric Association was titled "Hope." In this lecture, Menninger argued that engendering and building hope is essential in eliciting recovery from mental illness and called for increased scientific study of this construct, beginning with attempts at an operational definition. This lecture ignited a series of investigations that legitimized the study of hope as both a process and an outcome. Frank (1968, p. 285) noted that it had become possible to study hope "without damage to one's scientific or moral integrity." The primary aim of these investigations was to understand hope as a scientific variable such that it could eventually be manipulated and augmented to enhance lives (Orne, 1968).

Defining Hope: Emotion or Cognition?

Using a behavioral framework, Mowrer (1960) defined *hope* as an affective form of secondary reinforcement. According to this model, hope is an emotion that reinforces anticipatory behavior and is therefore associated with the expectation of pleasurable stimuli. Conversely, fear, the emotional antithesis of hope, is associated with dread of aversive stimuli. Accordingly, hope is an emotion that drives movement toward one's goals, whereas fear is an emotion that disrupts goal pursuits. In keeping with this model, Kirkland and Cunningham (2012) suggest that hope and fear are the emotions most strongly associated with predicting future outcome: Specifically, hope predicts that one's situation will improve, whereas fear predicts that the future will be worse than the present in some important way. Hope and fear are therefore hypothesized to result from the *prediction* of future outcomes, in contrast to other emotions that are hypothesized to result from observed outcomes (e.g., joy associated with desired outcomes, sadness associated with unwanted outcomes). Kirkland and Cunningham define *hope* as the emotion associated with the prediction that things may soon improve in comparison to one's current state.

In contrast to these models that highlight hope as an emotion, hope also has been conceptualized in terms of goal-relevant cognitions. In one of the earliest examples of this viewpoint, Erikson defined hope as "the enduring belief in the attainability of fervent wishes, in spite of dark urges and rages" (1964, p. 118). Stotland (1969) proposed that hope is the expectation that a goal has some possibility (i.e., a probability greater than zero) of being attained. Stotland further conceptualized hope as a mediating variable that explains the relationship between precipitating events and the associated emotional outcomes. According to this model, *hope* is defined as a cognitive interpretation of events that leads to a positive emotion (as opposed to a positive emotional state that leads to behaviors). In what might be considered an effort to synthesize these views, Staats and Stassen (1985) labeled hope as the "affective cognition," thus highlighting both the emotional and cognitive aspects of hope.

Snyder's Model of Hope

In the past two decades, Snyder's (1994) model of hope has emerged as the predominant framework for the vast majority of empirical work focused on hope. In this model, *hope* is defined as "a positive motivational state that is based on an interactively derived sense of successful (a) agency (goal-directed energy) and (b) pathways (planning to meet goals)" (Snyder, Irving, & Ander-

son, 1991, p. 287). Thus, hope comprises three parts: goals, pathways thinking, and agency thinking. We discuss each of these components and the empirical evidence to support their relevance to the overall hope construct in the following sections.

Goals

Goals, or the mental endpoints of purposeful activity, are the cornerstone of hope theory and have been explicitly highlighted in both Snyder's original conceptualization (1994) and the expanded model of hope (Snyder, 2002). An underlying assumption of hope theory is that all human behaviors are goal oriented (Snyder, 1994). That is, all effortful behavior is organized in order to attain, feel, experience, or excel at something; alternatively, behavior may be organized to avoid, decrease, or terminate something. In this sense, the hoped for "something" is the goal in hope theory. In the context of hope theory, goals are posited to vary in terms of importance to the individual, as well as the life domain within which the goal resides (Sympson, 1999). Six domains have been delineated in hope theory (see Lopez, Ciarlelli, Coffman, Stone, & Wyatt, 2000): social relationships (e.g., friendships, casual relationships), academics, romantic relationships, family life, work, and leisure activities (e.g., sports, music, arts, reading). Thus, goals that are set in domains that are important to the individual are more likely to be salient, to occupy conscious awareness, and to guide behavior. For example, someone might have the goals of getting into graduate school, developing romantic relationships, and training for a marathon. If the leisure and romantic domains are more important for this particular person than the academic domain, it is likely that this individual's day-to-day behavior would be spent perusing dating sites and running, as opposed to completing Graduate Record Exam (GRE) practice tests. As this tenet of the theory suggests, goals are likely to differ across people, time, and circumstances.

It is important to note that within Snyder's model, hopeful goals are not limited to improving unfavorable contingencies in some way. Some authors have argued that the label of "hope" only applies when a person is in a bad circumstance and expects that things will be better in the future (e.g., Kirkland & Cunningham, 2012; Lazarus, 1999); however, Snyder, Cheavens, and Michael (2005) suggested that hope incorporates both "repair" goals (i.e., improving on that which is unsatisfactory) and "enhancement" goals (i.e., maintaining or improving on that which is already satisfactory). In other words, one might hope to improve a difficult working environment to fit skills and needs better, and one might also hope that loving and satisfying relationships are maintained. Thus, there is nothing inherent in Snyder's (1994, 2002) definition of hope that requires an unwanted present circumstance for the development of a hopeful goal.

Goals vary in three important ways. First, they may have different temporal frames, spanning minutes (e.g., eating lunch) to years (e.g., obtaining a medical degree). The time frame for hopeful thought, however, is future-oriented. To some degree, the time frame associated with a goal may be related to the difficulty or breadth of a goal, with more difficult and broad goals requiring more time to complete. For example, one might have the goals to lose weight and to mow the lawn. Obviously, it will take more time to lose a significant amount of weight than to mow the lawn.

Second, goals may differ in the degree to which they are specified. For example, although someone may have "being happy" or "being true to myself" as stated goals, these would be considered vague goals, as no endpoint has been articulated and there is no specific way to measure progress toward (or final achievement of) these goals. Importantly, goals that are relatively unspecified are generally less likely to compel a person toward future behavior because planning for unspecified or loosely defined goals is difficult. Moreover, difficulty in knowing when vague goals have been achieved both attenuates the ability to experience the emotional satisfaction associated with goal attainment and precludes the disengagement from the goal pursuit that typically occurs once a goal has been achieved or once it is clear that adequate progress is not currently available. That is, goal seekers who are unsure of their specified targets have no metric by which to judge a particular goal as accomplished and may therefore continue working

toward an endpoint with no identifiable finish line. According to hope theory, people with higher hope are more likely to have well-specified goals (Snyder, 2002). Some important goals, such as being a good parent, partner, or employee, are unlikely to have obvious endpoints. In this way, focusing on subgoals and paying particular attention to the ways in which the form of the goal changes (e.g., what constitutes "good parenting" may differ for parents of toddlers vs. teenagers) increases the likelihood of engaging hopeful thought.

Third, goals can vary in level of probability of attainment. Presumably, goals with an intermediate probability of achievement—that is, goals that are slightly out of reach and therefore require effort but are attainable nonetheless—are most strongly associated with hope and positive emotions (Averill, Catlin, & Chon, 1990). Conversely, goals with guaranteed success may require less hopeful thought as they are considered pro forma and unlikely to spark the planning and excitement associated with hopeful thought. Similarly, goals with low probabilities of success may sap hopeful thought either through failure experiences (i.e., goal nonattainment, which tends to increase negative affect and reduce agentic thought) or difficulty in engaging hopeful thought due to the numerous and often substantial barriers associated with low probability goals. Importantly, individuals with high hope are more likely to choose to work on difficult goals, attribute difficulties in goal achievement to poorly chosen strategies rather than personal weaknesses, and redouble their efforts in the form of generating more pathways when given negative feedback about their goals (Snyder, Harris, et al., 1991). That is, they are more likely than individuals with low hope to respond to difficult goals and setbacks with a sense of energy and determination.

Pathways Thinking

"Pathways thinking" has been defined as the ability to develop routes that link the present circumstance to an imagined future (Rand & Cheavens, 2009). In other words, pathways thinking allows one to determine how to get from where one is to where one would like to be. Hopeful thought requires the generation of at least one primary pathway to a desired outcome, as well as the perception that the pathway is viable. Because most goals come with unexpected difficulties or blockages of some sort, hope is theorized to be associated with the ability to generate multiple routes and to respond flexibly to goal barriers. That is, when one pathway is blocked, individuals with high hope have the ability to perceive the goal blockage accurately, disengage from that pathway, and choose another route to goal attainment. Available evidence suggests that people with high hope are indeed able to generate multiple, workable pathways to goals (Irving, Snyder, & Crowson, 1998; Snyder, Harris, et al., 1991).

Agency Thinking

Agency, or the motivational component in hope theory, propels an individual along the pathways that have been generated toward desired goals. Specifically, agency involves self-referential thoughts about one's ability to successfully use the pathways generated and, on a more global level, to reach desired outcomes in one's life. Snyder, Lapointe, Crowson, and Early (1998) found that when given the choice, individuals with higher hope prefer self-statements reflecting strong agency thinking (e.g., "I can do this").

Snyder's conceptualization of agency overlaps to some degree with Bandura's (1997) construct of self-efficacy. Snyder suggests that agency is the belief or perception that one *will* successfully reach a goal through use of generated pathways, while Bandura highlights the situation-specific belief that one *can* engage in the necessary behavior to reach a goal. Thus, there are two primary differences in these conceptualizations. The first is the focus on intentions (i.e., hope) as opposed to abilities (i.e., self-efficacy). The second distinction is that hope is hypothesized to be a trait that represents one's goal-related proclivities; in contrast, Bandura suggests that self-efficacy is relevant for specific judgments about one's capabilities. Agency and self-efficacy are both conceptually and empirically related; however, there is evidence that they are separate constructs (Magaletta & Oliver, 1999). Although agency and pathways are discussed as separate constructs, they are theorized to transact iteratively over time with increases in one leading to increases in the other component.

Full Hope Model

In 2002, Snyder introduced the "elaborated" hope model, which incorporates two new elements: (1) the contextual contributions of past learning history and future consequences of goal-related behaviors; and (2) the role of emotions, expectations, and stressors in a hope-relevant event. Moving temporally across the model, the earliest factor thought to impact hope is one's goal-relevant learning history. Snyder (1994, 2002) hypothesized that we develop trait-like pathways and agency thoughts early in our developmental histories through lessons of causality (i.e., this leads to that) and through the recognition of the self as a causal agent (i.e., "I made that happen"). These pathways- and agency-generating lessons are presumed to transact iteratively over time to result in dispositional hope. For example, one might set a goal of becoming a better athlete, then develop the plan to try out for the soccer team as a primary pathway. Success in utilizing this pathway is hypothesized to increase agentic thinking, including thoughts such as "I meet the goals I set for myself," which in turn would promote later pathways thinking. The Trait Hope Scale (Snyder, Harris, et al., 1991) measures these long-standing hopeful thoughts and taps into one's general tendency to believe that one can generate and successfully use routes to important goals. The State Hope Scale (Snyder et al., 1996) was developed later to measure hopeful thought in shorter time spans and to allow for assessment of change in hope.

In this expanded model, Snyder (2002) also noted that enduring hopeful thinking is associated with trait-like affective tones, such that individuals with higher hope are likely to experience higher levels of positive affect and lower levels of negative affect, while those with lower levels of hope are less likely to experience positive affect and more likely to experience negative affect on a regular and sustained basis. As a corollary, Snyder posited that goal-directed thoughts and activities produce predictably valenced emotions; specifically, positive emotions follow perceived success or progress toward goals, and negative emotions follow perceived goal stagnation or failure. Accordingly, a history of successful or unsuccessful goal pursuits is thought to produce either a more positive or negative dispositional emotional set, respectively. Thus, a person with a history of successful goal pursuits is likely to approach goal-relevant situations with curiosity, interest, and enthusiasm, whereas a person with a history of unsuccessful goal pursuits is likely to experience reluctance, hopelessness, and apathy when faced with goal pursuits.

Taken together, individual goal pursuits happen within the context of this larger learning history. In an individual goal pursuit, an initial evaluation of the outcome of a particular goal is made. According to Snyder (2002), goals based on one's own values and standards will be assessed as more worthwhile and the associated hopeful thought will be greater for those goals. Additionally, if the goal is in a domain associated with past success experiences and positive emotions, that goal will be more closely aligned with hopeful thought. If the goal is determined to be valuable and important enough to warrant further attention and continued effort, goal pursuit is initiated. Within each individual goal pursuit, pathways and agency thoughts transact with one another, as well as with the interpretations about the progress (or lack thereof) of the goal pursuit and the emotions that arise from these evaluations of progress. This continued evaluation of goals is important, as the value of an anticipated outcome can change over time (particularly with long-term goals); additionally, it may be difficult to assess accurately the value of a given outcome before fully appreciating the effort associated with the goal pursuit. For example, imagine a woman who sets the goal of becoming a physician and starts medical school in pursuit of this goal. Over the course of medical school, she deems the costs associated with continued goal pursuit as too much given perceived progress (e.g., she is confronted with objective success or failure), changes in personal circumstances (e.g., she gives birth to twins), or interests (e.g., she determines that a law degree would better suit her goals). Without evaluation, she might complete medical school but no longer value this goal, thus, robbing herself of the positive affect associated with successful goal completion. In this elaborated model, Snyder proposed a feedback loop between goal-specific and trait-level hopeful thought, such that appraised success or failure of each particular goal sequence and

the associated emotions influence generalized hope; that is, trait hope could increase or decrease over time based on repeated successes or failures.

The last pieces of the elaborated hope model include stressors and surprise events (Snyder, 2002; Snyder et al., 2005). Within hope theory, a *stressor* is defined as any event or impediment that jeopardizes the likelihood of a successful goal pursuit. There is some evidence that individuals with higher hope may experience stressors as challenges, as opposed to threats (e.g., Snyder, Harris, et al., 1991). When stressors are encountered in the pursuit of an important, valued goal, those with high hope should be able to generate new pathways, use available pathways differently, or recast the stressors in a way that reduces negative emotion associated with the stressor. Similarly, surprise events are unplanned and personally relevant but, unlike stressors, occur outside the context of the particular goal pursuit (see Rand & Cheavens, 2009). Examples of surprise events include unexpectedly receiving a gift, being in a car accident, or regaining contact with someone from one's past. Surprise events may be positive or negative in the absolute sense and are likely to influence the ongoing goal pursuit by impacting both agency and pathways thinking, as well as outcome evaluations and emotions, in the moment.

Hope as a Unique Positive Psychology Construct

In describing positive psychology, Seligman (2002) described various levels of analysis that are relevant to the field, including subjective experiences, individual traits, and group-level virtues. For the most part, hope has been conceptualized at the levels of subjective experience and individual traits. Snyder's (1994, 2002) model specifically discusses hope as an individual trait and/or state that is positively associated with reinforcing subjective experiences such as well-being, happiness, joy, and meaning. Although there has been discussion of hope as a group-level virtue (see McCullough & Snyder, 2000), Shorey, Snyder, Rand, Hockemeyer, and Feldman (2002) argued that hope is value-neutral at the societal level but incorporates values at the individual level. The authors argued that when a specific goal is valued by society, higher hope would lead to an increased likelihood of successful goal attainment and the associated positive affect, self-esteem, and other markers of psychological health. Using this framework, conceptualizing hope at the societal or group level limits the utility of hope in understanding how people pursue daily goals. In other words, to understand why and how a person pursues goals, it is more useful to look to the values of the individual as opposed to the values of society or some other larger group.

Thus, hope conceptualized at the level of the individual involves positive interpretations of past goal pursuits and positive expectancies for the future. *Optimism*, as defined by Scheier and Carver (1985), is similar to hope both in terms of operational definitions and patterns of association with other psychological constructs (Aspinwall & Leaf, 2002). The primary theoretical difference between hope and optimism is the importance placed on personal agency; hope theory specifically highlights the role of the individual in enacting pathways that lead to positive outcomes in the future, whereas optimism includes positive outcomes that are dependent on external circumstances (e.g., the behavior of others, luck). In addition to these theoretical distinctions, several empirical investigations have demonstrated that hope and optimism are related yet distinct constructs (e.g., Bryant & Cvengros, 2004; Gallagher & Lopez, 2009; Magaletta & Oliver, 1999; Rand, 2009).

This evidence that hope and optimism are independent, albeit associated, constructs is complemented by findings that hope and optimism are differentially associated with and predictive of markers of success and psychological health. For example, Gallagher and Lopez (2009) used structural equation modeling to assess whether hope and optimism were distinct latent constructs and, if so, whether they were differentially related to well-being. They found that hope and optimism are distinct, obliquely related constructs ($r = .66$). Furthermore, they found that both constructs are related to well-being, but that the patterns of the relations differ, with hope being more strongly related to measures of well-being that stress autonomy and personal growth.

Similarly, Rand (2009) found that the relationship between hope and optimism is best explained in a model that accounts for both shared (a higher-order "goal attitude" factor) and unique variance for each construct.

Thus, hope is a member of the positive psychology nomological network in that it is related to, yet distinct from, other positive, future-oriented constructs. Hope confers a multitude of benefits across the lifespan, both in the short and the long term. There are some advantages that are inherent to having higher hope, such as well-defined goals, greater confidence in one's ability to map and use various routes to important goals, and more positive self-talk. In addition, individuals with high hope report several emotional and physical advantages compared to their low-hope counterparts in multiple life domains (for reviews, see Rand & Cheavens, 2009; Snyder, 2002). Based on the theoretical model, we would expect hope to be related to broad markers of psychological health and flourishing (e.g., positive affectivity, self-esteem, meaning) and negatively related to markers of psychological disorder and distress (e.g., depressive and anxiety symptoms, hopelessness). Research has generally supported these theoretical propositions. For example, higher hope is associated with greater well-being in both adults (e.g., Gallagher & Lopez, 2009) and school-age children (e.g., Snyder, Hoza, et al., 1997) and negatively associated with symptoms of psychopathology in both adults (e.g., Chang, 2003; Cramer & Dyrkacz, 1998; Geiger & Kwon, 2010) and school-age children (Snyder, Hoza, et al., 1997). In a longitudinal investigation, Arnau, Rosen, Finch, Rhudy, and Fortunato (2007) found that higher scores on the Agency subscale of the Hope Scale predicted lower levels of psychological difficulties 1 month later. Moreover, they found that symptom severity scores at time 1 did not impact hope scores at later time points, suggesting that hope is not lessened over time by symptoms of psychopathology (at least in the short run).

More recently, researchers have turned to more fine-tuned analyses of the relations between hope and specific indices of well-being, as well as the particular role that hopeful thought may play in the "good life." Additionally, recent research has examined the role that hope might play in buffering individuals from the difficult life events that befall us all. Here, we briefly review the evidence to date about the relations of hope and well-being, as well as hope in the context of difficult life events.

Hope and Well-Being: Affect, Life Satisfaction, and Meaning

"Subjective well-being" has been defined as "a broad concept that includes experiencing pleasant emotions, low levels of negative moods, and high life satisfaction" (Diener, Lucas, & Oishi, 2002, pg. 63). Magaletta and Oliver (1999) found that hope is related to the overall construct of well-being, as well as the three component parts of well-being articulated by Diener and colleagues (2002). Gallagher and Lopez (2009) found that hope is related to subjective (or hedonic), psychological (or eudaimonic) and social well-being. Relative to optimism, hope has a weaker association with subjective well-being (negative affect, life satisfaction) and a stronger association with psychological well-being (autonomy, growth, purpose in life). These data linking hope to specific aspects of well-being provide important directions for future research and add substantial clarification to our understanding of hope, as they highlight the relationship between hopeful thought and expectancies related to personal agency and mastery (as opposed to solely global positive expectancies). Several studies have also examined the relations between hope and the component parts of well-being, including affect, life satisfaction, and meaning.

Some of the first studies on the relation between hope and well-being demonstrated that higher hope is associated with reports of higher positive and lower negative affect (e.g., Snyder, Harris, et al., 1991). Within Snyder and colleagues' (1991) theoretical framework, hope and positive affect are hypothesized to be related in two ways: (1) Positive affect results from goal (and subgoal) successes and (2) over time, repeated successful goal pursuits tend to result in a consistent, positive mood disposition. More recently, researchers have begun to investigate the temporal relationship between hope and mood. Steffen and Smith (2013) examined the interplay of hope and affect with a sample of 84 firefighters using an elec-

tronic daily diary paradigm. After accounting for the impact of age, gender, education, income, and months in the fire service, they found that hope was significantly related to same-day reports of positive affect and significantly predicted next-day positive, but not negative, affect. The interaction between hope and stress was not significant, suggesting that the relation between hope and positive affect did not vary in relation to stress. Hope scores did interact with stress to predict both same-day and next-day negative affect, with individuals with higher hope having less same-day and next-day negative affect under periods of stress. The results from this study suggest that hopeful thought predicts positive affect (i.e., temporally preceded positive affect) and interacts with stress to predict less negative affect.

Positive affect is usually defined as a state, whereas life satisfaction is typically thought of as an overarching positive evaluation of one's life, either *in toto* or in specific domains (e.g., social relationships, work). Hope has received considerable attention in the research literature as a strong predictor of life satisfaction (Bailey, Eng, Frisch, & Snyder, 2007). In older adults, high hope is related to greater overall life satisfaction and perceived physical health (Wrobleski & Snyder, 2005). In youth samples, hope is positively correlated with global ratings of life satisfaction (Valle, Huebner, & Suldo, 2004); moreover, Valle and colleagues (2006) found that adolescents' levels of hope predicted global life satisfaction over a 1-year period, even after controlling for initial life satisfaction. In an effort to understand how hope is related to life satisfaction, above and beyond the associations between hope and other markers of psychological functioning, Halama (2010) examined the associations of both hope and the Big Five personality traits with life satisfaction. Results suggested that hope, Neuroticism, Extraversion, Agreeableness, and Conscientiousness were all significantly associated with life satisfaction. Furthermore, hope accounted for variance in life satisfaction after accounting separately for Neuroticism, Conscientiousness, and Extraversion. The direct effect between Extraversion and life satisfaction was no longer significant with hope in the model. Taken together, these results suggest that (1) hope is an important predictor of life satisfaction, both cross-sectionally and longitudinally, and (2) the relationship between hope and life satisfaction is robust, as indicated by the fact that significant findings remain even after controlling for powerful other variables.

If we were to think about positive markers of experience on a continuum from narrow and specific to broad and global constructs, positive affect would be at the specific end and meaning would be at the broad end of the scale. That is, meaning is the overarching sense that there is coherence in experiences, and that day-to-day life is related to something bigger than oneself. In a factor analysis that included the Hope Scale and three measures assessing perceived life coherence and meaning, Feldman and Snyder (2005) found that both hope and meaning in life loaded onto a single factor, suggesting that hope can be thought of as a major component of "life meaning." Moreover, all three Life Meaning scales used in this study were positively correlated with the Hope Scale. When assessing the relations among meaning in life and symptoms of anxiety and depression, controlling for hope attenuated the relations between these measures, indicating that hope and perceived success in goal pursuits might be important to having a meaningful life that is associated with lower levels of psychopathology. Similarly, Michael and Snyder (2005) found that hope is related to perceptions of meaning and psychological well-being in the context of bereavement, and it appears to confer benefit by keeping the bereaved individual focused on both present-oriented functioning and future-oriented goals. Overall, these findings suggest that hopeful thought may be an important part of perceiving one's life as having meaning, even in trying times.

Several other examples illustrate the positive association between hope and meaning; directionality of these relationships, however, remains unclear. In a study evaluating the relations among stress, psychological distress, hope, and meaning in a sample of college undergraduates, Mascaro and Rosen (2005) found that state hope and personal meaning in life (i.e., having a sense of purpose) were positively correlated. Additionally, they found that meaning in life scores predicted State Hope Scale scores 2 months later after accounting for variance associ-

ated with baseline State Hope Scale scores, personality variables, and symptoms of depression. Based on these findings, we might conclude that making meaning in life precedes hopeful thought; however, Bronk, Hill, Lapsley, Talib, and Finch (2009) found an opposite pattern of results. Replicating Feldman and Snyder (2005) and Mascaro and Rosen (2005), these authors found that both pathways and agency positively correlated with identified purpose and searching for purpose (two proposed components of meaning) in samples of adolescents and young adults. Agency, but not pathways, mediated the relationship between purpose in life and life satisfaction in adolescents and young adults, suggesting that the relationship between meaning and life satisfaction was best explained by an indirect path through hope for these samples. Thus, while it is clear that meaning and hope are strongly related to one another, and both are related to other markers of psychological health, the exact nature of these relations it is not yet clear.

Hope in the Context of Difficult Life Events

While a number of studies have demonstrated the strong, positive associations between hope and various measures of success (e.g., academic, athletic), psychological well-being (e.g., positive affect, life satisfaction, meaning), and less psychopathology (e.g., symptoms of depression and anxiety, Neuroticism), most of these studies have sampled college students and other healthy adults. It is one thing to see beneficial outcomes of hope when things are going well in one's life but may be quite another to examine how hope is related to various outcomes in times of duress. Several researchers have started to take on study designs that address this area of inquiry.

One type of stressor that might influence the relations between hope and outcomes is environmental. Glass, Flory, Hankin, Kloos, and Turecki (2009) surveyed 228 adult survivors of Hurricane Katrina between 2 and 9 months after landfall. Results indicated that hope was negatively related to both posttraumatic stress disorder (PTSD) symptoms and general psychological distress.

Furthermore, in a model including age, sex, race, time since hurricane, avoidant coping, problem-focused coping, social support, and hope, only hope (negatively) and avoidant coping (positively) were significantly related to PTSD symptoms. In a similar model, age, sex, avoidant coping, hope, and social support were related to general psychological distress. Specifically, hope moderated the relationship between avoidant coping and general psychological distress, such that avoidant coping was less problematic at higher than lower levels of hope.

Another type of environmental stressor is related to treatment by others in one's environment. Cooley and Ritschel (2012) recruited 223 adolescents from a low-income, urban high school and found that hope was generally protective for victimized youth. Specifically, they found that hope was inversely correlated with psychological distress, regardless of the intensity of peer victimization. Furthermore, high hope served a main protective effect against the development of depressive symptoms and emotion dysregulation at low to moderate (but not high) levels of peer victimization. Taken together, these two studies suggest that hopeful thought may play an important role in buffering against the effects of disruptive environmental stressors, with the caveat that this relation may weaken at the most powerful levels of the stressor. More research is needed in this important and understudied area.

Medical and health stressors are the most commonly studied examples of adverse situations in which hope has been studied. Hope has largely been found to be associated with better outcomes and functioning for those who experience significant medical stressors, either directly or indirectly. For example, Gum, Snyder, and Duncan (2006) found that hope was inversely correlated with depression scores 3 months after stroke; as in several other studies reviewed here, agency thinking was a stronger predictor of psychopathology than pathways thinking poststroke. Similarly, Parenteau, Gallant, Sarosiek, and McCallum (2006) found that higher hope prior to receiving a gastric pacemaker was correlated with better psychological outcomes on measures of depression and anxiety at baseline, and 3 and 6 months postsurgery. Billington, Simpson, Unwin, Bray, and Giles (2008) found that hope was a significant (negative) predictor of depression and anxiety in a sample of patients in end-stage renal failure (ESRF). Moreover, higher hope was related to better outcomes on a quality-of-life measure and postdiagnostic adjustment. The authors theorized that ESRF patients with higher hope may be better able to combat the fatigue associated with the disease, and are less likely than those with lower hope to perceive their diagnoses and physical limitations as overly burdensome. They noted that high hope was less strongly related to physical quality-of-life outcomes, suggesting that the relationship between hope and better outcomes is not accounted for by physical functioning.

Billington and colleagues (2008) examined the extent to which hope contributes to adjustment to physical illness by examining the relation between hope and psychological functioning after taking physical functioning into account. Kortte, Gilbert, Gorman, and Wegener (2010) furthered this line of research by comparing the effects of hope with several other psychological variables in a longitudinal study of patients with spinal cord injuries, and found that hope was positively associated with life satisfaction at both admission and 3 months postdischarge. At admission, hope remained significantly associated with life satisfaction after controlling for negative affect, avoidant coping, and depressive symptoms. Hope and positive affect (entered as a block) predicted life satisfaction 3 months later after controlling for demographic variables, negative affect, avoidant coping, and depressive symptoms. Thus, this study suggests that in addition to being related to better psychological functioning and outcomes, hope is a predictor of psychological functioning even after controlling for other powerful variables.

The previous studies all examined the relation of hope and functioning when the participant is the one with the stressor or challenge. Lloyd and Hastings (2009), however, examined parents of children with intellectual disabilities in their investigation of the association between hope and symptoms of psychopathology. They found that scores on the Hope Scale were significantly related to higher scores on measures of positive affect and lower scores on measures of depression and anxiety. Specifically, agency scores conferred resilience for both mothers and fathers on measures of psychological well-being; pathways scores were protective for mothers against depression (but not anxiety) and were unrelated to fathers' levels of psychopathology. These authors concluded that higher hope confers resiliency on parents of children with intellectual disabilities. In all, these studies can be taken to support the hypothesis that hope is related to and predictive of better psychological and physical outcomes even in the face of serious and sometimes chronic stressors.

Hope and Coping

One way that hope might be associated with these superior outcomes is by way of skillful and effective coping. In a sample of college students, Chang and DeSimone (2001) found that hope was positively correlated with engaged coping (e.g., "I worked on solving the problems in the situation") and negatively correlated with disengaged coping (e.g., "I avoided thinking or doing anything about the situation"). In a sample of children with sickle-cell disease, coping style moderated the significant relationship between hope and anxiety symptoms (Lewis & Kliewer, 1995). Specifically, high hope predicted low anxiety when the child reported engaging in more active (i.e., less avoidant) coping strategies. Drach-Zahavy and Somech (2001) examined the relationship between hope and constructive coping in a sample of college students with stressful health problems and found that (1) hope and constructive thinking/coping are distinct yet related constructs; (2) agency thinking is more strongly related to constructive thinking than pathways thinking; and (3) pathways thinking is more strongly related to resource allocation than agency thinking when coping with stress. In particular, they noted that high pathways thinkers were better able to deploy attentional resources to problem-relevant issues and to refocus attention to problem solving when attention wandered to off-task activities, negative affect, or self-regulatory cognitions. These findings suggest that those with high hope may be better able to cope with stressful life events because they are better able to keep their attention focused on problem-solving activities in the face of stressful stimuli.

In a daily diary study, Roesch, Duangado, Vaughn, Aldridge, and Villodas (2010) examined how dispositional hope predicted coping strategies over the course of 5 days with a sample of socioeconomically disadvantaged, minority high school students. The authors examined pathways and agency thinking separately in order to understand better how hopeful thought specifically predicts coping behaviors. Pathways thinking predicted increased use of problem solving, planning, positive thinking, religious coping, distracting actions, and overall use of coping strategies; this is to be anticipated given that higher pathways scores should be related to the perceived ability to generate and use many different coping strategies. Agency thinking was significantly related only to talking with others who have had similar stressful experiences. Thus, hope tends to be positively related to adaptive coping and negatively related to problematic coping. In addition, pathways thinking and agency thinking are differentially related to coping; pathways thinking is related to using a greater number of different kinds of coping strategies and resource allocation, whereas agency thinking is more strongly related to seeking support of others and constructive thinking.

Is Hope Malleable?

Given the numerous benefits associated with hope, it is not surprising that researchers have turned their attention to the development of interventions with the aim to increase hopeful thought. Two tracks have been pursued in the development of hope interventions. In the first, interventions are developed to bolster hope for those with evidence of successful goal pursuits, without particular regard to pretreatment hope levels. This is the classic positive psychology model in which interventions are designed to move people from an adequate or normal level of some construct (in this case, hope) to an optimal level of functioning. In the second track, a specific deficit is identified, and the aim of the intervention is to remedy this deficit, such that participants are brought back to a "normal" level of functioning. This model is in line with traditional treatment models in which individuals are identified on the basis of disorder (e.g., depression) or deficit (e.g., social skills) and, through participation in treatment, are expected to move into a typical range of functioning.

Positive Psychology Hope Interventions

An excellent example of a positive psychology intervention exists within the realm of athletics. Although National Collegiate Athletic Association (NCAA) Division I athletes are, by definition, successful in this domain of their lives, much attention is paid to attempts to find ways to engender optimal performance. In addition to flourishing in specific athletic realms, there is evidence that athletes have higher dispositional hope than nonathletes (Curry, Snyder, Cook, Ruby, & Rehm, 1997). Furthermore, Curry and colleagues found that hope (but not global self-esteem) is significantly related to academic and athletic performance, even after accounting for other powerful predictors of these outcomes. Thus, one could argue that hope is a strength for elite athletes, and that harnessing and increasing hopeful thought might lead to optimal performance in athletics and academics for these individuals.

In order to build on the high levels of hope in college athletes, Curry, Maniar, Sondag, and Sandstedt (1999) developed a 15-week (i.e., one semester) optimal performance curriculum based on hope theory. For the 143 student-athletes who participated in the class, hope scores significantly increased from pre- to postcourse, and these increases were maintained for the following year (Curry & Snyder, 2000). Additionally, hope significantly predicted semester grade point average (GPA) after controlling for both cumulative GPA and overall perceptions of self-worth (although self-worth was a nonsignificant predictor). The authors simultaneously collected data from a group of student-athletes that did not participate in the course ($N = 43$) to compare trajectories of hope and academic achievement. For the control group, hope scores did not change over the semester, and hope did not predict semester GPA after controlling for cumulative GPA. This suggests that the hope intervention further increased already high levels of hope, and that hope scores were associated with concurrent academic performance in a way that was not evident for those who

did not participate in the intervention. Rolo and Gould (2007), who conducted a similar study with a 6-week hope intervention, found that student-athletes randomized to the intervention condition had significantly greater increases in state hope compared to student-athletes in the control condition; there were no differences, however, in athletic or academic performance.

Treatment Model Hope Interventions

In one of the first attempts to use a hope-based intervention to treat psychopathology, Klausner and colleagues (1998) tested a hope-based group therapy in the treatment of geriatric depression. Thirteen older adults who had residual depressive symptoms despite at least 10 weeks of treatment (either pharmacotherapy or psychotherapy) were assigned, using stratified randomization, to either the hope-based group or a reminiscence group. Each group met for 1 hour each week for 11 weeks. The hope-based group resulted in lower observer-rated depressive symptoms and patient-rated hopelessness than the reminiscence group. Additionally, patients in the hope-based group had significant pre- to posttreatment reductions in all measures of depression, as well as measures of hopelessness, anxiety, and disability, with corresponding increases in overall hope and agency scores. The authors concluded that a hope-based, group treatment resulted in relatively large effect sizes and was likely to be efficacious in treating depression and perhaps anxiety in late life.

Following this trial, Cheavens, Feldman, Gum, Michael, and Snyder (2006) developed and implemented an 8-week (2 hours per session) group hope intervention. This trial was originally designed as a positive psychology intervention that was meant to increase hope scores for individuals without psychopathology. Approximately half of the recruited sample ($N = 39$, 32 treatment completers), however, met criteria for a current psychiatric diagnosis, and their scores on measures of depression and anxiety were in the clinically relevant range. Thus, this trial is better conceptualized as a treatment trial. Participants were randomized to either the group hope treatment or a wait-list control. Those in the hope group had significantly greater reductions in anxiety symptoms and increases in agency, self-esteem, and meaning in life than those in the wait-list group. Additionally, there were trends ($p = .07$) for those in the hope group to have greater increases in overall hope and decreases in depressive symptoms. In terms of change in depressive symptoms, both pretreatment hope scores and hope change scores significantly accounted for posttreatment depression scores after controlling for pretreatment depression scores. Thus, the intervention, which was designed to increase hopeful thought, was associated with increases in agency and trend level changes in overall hope; perhaps more importantly, changes in hope were related to decreases in depressive symptoms, suggesting that hope may be an important construct in ameliorating depressive symptoms.

In order to assess the immediate impact of intervening on hope, Berg, Snyder, and Hamilton (2008) recruited college students with low hope (defined as those scoring below the median) to participate in a 15-minute hope intervention. Given that the intervention was so brief and the goal was defined explicitly for all participants, this intervention might be considered a form of hope coaching. Participants were randomized to either the hope intervention or a control condition (i.e., reading a book on home organization) and were asked to tolerate a painful task (i.e., cold pressor) for as long as possible following the intervention. Those who participated in the hope intervention had a significantly greater increase in hope scores and tolerated pain significantly longer than those in the control condition. These results suggest that even this brief hope intervention resulted in hope changes in the moment, as well as increased successful goal behavior (i.e., pain tolerance in this case).

Taken together, this preliminary evidence suggests that the tenets of hopeful thinking can be taught, and the simplicity of the model allows for the development of interventions aimed at increasing hope across a variety of populations. Additionally, these results suggest that targeting hope in interventions may result in other beneficial outcomes, including reduced depression and anxiety symptoms, and increased pain/distress tolerance, self-esteem, and meaning in life. As reviewed earlier in this chapter, high hope is associated with many markers of the "good life" and positive emotion. Increasing hopeful thought may be one way to increase access to positive emotions and experiences, both for people who are already thriving and for those with more difficult circumstances and experiences.

Conclusion

Hope, as defined by Snyder (1994), is a set of goal-relevant thoughts that propel us toward important outcomes and the resultant positive emotions in our lives. Hope is positively related to positive affect, meaning in life, life satisfaction, academic and athletic achievement, and coping with adversity, and is negatively associated with negative affect, psychopathology, and other markers of distress. For many, the lessons of hope are learned early in life, and success in important life domains maintains and increases hope over the lifespan. There is also evidence that hope can be learned and strengthened through interventions targeted at augmenting agency and pathways thinking. Although there is a strong hope literature base, we are in need of more studies that provide information about the temporal unfolding of the hope model and also parse out the differential relations of hope with other positive psychology constructs. Additionally, we would benefit from a continued examination of how the component parts of hope (i.e., goals, pathways thinking, agency thinking) transact with one another and predict the benefits associated with hope. In summary, there have been important advances in the theoretical and empirical underpinnings of hope in the last two decades, and we are excited to see where new investigations will lead us in the decades to come.

References

Arnau, R. C., Rosen, D. H., Finch, J. F., Rhudy, J. L., & Fortunato, V. J. (2007). Longitudinal effects of hope on depression and anxiety: A longitudinal analysis. *Journal of Personality, 75*, 43–63.

Aspinwall, L. G., & Leaf, S. L. (2002). In search of the unique aspects of hope: Pinning our hopes on positive emotions, future oriented thinking, hard times, and other people. *Psychological Inquiry, 13*, 276–288.

Averill, J. R., Catlin, G., & Chon, K. K. (1990). *Rules of hope.* New York: Springer-Verlag.

Bailey, T. C., Eng, W., Frisch, M. B., & Snyder, C. R. (2007). Hope and optimism as related to life satisfaction. *Journal of Positive Psychology, 2*, 168–175.

Bandura, A. (1997). *Self-efficacy: The exercise of control.* New York: Freeman.

Berg, C. J., Snyder, C. R., & Hamilton, N. (2008). The effectiveness of a hope intervention in coping with cold pressor pain. *Journal of Health Psychology, 13*, 804–809.

Billington, E., Simpson, J., Unwin, J., Bray, D., & Giles, D. (2008). Does hope predict adjustment to end-stage renal failure and consequent dialysis? *British Journal of Health Psychology, 13*, 683–699.

Bronk, K. C., Hill, P. L., Lapsley, D. K., Talib, T. L., & Finch, H. (2009). Purpose, hope, and life satisfaction in three age groups. *Journal of Positive Psychology, 4*, 500–510.

Bryant, F. B., & Cvengros, J. A. (2004). Distinguishing hope and optimism: Two sides of a coin, or two separate coins? *Journal of Social and Clinical Psychology, 23*, 273–302.

Chang, E. C. (2003). A critical appraisal and extension of hope theory in middle-aged men and women: Is it important to distinguish agency and pathways components? *Journal of Social and Clinical Psychology, 22*, 121–143.

Chang, E. C., & DeSimone, S. L. (2001). The influence of hope on appraisals, coping, and dysphoria: A test of hope theory. *Journal of Clinical and Social Psychology, 20*, 117–129.

Cheavens, J. S., Feldman, D. B., Gum, A., Michael, S. T., & Snyder, C. R. (2006). Hope therapy in a community sample: A pilot investigation. *Social Indicators Research, 77*, 61–78.

Cooley, J. L., & Ritschel, L. A. (2012, August). *Hope as a protective factor against the effects of peer victimization.* Poster presented at the 120th Annual American Psychological Association Convention, Orlando, FL.

Cramer, K. M., & Dyrkacz, L. (1998). Differential prediction of maladjustment scores with the Snyder Hope subscales. *Psychological Reports, 83*, 1035–1041.

Curry, L. A., Maniar, S. D., Sondag, K. A., & Sandstedt, S. (1999). *An optimal performance academic course for university students and student-athletes.* Unpublished manuscript, University of Montana, Missoula.

Curry, L. A., & Snyder, C. R. (2000). Hope takes the field. In C. R. Snyder (Ed.), *Handbook of hope* (pp. 243–259). San Diego, CA: Academic Press.

Curry, L. A., Snyder, C. R., Cook, D. L., Ruby, B. C., & Rehm, M. (1997). The role of hope in student-athlete academic and sport achievement. *Journal of Personality and Social Psychology, 73*, 1257–1267.

Diener, E., Lucas, R. E., & Oishi, S. (2002). Subjective well-being: The science of happiness and life satisfaction. In C. R. Snyder & S. J. Lopez (Eds.), *Handbook of positive psychology* (pp. 63–73). Oxford, UK: Oxford University Press.

Drach-Zahavy, A., & Somech, A. (2001). Coping with health problems: The distinctive relationships of hope sub-scales with constructive thinking and resource allocation. *Personality and Individual Differences, 33*, 103–117.

Erikson, E. H. (1964). *Insight and responsibility.* New York: Norton.

Feldman, D. B., & Snyder, C. R. (2005). Hope and the meaningful life: Theoretical and empirical associations between goal-directed thinking and life meaning. *Journal of Social and Clinical Psychology, 24*, 401–421.

Frank, J. (1968). The role of hope in psychotherapy. *International Journal of Psychiatry, 5*, 393–395.

Gallagher, M. W., & Lopez, S. J. (2009). Positive expectancies and mental health: Identifying the unique contributions of hope and optimism. *Journal of Positive Psychology, 4*, 548–556.

Geiger, K. A., & Kwon, P. (2010). Rumination and depressive symptoms: Evidence for the moderating role of hope. *Personality and Individual Differences, 49*, 391–395.

Glass, K., Flory, K., Hankin, B. L., Kloos, B., & Turecki, G. (2009). Are coping strategies, social support, and hope associated with distress among Hurricane Katrina survivors? *Journal of Social and Clinical Psychology, 28*, 779–795.

Gum, A., Snyder, C. R., & Duncan, P. W. (2006). Hopeful thinking, participation, and depressive symptoms three months after stroke. *Psychology and Health, 21*, 319–334.

Halama, P. (2010). Hope as a mediator between personality traits and life satisfaction. *Studia Psychologica, 52*, 309–314.

Irving, L. M., Snyder, C. R., & Crowson, Jr., J. J. (1998). Hope and the negotiation of cancer facts by college women. *Journal of Personality, 66*, 195–214.

Kirkland, T. & Cunningham, W. A. (2012). Mapping emotions through time: How affective trajectories inform the language of emotion. *Emotion, 12,* 268–282.

Klausner, E. J., Clarkin, J. F., Spielman, L., Pupo, C., Abrams, R., & Alexopoulos, G. S. (1998). Late-life depression and functional disability: The role of goal-focused group psychotherapy. *International Journal of Geriatric Psychiatry, 13,* 707–716.

Kortte, K. B., Gilbert, M., Gorman, P., & Wegener, S. T. (2010). Positive psychological variables in the prediction of life satisfaction after spinal cord injury. *Rehabilitation Psychology, 55,* 40–47.

Lazarus, R. S. (1999). Hope: An emotion and vital resource against despair. *Social Research, 66,* 665–669.

Lewis, H. A., & Kliewer, W. (1995). Hope, coping, and adjustment among children with sickle cell disease: Tests of mediator and moderator models. *Journal of Pediatric Psychology, 21,* 25–41.

Lloyd, T. J., & Hastings, R. (2009). Hope as a psychological resilience factor in mothers and fathers of children with intellectual disabilities. *Journal of Intellectual Disability Research, 53,* 957–968.

Lopez, S. J., Ciarlelli, R., Coffman, L., Stone, M., & Wyatt, L. (2000). Diagnosing for strengths: On measuring hope building blocks. In C. R. Snyder (Ed.), *The handbook of hope: Theory, measures, and application* (pp. 57–85). San Diego, CA: Academic Press.

Magaletta, P. R., & Oliver, J. M. (1999). The hope construct, will, and ways: Their relations with self-efficacy, optimism, and general well-being. *Journal of Clinical Psychology, 55,* 539–551.

Mascaro, N., & Rosen, D. H. (2005). Existential meaning's role in the enhancement of hope and prevention of depressive symptoms. *Journal of Personality, 73,* 985–1013.

Menninger, K. (1959). The academic lecture: Hope. *American Journal of Psychiatry, 116,* 481–491.

McCullough, M., & Snyder, C. R. (2000). Classical sources of human strength: Revisiting an old home and building a new one. *Journal of Social and Clinical Psychology, 19,* 1–10.

Michael, S. T., & Snyder, C. R. (2005). Getting unstuck: The roles of hope, finding meaning, and rumination in the adjustment to bereavement among college students. *Death Studies, 29,* 435–458.

Mowrer, O. H. (1960). *Learning theory and behavior.* New York: Wiley.

Orne, M. (1968). On the nature of effective hope. *International Journal of Psychiatry, 5,* 403–410.

Parenteau, S. C., Gallant, S., Sarosiek, I., & McCallum, R. W. (2006). The role of hope in the psychological adjustment of gastropareutic patients receiving the gastric pacemaker: A longitudinal study. *Journal of Clinical Psychology in Medical Settings, 13,* 49–56.

Rand, K. L. (2009). Hope and optimism: Latent structures and influences on grade expectancy and academic performance. *Journal of Personality, 77,* 231–260.

Rand, K. L., & Cheavens, J. S. (2009). Hope theory. In S. J. Lopez (Ed.), *Oxford handbook of positive psychology* (2nd ed., pp. 323–334). Oxford, UK: Oxford University Press.

Roesch, S. C., Duangado, K. M., Vaughn, A. A., Aldridge, A. A., & Villodas, F. (2010). Dispositional hope and the propensity to cope: A daily diary assessment of minority adolescents. *Cultural Diversity and Ethnic Minority Psychology, 16,* 191–198.

Rolo, C., & Gould, D. (2007). An intervention for fostering hope, athletic, and academic performance in university student-athletes. *International Coaching Psychology Review, 2,* 44–61.

Seligman, M. E. P. (2002). Positive psychology, positive prevention, and positive therapy. In C. R. Snyder & S. J. Lopez (Eds.), *Handbook of positive psychology* (pp. 1–9). Oxford, UK: Oxford University Press.

Scheier, M. F., & Carver, C. S. (1985). Optimism, coping, and health: Assessment and implications of generalized outcome expectancies. *Health Psychology, 4,* 219–247.

Shorey, H. S., Snyder, C. R., Rand, K. L., Hockemeyer, J. R., & Feldman, D. B. (2002). Somewhere over the rainbow: Hope theory weathers its first decade. *Psychological Inquiry, 13,* 322–331.

Snyder, C. R. (1994). *The psychology of hope: You can get there from here.* New York: Free Press.

Snyder, C. R. (2002). Hope theory: Rainbows in the mind. *Psychological Inquiry, 13,* 249–275.

Snyder, C. R., Cheavens, J. S., & Michael, S. T. (2005). Hope theory: History and elaborated model. In J. Eliott (Ed.), *Interdisciplinary perspectives on hope* (pp. 101–118). New York: Nova Science.

Snyder, C. R., Harris, C., Anderson, J. R., Holleran, S. A., Irving, L. M., Sigmon, S. T., et al.

(1991). The will and the ways: Development and validation of an individual-differences measure of hope. *Journal of Personality and Social Psychology, 60,* 570–585.

Snyder, C. R., Hoza, B., Pelham, W. E., Rapoff, M., Ware, L., Danovsky, M., et al. (1997). The development and validation of the Children's Hope Scale. *Journal of Pediatric Psychology, 22,* 399–421.

Snyder, C. R., Irving, L., & Anderson, J. R. (1991). Hope and health: Measuring the will and the ways. In C. R. Snyder & D. R. Forsyth (Eds.), *Handbook of social and clinical psychology: The health perspective* (pp. 285–305). Elmsford, NY: Pergamon.

Snyder, C. R., Lapointe, A. B., Crowson, J. J., Jr., & Early, S. (1998). Preferences of high and low-hope people for self-referential input. *Cognition and Emotion, 12,* 807–823.

Snyder, C. R., Sympson, S. C., Ybasco, F. C., Borders, T. F., Babyak, M. A., & Higgins, R. L. (1996). Development and validation of the State Hope Scale. *Journal of Personality and Social Psychology, 70,* 321–335.

Staats, S. R., & Stassen, M. A. (1985). Hope: An affective cognition. *Social Indicators Research, 17,* 235–242.

Steffen, L. E., & Smith, B. W. (2013). The influence of between and within-person hope among emergency responders on daily affect in a stress and coping model. *Journal of Research in Personality, 47,* 738–747.

Stotland, E. (1969). *The psychology of hope.* San Francisco: Jossey-Bass.

Sympson, S. C. (1999).*Validation of the domain-specific Hope Scale.* Doctoral dissertation, University of Kansas, Lawrence.

Valle, M. F., Huebner, E. S., & Suldo, S. M. (2004). Further evaluation of the Children's Hope Scale. *Journal of Psychoeducational Assessment, 22,* 320–337.

Valle, M. F., Huebner, E. S., & Suldo, S. M. (2006). An analysis of hope as a psychological strength. *Journal of School Psychology, 44,* 393–406.

Wrobleski, K. K., & Snyder, C. R. (2005). Hopeful thinking in older adults: Back to the future. *Experimental Aging Research, 31,* 217–233.

PART V

Outcomes of Positive Emotions

CHAPTER 24

Health and Psychology

The Importance of Positive Affect

Judith Tedlie Moskowitz
Laura R. Saslow

The idea that our emotions have an impact on our physical health is now well ingrained in popular culture and has, in the past few decades, garnered significant empirical support. Initially, most research on the topic focused on how depression and other negative affective constructs were detrimental in terms of physical health, but more recently, attention has turned to positive affect as a unique predictor of better health and longer life. Alongside studies showing that positive affect has unique, beneficial social, cognitive, and behavioral effects (e.g., Fredrickson, 1998; Isen, Daubman, & Nowicki, 1987; Lyubomirsky, 2007), studies have begun to convincingly demonstrate that positive affect is associated with health-relevant constructs, including longer life and slower disease progression. As with any emerging literature, however, there are inconsistencies, controversies, challenges, and lessons to be learned. In this chapter, we provide an overview of the current state of the field regarding positive affect and physical health. We start by reviewing findings from recent meta-analyses on positive affect and health (e.g., Chida & Steptoe,

2008; Howell, Kern, & Lyubomirsky, 2007; Lamers, Bolier, Westerhof, Smit, & Bohlmeijer, 2012), then discuss the new findings that have been published subsequently. We consider potential psychological, biological, and behavioral pathways by which positive affect and related constructs may impact health, discuss some of the shortcomings in the literature, and, finally, suggest ways in which these findings can be translated into interventions to improve physical health via increases in positive affect.

Defining Positive Affect

We define "positive affect" as the subjective experience of positively valenced feelings, including lower activation feelings such as calm or satisfied, as well as higher activation feelings such as excited or thrilled. In our definition of affect we include both momentary emotional experience and longer-lasting moods. Many of the early findings regarding positive affect and health focused primarily on the physical health variables, making the selection of positive affect measure a matter of convenience or availability. Thus, the research literature includes a broad range of operationalizations of affect, which vary in the degree to which they overlap with this definition. In our view, the imprecise measurement of affect is one of the key issues in the literature on affect and health. Therefore, we make special note of how the positive affective constructs are measured and labeled as we review each study, and we discuss the issue of affect measurement in more detail at the end of the chapter.

Positive Affect and Longevity in Initially Healthy Samples

In recent decades a number of studies have demonstrated that people who have higher positive affect tend to live longer (Cohen & Pressman, 2006; Diener & Chan, 2011). Meta-analyses summarize these findings and confirm that the experience of positive affect predicts greater longevity in samples of healthy individuals (Chida & Steptoe, 2008; Howell et al., 2007). For example, Chida and Steptoe (2008) meta-analyzed 35 studies of initially healthy samples and found that positive affective constructs, including both trait-like constructs, such as optimism, and more state-like constructs, such as happiness, conferred a reduced risk of mortality. Controlling for negative affect had a negligible effect on the results, indicating that positive affect is uniquely associated with longevity, over and above any effect of negative affect.

In a study published since the Chida and Steptoe (2008) meta-analysis, Steptoe and Wardle (2011) examined average reported positive affect over the course of a day for over 3,500 individuals, ages 52 to 79, living in England. Individuals reported their positive affect ("happy," "excited," and "content") at four time periods over 1 day: just after waking, 30 minutes after waking, at 7:00 P.M., and at bedtime. The researchers then examined how positive affect averaged over the day, divided into tertiles, predicted all-cause mortality. Even after the researchers controlled for age, sex, smoking, physical activity, self-reported health, diagnoses of illness, indicators of depression, and negative affect, high positive affect was associated with a 35% decreased risk in mortality

over a 5-year follow-up period. This study is particularly provocative because of its measure of positive affect: the experience of happiness, excitement, and contentment at four time points over a single day.

Because of its widespread use in large epidemiological studies (Blazer & Hybels, 2004; Ostir, Markides, Black, & Goodwin, 2000; Ostir, Markides, Peek, & Goodwin, 2001) a number of researchers have relied on the Positive Affect subscale of the Center for Epidemiologic Studies Depression Scale (CES-D; Radloff, 1977) to explore associations between positive affect and health. The CES-D Positive Affect subscale comprises four items: "I felt I was just as good as other people," "I felt hopeful about the future," "I was happy," and "I enjoyed life." Participants consider what they have experienced over the past week, rating the items on a scale from 0 (rarely or none of the time, less than 1 day), to 1 (some or a little of the time, 1 to 2 days), to 2 (occasionally or a moderate amount of time, 3 to 4 days) to 3 (most or all of the time, 5 to 7 days). For example, Blazer and Hybels (2004) examined positive affect, measured with the CES-D subscale, in over 3,500 individuals between ages 65 and 105 in the United States. After they controlled for age, sex, ethnicity, marital status, education, income, cognitive impairment, functional impairment, and negative affect, positive affect predicted a reduced risk of all-cause mortality over a 10-year period. Moskowitz, Epel, and Acree (2008) examined the Positive Affect subscale among 2,673 people with no chronic conditions and found no significant association with mortality. However, when the sample was restricted to the 334 participants over the age of 65, the individual items "I enjoyed life" and "I was happy" were significantly associated with longevity, even when effects of negative affect were controlled. More recently, in the Netherlands, Krijthe and colleagues (2011) used the Positive Affect subscale of the CES-D to measure positive affect in over 4,000 adults between ages 61 and 102. For adults ages 61–70 at the start of the study, after the researchers controlled for age, sex, socioeconomic status, smoking, alcohol, health status (disability status and prevalent disease type), and negative affect, positive affect predicted greater survival over roughly 7 years. Interestingly, results were not significant for individuals over age 70.

Some studies have compared different operationalizations of positive affect in predicting longevity. For example, in Sweden, Lyyra, Törmäkangas, Read, Rantanen, and Berg (2006) examined life satisfaction and positive affect as predictors of 10-year mortality in a sample of 320 same-sex twins ages 80 and older (most below the age of 85). The researchers factor-analyzed the 13-item Life Satisfaction Index Z (LSI-Z; Wood, Wylie, & Sheafor, 1969), into three components. One component, called *zest*, appears to be a mixture of positive affect and future planning: "As I grow older, things seem better than I thought they would," "I am just as happy as when I was younger," "The things I do are as interesting to me as they ever were," and "I have made plans for things I'll be doing a month or a year from now." Another component, was called *life satisfaction* or *congruence* (as in congruence between desired and achieved goals): "I have gotten more breaks in life than most of the people I know," "As I look back on my life, I am fairly well satisfied," "When I think back over my life, I didn't get most of the important things I wanted," "I've gotten pretty much what I expected out of life." After controlling for age, sex, education, whether the individual lived alone, number of serious illnesses, physical functioning, social functioning, cognitive functioning, and depressive symptoms, positive affect (zest) was predictive of a lower risk of mortality over 10 years. No such effect was found for the life satisfaction (congruence) measure.

In contrast, Xu and Roberts (2010) came to the opposite conclusion—that life satisfaction but not positive affect is associated with longevity. These authors compared the differential associations of life satisfaction and positive affect with all-cause mortality in a sample of over 6,000 U.S. residents. Life satisfaction was measured with the items: "All in all, how happy are you these days?"; "On the whole life gives me a lot of pleasure"; and "I feel as good now as I ever have." These three items appear to tap into the experience of positive affect (happy, pleasure, feel good), rather than a more cognitive appraisal of life satisfaction (Diener, Emmons, Larsen, & Griffin, 1985). The so-called "positive affect measure" used

the items: "How often do you feel on top of the world?"; "How often do you feel particularly excited or interested in something"; and "How often do you feel pleased about having accomplished something." All items were from the Positive Feeling subscale of the Bradburn–Caplovitz Index (Bradburn & Caplovitz, 1965) and appear to be tapping high-arousal positive affect (elation, excitement) in addition to pleasure at accomplishment. After controlling for age, sex, education, and baseline health, so-called "life satisfaction" ("Happy," "Life gives me pleasure," and "I feel good") but not positive affect ("On top of the world," "Excited/interested," "Pleased at having accomplished something") predicted a lower relative risk of all-cause and natural-cause mortality over 28 years. As a side note, they found no link between "negative feelings" and longevity. Putting aside the labels applied to the constructs in this study, it appears that high-arousal positive affects are not associated with longevity, but somewhat lower-arousal positive affects that tap pleasure and enjoyment are predictive of longer life.

In another relatively recent study that included both positive affect and life satisfaction, Wiest, Schüz, Webster, and Wurm, 2011) also examined the impact on mortality in a broad sample of over 3,000 German adults between ages 40 and 85 years. Their measure of positive affect was the Positive subscale of the Positive and Negative Affect Schedule (PANAS; Watson, Clark, & Tellegen, 1988), which asks participants to rate how much they have felt "excited," "interested," "proud," "alert," "strong," and "active" over the past month. Some of these items, particularly "strong" and "active," may also be tapping into physical health, however, rather than just the experience of positive affect. Life satisfaction was assessed with the Satisfaction with Life Scale (Diener et al., 1985), a more cognitive assessment. Participants rate how much they agree with the statements: "In most ways my life is close to my ideal," "The conditions of my life are excellent," "I am satisfied with my life," "So far I have gotten the important things I want in life," and "If I could live my life over, I would change almost nothing." After controlling for age, sex, education, area of the country the individuals were living in, romantic partner status, and negative affect, the researchers found that both life satisfaction and positive affect had a positive relationship with longevity. Both life satisfaction and positive affect were simultaneously included in the statistical model, and both were significant, suggesting that they have independent, positive effects on longevity. The effect was stronger among those age 65 and older (Wiest et al., 2011).

Not all studies have used self-report to assess whether the experience of positive affect is related to longevity. One study measured the intensity of smiles in the official 1952 portraits of 230 male professional baseball players (Abel & Kruger, 2010). Researchers assessed smiling in the photographs from 1 (*no smiling*) to 2 (*partially smiling using just the mouth*) to 3 (*fully smiling using the mouth and the eyes*). After controlling for age, body mass index (BMI), factors related to their baseball careers, marital status, and college attendance, baseball players who were fully smiling were half as likely to die in any year, over a nearly 50-year period, as nonsmilers. In other words, momentary nonverbal expressions of positive affect were related to longevity. This finding is similar to Steptoe and Wardle's (2011) research, discussed earlier, in which momentary experiences of positive emotion on 1 day predicted later longevity.

Researchers have also found a relationship between positive affect words used in autobiographical writings and longevity. In a now classic study of 180 nuns, researchers measured positive affect in the women's autobiographies, written in their early 20s, just as they were entering the nunnery (Danner, Snowdon, & Friesen, 2001). For example, a nun with high levels of positive affect wrote, "The past year . . . has been a very happy one. Now I look forward with eager joy . . . " A nun using low levels of positive affect words wrote, "The year was spent . . . teaching. . . . I intend to do my best." Happiness, interest, love, hope, gratefulness, contentment, and accomplishment were some of the most frequently used positive affects. Even after researchers controlled for age, education, and negative affect usage in the autobiographies, positive affect words predicted longevity; compared to nuns in the bottom quartile, nuns in the top quartile of positive affect word usage had a 2.5 lower risk of dying between the ages of 75 and 95.

Pressman and Cohen (2012) also used autobiographical writings to measure the potential relationship between positive affect and longevity. Instead of grouping all positive affect together, they took into account levels of high versus low activation or arousal. The researchers measured how 88 well-known, now deceased psychologists wrote about themselves in a 1961 book entitled *A History of Psychology in Autobiography*. On average, the psychologists were age 67 at the time of writing the autobiography and lived another 12 years after the book's publication. Most were male and all were white. Even after controlling for their date of birth, age at publication, sex, a measure of health, whether the writing had been translated, and negative affect words, high-arousal positive affect words (*active, energetic, vigorous, alert, lively, activated, stimulated,* and *aroused*), humor and laughter words (*chuckle, laugh, funny, humor, giggle, hilarious, fun, hilarity, jolly,* and *silly*), and self-confidence–related words (*proud, strong, confident, bold, daring,* and *fearless*) predicted greater longevity. Negative affect words and low-arousal positive affect words (*peaceful, relaxed, contented, pleasant, comfortable, calm, restful,* and, oddly, the word *cheerful*) were not related to longevity. Importantly, this research by Pressman and Cohen (2012), distinguishing between high- and low-arousal positive affect, found only high-arousal positive emotion to be linked to longevity. However, some of the high-arousal positive affect words (*energetic, vigorous, alert,* and *strong*) were also measuring physical vigor, which could confound whether results are due to the experience of positive affect alone or to high-energy states related to better health. This study and Danner and colleagues' (2001) nun study suggest that how much positive affect people naturally express in self-relevant writing may be a valid way to assess experiences of positive affect.

In summary, some of the strongest evidence of an association between positive affect and longevity is in initially healthy samples of people. Despite use of a number of different measures of and labels for positive affect and a wide variety of control variables, the data strongly support the hypothesis that positive affect is uniquely associated with longer life, independent of any effect of negative affect. The majority of this work was with samples of adults over the age of 60, and there is some indication that the associations between positive affect and longevity may be stronger in older samples (e.g., Moskowitz et al., 2008). This may simply be a reflection of the higher risk of mortality associated with age, but this finding may also suggest a strong rationale for positive affect interventions in older samples (Chida & Steptoe, 2008). Finally, in these studies of positive affect and longevity in initially healthy samples, there is some suggestion that a discrete emotions perspective, in which researchers look beyond global positive affect to unique effects of individual emotions, may hold promise (Consedine & Moskowitz, 2007). A more fine-grained measurement approach that taps a number of discrete emotions, with appropriate controls for physical health, has the potential to uncover important differences and suggest particular target affects for future interventions (e.g., gratitude interventions; Emmons & McCullough, 2003).

Positive Affect and Longevity in Initially Ill Samples

There is also evidence that positive affect is related to longevity in samples of people living with serious illness, although this evidence is somewhat less consistent than the results in initially healthy samples. In a meta-analysis of 35 studies of initially ill populations (with individuals with cancer, renal failure, hematopoietic disease, chronic heart failure, chronic heart disease, spinal cord injury, or HIV, among others; Chida & Steptoe, 2008), positive affect again conferred a reduced risk of mortality, albeit a seemingly smaller one compared to the effect in healthy samples. The effect remained significant in the studies in which researchers controlled for negative affect. A more recent meta-analysis focused on positive affect and survival in ill populations (Lamers et al., 2012), including samples with chronic heart disease, coronary artery disease, congestive heart failure, chronic alveolar hypoventilation, cancer, spinal cord injury, and patients undergoing hemodialysis and those in a general medical ward. Although the meta-analysis indicated that positive affect is

related to longer life overall, few researchers controlled for negative affect, so the extent to which positive affect was a unique predictor of longevity is not clear.

As in the studies of initially healthy samples, a number of the studies in initially ill samples relied on the Positive Affect subscale of the CES-D (Radloff, 1977). For example, Moskowitz (2003) used this subscale to predict all-cause mortality in a sample of over 400 HIV-positive men, ages 25–53, living in the United States (California). After researchers controlled for physical health measures related to mortality and negative affect, positive affect predicted lower risk of mortality 1 and 2 years later. Similarly, in a study of over 700 individuals with diabetes, with an average age of 63 years, living in the United States, researchers (Moskowitz et al., 2008) again used the Positive Affect subscale of the CES-D (Radloff, 1977). Although bivariate analyses indicated that positive affect was associated with lower risk of mortality, after researchers controlled for age, race, health status, and physical activity, the Positive Affect subscale was no longer a significant predictor of longevity. However, when the four items on the CES-D Positive Affect subscale ("I was happy," "I enjoyed life," "I felt hopeful," and "I felt I was as good as other people") were analyzed separately, the "I enjoyed life" item remained related to longevity when the other significant predictors were included in the model.

As the Moskowitz and colleagues (2008) study suggests, "enjoyment" may be a key positive affect in predicting longevity of people living with serious illness. In Germany, Scherer and Herrmann-Lingen (2009) found that a single item from the Hospital Anxiety and Depression Scale (Zigmond & Snaith, 1983), "I still enjoy the things I used to enjoy," was related to 1-year survival in over 500 general medical ward patients with an average age of 59. Results held after researchers controlled for other measures related to mortality (physician ratings of health and diagnoses of other illnesses). It may be that "I still enjoy the things I used to enjoy" is confounded with physical health, however. It is likely that healthier people are able to continue to engage in and enjoy the things they used to enjoy and are also likely to live longer because of their good health. The fact that the authors controlled for physician ratings of health and diagnoses of other illnesses, however, diminishes this concern to some extent.

Birket-Smith, Hansen, Hanash, Hansen, and Rasmussen (2009) used the World Health Organization Well-Being Index (WHO-5; Bech, 1998) to measure positive affect in a sample of 86 cardiology outpatients and predicted mortality over a 6-year follow-up. Controlling for age, number of social contacts, cardiac diagnosis, somatic symptoms, depression, and anxiety, positive affect was significantly associated with lower risk of mortality. The WHO-5 measures positive affect over the past 2 weeks using the items "I have felt cheerful and in good spirits," "I have felt calm and relaxed," "My daily life has been filled with things that interest me," "I have felt active and vigorous," and "I woke up feeling fresh and rested." Unfortunately, this measure not only asks about the experience of positive emotion (cheerfulness, calm, and interest) but also taps into physical activity and vigor, as well as high-quality sleep, two measures likely confounded with physical health.

It has been suggested that positive affect may be differentially related to longevity, depending on the disease or condition (e.g., Pressman & Cohen, 2005). Chida and Steptoe (2008) looked at this question in their meta-analysis and compared effect sizes across studies of cardiovascular disease, cancer, renal failure, and HIV. They found that the biggest protective effects of positive affect were in samples with renal failure or HIV. The effect of positive affect on longevity in samples with cardiovascular disease was marginally significant, and in cancer it was nonsignificant. Pressman and Cohen (2005) hypothesized that positive affect is most beneficial for persons with diseases in which health behaviors may have an impact, and less beneficial (or perhaps even detrimental) in those with diseases in which short-term mortality is high. There is some evidence to support this hypothesis, although more extensive study is warranted; studies in patients with heart disease or diabetes, in which health behaviors likely play a large role in determining survival, demonstrate that positive affect is associated with lower risk of mortality (Birket-Smith et al., 2009; Moskowitz et al., 2008), and studies in patients with diseases with high short-term mortality indicate a less central role for

positive affect in predicting longevity (e.g., Brown, Levy, Rosberger, & Edgar, 2003).

Positive Affect and Illness Onset

The bulk of the evidence seems to support the idea that positive affect is associated with lower risk of mortality among people who are healthy or living with a serious illness. Other research has examined a related question: Does positive affect predict the onset of illnesses? For example, could positive affect prevent the flu or reduce one's likelihood of becoming diabetic?

To address this question of positive affect and illness onset, Cohen, Doyle, Turner, Alper, and Skoner (2003) exposed healthy volunteers to a cold virus, then assessed who became infected with the virus and developed cold symptoms. Positive affect was measured with nine positive affect items (adjectives) that were asked on three evenings per week for 2 weeks during the month before the actual study began, as well as the start of the study. Those nine adjectives measured vigor (*lively, full of pep*, and *energetic*), well-being (*happy, pleased*, and *cheerful*), and calm (*at ease, calm*, and *relaxed*). Participants rated how accurately the adjectives described how they had been feeling over the past day, rated on a scale from 0 (*not at all accurate*) to 4 (*extremely accurate*). After researchers controlled for sex, race, education, BMI, month of exposure, virus type, immune factors, and negative affect, positive affect was related to being less likely to develop a cold up to 5 days after exposure. In follow-up analyses, only vigor and well-being, but not calm, were protective against developing a cold. The vigor dimension is problematic, however, as it may in itself be an indirect measure of health. The well-being measure, however, appears to be a more pure measure of felt positive affect. The fact that low-arousal positive affect was not related to the health outcome is an important reminder of the necessity to separate out the effects of arousal on the link between positive affect and health.

In a replication of this study a few years later, Cohen, Alper, Doyle, Treanor, and Turner (2006) exposed 193 healthy volunteers to either a cold or a flu virus and examined whether average daily positive affect (vigor, well-being, and calm) over a 2-week period was associated with onset of a cold, controlling for negative affect (depression, anxiety, and hostility), type of virus, education, body mass index, race, gender, season of exposure, and self-rated health. In addition, they controlled for positive dispositional traits of mastery, optimism, self-esteem, life engagement, and Extraversion. As in the previous study, vigor and well-being were both significantly associated with fewer colds, but calm was not. Of the positive traits, only Extraversion was associated with colds, but when entered into the equation with positive affect, it was no longer a significant predictor, indicating that state positive affect may have a stronger link than trait Extraversion in this case.

A comparatively large body of research has examined the association between positive affect and the occurrence of stroke or incidence of heart disease. For example, Ostir and colleagues (2001) found that positive affect is associated with lower incidence of stroke. The researchers examined over 2,500 U.S. individuals age 65 years or older, measuring positive affect with a subscale of the CES-D (Radloff, 1977). After researchers controlled for age, income, education, marital status, BMI, smoking, other health factors, and negative affect, positive affect conferred a reduced risk of having a stroke over a 6-year period.

The 10-year incidence of heart disease has also been found to be lower among those with higher levels of positive affect (Davidson, Mostofsky, & Whang, 2010). As with the study of baseball players described earlier (Abel & Kruger, 2010), researchers examined nonverbal expressions of positive affect. Unlike the baseball study, which examined men's smiles in still photographs, this research examined naturally expressed positive emotion in a 12-minute interview about how the participants tended to react in anger-provoking and stressful situations. Positive affect was coded as both nonverbal behavior, such as smiling, and the tone of the responses, such as degree of cheerfulness. Coders rated the videos from 1 (*no positive affect expressed*) to 5 (*extremely high levels of positive affect expressed*). Participants included over 1,500 individuals living in Canada (Nova Scotia). After controlling for age, sex, cardiovascular risk factors, and self-reported negative affect, the researchers related positive affect to a lower incidence of heart disease over a 10-year period.

In a large study of over 85,000 Japanese adults between ages 50 and 69, researchers examined the relationship between positive affect and stroke, coronary heart disease, and total cardiovascular disease (Shirai et al., 2009). Positive affect was measured with one item "Are you enjoying your life?" rated at three levels, from low to medium to high. After researchers controlled for age, occupation, BMI, smoking, alcohol, physical activity, health variables, and negative affect (stress and Type A characteristics), positive affect was related to being less likely to develop or to die from stroke, coronary heart disease, or total cardiovascular disease over a 12-year period in men but not women.

Another study found an association of the discrete positive affects of hope and curiosity with the diagnosis of hypertension or diabetes. The study examined over 1,000 individuals, average age 62 years old, drawn from multispecialty medical practices in the United States (Richman et al., 2005). Researchers examined hope (how much participants generally felt "hopeful," "challenged," "confident, and "expectant"; Ellsworth & Smith, 1988) and curiosity (how much they agreed with statements such as "I feel like exploring my environment," "I feel curious," "I feel interested," "I feel inquisitive," "I feel eager," "I am in a questioning mood," "I feel stimulated," and "I feel mentally active"; Spielberger, 1986). After researchers controlled for age, sex, smoking, exercise, alcohol, subjective socioeconomic status, and negative affect, both hope and curiosity were related to being less likely to be diagnosed with hypertension or diabetes over a 2-year period.

Although the literature concerning positive affect and illness onset is small compared to the literature linking positive affect and mortality, the evidence points to a significant effect, at least in terms of cold or flu viruses, diabetes, and cardiovascular events.

Pathways Linking Positive Affect to Health-Relevant Outcomes

As the previously discussed findings show, convincing evidence suggests that positive affect is related to lower risk of mortality and likelihood of illness onset in both initially healthy and initially ill samples, independent of any association of negative affect and health. An important question that arises, then, is what mechanism or pathway might account for this association? Researchers in the field have suggested several possible routes through which positive affect may influence physical health. One possible pathway is *biological*, via direct influence on the immune, cardiovascular, or endocrine systems. A second possible pathway linking positive affect to health is *behavioral*, through improved health behaviors, such as adherence to medications. Finally, positive affect may influence physical health via the more *psychological* route of the stress and coping process. We discuss the literature supporting each of these links. For ease of presentation we focus on each path individually, but the true pathways are likely more complex.

Biological Mechanisms Linking Positive Affect and Health

In a meta-analysis of psychological well-being and health biomarkers (Howell et al., 2007), psychological well-being was related to better *immune* functioning (e.g., secretory immunoglobulin A concentration, natural killer cell activity), and *cardiovascular* functioning (e.g., heart rate variability and ischemic episodes that include stroke-like symptoms), as well as a decreased *endocrine* system response (e.g., cortisol, epinephrine, norepinephrine).

Positive Affect and Immune Function

Various immune parameters have been shown to be susceptible to influence by experimentally induced, as well as naturally occurring affective states (Futterman, Kemeny, Shapiro, & Fahey, 1994; Marsland, Pressman, & Cohen, 2007; Pressman & Cohen, 2005; Stone, Cox, Valdimarsdottir, & Jandorf, 1987). Brief positive mood inductions seem to improve immune function in healthy adults, and the tendency to feel positive emotions predicts greater antibody responses. For example, in a study of 84 healthy U.S. graduate students vaccinated for hepatitis B, higher levels of dispositional positive affect (self-ratings of "lively," "full of pep," "energetic," "happy," "pleased," "cheerful," "at ease," "calm," and "relaxed") were related to an index of

a healthy immune response (the amount of antibody response to the hepatitis B vaccination) after researchers controlled for age, sex, and BMI. The effect of positive affect was also generally independent of the impact of negative affect (Marsland, Cohen, Rabin, & Manuck, 2006). Unlike some other studies (Cohen et al., 2003; Cohen & Pressman, 2006; Pressman & Cohen, 2012), follow-up analyses did not find differential effects for high- versus low-arousal positive emotions.

In research on 60 healthy, U.S. young adults, half of participants were exposed to a speech-related stressor. In those exposed to the stressor, greater trait, high-activation positive affect (measured with the Positive subscale of the PANAS (Watson et al., 1988) was related to faster skin barrier recovery, an indicator of healthier immune functioning. Results held when also controlling for trait negative affect (Robles, Brooks, & Pressman, 2009). Similarly, in research on 124 first-year U.S. law students, increase in positive affect over a year was related to healthier immune responses (Segerstrom & Sephton, 2010). Positive affect was measured at several times over the year, using an average of the Positive subscale of an expanded PANAS (PANAS-X; Watson & Clark, 1994), which, unlike the original PANAS, included both low- and high-activation affect. Immune function was not related to negative affect, and results were not altered by sex, age, menstrual phase, prescription medications, alcohol, caffeine, smoking, exercise, cold symptoms, or allergy or asthma symptoms.

Positive Affect and Cardiovascular Function

A cardiovascular pathway that includes indicators such as blood pressure and heart rate variability may also mediate the association of positive affect with physical health. A number of studies have examined heart rate variability (also called vagal tone), a measure of the variability in the time between heartbeats. This variation is partially under the control of the parasympathetic nervous system, specifically the vagus system, which can slow heart rate. As greater heart rate variability is an index of physical health, it may be a process through which positive affect can increase physical well-being (Marsland et al., 2007; Steptoe, Dockray, & Wardle, 2009). For example, 67 British individuals with likely coronary heart disease were measured for 24 hours for heart rate variability (Bhattacharyya, Whitehead, Rakhit, & Steptoe, 2008). Their positive affect was measured using the day reconstruction method, in which participants thought about each episode of their day and rated them for how much they felt happy in each. The ratings were weighted by duration of the episode and then averaged. After researchers controlled for age, sex, health indices, medication use, smoking, BMI, physical activity, and depression, positive affect was related to greater heart rate variability during the day. Similarly, in a study of 68 heterosexual U.S. couples, for women only, resting heart rate variability was related to the average positive affect, measured daily for 3 weeks with the Positive subscale of the PANAS (Diamond, Hicks, & Otter-Henderson, 2011).

Naturally occurring positive affect may also help reduce cardiovascular arousal as measured through heart rate or blood pressure. Research with 33 adults in the Netherlands measured ambulatory heart rate and positive affect every hour for a day. If people were experiencing positive affect, their heart rate decreased in the 5-minute epoch following the initial heart rate measurement (Brosschot & Thayer, 2003). Positive affect was measured using a 5-point scale from 5 (negative valence) to 1 (positive valence).

Several studies have found that positive affect can help undo the negative effects of stress or anxiety on cardiovascular indices. In research on 60 female, U.S. college students, participants assigned to watch a short contentment-inducing or amusing film after a short fear-inducing film showed a faster cardiovascular recovery than those assigned to watch a neutral or sad film (Fredrickson & Levenson, 1998). In other words, the positive emotions of contentment or amusement helped the students recover physiologically from fear. In a follow-up study, results were replicated in a larger sample using a speech preparation task to induce anxiety, rather than a fear-inducing video (Fredrickson, Mancuso, Branigan, & Tugade, 2000). As before, the contentment-inducing and amusing films helped participants physiologically recover more quickly than a neutral or sad film.

A study of 203 female, U.S. nurses examined ambulatory blood pressure and positive affect every 20 minutes for 4 days. Researchers found that positive affect seemed to undo the deleterious effects of anxiety on diastolic blood pressure (Shapiro, Jamner, Goldstein, & Delfino, 2001). Participants rated their positive affect by rating how much they were feeling "happy," on a scale from 1 (none) to 5 (an extreme amount). In other words, positive affect helped reduce the higher blood pressure induced by anxiety.

In research on 72 healthy British men, diastolic blood pressure recovery from a laboratory stressor was more rapid for participants with higher positive affect (Steptoe, Gibson, Hamer, & Wardle, 2007). Positive affect was measured four times over 2 days as how much participants were feeling happiness in the past 5 minutes from 1 (low) to 5 (high). These ratings were then divided into quintiles, with the lowest almost never reporting happiness and the highest almost always reporting happiness. Thus, men who felt happier in their day-to-day life recovered more rapidly from a laboratory stressor.

Positive Affect and Endocrine Indices

The primary stress response system, the hypothalamic–pituitary–adrenal (HPA) axis, and cortisol in particular, has been a focus of study as a likely link between psychological variables such as positive affect and physical health (Steptoe, Wardle, & Marmot, 2005). Cortisol is released not only in response to acute stressors but also in a predictable pattern throughout the day, with the highest levels in the morning, peaking shortly after waking, and a steady decline until evening. Chronic or repeated stress can lead to alterations in daily cortisol secretion leading to a more maladaptive pattern—chronically elevated levels, or a flatter diurnal rhythm (Abercrombie et al., 2004; Bower et al., 2005; Sephton, Sapolsky, Kraemer, & Spiegel, 2000). A number of studies have demonstrated that positive affect is associated with a more adaptive cortisol level and diurnal pattern. For example, positive affect is associated with lower total levels of cortisol (Lindfors & Lundberg, 2002; Smyth et al., 1998; Steptoe et al., 2005). In a sample of 72 men (average age 33.6 years), Steptoe and colleagues (2007) found that average daily momentary assessments of positive affect (happiness) were associated with lower levels of cortisol earlier in the day. Specifically, the average cortisol awakening response over 2 days, controlling for age, BMI, time of waking in the morning, and negative affect was lower among participants with higher momentary positive affect compared to those with lower momentary positive affect. It is noteworthy, however, that retrospective reports of positive affect, as assessed with the PANAS, were not associated with the cortisol awakening response.

Quirin, Kazén, Rohrmann, and Kuhl (2009) used an implicit measure of affect to examine correlations of positive and negative affect with cortisol levels over the course of 2 days in a sample of 32 women ages 20–36. The implicit measure of affect paired nonsense words with either positive (happy, cheerful, energetic) or negative (helpless, tense inhibited) affect words and had participants indicate whether the nonsense word was positive or negative. The participant's tendency to rate the nonsense words as positive or negative was taken as an indication of his or her dispositional affect. Results indicated that participants who were more likely to rate the nonsense words as positive had lower levels of cortisol throughout the day. There was no association of implicit negative affect or explicit positive or negative affect (as measured with the PANAS) with cortisol.

The evidence relating positive affect to adaptive cortisol patterns is not entirely consistent, however. There is some contrary evidence demonstrating that positive affect is associated with a flattened diurnal cortisol rhythm (Lindfors & Lundberg, 2002; Polk, Cohen, Doyle, Skoner, & Kirschbaum, 2005). In their review of positive affect and health-relevant biological factors, Dockray and Steptoe (2010) suggest that the inconsistent evidence of the association between positive affect and cortisol may be attributable, in part, to age and gender differences across the samples. This possibility merits further study.

Positive Affect and Adaptive Health Behaviors

A second likely pathway linking positive affect to lower risk of morbidity and mortality is through improved health behaviors. Positive affect may facilitate attention to and processing of health-relevant informa-

tion, which is an important prerequisite for engagement in health-promoting behaviors. Salovey and Birnbaum (1989) randomly assigned participants who had a cold or flu to a positive, neutral or negative mood via an experimental mood manipulation. They then had participants report on symptoms and discomfort, and rate how confident they were that they could carry out a series of 26 health-promoting behaviors. Those participants in a positive mood reported significantly fewer aches and pains, less discomfort, and were significantly more confident that they could carry out the health-promoting behaviors. Reed and Aspinwall (1998) found that women who were given the opportunity to affirm a positive aspect of themselves (and presumably experience positive affect as a result) oriented to information regarding their risk of a serious illness more quickly than did those not given the opportunity to affirm another aspect of the self. They also found the information more convincing and recalled more of the risk-confirming information at a 1-week follow-up session. These findings suggest the possibility that increases in positive affect may help individuals attend to information regarding their health and perhaps facilitate more effective preventive care.

Although the bulk of the research regarding affect and adherence to medication and other health recommendations has focused on negative affect (DiMatteo, Lepper, & Croghan, 2000; Gordillo, del Amo, Soriano, & Gonzalez-Lahoz, 1999; Holzemer et al., 1999; Paterson et al., 2000), emergent findings are beginning to indicate that positive affect may be uniquely associated with better adherence. For example, Gonzales and colleagues (2004) found that positive states of mind (a measure of the ability to attain positive psychological states; Horowitz, Adler, & Kegeles, 1988) was associated with better antiretroviral adherence in a sample of 90 people living with HIV. Similarly, in a sample of 153 people newly diagnosed with HIV, Carrico and Moskowitz (in press) found that positive affect, as measured with the modified Differential Emotions Scale (Fredrickson, Tugade, Waugh, & Larkin, 2003) in the month after diagnosis was associated with a higher likelihood of linkage to medical care for HIV, and a greater likelihood of initiating and remaining on antiretroviral therapy. These effects were independent of negative affect.

A recent intervention that explicitly targeted positive affect resulted in significant improvements in adherence to medication in a sample of 256 African Americans with hypertension (Ogedegbe et al., 2012). Participants were randomized to receive an education booklet plus positive affect and self-affirmation intervention or an education booklet alone. Bimonthly, participants in the positive affect condition were reminded to savor small things in their lives that make them feel good and to consider times when they felt proud in situations that made adhering to their medical regimen difficult. They also received small, bimonthly gifts such as T-shirts. At the end of the 12-month trial, the participants in the positive affect condition had significantly better adherence compared to the education booklet only condition (42% of doses taken vs. 36% of doses taken). The authors did not, however, report whether increases in positive affect mediated the effect of the intervention on adherence. Another study by the same group of researchers (Peterson et al., 2012) found that the positive affect intervention was associated with a greater likelihood of achieving exercise recommendations in patients who had undergone coronary angioplasty. Compared to individuals in the control condition, those in the positive affect condition were 1.7 times more likely to meet the exercise goals over 12 months. The authors note that a change on the PANAS score predicted a change in the number of calories expended at 12 months, although they do not specify that the change was due to the Positive Affect subscale, Negative Affect subscale, or both, so it is not clear whether increased positive affect uniquely predicted adherence to exercise goals.

Positive Affect and Resources for Coping

Finally, the third major pathway potentially linking positive affect with improved physical health outcomes is via increased coping resources, such as social support, that enable the individual to cope better with stress in a variety of ways (Folkman & Moskowitz, 2000; Fredrickson, 1998; Tugade & Fredrickson, 2004), thus buffering the effect of stress on physical health. Consistent with

the idea that positive emotion may influence health via increased personal resources for coping, Fredrickson, Cohn, Coffey, Pek, and Finkel (2008) found that a meditation intervention that increased positive emotions also subsequently increased personal resources, including self-acceptance, positive relations with others, and mindful attention. These resources are hypothesized to support further adaptive coping efforts (Fredrickson & Levenson, 1998).

Social support is another important coping resource that has received research attention. Positive affect is hypothesized to facilitate social support, and social support has been shown to be associated with improved health outcomes (Cohen & Wills, 1985). When researchers control for negative affect and other potential confounders, positive affect is associated with greater social connectedness (Steptoe, O'Donnell, Marmot, & Wardle, 2008). Bonanno and Keltner (1997) found that bereaved individuals who showed genuine laughs or smiles (as determined by coding of facial expressions), while describing the relationship with their deceased spouse, elicited more positive affect and less frustration in observers than bereaved individuals who did not show the genuine laughs or smiles. Perhaps more importantly, untrained observers indicated that they would be more likely to offer comfort to those individuals who showed the genuine laughs or smiles. These findings suggest that individuals may elicit social support from others by their displays of positive affect.

Complexity of Meditational Pathways

The pathways mediating the association between positive affect and health outcomes are likely to be complex and multidimensional, not the simple unidirectional associations we described earlier. Instead, it may be that multiple pathways are in play, and that these pathways interact with each other and with contextual variables to influence physical health. For example, one likely scenario in HIV is that positive affect is associated with improved immune response (Ickovics et al., 2006) and better adherence to medication (Carrico & Moskowitz, in press). This in turn increases self-efficacy for engaging in further beneficial health behaviors (Reed & Aspinwall, 1998) and improves coping (Moskowitz, Hult, Bussolari, & Acree, 2009), which then buffers the response to subsequent stressors, and, finally, feeds back to increase positive affect.

Testing such complex associations among multiple variables can be resource and time intensive and presents a significant challenge to researchers. Any single study, no matter how large and long term, is unlikely to provide the final word in associations of positive affect; physical health; and the biological, behavioral, and psychological mediators. However, taken as a whole, a series of thoughtfully designed, systematically conducted, theory-guided studies will significantly advance our understanding of these associations.

Discussion

In this chapter we have reviewed a significant body of literature demonstrating that positive affect is associated with better health. A number of questions remain, however, and suggest several recommendations to help move the field forward. In our view, the key issues that need attention are measurement of positive affect, thoughtful inclusion of mediators and moderators, and randomized trials that test interventions to increase positive affect, enabling stronger causal conclusions regarding positive affect and physical health.

Measuring Positive Affect

Much of the research on positive affect and health has come out of medical or epidemiological studies with a focus on the physical health outcome rather than affective predictors. As a result, many studies have relied on measures of positive affect that have significant overlap with physical health by asking about vigor, energy, or strength (Birket-Smith et al., 2009; Cohen et al., 2003; Pressman & Cohen, 2012; Wiest et al., 2011). Research in emotion would benefit future studies by making several important contributions. First, emotions can be conceptualized as having both valence and arousal/activation. For example, "calm" is a positively valenced low-arousal emotion, whereas "ecstatic" is a positively valenced high-arousal emotion. Although most research on positive affect and health has ignored this potentially important distinction between high- and low-activation emotions, Cohen and Pressman's research (Cohen et al., 2003; Pressman & Cohen, 2012) has measured positive emotions with respect to their level of arousal. In both cases, higher- but not lower-arousal positive emotions were related to health. Thus, we recommend that research distinguish among high-arousal positive affect without physical vigor (enthusiastic, excited, and elated, but not vigorous, strong, and energetic), midlevel-arousal positive affect (happy, satisfied, and content), and low-arousal positive affect (calm, relaxed, peaceful, and serene).

Modern emotion researchers have also made great efforts to study discrete positive emotions, with some arguing that simply describing emotions using valence and arousal greatly oversimplifies our emotional experiences (Ekman, 1992; Oatley, Keltner, & Jenkins, 2006). Happiness, pride, hope, relief, love, compassion, thankfulness, amusement, curiosity, moral uplift (or elevation), contentment, and awe are all positive emotions that can be measured and distinguished from one another (Goldberg et al., 2006; Park, Peterson, & Seligman, 2004; Shiota, Keltner, & John, 2006). Currently we know very little about how discrete positive emotions may be differentially related to health. However, measuring these discrete positive emotions may open up a host of possible pathways through which positive affect influences physical health (Consedine & Moskowitz, 2007).

Given the resource-intensive nature of the large epidemiological studies required to provide reliable data to address questions about the association between positive affect and mortality and morbidity in general population samples, space on questionnaires is often at a premium. If researchers have space for only one item related to positive affect, however, they might consider asking about enjoyment. In three different studies, a question about enjoyment predicted greater longevity (Moskowitz et al., 2008; Scherer & Herrmann-Lingen, 2009; Shirai et al., 2009), although measured slightly differently in each of the three: "I enjoyed life" (in the past week); "Are you enjoying your life?"; or "I still enjoy the things I used to enjoy." A problem with a single "enjoyment" measure is that it may be confounded with physical health and simply differentiate between those healthy enough to enjoy life and those who are not. Careful control for baseline physical health will help address this concern and enable researchers to determine whether enjoyment, independent of functional status or other indicators of physical health, is significantly predictive of morbidity and mortality.

Mediators, Moderators, and Confounders

Our review of the literature reveals that researchers often statistically control for a number of constructs, including some of the variables that are hypothesized as potential mediators of the association between positive affect and health. For example, several of the studies we reviewed controlled for social support by including marital status (Abel & Kruger, 2010; Blazer & Hybels, 2004; Wiest et al., 2011), whether the participant lived alone (Lyyra et al., 2006), or number of social contacts (Birket-Smith et al., 2009) in the analysis. Similarly, researchers have controlled for health behaviors, including smoking (Krijthe et al., 2011; Shirai et al., 2009; Steptoe & Wardle, 2011) and physical activity (Shirai et al., 2009; Steptoe & Wardle, 2011). On the one hand, the fact that inclusion of these variables did not significantly decrease the association between positive affect and health indicates that they are unlikely to be the sole factor linking affect and physical health. However, a careful meditational analysis in which each of these variables was systematically tested individually, and then in combination with other potential mediators, would significantly advance our understanding of the true nature of the associations.

There are a number of likely moderators of the association of positive affect and health that merit careful consideration. Age has shown to be critical, with some research demonstrating a stronger association between positive affect and mortality in older samples (Moskowitz et al., 2008). There are exceptions to this finding, however (Krijthe et al., 2011), that indicate the importance of studying samples with a wide age range. Other possible moderators include the baseline stress level of the

individual (Zautra, 2003) and personality (Emmons & Diener, 1985).

Culture, too, may be important in terms of the differential value placed on positive affect and well-being in different cultures (Tsai, Knutson, & Fung, 2006; Uchida & Kitayama, 2009). Regarding cultural differences in the association of positive affect and health, future work could draw on ideas developed by Tsai and colleagues (e.g., 2006), who have found that not only do people make distinctions between arousal levels of positive affect but these levels are also differentially valued. In the United States and Europe, high-arousal positive affect is often more valued, whereas in Asia, low arousal positive affect is often more valued. Future research could examine whether culture alters the impact of high- versus low-arousal positive affect on health. For example, researchers could test whether it is healthier to feel culturally appropriate versus inappropriate positive affect.

A potentially important confounding factor that is often overlooked is sleep. Sleep is important for health (for a review, see Alvarez & Ayas, 2004) and is tied to the experience of positive affect (Berger, Miller, Seifer, Cares, & Lebourgeois, 2012; Kaida, Takahashi, & Otsuka, 2007; Lamarche, Driver, Forest, & De Koninck, 2010; Luo & Inoué, 2000; Robles et al., 2009), attention toward positive stimuli (Gujar, McDonald, Nishida, & Walker, 2011), and memory for positive events (Walker & van der Helm, 2009). There is likely a bidirectional association between positive affect and sleep, such that an individual who sleeps better will likely experience more positive affect and better health; or, it may be that happier individuals sleep better, therefore improving their own health. Yet again, poor health may disturb sleep and positive affect. Future research needs to do a better job of measuring and understanding the role of sleep in the link between positive affect and health.

At minimum, we recommend that all analyses of positive affect and health control for negative affect and baseline physical health. Even though positive affect and negative affect differentially predict physical health outcomes, their effects are not entirely independent, and it is important to control for negative affect in order to demonstrate that presence of positive affect is not the same as absence of negative affect (Pressman & Cohen, 2005). Similarly, it is important to control for indicators of physical health status in order to ensure that positive affect is not simply a reflection of poor health instead of a predictor of future morbidity and mortality.

Positive Affect Interventions: The Next Big Frontier?

The majority of the studies on positive affect and physical health are observational. Although these studies provide critical data on naturally occurring positive affect, without experimental studies that manipulate positive affect and demonstrate effects on health-relevant outcomes, the link between positive affect and health is open to question, particularly regarding the direction of causality and influence of potential unmeasured variables (Coyne, Tennen, & Ranchor, 2010).

The next critical step for the field is the development and testing of positive affect interventions to address questions of causality more definitely. Several existing interventions appear to influence positive affect (Moskowitz, 2010a). Numerous research groups are currently testing such interventions with people who cope with serious illness, and are exploring the impact of the intervention on health-relevant outcomes. For example, as described earlier, a cluster of three different randomized trials designed to increase positive affect and self-efficacy, in order to increase medication adherence or physical activity, have shown some promise (Mancuso et al., 2012; Ogedegbe et al., 2012; Peterson et al., 2012).

We are currently conducting a trial of a positive affect intervention for people newly diagnosed with HIV and are looking at effects of the intervention on health behaviors, resources for coping, as well as direct effects on biological indicators of HIV progression (CD4 and viral load). The theoretically based intervention comprises eight skills that are hypothesized to increase the daily experience of positive affect and, ultimately, result in improvements in health-relevant outcomes. Pilot studies indicate that the intervention is feasible and acceptable, and preliminary data for the intervention were promising in terms of efficacy

for increasing positive affect (Moskowitz, 2010b; Moskowitz et al., 2012). We have also begun pilot tests of the intervention in samples coping with advanced breast cancer and type 2 diabetes. Finally, we are also developing the intervention for people coping with general life stress: high school students and university employees. We are exploring associations with outcomes such as substance use (in the students) and work burnout (in the employees).

Conclusion

A recently published study provided convincing evidence that the association between positive affect and health is widespread. Researchers examined the association of observer-rated positive affect and longevity in 150 individuals and found that those subjects who displayed more positive affect lived significantly longer (Weiss, Adams, & King, 2011). This may not seem particularly noteworthy given the numerous other studies we reviewed demonstrating this link. What is surprising, however, is that the participants were orangutans. It is possible to measure positive emotion in many other species (Boissy et al., 2007), for example, through play behavior or positive vocalizations, such as purring in cats (Yeates & Main, 2008). Moreover, in a recent review on improving farm animal welfare, it was noted that socially enriched environments with known conspecifics can help animals cope with stress and recover more quickly from health problems. These results mirror those found in humans (Rault, 2012). In other words, positive affect may be beneficial for health across species.

The field of health psychology is clearly poised for a shift away from a narrow, negative-affect-only focus toward a broader view that includes positive affect as well. This is not to say that negative affect is not important. We are not advocating a simplistic positive-affect-only approach to improved physical health. Clearly negative emotions serve important adaptive functions and at sustained or extreme levels, need to be addressed directly. However, we argue that positive affect is a key factor in the effect of psychology on physical health, and it is a worthy focus of further research and intervention.

References

Abel, E. L., & Kruger, M. L. (2010). Smile intensity in photographs predicts longevity. *Psychological Science, 21*(4), 542–544.

Abercrombie, H. C., Giese-Davis, J., Sephton, S., Epel, E. S., Turner-Cobb, J. M., & Spiegel, D. (2004). Flattened cortisol rhythms in metastatic breast cancer patients. *Psychoneuroendocrinology, 29*(8), 1082–1092.

Alvarez, G. G., & Ayas, N. T. (2004). The impact of daily sleep duration on health: A review of the literature. *Progress in Cardiovascular Nursing, 19*(2), 56–59.

Bech, P. (1998). *Quality of life in the psychiatric patient.* London: Mosby-Wolfe.

Berger, R., Miller, A., Seifer, R., Cares, S., & Lebourgeois, M. (2012). Acute sleep restriction effects on emotion responses in 30-to 36-month-old children. *Journal of Sleep Research, 21*(3), 235–246.

Bhattacharyya, M. R., Whitehead, D. L., Rakhit, R., & Steptoe, A. (2008). Depressed mood, positive affect, and heart rate variability in patients with suspected coronary artery disease. *Psychosomatic Medicine, 70*(9), 1020–1027.

Birket-Smith, M., Hansen, B. H., Hanash, J. A., Hansen, J. F., & Rasmussen, A. (2009). Mental disorders and general well-being in cardiology outpatients—6-year survival. *Journal of Psychosomatic Research, 67*(1), 5–10.

Blazer, D. G., & Hybels, C. F. (2004). What symptoms of depression predict mortality in community-dwelling elders? *Journal of the American Geriatric Society, 52,* 2052–2056.

Boissy, A., Manteuffel, G., Jensen, M. B., Moe, R. O., Spruijt, B., Keeling, L. J., et al. (2007). Assessment of positive emotions in animals to improve their welfare. *Physiology and Behavior, 92*(3), 375–397.

Bonanno, G. A., & Keltner, D. (1997). Facial expressions of emotion and the course of conjugal bereavement. *Journal of Abnormal Psychology, 106,* 126–137.

Bower, J. E., Ganz, P. A., Dickerson, S. S., Petersen, L., Aziz, N., & Fahey, J. L. (2005). Diurnal cortisol rhythm and fatigue in breast cancer survivors. *Psychoneuroendocrinology, 30*(1), 92–100.

Bradburn, N., & Caplovitz, D. (1965). *Reports on happiness: A pilot study of behavior related to mental health.* Chicago: Aldine.

Brosschot, J. F., & Thayer, J. F. (2003). Heart rate response is longer after negative emotions than after positive emotions. *International Journal of Psychophysiology, 50*(3), 181–187.

Brown, K. W., Levy, A. R., Rosberger, Z., & Edgar, L. (2003). Psychological distress and cancer survival: A follow-up 10 years after diagnosis. *Psychosomatic Medicine, 65*(4), 636–643.

Carrico, A. W., & Moskowitz, J. T. (in press). Positive affect promotes engagement in care following HIV diagnosis. *Health Psychology.*

Chida, Y., & Steptoe, A. (2008). Positive psychological well-being and mortality: A quantitative review of prospective observational studies. *Psychosomatic Medicine, 70,* 741–756.

Cohen, S., Alper, C. M., Doyle, W. J., Treanor, J. J., & Turner, R. B. (2006). Positive emotional style predicts resistance to illness after experimental exposure to rhinovirus or influenza A virus. *Psychosomatic Medicine, 68,* 809–815.

Cohen, S., Doyle, W. J., Turner, R. B., Alper, C. M., & Skoner, D. P. (2003). Emotional style and susceptibility to the common cold. *Psychosomatic Medicine, 65,* 652–657.

Cohen, S., & Pressman, S. D. (2006). Positive affect and health. *Current Directions in Psychological Science, 15*(3), 122–125.

Cohen, S., & Wills, T. A. (1985). Stress, social support, and the buffering hypothesis. *Psychological Bulletin, 98*(2), 310–357.

Consedine, N. S., & Moskowitz, J. T. (2007). The role of discrete emotions in health outcomes: A critical review. *Applied and Preventive Psychology, 12,* 59–75.

Coyne, J. C., Tennen, H., & Ranchor, A. V. (2010). Positive psychology in cancer care: A story line resistant to evidence. *Annals of Behavioral Medicine, 39*(1), 35–42.

Danner, D. D., Snowdon, D. A., & Friesen, W. V. (2001). Positive emotions in early life and longevity: Findings from the nun study. *Journal of Personality and Social Psychology, 80,* 804–813.

Davidson, K. W., Mostofsky, E., & Whang, W. (2010). Don't worry, be happy: Positive affect and reduced 10-year incident coronary heart disease: The Canadian Nova Scotia Health Survey. *European Heart Journal, 31*(9), 1065–1070.

Diamond, L. M., Hicks, A. M., & Otter-Henderson, K. D. (2011). Individual differences in vagal regulation moderate associations between daily affect and daily couple interactions. *Personality and Social Psychology Bulletin, 37*(6), 731–744.

Diener, E., & Chan, M. Y. (2011). Happy people

live longer: Subjective well-being contributes to health and longevity. *Applied Psychology: Health and Well-Being, 3*(1), 1–43.

Diener, E., Emmons, R. A., Larsen, R. J., & Griffin, S. (1985). The Satisfaction with Life Scale. *Journal of Personality Assessment, 49*(1), 71–75.

DiMatteo, M. R., Lepper, H. S., & Croghan, T. W. (2000). Depression is a risk factor for noncompliance with medical treatment: meta-analysis of the effects of anxiety and depression on patient adherence. *Archives of Internal Medicine, 160*(14), 2101–2107.

Dockray, S., & Steptoe, A. (2010). Positive affect and psychobiological processes. *Neuroscience and Biobehavioral Reviews, 35*(1), 69–75.

Ekman, P. (1992). An argument for basic emotions. *Cognition and Emotion, 6*(3/4), 169–200.

Ellsworth, P. C., & Smith, C. A. (1988). Shades of joy: Patterns of appraisal differentiating pleasant emotions. *Cognition and Emotion, 2*(4), 301–331.

Emmons, R. A., & Diener, E. (1985). Personality correlates of subjective well-being. *Personality and Social Psychology Bulletin, 11*(1), 89–97.

Emmons, R. A., & McCullough, M. E. (2003). Counting blessings versus burdens: An experimental investigation of gratitude and subjective well-being in daily life. *Journal of Personality and Social Psychology, 84*, 377–389.

Folkman, S., & Moskowitz, J. T. (2000). Positive affect and the other side of coping. *American Psychologist, 55*, 647–654.

Fredrickson, B. L. (1998). What good are positive emotions? *Review of General Psychology, 2*, 300–319.

Fredrickson, B. L., Cohn, M. A., Coffey, K. A., Pek, J., & Finkel, S. M. (2008). Open hearts build lives: Positive emotions, induced through meditation, build consequential personal resources. *Journal of Personality and Social Psychology, 95*, 1045–1062.

Fredrickson, B. L., & Levenson, R. W. (1998). Positive emotions speed recovery from the cardiovascular sequelae of negative emotions. *Cognition and Emotion, 12*(2), 191–220.

Fredrickson, B. L., Mancuso, R. A., Branigan, C., & Tugade, M. M. (2000). The undoing effect of positive emotions. *Motivation and Emotion, 24*(4), 237–258.

Fredrickson, B. L., Tugade, M. M., Waugh, C. E., & Larkin, G. R. (2003). What good are positive emotions in crises?: A prospective study of resilience and emotions following the terrorist attacks on the United States on September 11th, 2001. *Journal of Personality and Social Psychlogy, 84*, 365–376.

Futterman, A. D., Kemeny, M. E., Shapiro, D., & Fahey, J. L. (1994). Immunological and physiological changes associated with induced positive and negative mood. *Psychosomatic Medicine, 56*, 499–511.

Goldberg, L. R., Johnson, J. A., Eber, H. W., Hogan, R., Ashton, M. C., Cloninger, C. R., et al. (2006). The International Personality Item Pool and the future of public-domain personality measures. *Journal of Research in Personality, 40*(1), 84–96.

Gonzalez, J. S., Penedo, F. J., Antoni, M., Duran, R. E., Fernandez, M. I., McPherson-Baker, S., et al. (2004). Social support, positive states of mind, and HIV treatment adherence in men and women living with HIV/AIDS. *Health Psychology, 23*, 413–418.

Gordillo, V., del Amo, J., Soriano, V., & Gonzalez-Lahoz, J. (1999). Sociodemographic and psychological variables influencing adherence to antiretroviral therapy. *AIDS, 13*, 1763–1769.

Gujar, N., McDonald, S. A., Nishida, M., & Walker, M. P. (2011). A role for REM sleep in recalibrating the sensitivity of the human brain to specific emotions. *Cerebral Cortex, 21*(1), 115–123.

Holzemer, W. L., Corless, I. B., Nokes, K. M., Turner, J. G., Brown, M. A., Powell-Cope, G. M., et al. (1999). Predictors of self-reported adherence in persons living with HIV disease. *AIDS Patient Care and STDs, 13*(3), 185–197.

Horowitz, M. J., Adler, N., & Kegeles, S. (1988). A scale for measuring the occurrence of positive states of mind: A preliminary report. *Psychosomatic Medicine, 50*(5), 477–483.

Howell, R. T., Kern, M. L., & Lyubomirsky, S. (2007). Health benefits: Meta-analytically determining the impact of well-being on objective health outcomes. *Health Psychology Review, 1*, 83–136.

Ickovics, J. R., Milan, S., Boland, R., Schoenbaum, E., Schuman, P., & Vlahov, D. (2006). Psychological resources protect health: 5-year survival and immune function among HIV-infected women from four US cities. *AIDS, 20*(14), 1851–1860.

Isen, A. M., Daubman, K. A., & Nowicki, G. P. (1987). Positive affect facilitates creative problem solving. *Journal of Personality and Social Psychology, 52*, 1122–1131.

Kaida, K., Takahashi, M., & Otsuka, Y. (2007).

A short nap and natural bright light exposure improve positive mood status. *Industrial Health, 45*(2), 301–308.

Krijthe, B. P., Walter, S., Newson, R. S., Hofman, A., Hunink, M. G., & Tiemeier, H. (2011). Is positive affect associated with survival? A population-based study of elderly persons. *American Journal of Epidemiology, 173*(11), 1298–1307.

Lamarche, L. J., Driver, H. S., Forest, G., & De Koninck, J. (2010). Napping during the late-luteal phase improves sleepiness, alertness, mood and cognitive performance in women with and without premenstrual symptoms. *Sleep and Biological Rhythms, 8*(2), 151–159.

Lamers, S. M. A., Bolier, L., Westerhof, G. J., Smit, F., & Bohlmeijer, E. T. (2012). The impact of emotional well-being on long-term recovery and survival in physical illness: A meta-analysis. *Journal of Behavioral Medicine, 35*(5), 538–547.

Lindfors, P., & Lundberg, U. (2002). Is low cortisol release an indicator of positive health? *Stress and Health, 18*, 153–160.

Luo, Z., & Inoué, S. (2000). A short daytime nap modulates levels of emotions objectively evaluated by the emotion spectrum analysis method. *Psychiatry and Clinical Neurosciences, 54*(2), 207–212.

Lyubomirsky, S. (2007). *The how of happiness.* New York: Penguin.

Lyyra, T. M., Törmäkangas, T. M., Read, S., Rantanen, T., & Berg, S. (2006). Satisfaction with present life predicts survival in octogenarians. *Journals of Gerontology B: Psychological Sciences and Social Sciences, 61*(6), P319–P326.

Mancuso, C. A., Choi, T. N., Westermann, H., Wenderoth, S., Hollenberg, J. P., Wells, M. T., et al. (2012). Increasing physical activity in patients with asthma through positive affect and self-affirmation: A randomized trial. *Archives of Internal Medicine, 172*(4), 337–343.

Marsland, A. L., Cohen, S., Rabin, B. S., & Manuck, S. B. (2006). Trait positive affect and antibody response to hepatitis B vaccination. *Brain, Behavior, and Immunity, 20*(3), 261–269.

Marsland, A. L., Gianaros, P. J., Prather, A. A., Jennings, J. R., Neumann, S. A., & Manuck, S. B. (2007). Stimulated production of proinflammatory cytokines covaries inversely with heart rate variability. *Psychosomatic Medicine, 69*(8), 709–716.

Marsland, A. L., Pressman, S., & Cohen, S. (2007). Positive affect and immune function. *Psychoneuroimmunology, 4*, 761–779.

Moskowitz, J. T. (2003). Positive affect predicts lower risk of AIDS mortality. *Psychosomatic Medicine, 65*, 620–626.

Moskowitz, J. T. (2010a). Coping interventions and the regulation of positive affect. In S. Folkman (Ed.), *The Oxford handbook of stress, health, and coping* (pp. 407–427). New York: Oxford University Press.

Moskowitz, J. T. (2010b). Positive affect at the onset of chronic illness: Planting the seeds of resilience. In J. W. Reich, A. J. Zautra, & J. Hall (Eds.), *Handbook of adult resilience* (pp. 465–483). New York: Guilford Press.

Moskowitz, J. T., Epel, E. S., & Acree, M. (2008). Positive affect uniquely predicts lower risk of mortality in people with diabetes. *Health Psychology, 27*, S73–S82.

Moskowitz, J. T., Hult, J. R., Bussolari, C., & Acree, M. (2009). What works in coping with HIV?: A meta-analysis with implications for coping with serious illness. *Psychological Bulletin, 135*, 121–141.

Moskowitz, J. T., Hult, J. R., Duncan, L. G., Cohn, M. A., Maurer, S. A., Bussolari, C., et al. (2012). A positive affect intervention for people experiencing health-related stress: Development and non-randomized pilot test. *Journal of Health Psychology, 17*(5), 676–692.

Oatley, K., Keltner, D., & Jenkins, J. M. (2006). *Understanding emotions.* Wiley-Blackwell.

Ogedegbe, G. O., Boutin-Foster, C., Wells, M. T., Allegrante, J. P., Isen, A. M., Jobe, J. B., et al. (2012). A randomized controlled trial of positive-affect intervention and medication adherence in hypertensive African Americans. *Archives of Internal Medicine, 172*(4), 322–326.

Ostir, G. V., Markides, K. S., Black, S. A., & Goodwin, J. S. (2000). Emotional well-being predicts subsequent functional independence and survival. *Journal of the American Geriatrics Society, 48*, 473–478.

Ostir, G. V., Markides, K. S., Peek, M. K., & Goodwin, J. S. (2001). The association between emotional well-being and the incidence of stroke in older adults. *Psychosomatic Medicine, 63*(2), 210–215.

Park, N., Peterson, C., & Seligman, M. E. P. (2004). Strengths of character and well-being. *Journal of Social and Clinical Psychology, 23*(5), 603–619.

Paterson, D. L., Swindells, S., Mohr, J., Brester, M., Vergis, E. N., Squier, C., et al. (2000). Adherence to protease inhibitor therapy and outcomes in patients with HIV infection. *Annals of Internal Medicine, 133*(1), 21–30.

Peterson, J. C., Charlson, M. E., Hoffman, Z., Wells, M. T., Wong, S. C., Hollenberg, J. P., et al. (2012). Randomized controlled trial of positive affect induction to promote physical activity after percutaneous coronary intervention. *Archives of Internal Medicine,172*(4), 329–336.

Polk, D. E., Cohen, S., Doyle, W. J., Skoner, D. P., & Kirschbaum, C. (2005). State and trait affect as predictors of salivary cortisol in healthy adults. *Psychoneuroendocrinology, 30*(3), 261–272.

Pressman, S. D., & Cohen, S. (2005). Does positive affect influence health? *Psychological Bulletin, 131*(6), 925–971.

Pressman, S. D., & Cohen, S. (2012). Positive emotion word use and longevity in famous deceased psychologists. *Health Psychology, 31*(3), 297–305.

Quirin, M., Kazén, M., Rohrmann, S., & Kuhl, J. (2009). Implicit but not explicit affectivity predicts circadian and reactive cortisol: Using the Implicit Positive and Negative Affect Test. *Journal of Personality, 77*(2), 401–426.

Radloff, L. S. (1977). The CES-D Scale. *Applied Psychological Measurement, 1*(3), 385–401.

Rault, J. L. (2012). Friends with benefits: Social support and its relevance for farm animal welfare. *Applied Animal Behaviour Science, 136*, 1–14.

Reed, M. B., & Aspinwall, L. G. (1998). Self-affirmation reduces biased processing of health-risk information. *Motivation and Emotion, 22*, 99–132.

Richman, L. S., Kubzansky, L., Maselko, J., Kawachi, I., Choo, P., & Bauer, M. (2005). Positive emotion and health: Going beyond the negative. *Health Psychology, 24*(4), 422–429.

Robles, T. F., Brooks, K. P., & Pressman, S. D. (2009). Trait positive affect buffers the effects of acute stress on skin barrier recovery. *Health Psychology, 28*(3), 373–378.

Salovey, P., & Birnbaum, D. (1989). Influence of mood on health-relevant cognitions. *Journal of Personality and Social Psychology, 57*(3), 539–551.

Scherer, M., & Herrmann-Lingen, C. (2009). Single item on positive affect is associated with 1-year survival in consecutive medical inpatients. *General Hospital Psychiatry, 31*(1), 8–13.

Segerstrom, S. C., & Sephton, S. E. (2010). Optimistic expectancies and cell-mediated immunity. *Psychological Science, 21*(3), 448–455.

Sephton, S. E., Sapolsky, R. M., Kraemer, H. C., & Spiegel, D. (2000). Diurnal cortisol rhythm as a predictor of breast cancer survival. *Journal of the National Cancer Institute, 92*(12), 994–1000.

Shapiro, D., Jamner, L. D., Goldstein, I. B., & Delfino, R. J. (2001). Striking a chord: Moods, blood pressure, and heart rate in everyday life. *Psychophysiology, 38*(2), 197–204.

Shiota, M. N., Keltner, D., & John, O. P. (2006). Positive emotion dispositions differentially associated with Big Five personality and attachment style. *Journal of Positive Psychology, 1*(2), 61–71.

Shirai, K., Iso, H., Ohira, T., Ikeda, A., Noda, H., Honjo, K., et al. (2009). Perceived level of life enjoyment and risks of cardiovascular disease incidence and mortality. *Circulation, 120*(11), 956–963.

Smyth, J., Ockenfels, M. C., Porter, L., Kirschbaum, C., Hellhammer, D. H., & Stone, A. A. (1998). Stressors and mood measured on a momentary basis are associated with salivary cortisol secretion. *Psychoneuroendocrinology, 23*(4), 353–370.

Spielberger, C. D. (1986). *Preliminary manual for the State–Trait Personality Inventory (STPI).* Unpublished manuscript, University of South Florida, Tampa.

Steptoe, A., Dockray, S., & Wardle, J. (2009). Positive affect and psychobiological processes relevant to health. *Journal of Personality, 77*(6), 1747–1776.

Steptoe, A., Gibson, E. L., Hamer, M., & Wardle, J. (2007). Neuroendocrine and cardiovascular correlates of positive affect measured by ecoogical momentary assessment and by questionnaire. *Psychoneuroendocrinology, 32*, 56–64.

Steptoe, A., O'Donnell, K., Marmot, M., & Wardle, J. (2008). Positive affect and psychosocial processes related to health. *British Journal of Psychology, 99*(2), 211–227.

Steptoe, A., & Wardle, J. (2011). Positive affect measured using ecological momentary assessment and survival in older men and women. *Proceedings of the National Academy of Sciences USA, 108*(45), 18244–18248.

Steptoe, A., Wardle, J., & Marmot, M. (2005). Positive affect and health-related neuroendocrine, cardiovascular, and inflammatory processes. *Proceedings of the National Academy of Sciences USA, 102*(18), 6508–6512.

Stone, A. A., Cox, D. S., Valdimarsdottir, H., & Jandorf, L. (1987). Evidence that secretory IgA antibody is associated with daily mood. *Journal of Personality and Social Psychology, 52*(5), 988–993.

Tsai, J. L., Knutson, B., & Fung, H. H. (2006). Cultural variation in affect valuation. *Journal of Personality and Social Psychology, 90*(2), 288–307.

Tugade, M. M., & Fredrickson, B. L. (2004). Resilient individuals use positive emotions to bounce back from negative emotional experiences. *Journal of Personality and Social Psychlogy, 86*, 320–333.

Uchida, Y., & Kitayama, S. (2009). Happiness and unhappiness in east and west: Themes and variations. *Emotion, 9*(4), 441–456.

Walker, M. P., & van der Helm, E. (2009). Overnight therapy?: The role of sleep in emotional brain processing. *Psychological Bulletin, 135*(5), 731–748.

Watson, D., & Clark, L. A. (1994). *The PANAS-X: Manual for the Positive and Negative Affect Schedule—Expanded Form.* Ames: University of Iowa.

Watson, D., Clark, L. A., & Tellegen, A. (1988). Development and validation of brief measures of positive and negative affect: the PANAS scales. *Journal of Personality and Social Psychology, 54*(6), 1063–1070.

Weiss, A., Adams, M. J., & King, J. E. (2011). Happy orang-utans live longer lives. *Biology Letters, 7*(6), 872–874.

Wiest, M., Schüz, B., Webster, N., & Wurm, S. (2011). Subjective well-being and mortality revisited: Differential effects of cognitive and emotional facets of well-being on mortality. *Health Psychology, 30*(6), 728–735.

Wood, V., Wylie, M. L., & Sheafor, B. (1969). An analysis of a short self-report measure of life satisfaction: Correlation with rater judgments. *Journal of Gerontology, 24*(4), 465–469.

Xu, J., & Roberts, R. E. (2010). The power of positive emotions: It's a matter of life or death—subjective well-being and longevity over 28 years in a general population. *Health Psychology, 29*(1), 9–19.

Yeates, J., & Main, D. (2008). Assessment of positive welfare: A review. *Veterinary Journal, 175*(3), 293–300.

Zautra, A. (2003). *Emotions, stress, and health.* New York: Oxford University Press.

Zigmond, A. S., & Snaith, R. (1983). The Hospital Anxiety and Depression Scale. *Acta Psychiatrica Scandinavica, 67*(6), 361–370.

CHAPTER 25

■ ■ ■ ■ ■ ■ ■ ■ ■

Positive Emotion Disturbance across Clinical Disorders

June Gruber
Sunny J. Dutra
Aleena C. Hay
Hillary C. Devlin

I wanted change and excitement and to shoot off in all
directions myself, like the colored arrows from a Fourth
of July rocket.
—Sylvia Plath (1971)

The experience of happiness, and positive emotions more generally, is a basic building block of human nature (e.g., Myers & Diener, 1995). Positive emotions motivate us to pursue important goals, allow us to savor important experiences, and reinforce adaptive behavior patterns. It is no surprise that we see an overflowing amount of popular and scientific emphasis on understanding happiness, with an increasing interest in motivational speakers, psychotherapists, and scientific enterprises focused on ways to attain and maximize feelings of positive emotion and happiness (for reviews, see Lyubomirsky, King, & Diener, 2005; Lyubomirsky, Sheldon, & Schkade, 2005; Seligman & Csikszentmihalyi, 2000). From this robust body of work emerges a clear theme that positive emotion is a vital ingredient of our well-being and ability to flourish.

Although the benefits of positive emotion are clear, it is less clear whether positive emotions may, in certain contexts, be maladaptive (e.g., Gruber, Mauss, & Tamir, 2011). In other words, can feeling too good ever be bad or unmanageable, as alluded to in the opening quotation? In this chapter, we raise an intriguing and underexplored question: Is positive emotion always good for us, or can positive emotion sometimes go awry? One approach to explore this possibility further is to examine individuals with psychological disorders who exhibit notable absences, extremes, or perturbations in positive emotion functioning. Intuitively, it would seem that people who experience a relative dearth of positive emotion would encounter difficulties in attaining goals, forming strong social bonds, and general well-being. It is less intuitive, however, to consider the scenario of how and for whom experiencing too much positive emotion might yield maladaptive emotional and social outcomes.

Psychopathology as a Window into Positive Emotion

We suggest that exploring emotional disorders provides an important window into positive emotion disturbance and function. Specifically, examining individuals characterized by positive emotion disturbance enables a better understanding of how the normative function of positive emotion can break down, affording a view of the associated cognitive, biological, and social consequences of positive emotion dysfunction. For example, recent discoveries concerning relationships between autism and deficits in the self-conscious emotions (e.g., Heerey, Keltner, & Capps, 2003) point to likely origins of this disorder in theory of mind deficits, as well as provide means for identifying and possibly treating at-risk children. At the same time, studies of positive emotion dysfunction reveal systematic outcomes associated with deficits or excesses in positive emotion, thus informing claims about the basic function of positive emotion. Such investigations are an important step forward in identifying emotion-related deficits in clinical disorders, and provide insight into the normative function of positive emotion.

In this chapter, we aim to provide insight into the nature of positive emotion disturbance associated with psychopathology. We do so by highlighting three key positive emotion processes likely to be impacted by emotion disturbance: positive emotion *reactivity, anticipation* of positive outcomes, and *regulation* of positive emotion. We conclude by discussing social outcomes that result from dysfunction in these three process domains. In order to illustrate how these three processes are disrupted in psychopathology, we focus on two emotional disorders characterized by disturbance in positive emotion: bipolar disorder (BD), marked by relative excesses of positive emotion, and major depressive disorder (MDD), marked by relative absences of positive emotion. We conclude with implications across other clinical disorders and a road map for future research.

Key Process I. Positive Emotion Reactivity

Emotion reactivity refers to the change in emotion state that occurs in response to a salient stimulus, including coordinated changes in subjective experience, facial display, and physiology (Gross, Sutton, & Ketelaar, 1998). Thus, *positive emotion reactiv-*ity refers to a specific change or increase in positive emotion response. In this section we explore the differences and consequences of positive emotion in mood disorders characterized by putative excesses (BD) and deficits (MDD) in responding to positive stimuli.

BD and Heightened Positive Emotion Reactivity

A prominent view is that BD is associated with excessive positive emotional reactions in response to rewarding stimuli (e.g., Gruber, 2011; Johnson, 2005). Supportive evidence has documented that individuals with BD exhibit greater positive emotional reactivity compared to healthy controls, independent of current symptom levels (Johnson, 2005; Johnson, Gruber, & Eisner, 2007). With respect to self-reported emotion experience, increases in self-reported positive emotion after earning a monetary reward have been associated with higher levels of manic symptoms in a college sample (Johnson, Ruggero, & Carver, 2005). *Euthymic* (i.e., neither currently manic nor depressed) individuals with BD report greater positive affect (PA) in response to neutral photos (M'Bailara et al., 2009) and at the prospect of earning rewards in their daily lives (Meyer, Johnson, & Winters, 2001). Two experimental studies found that individuals at high risk for, and diagnosed with, BD reported greater positive emotion across a variety of contexts, such as when viewing positive, negative, and neutral films (Gruber, Harvey, & Purcell, 2011; Gruber, Johnson, Oveis, & Keltner, 2008). Individuals at risk for BD have also been found to report greater PA in response to false success feedback (Meyer & Baur, 2009). Furthermore, two experience-sampling studies suggest that individuals at high risk for mania (Hofmann & Meyer, 2006) and those exhibiting bipolar spectrum disorders (Lovejoy & Steuerwald, 1995) report elevated levels of PA across varied daily life circumstances. This suggests that individuals at risk for, and diagnosed with, BD report increased PA in response to emotional stimuli regardless of the context (Gruber, 2011).

Research investigating physiological responses to positive stimuli yields some data suggestive of pervasive positive emotional responding across contexts. First, one startle eyeblink study demonstrated that individuals at risk for, and diagnosed with, BD exhibited more attenuated startle response (an indirect marker of positive emotion) while viewing photos of peaceful landscapes and pleasant imagery (Sutton & Johnson, 2002), though clinically diagnosed participants with BD were not found to exhibit differences in their startle response to positive photos (M'Bailara et al., 2009). Another study assessing autonomic responses to emotional film clips indicated that those at high risk for BD demonstrated elevated levels of cardiac vagal tone, which is a putative parasympathetic marker of positive emotionality and resilience (e.g., Porges, 1991), in response to positive, negative, and even neutral film clips compared to low-risk participants (Gruber, Johnson, et al., 2008). Neuroimaging studies further suggest that patients with BD, compared to healthy controls, exhibit increased activity in the amygdala, putamen, and orbitofrontal cortex (OFC) in response to photos of human smiles (cf. Almeida, Versace, Hassel, Kupfer, & Phillips, 2010; Elliott et al., 2004; Lawrence et al., 2004; Yurgelun-Todd et al., 2000). In addition, Bermpohl and colleagues (2009) found that currently manic patients with BD demonstrated elevated left amygdala activity in response to positive pictures. Activity in the amygdala and putamen (part of the basal ganglia) has been associated with the experience of PA and reward (e.g., Phillips & Vieta, 2007).

Taken together, these results suggest that BD is associated with greater physiological responses indicative of positive emotion across a variety of emotional (positive, negative, and neutral) contexts. This feature appears to be a trait-like marker of BD. As such, results from these studies diverge from the perspective that BD is associated with elevated positive emotion *only* in response to positive stimuli (e.g., Johnson, 2005). Rather, they suggest that BD may be associated with elevated positive emotion regardless of stimulus valence, and that this pattern of positive emotional responding is chronic across manic and remitted phases of BD (Gruber, 2011). These findings are consistent with work in MDD suggesting a *context-insensitive* pattern of emotional responding that does not depend on the emotional content of the stimulus or environmental context (e.g., Rottenberg, Gross, & Gotlib, 2005).

MDD and Diminished Positive Emotion Reactivity

Anhedonia, or deficits in the ability to experience positive emotion, is a core symptom of MDD (American Psychiatric Association, 2013). Positive emotional disturbances play a central role in current theories of depression; indeed, depression and positive emotion are often viewed as opposing ends along a single continuum (e.g., Joseph, 2006). As such, numerous studies have investigated and characterized reduced emotional responding to positive stimuli in MDD across subjective, behavioral, and neuroimaging levels of analysis. These findings suggest that MDD is characterized by diminished positive emotion at both trait and state levels.

Empirical research has generally found reduced PA in the daily lives of depressed patients. One experience-sampling study found that MDD patients reported reduced PA in daily life compared with healthy controls (Bylsma, Taylor-Clift, & Rottenberg, 2011). In addition, Lovejoy and Steurwald (1995) found that participants with clinical diagnoses of intermittent depression report lower levels of PA across a 28-day period compared to both BD spectrum and control participants. Similarly, Peeters, Nicholson, & Berkhof (2003) found that participants with MDD reported lower PA across a 6-day period, relative to a control group. Researchers have also found associations between decreased trait PA and MDD (Tellgen & Waller, 1992). Individuals with MDD also demonstrate reduced reactivity to positive emotional stimuli in laboratory settings (for review, see Bylsma, Morris, & Rottenberg, 2008). For example, those with MDD report decreased PA in response to positive films (Gruber, Oveis, Keltner, & Johnson, 2011; Rottenberg, Kaasch, Gross, & Gotlib, 2002) and positive pictures (Dunn, Dalgleish, Lawrence, Cusack, & Ogilvie, 2004; Sloan, Strauss, & Wisner, 2001). Facial behavior in response to positive stimuli has also been found to differentiate individuals with MDD from healthy controls. Berenbaum and Oltmanns (1992) found that depressed patients displayed fewer positive facial expressions in response to sweet-tasting drinks and a stand-up comedy clip. Similarly, MDD patients were found to display reduced facial muscle activity while imagining both happy and sad situations, as compared to healthy controls (Gehricke & Shapiro, 2000). Thus, diminished positive emotion reactivity in MDD is evident across experiential and behavioral channels.

Several neuroimaging studies converge with this growing body of work suggesting diminished positive emotion reactivity, indicating that individuals with MDD exhibit reduced activity in reward- and emotion-related brain regions in response to positive stimuli. For example, patients with MDD display reduced activation in the medial prefrontal cortex (mPFC), putamen, and insula (Knutson, Bhanji, Cooney, Atlas, & Gotlib, 2008), as well as the left nucleus accumbens (NAcc) and bilateral caudate in response to positive cues such as monetary rewards, compared to controls (Pizzagalli et al., 2009). Epstein and colleagues (2006) reported reduced NAcc and thalamus activation in MDD participants compared to controls in response to positive words. Furthermore, MDD has been associated with decreased left, as compared to right, frontal lobe activation associated with reduced positive emotion (e.g., Davidson, Abercrombie, Nitschke, & Putnam, 1999; Davidson, Pizzagalli, Nitschke, & Putnam, 2002). Taken together, these findings suggest that individuals with MDD display reduced subjective, behavioral, and neural reactivity in response to positive emotional stimuli.

We have seen that individuals with BD display heightened positive emotion reactivity across across positive, negative, and neutral stimuli, whereas those with MDD display a diminution in positive emotion reactivity. Findings from both groups converge across state and trait levels of emotion assessment, suggesting that BD and MDD may be prime candidates to study the two extremes of the spectrum of positive emotion reactivity.

Key Process II. On the Edge of Glory?: Anticipation of Positive Outcomes

From an evolutionary standpoint, an important function of an emotion is to define goals based on cues from the environment, such as the odor of a desired food (Cosmides &

Tooby, 2000). When cues are associated with rewards or pleasurable outcomes (e.g., enjoyment of the desired food), the cues can attain a motivational quality of their own, termed *incentive salience* (Berridge & Aldridge, 2008). When incentive salience is high, these cues can elicit anticipation of positive outcomes, as well as motivation to pursue these outcomes, termed *incentive motivation*. This anticipation, in combination with the motivation to pursue positive outcomes, has been described as *wanting* (Berridge, Robinson, & Aldridge, 2009). This anticipatory or wanting state is crucial to enabling the pursuit of both immediate (e.g., food) and long-term (e.g., a college degree) goals. This section explores anticipatory processes in BD, which, we posit, are marked by heightened anticipation of positive outcomes. This will be contrasted with MDD, which, we suggest, is marked by diminished anticipation of positive outcomes.

BD and Heightened Anticipation

Criterion for the diagnosis of BD include increases in reward- and pleasure-seeking activities, such as unrestrained buying sprees, sexual liaisons, and pursuit of overly ambitious goals (American Psychiatric Association, 2013). Psychosocial models of BD stress increased anticipation and pursuit of potential rewards or positive outcomes as a core characteristic of BD linked to the onset and maintenance of the disorder (e.g., Johnson, 2005). As such, recent studies have revealed that individuals at risk for, and diagnosed with, BD exhibit increased emotional response when anticipating future positive outcomes or rewards (Abler, Greenhouse, Ongur, Walter, & Heckers, 2008; Bermpohl et al., 2010; Meyer et al., 2001). For example, individuals at risk for, or with a history of BD display heightened neural activity in response to potential future rewards, such as monetary gains (Abler et al., 2008; Bermpohl et al., 2010). Furthermore, neuroimaging research documents heightened engagement of reward-related neural circuitry during anticipation of positive outcomes in BD, including increased activity in the OFC, associated with the experience of reward and pleasure, as well as the NAcc, associated with anticipating reward. For example, when anticipating monetary rewards, currently manic patients with BD exhibit increased OFC activity (Bermpohl et al., 2010). Another study found increased activation in the NAcc at baseline, suggesting chronic overactivity in reward-related circuitry even when a future positive outcome or reward cue was not present (Abler et al., 2008). Clinically, increased emotional responding to future positive outcomes has been implicated in the etiology of BD, such that it predicts the onset and recurrence of symptoms (e.g., Johnson, 2005). For example, endorsement of items tapping into anticipation of positive outcomes on the Behavioral Activation and Inhibition Scale (e.g., "If I see a chance to get something I want, I move on it right away"; Carver & White, 1994) prospectively predicts future manic symptoms in adults diagnosed with BD (Meyer et al., 2001).

A second line of evidence suggests that BD is associated with not only heightened anticipation of positive outcomes but also a tendency behaviorally to pursue future positive outcomes. For example, individuals at risk for, and diagnosed with BD demonstrate heightened levels of ambitious goal setting and achievement motivation (e.g., Johnson, 2005). For example, risk for developing BD is associated with overly ambitious goal setting for fame, wealth, and political influence (Gruber & Johnson, 2009; Johnson & Carver, 2006), as well as increased striving for rewarding goals (e.g., Nusslock, Abramson, Harmon-Jones, Alloy, & Hogan, 2007). Clinically, this increased ambitious goal setting and striving for future positive outcomes prospectively predicts increases in manic symptoms (Johnson, Cuellar, et al., 2008; Johnson, Meyer, Winett, & Small, 2000).

MDD and Diminished Anticipation

Core criteria for a diagnosis of MDD includes diminished anticipation of positive outcomes and decreased motivation to pursue these outcomes. For example, this includes decreased pleasure in everyday activities, referred to as *anhedonia* (American Psychiatric Association, 2013). These clinical observations are consistent with empirical work documenting reduced expectation of future positive outcomes and decreased

behavioral pursuit of potential positive outcomes in MDD (Alloy & Ahrens, 1987). For example, when asked to predict the likelihood of positive future events, individuals with MDD tend to predict fewer successes and more failures for themselves and others compared to healthy adults (Alloy & Ahrens, 1987). Although efforts to locate the neural underpinnings of reward anticipation have not been consistent (e.g., Knutson et al., 2008; Pizzagalli et al., 2009), some promising results have emerged. For example, in one study, during anticipation of monetary gains, researchers found no differences between MDD and control groups in the basal ganglia (Pizzagalli et al., 2009) or NAcc (Knutson et al., 2008), two brain regions associated with emotion and reward. However, in another decision-making task involving anticipation of monetary rewards, participants with MDD displayed reduced basal ganglia activity associated with reward prediction compared with healthy participants (Smoski et al., 2009). Future work is warranted to isolate more clearly the neural mechanisms associated with positive outcome anticipation in MDD.

Clinically, reduced anticipation of positive outcomes in MDD has been shown to result in poor treatment outcome. Specifically, individuals who are more pessimistic regarding treatment at the outset of a group program for depression were found to have significantly poorer treatment outcomes (Hoberman, Lewinsohn, & Tilson, 1988). Moreover, *depressive pessimism*, or the tendency to estimate that negative future events are likely and positive events are not, is associated with increased depression severity (Andersen, 1990).

In summary, individuals with BD display heightened response to cues signaling future positive outcomes, whereas responses of those with MDD to these cues are relatively diminished. With respect to anticipation of positive outcomes, individuals with BD have been found to display more intense responses to reward cues, as well as behavioral manifestations of this reactivity in the form of excessive reward-focused goal setting and goal striving. Conversely, those with MDD demonstrate the reverse pattern of diminished incentive–motivation. In this way, BD and MDD may be characterized as sharing a core deficit in the ability to respond adaptively to incentives in the environment. These findings also point to the broader possibility that positive outcome anticipation exists along a continuum, with blunted responding to such cues characteristic of MDD at one end, and exaggerated responsivity to potential cues of pleasure or reward in BD at the other extreme.

Key Process III.
Positive Emotion Regulation

Emotion regulation has been defined as "the process by which individuals influence which emotions they have, when they have them, and how they experience and express those emotions" (Gross, 1998, p. 227). The ability to regulate emotion adaptively has been linked to favorable health outcomes, including greater well-being and social adjustment (Tamir, John, Srivastava, & Gross, 2007). Specifically, the ability to regulate positive emotions may sustain, and perhaps even improve, mental health outcomes (e.g., Folkman & Moskowitz, 2000; Tugade & Fredrickson, 2004). Given the multitude of benefits associated with adaptive emotion regulation, psychological disorders characterized by positive emotion dysregulation, such as BD and MDD, necessitate a better understanding. In this section, we first examine positive emotion regulation in BD, followed by an exploration of positive emotion regulation in MDD.

BD and Positive Emotion Regulation

An inability to regulate positive emotion is fundamental to BD (Green, Cahill, & Mahli, 2007; Johnson et al., 2007; Kring & Werner, 2004; Leibenluft, Charney, & Pine, 2003). First, individuals with BD have difficulties down-regulating positive emotions (Farmer et al., 2006), and exhibit a tendency to up-regulate positive emotions after being presented with emotional stimuli, instead of returning to a baseline state (Gruber, Harvey, & Johnson, 2009; Gruber, Mauss, et al., 2011). Indeed, euthymic individuals with BD self-report prolonged happiness compared with healthy controls after a positive mood induction (Farmer et al., 2006). Additionally, individuals with BD often employ maladaptive emotion regulation strategies

with unsuccessful results (Gruber, Eidelman, & Harvey, 2008; Johnson, McKenzie, & McMurrich, 2008).

Not only do individuals with BD have difficulties down-regulating positive emotional responses, but evidence also suggests these individuals have a tendency to up-regulate or heighten their responses to positive stimuli, referred to as *positive rumination*. Several studies suggest that individuals with BD engage in positive rumination in response to emotional stimuli (e.g., Gruber et al., 2009). Individuals with BD report greater trait positive rumination relative to healthy controls (Gruber, Eidelman, Johnson, Smith, & Harvey, 2011), and positive rumination is associated with greater lifetime frequency of depressive and manic episodes in individuals with BD. Interestingly, when individuals are instructed to utilize positive rumination, they show increased positive thoughts, PA, and heart rate compared to when they are instructed to utilize a reflective strategy that requires a more distanced perspective (Gruber et al., 2009). This experimental induction of positive rumination lends support to the notion that positive rumination is a key factor in the up-regulation of responses to emotional stimuli. Thus, positive rumination distinguishes individuals with BD from individuals with MDD and healthy controls (Gruber, Eidelman, et al., 2011; Johnson, McKenzie, et al., 2008).

Individuals with BD have also been found to use conflicting and sometimes inconsistent emotion regulation strategies, potentially contributing to impairments in effectively regulating emotional responses. For example, in one study, BD individuals utilized more spontaneous suppression and reappraisal while watching positive, neutral, and negative film clips compared with healthy control participants, but ultimately were found to be less successful in their emotion regulatory efforts (Gruber, Harvey, & Gross, 2012). These findings indicate that individuals with BD utilize diffuse and nonspecific emotion regulation strategies, which, despite the substantial amount of effort they put into these attempts, are often unsuccessful. Heightened implementation of emotion regulation strategies in BD may denote an attempt to neutralize the frequent and intense moods experienced by these individuals. It may be the case that these individuals recruit multiple, often conflicting, strategies in part because they do not have clear insight into how to implement emotion regulation strategies that are context-appropriate.

MDD and Positive Emotion Regulation

MDD also centrally features disruptions in emotion regulation (Gruber, 2011; Rottenberg et al., 2005). Individuals with MDD exhibit unique difficulties with positive emotion regulation. For example, those with MDD report a tendency to up-regulate negative emotions (Nolen-Hoeksema, 1991) but a failure to increase or up-regulate positive emotions (Garnefski & Kraaij, 2006; Sloan et al., 2001). Furthermore, individuals with MDD across the lifespan exhibit a decreased ability to sustain and promote positive emotions (Forbes & Dahl, 2005; McMakin, Santiago, & Shirk, 2009). One study examining currently depressed individuals with MDD, remitted depressed individuals with MDD, and healthy control groups found that recall of positive memories did not improve mood in formerly depressed MDD groups (Joormann, Siemer, & Gotlib, 2007). Furthermore, currently depressed individuals with MDD even experienced a decrease in positive emotion following the positive memory recall. Neuroimaging evidence further indicates that when attempting to up-regulate positive emotion, depressed individuals were unable to maintain activity in the NAcc (Heller et al., 2009), suggesting that individuals with MDD have a decreased ability to sustain engagement of neural structures centrally involved in PA. Additionally, individuals experiencing *dysphoria* (i.e., mild depression) demonstrate a decreased period of positive emotion following a positive film clip (McMakin et al., 2009). Taken together, this evidence provides support for the notion that individuals with MDD have trouble increasing and sustaining positive emotions.

Individuals with MDD have a tendency to increase negative emotion through a process called *rumination* (Nolen-Hoeksema, 1991), defined as a repetitive focus on the causes and consequences of one's current mood in a manner that is not conducive to problem solving, and that is associated with greater concurrent and prospective depressive symptom severity (e.g., Nolen-

Hoeksema, Parker, & Larson, 1994). Not only do those with MDD exhibit a tendency to increase negative emotion through rumination, but they also fail to increase positive emotion (Garnefski & Kraaij, 2006). One study in an adult sample with MDD showed that symptoms of depression were associated with decreases in the reported utility of positive emotion regulation strategies (i.e., positive refocusing, planning, positive reappraisal, putting into perspective; Garnefski & Kraaij, 2006). Individuals with MDD are also slower to identify the valence of positive stimuli than are nondepressed individuals (Siegle, Granholm, Ingram, & Matt, 2001). Finally, a study assessing negative rumination and positive rumination in a nonclinical sample at 3- and 5-month time periods demonstrated that decreasing positive mood directly using dampening regulation strategies predicted increased symptoms of depression prospectively (Raes, Smets, Nelis, & Schoofs, 2012). Taken together, these findings demonstrate that individuals with MDD demonstrate difficulty maintaining and increasing positive emotions.

Getting Social with Positive Emotion: Function and Dysfunction

Thus far, we have discussed how three key positive emotion processes (i.e., positive emotion *reactivity, anticipation* of positive outcomes, positive emotion *regulation*) can go awry in two important clinical disorders—BD and MDD. In individuals with these disorders, the disruption of these positive emotion processes does not occur in a vacuum, but rather often unfolds in the course of interacting with others, and so has critical social implications. Below, we focus on the social consequences of positive emotion dysregulation.

The vital role of positive emotion in social functioning has been evidenced through a robust line of work examining positive emotion in social contexts using healthy samples. Positive emotions have been found to build interpersonal resources and facilitate adaptive social processes (e.g., Fredrickson, 1998). More specifically, positive emotions appear to enhance relationship commitment and trust (Gonzaga, Keltner, Londahl, & Smith, 2001), increase prosociality (e.g.,

Isen, 1999), and heighten feelings of social connection (Algoe, Gable, & Maisel, 2010).

However, positive emotions can also be a source of interpersonal dysfunction. Psychological disorders, such as BD and MDD, provide a useful window to examine the links between positive emotion disturbance and social impairment (Gruber, 2011; Gruber & Keltner, 2011; Keltner & Kring, 1998). Many of the social difficulties associated with these disorders are partly a function of positive emotion dysregulation— either from an excess (i.e., BD) or severe lack (i.e., MDD) of positive emotion. Specifically, we discuss how these disruptions in positive emotion processes impact social outcomes across the development and maintenance of social networks, the perception of others' emotions, and responses to others' emotions.

Positive Emotion and Social Dysfunction in BD

Social dysfunction is a common feature of BD (American Psychological Association, 2000). Individuals with BD often report dysfunction in initiating and sustaining high-quality relationships (e.g., Coryell et al., 1993; Romans & McPherson, 1992). For example, they report less social support and social interaction than do nonclinical controls (Beyer et al., 2003). Individuals with BD also report greater social strain and impaired social relationships (Romans & McPherson, 1992). Furthermore, these relationship strains were found to be more prominent in individuals with a predominance of manic episodes, suggesting that persistent positive emotion may be a primary source of the social dysfunction associated with BD.

One form of positive emotion dysregulation associated with BD, namely, persistent positive emotion, may be an especially important factor in the development and maintenance of these interpersonal difficulties (Gruber, 2011). For example, individuals at risk for BD exhibit overly positive biases as they interpret and respond to the behavior of others (e.g., Piff, Purcell, Gruber, Hertenstein, & Keltner, 2012; Trevisani, Johnson, & Carver, 2008). Additionally, across a variety of contexts, these individuals may exhibit persistent positive emotion (Gruber, 2011) that results in inappropriate affect

displays in social settings. For example, individuals with BD rate themselves higher on dysfunctional social traits and behaviors, including inappropriate assertiveness, impulsivity, overconfidence, jealousy, and withdrawal (Goldstein, Miklowitz, & Mullen, 2006). Taken together, these examples highlight how an excess of positive emotion may negatively impact the formation and maintenance of healthy relationships in individuals with BD.

Accurate identification of others' emotions is one important social process that enhances interpersonal interaction and facilitates adaptive responses to others (Rich et al., 2008). BD is associated with overly positive biases in interpreting the emotions of others (Gruber & Keltner, 2011). For example, individuals with BD exhibit a heightened attunement to positive emotional expressions (Trevisani et al., 2008) and sometimes inaccurately perceive others' current emotional state as more positive than it actually is (Piff et al., 2012). This has been supported by work on the detection of emotion through facial displays. For example, individuals at risk for BD exhibit heightened abilities in identifying positive emotion (i.e., happiness) in others (Trevisani et al., 2008). These overly positive biases can also impact the detection of negative affect because individuals with BD attribute more positive emotion to others' displays of negative emotion (Lembke & Ketter, 2002). Furthermore, research indicates that individuals at risk for BD attribute increased prosociality and positive emotions (e.g., love) to a variety of touches received from a stranger (Piff et al., 2012). Therefore, individuals with BD may overestimate experiences of positive emotion in others based partly on their own positive emotional experience, and this overestimation may have negative consequences for social behavior and connecting with others.

Just as individuals with BD exhibit impairments in perceiving others' emotions, they also display dysfunction in responding to others' emotions. In comparison to healthy controls, individuals with BD report lower levels of *cognitive empathy*, defined as the ability to take someone else's perspective (Cusi, MacQueen, & McKinnon, 2010). Interruptions in empathic response appear to predict negative social outcomes across various contexts (e.g., familial, occupational). For example, a decreased ability to understand someone else's perspective may impair social communication in BD (Cusi et al., 2010). Last, the persistent positive emotion associated with BD may lead to experiences of positive emotion at inappropriate times (Gruber, 2011), such as when hearing the news of a negative event. In summary, it seems that disrupted positive emotion processes in individuals with BD can adversely affect the ways they respond to others' emotions.

Positive Emotion and Social Dysfunction in MDD

Individuals with MDD experience significant social difficulties related to relative *deficits* in positive emotion. For example, clinically depressed individuals derive less pleasure from social activity (Nezlek, Hampton, & Shean, 2000) and display less positive behaviors during interpersonal interactions (Biglan et al., 1985). In this section we discuss how a severe lack of positive emotion in MDD can impact the development and maintenance of social networks, the perception of others' emotions, and responses to others' emotions.

Individuals with MDD experience difficulties in initiating and sustaining social networks. These individuals report fewer social contacts and less social interaction (e.g., Gotlib & Lee, 1989), and often perceive their networks as less supportive (Gotlib, 1992). Individuals with MDD also find their interactions with others to be less enjoyable (Nezlek et al., 2000). For example, research indicates that depressed mothers display less PA during interactions with their infants and family members (e.g., Hops et al., 1987; Sheeber & Sorenson, 1998). Fathers who are depressed also show deficits in the expression of positivity during family communication (Jacob & Johnson, 2001). Moreover, individuals with MDD smile less frequently at their romantic partners (Rehman, Gollan, & Mortimer, 2008). This body of work sheds light on how deficient positive emotion can impair the relationships of individuals with MDD.

Individuals with MDD are less adept than nondepressed individuals at accurately identifying expressions of positive emotion (e.g., happiness) in others (e.g., Gotlib

et al., 2004; LeMoult, Joormann, Sherdell, Wright, & Gotlib, 2009; Surguladze et al., 2004). Depressive symptoms can also have a significant impact on *empathic accuracy* (Gadassi, Mor, & Rafaeli, 2011), which is defined as the ability to perceive accurately the dynamic changes in another person's emotions (Zaki, Bolger, & Ochsner, 2008). In a study of romantic couples, increased symptoms of depression in women were associated with less empathic accuracy for the negative emotions (but not positive emotions) of their partners (Gadassi et al., 2011). In summary, it appears that a lack of positive emotion in MDD can decrease one's ability to detect emotions of others accurately.

Individuals with MDD also experience difficulties in responding to the emotional displays of others. For example, depressed individuals direct more attention toward faces with negative expressions (as compared to neutral faces) during a dot-probe task (Gotlib et al., 2004), which suggests that they may be less attentive to individuals who are not distressed. Facial displays in response to others' emotions also appear to be impacted by depressive symptoms. After viewing facial expressions of happiness, depressed individuals are significantly less likely to exhibit zygomatic major facial muscle activity, which is an indicator of felt positive emotion (Sloan, Bradley, Dimoulas, & Lang, 2002). MDD is also associated with deficits in empathic responsiveness. For example, individuals with MDD report heightened levels of personal distress and decreased perspective taking in response to the personal suffering of others (O'Connor, Berry, Weiss, & Gilbert, 2002). These findings illustrate the social difficulties that can result from positive emotion deficits in MDD.

However, another line of work has found that depression does not always result in unfavorable social outcomes. Some researchers have found that depressed individuals are just as likely as healthy controls to be responsive to the suffering of others (Gruber, Oveis, et al., 2008). Furthermore, other researchers suggest that there may even be social strengths associated with MDD, which perhaps result from a heightened interpersonal sensitivity toward others who are suffering. For example, depressive symptoms have been associated with a greater interest in gaining an understanding of one's own social environment (Gleicher & Weary, 1991) and higher levels of self-reported altruism (O'Connor et al., 2002). Therefore, it seems plausible that heightened awareness of others' negative emotions could in some ways have potential to enhance the empathic abilities of individuals with MDD.

Taken together, the evidence reviewed previously suggests that the social dysfunction present in both BD and MDD may be explained in part by the disrupted positive emotion processes associated with each disorder. Impaired social functioning can be particularly problematic for these clinical populations because social support acts as a valuable buffer against mental illness. For example, inadequate social support often hinders recovery and worsens illness progression in both BD and MDD (Johnson, Winett, Meyer, Greenhouse, & Miller, 1999; Johnson et al., 2000). Therefore, it is important that the social difficulties associated with these disorders be examined carefully and understood because this information has important implications for fostering positive clinical outcomes.

Positive Emotion and Psychopathology: Where to Go Next?

In this chapter, we have detailed several promising lines of research relating positive emotion dysfunction with different psychological disorders. Specifically, we concentrated on three conceptual themes that illustrate the relationship between aberrant forms of positive emotion and psychopathology. These themes include anticipation of positive cues, emotional responses to positive stimuli, and the management or regulation of positive emotions. We did this across two populations centrally associated with relative excesses (i.e., BD) and deficits (i.e., MDD) in positive emotion. We concluded by focusing on social functioning and consequences of positive emotion in these clinical populations.

This body of work points to likely etiologies and treatments of different disorders, underscoring the importance of adopting a transdiagnostic approach to exploring the contribution of disrupted positive emotion to mental health outcomes across a variety of populations (e.g., Kring, 2008). In fact, recent work suggests that when experiencing extreme degrees of positive emotion, individuals are more inclined to engage in problematic behaviors, such as alcohol consumption, binge eating, drug use, and risk taking (Cyders & Smith, 2008). This highlights the importance of adopting a transdiagnostic approach in future research. A growing body of work has also drawn attention to disrupted positive emotion in other disorders, including schizophrenia and substance abuse. For example, in schizophrenia, a failure to anticipate positive emotional experiences appropriately plays an important role in mental health outcomes, even in light of otherwise intact consummatory pleasant feelings in the moment (e.g., Cohen & Minor, 2010; Kring & Moran, 2008). In addition, models of substance abuse highlight the centrality of exaggerated anticipation or desire for reward-related substance cues (American Psychiatric Association, 2013). This positive emotion–seeking behavior is a common reason for substance abuse, as well as relapse, and it has been found to predict increased severity in alcohol consumption and drinking-related impairment (Cooper, Frone, Russell, & Mudar, 1995). Future work is warranted to understand better the nature of positive emotion disturbance across a host of psychopathologies, and the extent to which it represents a core component in the etiology and maintenance of the disorders.

In conclusion, we return to the central theme guiding this chapter by focusing on the intersection of emotion and psychopathology. Empirical research on this intersection offers the promise of several conceptual gains in the respective fields (e.g., Keltner & Kring, 1998; Kring & Sloan, 2009). For affective scientists, the study of the relation between emotions and psychopathology still remains one of the clearest routes to understanding the function of a particular emotion. For clinical scientists, the kind of research we have detailed in this chapter offers similar promise for understanding the social expression and underpinnings of different disorders. More generally, individual differences in emotional behavior, which present early in life, may help to explain the life course of the individual, as well as relational difficulties and other problems that the person systematically encounters (e.g., Malatesta, 1990). More broadly, this research offers answers to an abiding question concerning the boundary conditions of how and in what manner positive emotion can go awry.

References

Abler, B., Greenhouse, I., Ongur, D., Walter, H., & Heckers, S. (2008). Abnormal reward system activation in mania. *Neuropsychopharmacology, 33,* 2217–2227.

Algoe, S. B., Gable, S. L., & Maisel, N. (2010). It's the little things: Everyday gratitude as a booster shot for romantic relationships. *Personal Relationships, 17,* 217–233.

Alloy, L. B., & Ahrens, A. H. (1987). Depression and pessimism for the future: Biased use of statistically relevant information in predictions for self versus others. *Journal of Personality and Social Psychology, 52,* 366–378.

Almeida, J. R. C., Versace, A., Hassel, S., Kupfer, D. J., & Phillips, M. L. (2010). Elevated amygdala activity to sad facial expressions: A state marker of bipolar but not unipolar depression. *Biological Psychiatry, 67,* 414–421.

American Psychiatric Association. (2013). *Diagnostic and statistical manual of mental disorders* (5th ed.). Arlington VA: Author.

Andersen, S. M. (1990). The inevitability of future suffering: The role of depressive predictive certainty in depression. *Social Cognition, 8,* 203–228.

Berenbaum, H., & Oltmanns, T. F. (1992). Emotional experience and expression in schizophrenia. *Journal of Abnormal Psychology, 101,* 37–44.

Bermpohl, F., Dalanay, U., Kahnt, T., Sajonz, B., Heimann, H., Ricken, R., et al. (2009). A preliminary study of increased amygdale activation to positive affective stimuli in mania. *Bipolar Disorders, 11,* 70–75.

Bermpohl, F., Kahnt, T., Dalanay, U., Hagele, C., Sajonz, B., Wegner, T., et al. (2010). Altered representation of expected value in the orbitofrontal cortex in mania. *Human Brain Mapping, 31,* 958–969.

Berridge, K. C., & Aldridge, J. W. (2008). Decision utility, incentive salience and cue-triggered "wanting." In E. Morsella, J. A. Bargh, & P. M. Gollwitzer (Eds.), *Oxford handbook of human action* (pp. 509–532). New York: Oxford University Press.

Berridge, K. C., Robinson, T. E., & Aldridge, J. W. (2009). Dissecting components of reward: "Liking," "wanting," and learning. *Current Opinion in Pharmacology, 9,* 65–73.

Beyer, J. L., Kuchibhatla, M., Looney, C., Engstrom, E., Cassidy, F., & Krishnan, K. R. R. (2003). Social support in elderly patients with bipolar disorder. *Bipolar Disorders, 5,* 22–27.

Biglan, A., Hops, H., Sherman, L., Friedman, L. S., Arthur, J., & Osteen, V. (1985). Problem-solving interactions of depressed women and their husbands. *Behavior Therapy, 16,* 431–451.

Bylsma, L. M., Morris, B. H., & Rottenberg, J. (2008). A meta-analysis of emotional reactivity in major depressive disorder. *Clinical Psychology Review, 28,* 676–691.

Bylsma, L. M., Taylor-Clift, L., & Rottenberg, J. (2011). Emotional reactivity to daily events in major and minor depression. *Journal of Abnormal Psychology, 120,* 155–167.

Carver, C. S., & White, T. L. (1994). Behavioral inhibition, behavioral activation, and affective responses to impending reward and punishment: The BIS/BAS scales. *Journal of Personality and Social Psychology, 67,* 319–333.

Cohen, A. S., & Minor, K. S. (2010). Emotional experience in patients with schizophrenia revisited: Meta-analysis of laboratory studies. *Schizophrenia Bulletin, 36,* 143–150.

Cooper, M. L., Frone, M. R., Russell, M., & Mudar, P. (1995). Drinking to regulate positive and negative emotions: A motivational model of alcohol use. *Journal of Personality and Social Psychology, 69,* 990–1005.

Coryell, W., Scheftner, W., Keller, M., Endicott, J., Maser, J., & Klerman, G. L. (1993). The enduring psychosocial consequences of mania and depression. *American Journal of Psychiatry, 150,* 720–727.

Cosmides, L., & Tooby, J. (2000). Evolutionary psychology and the emotions. In M. Lewis & J. M. Haviland-Jones (Eds.), *Handbook of emotions* (2nd ed., pp. 91–115). New York: Guilford Press.

Cusi, A., MacQueen, G. M., & McKinnon, M. C. (2010). Altered self-report of empathic responding in patients with bipolar disorder. *Psychiatry Research, 178,* 354–358.

Cyders, M. A., & Smith, G. T. (2008). Emotion-based dispositions to rash action: Positive and negative urgency. *Psychological Bulletin, 134,* 807–828.

Davidson, R. J., Abercrombie, H., Nitschke, J. B., & Putnam, K. (1999). Regional brain function, emotion, and disorders of emotion. *Current Opinion in Neurobiology, 9,* 228–234.

Davidson, R. J., Pizzagalli, D., Nitschke, J. B., & Putnam, K. (2002). Depression: Perspectives from affective neuroscience. *Annual Review of Psychology, 53,* 545–574.

Dunn, B., Dalgleish, T., Lawrence, A., Cusack, R., & Ogilvie, A. (2004). Categorical and dimensional reports of experienced affect to emotion-inducing pictures in depression. *Journal of Abnormal Psychology, 113,* 654–660.

Elliott, R., Ogilvie, A., Rubinsztein, J. S., Calderon, G., Dolan, R., & Sahakian, B. J. (2004). Abnormal ventral frontal response during performance of an affective go/no go task in patients with mania. *Biological Psychiatry, 55,* 1163–1170.

Epstein, J., Pan, H., Kocsis, J. H., Yang, Y., Butler, T., Chusid, J., et al. (2006). Lack of ventral striatal response to positive stimuli in depressed versus normal subjects. *American Journal of Psychiatry, 163,* 1784–1790.

Farmer, A., Lam, D., Sahakian, B., Roiser, J., Burke, A., O'Neill, N., et al. (2006). A pilot study of positive mood induction in euthymic bipolar subjects compared with healthy controls. *Psychological Medicine, 36,* 1213–1218.

Folkman, S., & Moskowitz, J. T. (2000). Positive affect and the other side of coping. *American Psychologist, 55,* 647–654.

Forbes, E. E., & Dahl, R. E. (2005). Neural systems of positive affect: Relevance to understanding child and adolescent depression? *Development and Psychopathology, 17,* 827–850.

Fredrickson, B. L. (1998). What good are positive emotions? *Review of General Psychology, 2,* 300–319.

Gadassi, R., Mor, N., & Rafaeli, E. (2011). Depression and empathic accuracy in couples: An interpersonal model of gender differences in depression. *Psychological Science, 22,* 1033–1041.

Garnefski, N., & Kraaij, V. (2006). Cognitive Emotion Regulation Questionnaire—development of a short 18-item version (CERQ-Short). *Personality and Individual Differences, 41,* 1045–1053.

Gehricke, J., & Shapiro, D. (2000). Reduced facial expression and social context in major depression: Discrepancies between facial muscle activity and self-reported emotion. *Psychiatry Research, 21,* 157–167.

Gleicher, F., & Weary, G. (1991). Effects of depression on quantity and quality of social inferences. *Journal of Personality and Social Psychology, 61,* 105–114.

Goldstein, T. R., Miklowitz, D. J., & Mullen, K. (2006). Social skills knowledge and performance among adolescents with bipolar disorder. *Bipolar Disorders, 8,* 350–361.

Gonzaga, G. C., Keltner, D., Londahl, E. A., & Smith, M. D. (2001). Love and the commitment problem in romantic relations and friendship. *Journal of Personality and Social Psychology, 81,* 247–262.

Gotlib, I. H. (1992). Interpersonal and cognitive aspects of depression. *Current Directions in Psychological Science, 1,* 149–154.

Gotlib, I. H., Kasch, K. L., Traill, S., Joormann, J., Arnow, B. A., & Johnson, S. L. (2004). Coherence and specificity of information-processing biases in depression and social phobia. *Journal of Abnormal Psychology, 113,* 386–398.

Gotlib, I. H., & Lee, C. M. (1989). The social functioning of depressed patients: A longitudinal assessment. *Journal of Social and Clinical Psychology, 8,* 223–237.

Green, M. J., Cahill, C. M., & Malhi, G. S. (2007). The cognitive and neurophysiological basis of emotion dysregulation in bipolar disorder. *Journal of Affective Disorders, 103,* 29–42.

Gross, J. J. (1998). Antecedent- and response-focused emotion regulation: Divergent consequences for experience, expression, and physiology. *Journal of Personality and Social Psychology, 74,* 224–237.

Gross, J. J., Sutton, S. K., & Ketelaar, T. (1998). Relations between affect and personality: Support for the affect-level and affective reactivity views. *Personality and Social Psychology Bulletin, 24,* 279–291.

Gruber, J. (2011). When feeling good can be bad: Positive emotion persistence (PEP) in bipolar disorder. *Current Directions in Psychological Science, 20*(4), 217–221.

Gruber, J., Eidelman, P., & Harvey, A. G. (2008). Transdiagnostic emotion regulation processes in bipolar disorder and insomnia. *Behaviour Research and Therapy, 46,* 1096–1100.

Gruber, J., Eidelman, P., Johnson, S. L., Smith, B., & Harvey, A. G. (2011). Hooked on a feeling: Rumination about positive and negative emotion in inter-episode bipolar disorder. *Journal of Abnormal Psychology, 120*(4), 956–961.

Gruber, J., Harvey, A. G., & Gross, J. J. (2012). When trying is not enough: Emotion regulation and the effort-success gap in bipolar disorder. *Emotion, 12*(5), 997–1003.

Gruber, J., Harvey, A. G., & Johnson, S. L. (2009). Reflective and ruminative processing of positive emotional memories in bipolar disorder and healthy controls. *Behaviour Research and Therapy, 47,* 697–704.

Gruber, J., Harvey, A. G., & Purcell, A. (2011). What goes up can come down?: A preliminary investigation of emotion reactivity and emotion recovery in bipolar disorder. *Journal of Affective Disorders, 133,* 457–466.

Gruber, J., & Johnson, S. L. (2009). Positive emotional traits and ambitious goals among people at risk for mania: The need for specificity. *International Journal of Cognitive Therapy, 2,* 176–187.

Gruber, J., Johnson, S. L., Oveis, C., & Keltner, D. (2008). Risk for mania and positive emotional responding: Too much of a good thing? *Emotion, 8*(1), 23–33.

Gruber, J., & Keltner, D. (2011). Too close for comfort?: Lessons from excesses and deficits of compassion in psychopathology. In S. Brown, M. Brown, & L. Penner (Eds.), *Moving beyond self-interest: Perspectives from Evolutionary biology, neuroscience, and the social sciences* (pp. 199–210). New York: Oxford University Press.

Gruber, J., Mauss, I. B., & Tamir, M. (2011). A dark side of happiness?: How, when, and why happiness is not always good. *Perspectives on Psychological Science, 6,* 222–233.

Gruber, J., Oveis, C., Keltner, D., & Johnson, S. L. (2011). A discrete emotions approach to positive emotion disturbance in depression. *Cognition and Emotion, 25,* 40–52.

Heerey, E. A., Keltner, D., & Capps, L. M. (2003). Making sense of self-conscious emotion: Linking theory of mind and emotion in children with autism. *Emotion, 3,* 394–400.

Heller, A. S., Johnstone, T., Shackman, A. J., Light, S. N., Peterson, M. J., Kolden, G. G., et al. (2009). Reduced capacity to sustain positive emotion in major depression reflects diminished maintenance of fronto-striatal brain activation. *Proceedings of the National Academy of Sciences, 106,* 22445–22450.

Hoberman, H. M., Lewinsohn, P. M., & Tilson, M. (1988). Group treatment of depression: Individual predictors of outcome. *Journal of Consulting and Clinical Psychology, 56,* 393–398.

Hofmann, B. U., & Meyer, T. D. (2006). Mood fluctuations in people putatively at risk for bipolar disorders. *British Journal of Clinical Psychology, 45,* 105–110.

Hops, H., Biglan, A., Sherman, L., Arthur, J., Friedman, L., & Osteen, V. (1987). Home observations of family interactions of depressed women. *Journal of Consulting and Clinical Psychology, 55,* 341–346.

Isen, A. M. (1999). Positive affect. In T. Dalgeish & M. J. Power (Eds.), *Handbook of cognition and emotion* (pp. 521–539). New York: Wiley.

Jacob, T., & Johnson, S. L. (2001). Sequential interactions in the parent–child communications of depressed fathers and depressed mothers. *Journal of Family Psychology, 15,* 38–52.

Johnson, S. L. (2005). Mania and dysregulation in goal pursuit: A review. *Clinical Psychology Review, 25,* 241–262.

Johnson, S. L., & Carver, C. S. (2006). Extreme goal setting and vulnerability to mania among undiagnosed young adults. *Cognitive Therapy and Research, 30,* 377–395.

Johnson, S. L., Cuellar, A. K., Ruggero, C., Winett-Perlman, C., Goodnick, P., White, R., et al. (2008). Life events as predictors of mania and depression in bipolar I disorder. *Journal of Abnormal Psychology, 117,* 268–277.

Johnson, S. L., Gruber, J., & Eisner, L. (2007). Emotion in bipolar disorder. In J. Rottenberg & S. L. Johnson (Eds.), *Emotion and psychopathology: Bridging affective and clinical science* (pp. 123–150). Washington, DC: American Psychological Association.

Johnson, S. L., McKenzie, G., & McMurrich, S. (2008). Ruminative responses to positive and negative affect among students diagnosed with bipolar disorder and major depressive disorder. *Cognitive Therapy and Research, 32*(5), 702–713.

Johnson, S. L., Meyer, B., Winett, C., & Small, J. (2000). Social support and self-esteem predict changes in bipolar depression but not mania. *Journal of Affective Disorders, 58,* 79–86.

Johnson, S. L., Ruggero, C. J., & Carver, C. S. (2005). Cognitive, behavioral, and affective responses to reward: Links with hypomanic symptoms. *Journal of Social and Clinical Psychology, 24,* 894–906.

Johnson, S. L., Winett, C. A., Meyer, B., Greenhouse, W. J., & Miller, I. (1999). Social support and the course of bipolar disorder. *Journal of Abnormal Psychology, 108,* 558–566.

Joorman, J., Siemer, M., & Gotlib, I. H. (2007). Mood regulation in depression: Differential effects of distraction and recall of happy memories on sad mood. *Journal of Abnormal Psychology, 116,* 484–490.

Joseph, S. (2006). Measurement in depression: positive psychology and the statistical bipolarity of depression and happiness. *Measurement: Interdisciplinary Research and Perspectives, 4,* 156–160.

Keltner, D., & Kring, A. M. (1998). Emotion, social function, and psychopathology. *Review of General Psychology, 2,* 320–342.

Knutson, B., Bhanji, J. P., Cooney, R. E., Atlas, L. Y., & Gotlib, I. H. (2008). Neural responses to monetary incentives in major depression. *Biological Psychiatry, 63,* 686–692.

Kring, A. M. (2008). Emotion disturbances as transdiagnostic processes in psychopathology. In M. Lewis, J. M. Haviland-Jones, & L. F. Barrett (Eds.), *Handbook of emotion* (3rd ed., pp. 691–705). New York: Guilford Press.

Kring, A. M., & Moran, E. K. (2008). Emotional response deficits in schizophrenia. *Schizophrenia Bulletin, 34,* 819–834.

Kring, A. M., & Sloan, D. S. (Eds.). (2009). *Emotion regulation and psychopathology: A transdiagnostic approach to etiology and treatment.* New York: Guilford Press.

Kring, A. M. & Werner, K. H. (2004). Emotion regulation in psychopathology. In P. Philippot & R. S. Feldman (Eds.), *The regulation of emotion* (pp. 359–385). New York: Erlbaum.

Lawrence, N. S., Williams, A. M., Surguladze, S., Giampietro, V., Brammer, M. J., Andrew, C., et al. (2004). Subcortical and ventral prefrontal cortical neural responses to facial expressions distinguish patients with bipolar disorder and major depression. *Biological Psychiatry, 15,* 578–587.

Leibenluft, E., Charney, D. S., & Pine, D. S. (2003). Researching the pathophysiology of pediatric bipolar disorder. *Biological Psychiatry, 53,* 1009–1020.

Lembke, A., & Ketter, T. A. (2002). Impaired recognition of facial emotion in mania. *American Journal of Psychiatry, 159,* 302–304.

LeMoult, J., Joormann, J., Sherdell, L., Wright, Y., & Gotlib, I. H. (2009). Identification of emotional facial expressions following recovery from depression. *Journal of Abnormal Psychology, 118,* 34–43.

Lennox, B. R., Jacob, R., Calder, A. J., Lupson, V., & Bullmore, E. T. (2004). Behavioural and neurocognitive responses to sad facial affect

are attenuated in patients with mania. *Psychological Medicine, 34,* 795–802.

Lovejoy, M. C., & Steuerwald, B. L. (1995). Subsyndromal unipolar and bipolar disorders: Comparisons on positive and negative affect. *Journal of Abnormal Psychology, 104,* 381–384.

Lyubomirsky, S., King, L. A., & Diener, E. (2005). The benefits of frequent positive affect: Does happiness lead to success? *Psychological Bulletin, 131,* 803–855.

Lyubomirsky, S., Sheldon, K. M., & Schkade, D. (2005). Pursuing happiness: The architecture of sustainable change. *Review of General Psychology, 9,* 111–131.

Malatesta, C. Z. (1990). The role of emotions in the development and organization of personality. In A. T. Ross (Ed.), *Nebraska Symposium on Motivation* (Vol. 36, pp. 1–56). Lincoln: University of Nebraska Press.

M'Bailara, K. M., Demotes-Mainard, J., Swendsen, J., Mathieu, F., Leboyer, M., & Henry, C. (2009). Emotional hyper-reactivity in normothymic bipolar patients. *Bipolar Disorders, 11,* 63–69.

McMakin, D. L., Santiago, C. D., & Shirk, S. R. (2009). The time course of positive and negative emotion in dysphoria. *Journal of Positive Psychology, 4(2),* 182–192.

Meyer, B., Johnson, S. L., & Winters, R. (2001). Responsiveness to threat and incentive in bipolar disorder: Relations of the BIS/BAS scales with symptoms. *Journal of Psychopathology and Behavioral Assessment, 23,* 133–143.

Meyer, T. D., & Baur, M. (2009). Positive and negative affect in individuals at high and low risk for bipolar disorders. *Journal of Individual Differences, 30,* 169–175.

Myers, D. G., & Diener, E. (1995). Who is happy? *Psychological Science, 6,* 10–19.

Nezlek, J. G., Hampton, C. P., & Shean, G. D. (2000). Clinical depression and day-to-day social interaction in a community sample. *Journal of Abnormal Psychology, 109,* 11–19.

Nolen-Hoeksema, S. (1991). Responses to depression and their effects on duration of depressive episodes. *Journal of Abnormal Psychology, 100,* 569–582.

Nolen-Hoeksema, S., Parker, L., & Larson, J. (1994). Ruminative coping with depressed mood following loss. *Journal of Personality and Social Psychology, 67,* 92–104.

Nusslock, R., Abramson, L. Y., Harmon-Jones, E., Alloy, L. B., & Hogan, M. E. (2007). A goal-striving life event and the onset of hypomanic and depressive episodes and symptoms: Perspective from the behavioral approach system (BAS) dysregulation theory. *Journal of Abnormal Psychology, 116,* 105–115.

O'Connor, L. E., Berry, J.W., Weiss, J., & Gilbert, P. (2002). Guilt, fear, submission, and empathy in depression. *Journal of Affective Disorders 71,* 19–27.

Peeters, F., Nicholson, N. A., & Berkhof, J. (2003). Cortisol responses to daily events in major depressive disorder. *Psychosomatic Medicine, 65,* 836–841.

Phillips, M. L., & Vieta, E. (2007). Identifying functional neuroimaging biomarkers of bipolar disorder: Toward DSM-IV. *Schizophrenia Bulletin, 33,* 893–904.

Piff, P. K., Purcell, A., Gruber, J., Hertenstein, M., & Keltner, D. (2012). Contact high: Mania proneness and positive perception of emotional touches. *Cognition and Emotion, 26*(6), 1116–1123.

Pizzagalli, D. A., Holmes, A. J., Dillon, D. G., Goetz, E. L., Birk, J. L., Bogdan, R., et al. (2009). Reduced caudate and nucleus accumbens response to rewards in unmedicated subjects with major depressive disorder. *American Journal of Psychiatry, 166,* 702–710.

Porges, S. W. (1991). Vagal tone: An autonomic mediator of affect. In J. Garber & K. A. Dodge (Eds.), *The development of emotion regulation and dysregulation* (pp. 111–128). New York: Cambridge University Press.

Raes, F., Smets, J., Nelis, S., & Schoofs, H. (2012). Dampening of positive affect prospectively predicts depressive symptoms in nonclinical samples. *Cognition and Emotion, 26*(1), 75–82.

Rehman, U. S., Gollan, J., & Mortimer, A. R. (2008). The marital context of depression: Research, limitations, and new directions. *Clinical Psychology Review, 28,* 179–198.

Rich, B. A., Fromm, S. J., Berghorst, L. H., Dickstein, D. P., Brotman, M. A., Pine, D. S., et al. (2008). Neural connectivity in children with bipolar disorder: impairment in the face emotion processing circuit. *Journal of Child Psychology and Psychiatry 49,* 88–96.

Romans, S. I., & McPherson, H. M. (1992). The social networks of bipolar affective disorder patients. *Journal of Affective Disorders, 25,* 221–228.

Rottenberg, J., Gross, J. J., & Gotlib, I. H. (2005). Emotion context insensitivity in major depressive disorder. *Journal of Abnormal Psychology, 114,* 627–639.

Rottenberg, J., Kaasch, K. L., Gross, J. J., & Gotlib, I. H. (2002). Sadness and amusement reactivity differentially predict concurrent and prospective functioning in major depressive disorder. *Emotion, 2,* 135–146.

Seligman, M. E. P., & Csikszentmihalyi, M. (2000). Positive psychology: An introduction. *American Psychologist, 55,* 5–14.

Sheeber, L., & Sorenson, E. (1998). Family relationships of depressed adolescents: A multimethod assessment. *Journal of Clinical Child Psychology, 27,* 268–277.

Siegle, G. J., Granholm, E., Ingram, R. E., & Matt, G. E. (2001). Pupillary and reaction time measures of sustained processing of negative information in depression. *Biological Psychiatry, 49,* 624–636.

Sloan, D. M., Bradley, M. M., Dimoulas, E., & Lang, P. J. (2002). Looking at facial expressions: Dysphoria and facial EMG. *Biological Psychology, 60,* 79–90.

Sloan, D. M., Strauss, M. E., & Wisner, K. L. (2001). Diminished response to pleasant stimuli by depressed women. *Journal of Abnormal Psychology, 110,* 488–493.

Smoski, M. J., Felder, J., Bizzell, J., Green, S. R., Ernst, M., Lynch, T. R., et al. (2009). fMRI alterations in reward selection, anticipation, and feedback in major depressive disorder. *Journal of Affective Disorders, 118,* 69–78.

Surguladze, S. A., Young, A. W., Senior, C., Brebion, G., Travis, M. J., & Phillips, M. L. (2004). Recognition accuracy and response bias to happy and sad facial expressions in patients with major depression. *Neuropsychology, 18,* 212–218.

Sutton, S. K., & Johnson, S. J. (2002). Hypomanic tendencies predict lower startle magnitudes during pleasant pictures. *Psychophysiology, 39*(Suppl.), 80.

Tamir, M., John, O. P., Srivastava, S., & Gross, J. J. (2007). Implicit theories of emotion: Affective and social outcomes across a major life transition. *Journal of Personality and Social Psychology, 92,* 731–744.

Tellegen, A., & Waller, N. G. (1992). *Exploring personality through test construction: Development of the Multi-Dimensional Personality Questionnaire (MPQ).* Unpublished manuscript, Department of Psychology, University of Minnesota.

Trevisani, D., Johnson, S. L., & Carver, C. S.

(2008). Positive mood induction and facial affect recognition among students at risk for mania. *Cognitive Therapy and Research, 32,* 639–650.

Tugade, M. M., & Fredrickson, B. L. (2004). Resilient individuals use positive emotions to bounce back from negative emotional experiences. *Journal of Personality and Social Psychology, 86,* 320–333.

Yurgelun-Todd, D. A., Gruber, S. A., Kanayama, G., Killgore, W. D. S., Baird, A. A., & Young, A. D. (2000). fMRI during affect discrimination in bipolar affective disorder. *Bipolar Disorders, 2,* 237–248.

Zaki, J., Bolger, N. & Ochsner, K. (2008). It takes two: The interpersonal nature of empathic accuracy. *Psychological Science, 19*(4), 399–404.

CHAPTER 26

Positive Emotions in Organizations

Stéphane Côté

Positive emotions facilitate success in various spheres of life, including organizations (Lyubomirsky, King, & Diener, 2005). Research has revealed some of the specific effects of positive emotions in organizations that explain these broad patterns. This research has specifically explored which workplace criteria are associated with positive emotions, and which mechanisms underlie these effects. This research has also identified some organizational contexts in which positive emotions do not facilitate performance, or may even hurt performance. In this chapter, I summarize the research on positive emotions in organizations, identifying when positive emotions help and also when they may impede success.

This chapter is divided into four parts. The research reviewed in the first part focuses on how the positive emotions of organization members relate to their own outcomes, such as their own performance. I refer to these effects as "intrapersonal effects." This research has the longest history in organizational behavior and has been reviewed to some extent previously (Barsade & Gibson, 2007; Brief & Weiss, 2002; Isen & Baron, 1991). The second part of this chapter extends past reviews of emotions in organizations in particular by summarizing more recent investigations of the social effects of

positive emotions in organizations, and the third part includes research on the positive affective tone of groups. I end this chapter by reviewing other recent developments that concern the role of discrete positive emotions, how positive emotions can be conceptualized at the group and organizational levels of analysis, and interventions to increase positive emotions and their benefits in organizations.

Researchers have drawn distinctions between the terms "emotion," "mood," and "affect" (cf. Barsade & Gibson, 2007; Rosenberg, 1998). Affect is typically construed as the broader term that includes emotions, which are relatively short in duration and more strongly tied to events, and moods, which last longer and become less tied to events over time. For the purposes of this chapter, I use the term "emotions" to refer to all positive affective states, including positive emotions and moods. This is because the conceptual mechanisms that link positive emotions and positive moods to the criteria described in this chapter are similar, and the measures of positive emotions and positive moods are also similar. In addition, at times I also refer to "dispositional positive emotions," a term that refers to the stable, trait-like tendency to feel positive emotions across situations and over time (Rosenberg, 1998).

The Intrapersonal Effects of Positive Emotions in Organizations

Emotions exert important influences on how people think and act via several mechanisms. Emotions include action tendencies that prepare individuals to respond to the social world in certain ways (Frijda, 1986). Past findings suggest that, at a general level, positive emotions are associated with approach action tendencies; they facilitate approach behaviors (Frijda, Kuipers, & ter Schure, 1989). When individuals feel positive emotions, they are more likely to want to be close to others. In addition, positive emotions generally signal to individuals that the environment is benign (Schwarz & Clore, 1996). As such, positive emotions encourage creative and novel behaviors that individuals have the luxury of doing when conditions are safe (Fredrickson, 1998; Isen, Daubman, & Nowicki, 1987).

Positive emotions also have effects on how people think—their judgments and decisions—by sending signals to individuals about conditions they encounter via a "feelings-as-information" mechanism (Schwarz & Clore, 2007). At times, positive emotions are relevant, or integral, to the judgment or decision at hand (Loewenstein & Lerner, 2003). Incidental emotions are unrelated to the judgment or decision at hand, yet they often exert the same effects because individuals often incorrectly attribute their emotions to the decision or judgment. This process has been labeled the "How do I feel about it?" heuristic by Schwarz and Clore (2007).

A core focus of the research on positive emotions in organizations concerns whether integral and incidental positive emotions predict various behaviors and attitudes of importance in organizations (Brief & Weiss, 2002). Because they shape the way individuals act and think, positive emotions are related to criteria such as job satisfaction and job performance.

Job Satisfaction

One of the most proximal consequences of positive emotions at work is job satisfaction, a relatively stable attitude that reflects employees' evaluations of their jobs (Wagner & Ilies, 2008). Job satisfaction has both cognitive and affective components. Researchers have proposed that the emotions that employees feel on the job feed into their attitudes about their jobs, including their job satisfaction (e.g., Weiss & Cropanzano, 1996). The evidence supports this intuition.

Several of the relevant studies on positive emotions and job satisfaction are experience-sampling studies in which employees completed multiple measures of their moods. In one study, managers reported their positive emotions four times a day and, at a separate time, completed a standard measure of job satisfaction (Weiss, Nicholas, & Daus, 1999). The researchers aggregated the reports of positive emotions to form an aggregate measure of how much positive emotion managers felt in their work. The more positive emotions managers felt, on average, the more satisfied they were with their jobs.

In another study, employees completed multiple daily reports of both their positive emotions and their job satisfaction (Ilies & Judge, 2002). Researchers analyzed the relations between these variables both within and between individuals. The findings, with measures aggregated over the duration of the study, showed that employees who tended to feel more positive emotions were also more satisfied with their jobs, replicating previous research. Plus, in within-individual analyses, employees who felt less positive emotions were more satisfied with their jobs than when they felt more positive emotions. Similar conclusions were reached by Fuller and her colleagues (2003) in a study of administrative and staff members of a university. Controlling for serial dependencies in event-sampling data, the more employees felt positive emotions, the more they reported feeling satisfied with their jobs on the same day, and also on the next day.

These studies did not identify the source of the positive emotions that feed into job satisfaction judgments. As such, the findings could be interpreted as showing that integral positive emotions—positive emotions that are the result of aspects of their jobs—cause employees to become more satisfied. An experiment showed, however, that a temporary, brief induction of positive emotions influences job satisfaction judgments, even when this induction is unrelated to work (e.g., receiving a cookie) (Brief, Butcher, & Roberson, 1995). This reveals that job satisfaction judgments are shaped by a variety of positive emotions, including momentary positive emotions that are unrelated to work.

Taken together, the results support an association between positive emotions and job satisfaction. Not surprisingly, the more positive emotions employees feel at work, the more favorably they evaluate their jobs.

Job Performance

Research on positive emotions and job performance has focused on testing the happy–productive worker hypothesis (Staw, Sutton, & Pelled, 1994; Weiss & Cropanzano, 1996; Wright & Staw, 1999). The early studies did not measure positive emotions specifically. Instead, these studies used job satisfaction as a proxy for positive emotions, and correlated job satisfaction with job performance. The results of these studies revealed a weak or no relationship between job satisfaction and job performance (Brayfield & Crockett, 1955; see Iaffaldano & Muchinsky, 1985, for meta-analytic estimates). Researchers have argued that these relationships are weak or inconsistent because job satisfaction cannot be equated with positive emotions. Rather, as an attitude, job satisfaction is a composite of both emotions and cognitions. Subsequent refinements in the conceptualization and measurement of emotions at work have produced more conclusive findings.

One study tested the association between dispositional positive emotions and several dimensions of the performance of employees of three organizations (a hospital and two manufacturing companies). Higher dispositional positive emotions were associated with more positive change over the duration of the study in evaluations of performance by supervisors, pay, and support received from supervisors (Staw et al., 1994). In a related study, dispositional positive emotions were associated with more positive change over the duration of the study in supervisory evaluations of the performance of employees of two governmental organizations (Wright & Staw, 1999). These researchers examined how dispositional positive emotions at time 1 predicted job performance at time 2, con-

trolling for job performance at time 1, to alleviate some concerns about the direction of causality between the constructs.

To examine how positive emotions are associated with more objectively assessed workplace performance, Staw and Barsade (1993) examined the association between dispositional positive emotions and the performance of MBA (Master of Business Administration) students on a number of simulations of managerial performance. MBA students with higher dispositional positive emotions (1) made more accurate decisions in an in-basket exercise in which participants assumed the role of a plant manager tasked with making several important decisions, (2) performed better (in terms of quality and quantity) in a leaderless group discussion exercise, and (3) were rated as having more potential as managers than those with lower dispositional positive emotions.

A separate study examined the mechanisms underlying the associations between positive emotions at work and high job performance in a sample of sales agents (Tsai, Chen, & Liu, 2007). Tsai and colleagues (2007) found evidence for two paths linking positive emotions to high sales. The first path focused on interpersonal dynamics: Positive emotions were associated with more helping behaviors between sales agents and their coworkers, and increased help in turn was related to higher sales. The second path focused on intrapersonal dynamics: Positive emotions were associated with higher self-efficacy and higher persistence, which were both related to higher sales.

In a study of a new direction extending basic research on implicit emotions, dispositional positive emotions measured implicitly (with a word-fragment task) were associated with higher job performance, assessed by supervisors, even when researchers controlled for explicit dispositional positive emotions measured with a traditional self-report measure (Johnson, Tolentino, Rodopman, & Cho, 2010).

The preceding evidence provides converging evidence that positive emotions are related to higher job performance. Researchers have identified jobs in which feeling and displaying positive emotions are hurtful to performance. A qualitative study examined display rules in a bill collection agency, identifying which emotions collectors were encouraged to display to increase their chances of garnering payment (Sutton, 1991). The study found that bill collectors tend to feel different emotions depending on the behaviors of the debtors. Friendly or despondent debtors tended to elicit sympathy from the bill collectors. To increase chances of garnering payment and attaining high performance, however, bill collectors were encouraged to show irritation or anger to these debtors. By contrast, angry debtors tended to elicit anger, but bill collectors were encouraged to be neutral or show calmness to these debtors. Thus, positive emotions were sometimes helpful, but sometimes unhelpful to performance, depending on the demeanor of the debtors.

Another study examined the effectiveness of a "good cop–bad cop" strategy in which two police interrogators alternated between displays of negative and positive emotions. This strategy elicited more confessions from criminal suspects than displays of positive or negative emotions alone (Rafaeli & Sutton, 1991). This is because suspects were inclined to admit wrongdoings to the good cop to escape dealings with the bad cop, or to reciprocate the perceived kindness of the good cop. Thus, it was effective for one interrogator to feel and show positive emotions; the other interrogator had to show contrasting, negative emotions to boost performance.

The preceding discussion suggests that positive emotions can facilitate job performance in many occupations, but it also indicates that the role of positive emotions is more complex for some jobs that, at times, call for feelings and displays of neutral or even negative emotions.

Creativity

Positive emotions signal to individuals that the environment is benign, and that there is little risk in trying new approaches and ideas (Fredrickson, 1998; Schwarz & Clore, 1983). Indeed, basic research on positive emotions and creativity demonstrated that organization members tend to be more creative when feeling positive emotions (see Isen & Baron, 1991, for a review).

Organizational researchers have tested the proposition that positive emotions enhance the creativity of employees more than neutral or negative emotions. In the most extensive investigation of this effect, Amabile, Barsade, Mueller, and Staw (2005) examined the association between positive emotions and creativity in a sample of employees of companies in the chemicals, high-tech, and consumer products industries. Employees reported on their positive emotions in a diary that they completed at the end of each day. In addition, expert raters coded the degree to which employees reported creative thoughts in response to an open-ended question answered daily, in which they described an event from the day that stood out in their minds as relevant to their work on a target project. The findings showed that at the within-individual level of analysis, employees were more creative when they felt positive emotions.

As with performance, there might be some organizational contexts in which positive emotions are unrelated to or even undermine creativity. George and Zhou (2002) found some evidence that positive moods can impede creativity in some circumstances. They studied the creativity of employees of a manufacturing company whose tasks involved creating new designs and manufacturing techniques. Creativity was rated by supervisors. The results show that when employees perceived creativity to be directly rewarded, and they were clear about their feelings, higher positive emotions reported by the employees were associated with less creativity. This, presumably, is because in these conditions, employees' positive emotions signaled that they were doing well and that they would be rewarded, consistent with the logic of the mood-as-input model (Martin, Ward, Achee, & Wyer, 1993). Hence, positive employees exerted less effort to be creative in these conditions.

Organizational Citizenship Behavior

Organizational researchers have presented the premise that employees who feel good are more likely to be prosocial (George & Brief, 1992). In organizational settings, prosocial action is manifest in organizational citizenship or spontaneity behaviors—behaviors that facilitate the attainment of organizational objectives, yet are not included in formal job descriptions (Organ, 1988). These behaviors include helping coworkers who are in need (e.g., because they have missed a day of work due to illness) and promoting the organization (e.g., by talking positively about the organization when not at work) (George & Brief, 1992; Lee & Allen, 2002; Organ, 1988).

There is support for this proposition. In one study, George (1991) examined the relation between the positive emotions of salespeople and their citizenship behaviors, evaluated by their superiors, and found a positive association. In another investigation, nurses who felt more positive emotions exhibited more citizenship behaviors, evaluated by their coworkers (Lee & Allen, 2002).

These findings indicate that employees who tend to feel the most positive emotions at work, on average, are those who tend to exhibit the most citizenship behaviors. Results of this research at the between-persons level of analysis cannot necessarily be extrapolated to the within-persons levels of analysis (Ostroff, 1993). Specifically, we cannot conclude from an association between positive emotions and citizenship behaviors at the between-persons level of analysis that when a specific employee feels positive emotions, that employee is more prosocial than when he or she feels neutral (at the within-person level of analysis). A positive association at one level of analysis can be nonexistent or even negative at a different level of analysis (Ostroff, 1993).

Ilies, Scott, and Judge (2006) tested the association between positive emotions and organizational citizenship behaviors at the within-person level of analysis, with multiple measures of both constructs for each employee. They found that employees exhibited more citizenship on days when they felt more positive emotions than on days when they felt less positive emotions. They also found that this association was less strong for employees with higher rather than lower levels of agreeableness. Agreeable employees were more likely to engage in citizenship behaviors regardless of their positive emotions because these employees behaved prosocially by default. By contrast, positive emotions were more strongly linked to the citizenship behaviors of employees low on agreeableness.

Cooperation

Via processes similar to those linking positive emotions to organizational citizenship behaviors, positive emotions may also produce more cooperative mindsets in individuals. In particular, positive emotions may influence individuals' approaches toward conflict resolution and, specifically, their tendencies to cooperate rather than compete with others. An early investigation found that participants were more likely to indicate willingness to collaborate to resolve future conflicts after they were exposed to a positive emotion induction, compared to a negative emotion induction (Baron, 1984). In another study, eliciting positive emotions led negotiators to adopt a more collaborative approach, to be more likely to adopt the point of view of their adversary, and to reach more integrative solutions, compared to negotiators who had not been subjected to this induction (Carnevale & Isen, 1986).

Performance Appraisal

Positive emotions have been found to produce favorable judgments. The mood-as-information model proposes that individuals can misattribute their emotions to the judgment task at hand, relying on a "How do I feel about it?" heuristic to make judgments (Schwarz & Clore, 1996). Consistent with this model, research has found that experiencing positive emotions toward an employee—indexed by liking of the employee—enhances evaluations of that employee's performance, all else being equal (Cardy & Dobbins, 1986; Tsui & Barry, 1986).

Although this effect represents a source of bias, positive emotions may also de-bias some judgments about performance. In one study (Keller et al., 2005), participants were asked to evaluate the performance of a job candidate, which was described in two paragraphs. In the first paragraph of information about the candidate, participants were presented with either some positive information about the candidate or some negative information. Participants who read positive information in the first paragraph read negative information in the second paragraph, and vice versa. Inducing positive emotions reduced participants' susceptibility to first impression effects, so that participants who read positive information first provided more nuanced evaluations of the candidate that reflected more openness to the latter information, compared to control participants. This result presumably reflects the broadening effect of positive emotions (Fredrickson, 1998).

Network Ties

There is a stream of research that examines the degree to which organization members' decisions about whom to associate and work with is determined by how they feel toward their coworkers. In a demonstration of this effect, the emotions that organization members felt toward their coworkers trumped perceived competence of coworkers as predictors of workplace interactions that specifically involved work tasks (Casciaro & Lobo, 2008). To perform their work tasks, organization members were more likely to choose to associate with coworkers toward whom they felt positive emotions, especially if these coworkers were also perceived to be competent. By contrast, organization members avoided coworkers toward whom they felt negative emotions, even when these coworkers were perceived to be highly competent. This effect, found in three different companies, provides convincing support for the idea that emotions shape social network structures in organizations and influence who will reach central and powerful positions.

Summary

The research summarized in the preceding section indicates that employees act and think differently when they feel positive emotions than when they feel neutral or negative emotions. Positive emotions have potent intrapersonal effects on employees; employees perform better on a number of tasks, are more creative, are more helpful to others, and have a more cooperative mindset when they feel positive emotions. For certain tasks, however, positive emotions are detrimental to performance. There is also evidence that positive emotions not only produce particularly lenient evaluations of the performance of other people but also broaden the set of information that individuals use when making these judgments.

The Interpersonal Effects of Positive Emotions in Organizations

In organizations, displays of emotions are particularly potent given that organizations encourage employees to display certain emotions and hide others (Hochschild, 1983; Rafaeli & Sutton, 1987), and that expressed emotions are used strategically to influence others (Andrade & Ho, 2009). Thus, in addition to their intrapersonal effects, research has also identified interpersonal, or social effects, of positive emotions in organizations.

These interpersonal effects are based on the social functions of emotions. Social-functional accounts of emotions posit that individuals attend to others' displays of emotions because these displays provide important information about the behavior they might expect from others (Côté, 2005; Frijda & Mesquita, 1994; Keltner & Haidt, 1999; Van Kleef, 2009). Individuals rapidly identify and respond to others' displays of emotions. They may catch the emotions that other people feel and display through a contagion process (Hatfield, Cacioppo, & Rapson, 1994), or like or dislike someone more depending on the emotions he or she expresses (Van Kleef, 2009). Individuals also draw inferences from others' displays of emotions, and these inferences, in turn, shape how perceivers think, act, and feel (Van Kleef, 2009).

Social-functional accounts of emotions are supported by evidence that basic emotions are characterized by specific facial displays involving distinct muscle movements (Ekman, 2003) and specific vocal expressions involving distinct acoustic features (Juslin & Scherer, 2005) that are similar across cultures. In addition, research shows that individuals are particularly attuned to identify information about emotions in their environments (MacLeod, Mathews, & Tata, 1986; Mogg & Bradley, 1999). Displays of emotions that are shown subliminally—outside of the conscious awareness of observers—elicit corresponding muscle movements in observers, suggesting that emotions cues have evolutionary significance (Dimberg, Thunberg, & Elmehed, 2000).

In addition, displays of emotions have systematic effects on the attitudes and behaviors of people who observe them. For instance, people infer the dispositions of other individuals, such as their dominance and affiliation, from their displays of emotions (Knutson, 1996). In one study, displays of positive emotions in yearbook photographs of women graduating from a private college were associated with naive observers' evaluations of both competence and affiliation, and with the women's marital satisfaction and well-being 40 years later (Harker & Keltner, 2001).

Organizational research has drawn from the social-functional approach to emotions to suggest that the emotions displayed by organization members influence the attitudes and behaviors of those who view these displays of emotions in various organizational contexts. In this section, I review the literature on the interpersonal effects of emotions in organizations—the effects of organization members' emotions on the attitudes, inferences, and behaviors of perceivers who are members of the organization or outsiders.

Leadership

Research has examined how the positive emotions of leaders are related to the emotions and performance of their followers. George (1995) examined how the positive emotions of leaders are associated with the level of customer service provided by salespeople. The results show that the teams of leaders who experience more positive emotions offer better service than the teams of leaders who experience less positive emotions. A related study found that teams of salespeople with leaders who felt more positive emotions exhibited more citizenship behaviors, had less voluntary turnover, and sold more than teams whose leaders had less positive mood (George & Bettenhausen, 1990). Bono and Ilies (2006) found that leaders who expressed more positive emotions were perceived to be more effective than leaders who expressed neutral emotions.

Other researchers examined the mechanisms that link positive emotions of leaders and worker performance. In one study, leaders who were induced to feel positive emotions had groups that exhibited better coordination, but less effort, than leaders induced to feel negative emotions (Sy, Côté, & Saavedra, 2005). The effects of the leaders' emotions on the teams occurred via two paths. The positive emotions of leaders were associated with higher team coordination through the positive emotions of the team members. Specifically, the positive emotions of leaders were caught by the members of the teams they led, and team members' positive emotions in turn were positively associated with the cooperation they exhibited (consistent with the findings on positive emotions and cooperation by Carnevale & Isen, 1986, described earlier). By contrast, the association between the positive emotions of leaders and the (reduced) effort of teams was not mediated by the positive emotions of team members. Instead, this effect may have occurred via an inferential process (Van Kleef, 2009). Presumably, team members inferred from their leaders' positive emotions that their performance was satisfactory, so no additional effort was needed.

A related study showed that these effects depend on the personality of the followers and, more specifically, their "epistemic motivation," which reflects the degree to which a person is motivated to develop a complex understanding of situations (Kruglanski, 1989). Van Kleef and his associates (2009) found that teams with higher epistemic motivation performed better when the leader displayed negative rather than positive emotions because negative emotions presumably indicated that the leader was not satisfied with the current progress. Teams with lower epistemic motivation, however, performed better when the leader displayed positive rather than negative emotions because these teams simply caught positive emotions that, in turn, enhanced their cooperative behavior.

Another study revealed that the effects of leaders' positive emotions depend on followers' desire for social harmony, operationalized in terms of individual differences in agreeableness (Van Kleef, Homan, Beersma, & Van Knippenberg, 2010). In this investigation, teams comprising highly agreeable followers performed better when the leader expressed happiness, but this effect was not found in teams comprising low-agreeable followers.

Negotiations

Positive emotions also have social effects in the domain of negotiations. Research in this domain has shown that displayed emotions influence the attitudes and behaviors of counterparts. These studies suggest that expressions of anger communicate toughness and high limits (Sinaceur & Tiedens, 2006; Van Kleef et al., 2004), whereas happiness communicates satisfaction with the current state of affairs (Van Kleef et al., 2004). In turn, expressions of happiness by one counterpart produce higher demands from opponents compared to neutral (Sinaceur & Tiedens, 2006) and angry emotional expressions (Van Kleef et al., 2004).

In another series of studies, Kopelman, Rosette, and Thompson (2006) found that (1) in a dispute setting, the counterparts of negotiators who displayed positive rather than negative or neutral emotions were more likely to desire future interaction; (2) in an ultimatum setting, negotiators who displayed positive rather than negative emotions were more likely to close a deal; and (3) in a distributive negotiation setting, negotiators placed higher demands on opponents displaying negative rather than positive emotions.

This research has almost exclusively focused on steady-state emotions that did not vary over time. However, in negotiations, as in other organizational contexts, the emotions that individuals show often vary over time. Filipowicz, Barsade, and Melwani (2011) examined the effects of switching from a display of happiness to one of anger, and vice versa, during negotiations. They found that displaying anger first, followed by happiness, led negotiation partners to develop worse impressions than did consistently displaying happiness. In the former case, (1) perceivers were more likely to attribute the happiness to the situation rather than the other person; also, (2) perceivers caught the other person's anger, and this caught anger, in turn, led them to react less favorably.

A related investigation examined how the effects of displayed "emotional ambivalence"—the simultaneous display of positive and negative emotions—differ from those of simpler displays of emotions (Rothman, 2011). Perceivers evaluated others whose displays were ambivalent as more deliberative and submissive, and perceivers were more dominant toward them than toward a simply happy other. These studies make the important point that the effects of displayed emotions are interpreted in context rather than in isolation. This point is particularly important to understanding the social effects of positive emotions in context-rich organizational settings.

Customer Service

Research on customer service has examined whether the emotions expressed by service agents influence customer judgments and behaviors. Customer service agents regulate their emotions to conform to organizational display rules (Hochschild, 1983; Rafaeli & Sutton, 1987) and, ultimately, influence the behavior and attitudes and customers. In customer service, agents typically up-regulate positive emotions and down-regulate negative emotions.

Several studies have found that displays of positive emotions by service agents have positive effects for organizations in various customer service settings. For example, Pugh (2001) found that bank tellers' positive emotional displays were related to clients' positive emotions following the service interaction and to positive customer evaluations of service quality. Research by Tsai (2001) and Tsai and Huang (2002) showed that retail employees' positive emotional displays increased customers' satisfaction with the quality of the service, and their willingness to return to the store and to make positive comments to friends.

Research on positive emotions in customer service has examined whether these effects occur for displays of positive emotions that are both authentic and inauthentic. In one study, authentic displays of positive emotions resulted in perceptions of friendliness and favorable performance judgments, but inauthentic displays of positive emotions—displays that are not accompanied by subjective positive emotions—did not show this effect (Grandey et al., 2005). In other studies, service agents who displayed authentic positive emotions were rated as performing better than those whose emotions were inauthentic (Grandey, 2003; Groth et al., 2009). These studies show that authenticity of displays of positive emotions plays an important role.

Sutton and Rafaeli (1988) found that employees' displays of pleasant emotions were negatively related to sales in convenience stores. To further investigate this unexpected result, the authors conducted some qualitative analyses. These analyses showed that employees of stores with high levels of sales were busier and, in turn, less likely to display positive emotions than employees in slow-paced stores, who had time and resources to devote to displaying positive emotions. This study shows that some powerful organizational contexts can reduce or eliminate the effects of positive emotions.

Summary

Research on the interpersonal effects of positive emotions reveals a pattern whereby organization members who observe others' displays of positive emotions infer they are satisfied with the state of affairs (especially in leadership and negotiation contexts) and willing to help (especially in customer service contexts). Thus, displaying positive emotions may sometimes hurt organization members by signaling to others that no additional efforts are needed, and that others can expect cooperation from displayers. The research on the interpersonal effects of positive emotions also highlights the importance of authenticity. Inauthentic displays of positive emotions elicit different responses in observers than do authentic displays.

Group-Level Positive Affect

Organizational researchers are often interested in predicting criteria at the group level of analysis, such as the performance of teams. The premise of this research is that positive emotions can be treated as a group-level property that predicts the outcomes of groups. One specific construct that has been examined in this literature is positive affective tone (George, 1990).

Positive Affective Tone

George (1990) defined "group affective tone" as "consistent or homogeneous affective reactions within a group" (p. 108). It is an aggregate of the moods of the individual members of the group and refers to mood at the group level of analysis. If the moods of individual group members are consistent, then group affective tone can be treated as a group property (George, 1990). Past research indicates that a majority of groups possess an affective tone (see George, 1996, for a review). Several mechanisms can produce consistent emotions within a group, including the selection and composition of group members, the socialization of group members, and exposure of group members to the same emotion-inducing events, such as task demands and outcomes (George, 1996; Weiss & Cropanzano, 1996). In addition, emotions tend to be shared among group members through processes such as emotional contagion (Hatfield et al., 1994) and impression management (Kelly & Barsade, 2001).

Research has found that positive affective tone is associated with meaningful group-level criteria. A study of salespeople found that there were fewer absences in groups with a higher positive affective tone than in groups with a lower positive affective tone (George, 1990). In addition, positive affective tone was not related to the amount of prosocial behavior exhibited by the group, but a higher negative affective tone was related to less prosocial behavior (George, 1990).

A previously mentioned study found that higher positive affective tone in groups was associated with better coordination among group members, but it was also related to reduced effort (Sy et al., 2005). When team members felt positive emotions, they were presumably more willing to cooperate with others, consistent with past research on emotions and cooperation (Carnevale & Isen, 1986; George, 1990). But positive emotions may inform team members that they have attained a high level of performance, signaling that no additional effort is necessary (Sy et al., 2005).

Summary

The research on positive affective tone reveals additional (mostly positive) consequences of positive emotions in organizations. Positive emotions are not just related to individual-level outcomes such as the job performance of employees. In addition, the average level of positive emotions in groups is associated with group-level outcomes such as absenteeism and cooperation.

New Research Developments

Discrete Positive Emotions

Almost all of the research described so far has focused on positive emotions as a broad construct. Research has only begun to explore the consequences of different discrete positive emotions in organizations. It is likely that different positive emotions, such as pride, interest, happiness, and awe, have different consequences for organization members, just as they do outside of organizations (Fredrickson, 1998; Shiota, Keltner, & John, 2006).

One investigation examined the role of pride in the commitment of volunteers (Boezeman & Ellemers, 2007). The more pride the volunteers felt, the more likely they were to indicate they would continue to volunteer for their organization, and that they were committed to their organization. This research highlights a positive aspect of pride: Pride in one's work increases commitment and, presumably, other outcomes, such as job performance.

Other research indicates that pride may also have nefarious effects on organizational outcomes. Oveis, Horberg, and Keltner (2010) found that pride increases the degree to which individuals feel similar to strong others and decreases the degree to which they feel similar to weak others. Thus, pride may guide organization members' decisions about whom they choose to work with and to hire. Furthermore, research has identified a distinct expression of pride that involves expanded posture, arms above the head or hands of hips, and the head tilted slightly back (Tracy & Robins, 2004). This display may have important social effects in organizations; those who observe displays of pride may infer that those who show pride have excelled at their work, which could shape how observers treat them, over and above any effect of actual performance. These questions await further research.

In addition, a small literature on compassion in organizations explores how compassion is triggered and how it influences individual and collective outcomes (Dutton, Worline, Frost, & Lilius, 2006; Lilius et al., 2008; Lilius, Worline, Dutton, Kanov, & Maitlis, 2011). This research has focused on compassion as an organizational-level construct, a topic to which I now turn.

The Emergence of Organizational-Level Positive Emotions

Researchers have devised several composition models to theorize about the meaning of group- or organizational-level constructs (e.g., Chan, 1998). The affective tone construct described earlier relies on averaging the levels of positive emotions experienced by the members of a group or the employees of the organization (to the extent that they are similar; George, 1990).

Other composition models are possible. One alternative model emphasizes the concept of "emotional capability," which is the degree to which members of organizations typically try to recognize, monitor, discriminate, and attend to each other's emotions (Huy, 1999; Reus & Liu, 2004). Groups with higher levels of emotional capability perform emotion-related organizational routines to achieve specific organizational goals, whereas groups with lower emotional capability do not. In particular, groups with higher emotional capability may enact actions that arouse positive emotions, such as hope, which motivates collective action, or empathy, which increases receptivity to major changes. Via these processes, emotional capabilities related to positive emotions may predict some of the outcomes of the organization.

Other researchers have examined another type of group construct: the amount of variability in positive emotions within groups. Barsade, Ward, Turner, and Sonnenfeld (2000) examined "affective diversity" in top management teams of companies, defined as the degree to which the emotions of the members of the teams varied from each other. In one set of analyses, the degree to which one team member's emotions matched those of the other team members predicted team member's attitudes about the group, and how much the team member perceived him- or herself to be influential in the team. In another set of analyses, teams with diverse levels of positive emotions exhibited the most conflict and the least cooperation, when the average level of positive emotion in the team was relatively low. These results suggest that whether all the members of a team experience positive emotions, or whether only some members feel positive emotions may have important consequences for organizational processes.

Another form of theorizing about organizational-level positive emotions involves more complex compositional models that are grounded in an emergence perspective (Kozlowski & Klein, 2000; Thiétart & Forgues, 1995). According to this perspective, collective phenomena are often more than the sum of their parts. Theories of emergence describe the patterns of interpersonal interaction that are involved in collective phenomena. Dutton and colleagues (2006) described the routines in organizations that facilitate general feelings of compassion by organization members. They found through qualitative research that behaviors such as improvisation and the enabling of attention to those who are suffering facilitated the emergence of compassion in an organization.

Interventions to Increase Positive Emotions

The evidence that positive emotions provide a host of benefits for organization members invites questions about whether positive emotions can be increased through intervention. Preliminary research provides some evidence that interventions may be successful if they are designed correctly and participants commit to them. In one investigation, participants assigned to express optimism and gratitude reported higher subjective well-being at the end of the 8-month intervention than did participants in a control group, particularly if they committed personal effort toward the intervention (Lyubomirsky, Dickerhoof, Boehm, & Sheldon, 2011).

Another investigation in an organization lends further credence to the proposition that interventions can boost positive emotions and their benefits (Fredrickson, Cohn, Coffey, Pek, & Finkel, 2008). Employees at a business software and information technology services company underwent an 8-week loving-kindness meditation intervention. The meditation involved directing love and compassion toward the self, loved ones, acquaintances, strangers, and all living beings. The results showed that the employees in the intervention group felt more positive emotions at the conclusion of the intervention than did a control group. In turn, increased positive emotions were associated with benefits such as decreased illness symptoms and higher social support. Although research in this area is preliminary, the findings suggest that interventions that boost positive emotions in organizational settings and provide the benefits associated with positive emotions may be successful.

Conclusion

The research described in this chapter reveals that positive emotions play important roles in organizations. Positive emotions shape organization members' behaviors and attitudes at work. Furthermore, because organizations are inherently interpersonal, positive emotions also shape organizational dynamics through social effects. Specifically, displays of positive emotions by organization members guide the behaviors and attitudes of others who view them in domains such as leadership and negotiation.

Many of the findings about positive emotions in organizations are consistent with the basic research described in other chapters of this volume. Organizational research, however, makes important contributions to our knowledge of positive emotions. This research identified organizational conditions that modify the effects of positive emotions, so that positive emotions can sometimes be hurtful to performance (depending on what is expected in the job), and displaying positive emotions can sometimes backfire (e.g., by signaling that the effort shown so far meets the expected standards). Thus, examining positive emotions in organizational contexts improves our understanding of their effects. In addition, organizational research examines the consequences of positive emotions as a collective property, such as the average level of positive emotion in the group or the diversity of positive emotional experiences. This research also expands our understanding of the manifestations of positive emotions in social life.

References

Amabile, T. M., Barsade, S. G., Mueller, J. S., & Staw, B. M. (2005). Affect and creativity at work. *Administrative Science Quarterly, 50,* 367–403.

Andrade, E. B., & Ho, T-H. (2009). Gaming emotions in social interactions. *Journal of Consumer Research, 36,* 539–551.

Baron, R. A. (1984). Reducing organizational conflict: An incompatible response approach. *Journal of Applied Psychology, 69,* 272–279.

Barsade, S., & Gibson, D. E. (2007). Why does affect matter in organizations? *Academy of Management Perspectives, 21,* 36–59.

Barsade, S. G., Ward, A. J., Turner, J. D. F., & Sonnenfeld, J. A. (2000). To your heart's content: A model of affective diversity in top management teams. *Administrative Science Quarterly, 45,* 802–836.

Boezeman, E. J., & Ellemers, N. (2007). Volunteering for charity: Pride, respect, and the commitment of volunteers. *Journal of Applied Psychology, 92,* 771–785.

Bono, J. E., & Ilies, R. (2006). Charisma, positive emotions and mood contagion. *Leadership Quarterly, 17,* 317–334.

Brayfield, A. H., & Crockett, W. H. (1955). Employee attitudes and employee performance. *Psychological Bulletin, 52,* 396.

Brief, A. P., Butcher, A. H., & Roberson, L. (1995). Cookies, disposition, and job attitudes: The effects of positive mood-inducing events and negative affectivity on job satisfaction in a field experiment. *Organizational Behavior and Human Decision Processes, 62,* 55–62.

Brief, A. P., & Weiss, H. M. (2002). Organizational behavior: Affect in the workplace. *Annual Review of Psychology, 53,* 279–307.

Cardy, R. L., & Dobbins, G. H. (1986). Affect and appraisal accuracy: Liking as an integral dimension in evaluating performance. *Journal of Applied Psychology, 71,* 672–678.

Carnevale, P. J., & Isen, A. M. (1986). The influence of positive affect and visual access on the discovery of integrative solutions in bilateral negotiation. *Organizational Behavior and Human Decision Processes, 37,* 1–13.

Casciaro, T., & Lobo, M. S. (2008). When competence is irrelevant: The role of interpersonal affect in task-related ties. *Administrative Science Quarterly, 53,* 655–684.

Chan, D. (1998). Functional relations among constructs in the same content domain at different levels of analysis: A typology of composition models. *Journal of Applied Psychology, 83,* 234–246.

Côté, S. (2005). A social interaction model of the effects of emotion regulation on work strain. *Academy of Management Review, 30,* 509–530.

Dimberg, U., Thunberg, M., & Elmehed, K. (2000). Unconscious facial reactions to emotional facial expressions. *Psychological Science, 11,* 86–89.

Dutton, J., Worline, M., Frost, P., & Lilius, J. (2006). Explaining compassion organizing. *Administrative Science Quarterly, 51,* 59–96.

Ekman, P. (2003). *Emotions revealed.* New York: Henry Holt.

Filipowicz, A., Barsade, S., & Melwani, S. (2011). Understanding emotional transitions: The interpersonal consequences of changing emotions in negotiations. *Journal of Personality and Social Psychology, 101,* 541–556.

Fredrickson, B. L. (1998). What good are positive emotions? *Review of General Psychology, 3,* 300–319.

Fredrickson, B. L., Cohn, M. A., Coffey, K. A., Pek, J., & Finkel, S. M. (2008). Open hearts build lives: Positive emotions, induced through loving-kindness meditation, build consequential personal resources. *Journal of Personality and Social Psychology, 95,* 1045–1062.

Frijda, N. H. (1986). *The emotions.* Cambridge, UK: Cambridge University Press.

Frijda, N. H., Kuipers, P., & ter Schure, E. (1989). Relations among emotions, appraisal, and emotional action tendencies. *Journal of Personality and Social Psychology, 57,* 212–228.

Frijda, N. H., & Mesquita, B. (1994). The social roles and functions of emotions. In S. Kitayama & H. R. Markus (Eds.), *Emotion and culture: Empirical studies of mutual influence* (pp. 51–87). Washington, DC: American Psychological Association.

Fuller, J. A., Stanton, J. M., Fisher, G. G., Spitzmüller, C., Russell, S. S., & Smith, P. C. (2003). A lengthy look at the daily grind: Time series analysis of events, mood, stress, and satisfaction. *Journal of Applied Psychology, 88,* 1019–1033.

George, J. M. (1990). Personality, affect, and behavior in groups. *Journal of Applied Psychology, 75,* 107–116.

George, J. M. (1991). State or trait: Effects of positive mood on prosocial behaviors at work. *Journal of Applied Psychology, 76,* 299–307.

George, J. M. (1995). Leader positive mood and group performance: The case of customer service. *Journal of Applied Social Psychology, 25,* 778–794.

George, J. M. (1996). Group affective tone. In M. West (Ed.), *Handbook of work group psychology* (pp. 77–93). New York: Wiley.

George, J. M., & Bettenhausen, K. (1990). Understanding prosocial behavior, sales performance, and turnover: A group level analysis in a service context. *Journal of Applied Psychology, 75,* 698–709.

George, J. M., & Brief, A. P. (1992). Feeling good-doing good: A conceptual analysis of the mood at work-organizational spontaneity relationship. *Psychological Bulletin, 112,* 310–329.

George, J. M., & Zhou, J. (2002). Understanding when bad moods foster creativity and good ones don't: The role of context and clarity of feelings. *Journal of Applied Psychology, 87,* 687–697.

Grandey, A. A. (2003). When "the show must go on": Surface and deep acting as determinants of emotional exhaustion and peer-rated service delivery. *Academy of Management Journal, 46,* 86–96.

Grandey, A. A., Fisk, G. M., Mattila, A. S., Jansen, K. J., & Sideman, L. A. (2005). Is "service with a smile" enough?: Authenticity of positive displays during service encounters. *Organizational Behavior and Human Decision Processes, 96,* 38–55.

Groth, M., Hennig-Thurau, T., & Walsh, G, (2009). Customer reactions to emotional labor: The roles of employee acting strategies and customer detection accuracy. *Academy of Management Journal, 52,* 958–974.

Harker, L., & Keltner D. (2001). Expressions of positive emotion in women's college yearbook pictures and their relationship to personality and life outcomes across adulthood. *Journal of Personality and Social Psychology, 80,* 112–124.

Hatfield, E., Cacioppo, J. T., & Rapson, R. L. (1994). *Emotional contagion.* New York: Cambridge University Press.

Hochschild, A. R. (1983). *The managed heart.* Berkeley: University of California Press.

Huy, Q. N. (1999). Emotional capability, emotional intelligence, and radical change. *Academy of Management Review, 24,* 325–349.

Iaffaldano, M. T., & Muchinsky, P. M. (1985). Job satisfaction and job performance: A meta-analysis. *Psychological Bulletin, 97,* 251–273.

Ilies, R., & Judge, T. A. (2002). Understanding the dynamic relationships among personality, mood, and job satisfaction: A field experience-sampling study. *Organizational Behavior and Human Decision Processes, 89,* 1119–1139.

Ilies, R., Scott, B. A., & Judge, T. A. (2006). The interactive effects of personal traits and experienced states on intraindividual patterns of citizenship behavior. *Academy of Management Journal, 49,* 561–575.

Isen, A. M., & Baron, R. A. (1991). Positive affect as a factor in organizational behavior. *Research in Organizational Behavior, 13,* 1–53.

Isen, A. M., Daubman, K. A., & Nowicki, G. P. (1987). Positive affect facilitates creative problem solving. *Journal of Personality and Social Psychology, 52,* 1122–1131.

Johnson, R. E., Tolentino, A. L., Rodopman, O. B., & Cho, E. (2010). We (sometimes) know not how we feel: Predicting work behaviors with an implicit measure of trait affectivity. *Personnel Psychology, 63,* 197–219.

Juslin, P. N., & Scherer, K. R. (2005). Vocal expression of affect. In J. A. Harrigan, R. Rosenthal, & K. R. Scherer (Eds.), *The new handbook of methods in nonverbal behavior research* (pp. 65–135). New York: Oxford University Press.

Kelly, J. R., & Barsade, S. G. (2001). Moods and emotions in small groups and work groups. *Organizational Behavior and Human Decision Processes, 86,* 99–130.

Keller, M. C., Fredrickson, B. L., Ybarra, O., Côté, S., Johnson, K., Mikels, J., et al. (2005). Research article. A warm heart and a clear head: The contingent effects of weather on mood and cognition. *Psychological Science, 16,* 724–731.

Keltner, D., & Haidt, J. (1999). Social functions of emotions at four levels of analysis. *Cognition and Emotion, 13,* 505–521.

Knutson, B. (1996). Facial expressions of emotion influence interpersonal trait inferences. *Journal of Nonverbal Behavior, 20,* 165–182.

Kopelman, S., Rosette, A., & Thompson, L. (2006). The three faces of eve: Strategic displays of positive negative and neutral emotions in negotiations. *Organizational Behavior and Human Decision Processes, 99,* 81–101.

Kozlowski, S. W. J., & Klein, K. J. (2000). A multilevel approach to theory and research in organizations: Contextual, temporal, and emergent processes. In K. J. Klein & S. W. J. Kozlowski (Eds.), *Multilevel theory, research, and methods in organizations* (pp. 3–90). San Francisco: Jossey-Bass.

Kruglanski, A. W. (1989). *Lay epistemics and human knowledge: Cognitive and motivational bases.* New York: Plenum Press.

Lee, K., & Allen, N. J. (2002). Organizational citizenship behavior and workplace deviance: The role of affect and cognitions. *Journal of Applied Psychology, 87,* 131.

Lilius, J., Worline, M., Dutton, J., Kanov, J., & Maitlis, S. (2011). Understanding compassion capability. *Human Relations, 64,* 873–891.

Lilius, J., Worline, M., Maitlis, S., Kanov, J., Dutton, J., & Frost, P. (2008). Contours of compassion at work. *Journal of Organization Behavior, 29,* 193–218.

Loewenstein, G., & Lerner, J. S. (2003). The role of affect in decision making. In R. Davidson, H. Goldsmith, & K. Scherer (Eds.), *Handbook of affective science* (pp. 619–642). Oxford, UK: Oxford University Press.

Lyubomirsky, S., Dickerhoof, R., Boehm, J. K., & Sheldon, K. M. (2011). Becoming happier takes both a will and a proper way: An experimental longitudinal intervention to boost well-being. *Emotion, 11,* 391–402.

Lyubomirsky, S., King, L. A., & Diener, E. (2005). The benefits of frequent positive affect. *Psychological Bulletin, 131,* 803–855.

MacLeod, C., Mathews, A., & Tata, P. (1986). Attentional bias in emotional disorders. *Journal of Abnormal Psychology, 95,* 15–20.

Martin, L. L., Ward, D. W., Achee, J. W., & Wyer, R. S., Jr. (1993). Mood as input: People have to interpret the motivational implications of their moods. *Journal of Personality and Social Psychology, 64,* 317–326.

Mogg, K., & Bradley, B. P. (1999). Orienting of attention to threatening facial expressions presented under conditions of restricted awareness. *Cognition and Emotion, 13,* 713–740.

Organ, D. W. (1988). *Organizational citizenship behavior: The good soldier syndrome.* Lexington, MA: Lexington Books.

Ostroff, C. (1993). Comparing correlations based on individual-level and aggregated data. *Journal of Applied Psychology, 78,* 569–582.

Oveis, C., Horberg, E. J., & Keltner, D. (2010). Compassion, pride, and social intuitions of self–other similarity. *Journal of Personality and Social Psychology, 98,* 618–630.

Pugh, S. D. (2001). Service with a smile: Emotional contagion in the service encounter. *Academy of Management Journal, 44,* 1018–1027.

Rafaeli, A., & Sutton, R. I. (1987). Expression of emotion as part of the work role. *Academy of Management Review, 12,* 23–37.

Rafaeli, A., & Sutton, R. I. (1991). Emotional contrast strategies as means of social influence: Lessons from criminal interrogators and bill collectors. *Academy of Management Journal, 34,* 749–775.

Reus, T. H., & Liu, Y. (2004). Rhyme and reason: Emotional capability and the performance of knowledge-intensive work groups. *Human Performance, 17,* 245–266.

Rosenberg, E. L. (1998). Levels of analysis and the organization of affect. *Review of General Psychology, 2,* 247–270.

Rothman, N. B. (2011). Steering sheep: How expressed emotional ambivalence elicits dominance in interdependent decision-making contexts. *Organizational Behavior and Human Decision Processes, 116,* 66–82.

Schwarz, N., & Clore, G. L. (1983). Mood, misattribution, and judgments of well-being: Informative and directive functions of affective states. *Journal of Personality and Social Psychology, 45,* 513–523.

Schwarz, N., & Clore, G. L. (1996). Feelings and phenomenal experiences. In E. T. Higgins & A. Kruglanski (Eds.), *Social psychology: Handbook of basic principles* (pp. 433–465). New York: Guilford Press.

Schwarz, N., & Clore, G. L. (2007). Feelings and phenomenal experiences. In A. W. Kruglanski & E. T. Higgins (Eds.), *Social psychology: Handbook of basic principles* (2nd ed., pp. 385–407). New York: Guilford Press.

Shiota, M. N., Keltner, D., & John, O. P. (2006). Positive emotion dispositions differentially associated with Big Five personality and attachment style. *Journal of Positive Psychology, 1,* 61–71

Sinaceur, M., & Tiedens, L. Z. (2006). Get mad and get more than even: When and why anger expression is effective in negotiations. *Journal of Experimental Social Psychology, 42,* 314–322.

Staw, B. M., & Barsade, S. G. (1993). Affect and managerial performance: A test of the sadder-but-wiser vs. happier-and-smarter hypotheses. *Administrative Science Quarterly, 38,* 304–331.

Staw, B. M., Sutton, R. I., & Pelled, L. H. (1994). Employee positive emotion and favorable outcomes at the workplace. *Organization Science, 5,* 51–71.

Sutton, R. I. (1991). Maintaining norms about expressed emotions: The case of bill collectors. *Administrative Science Quarterly, 36,* 245–268.

Sutton, R. I., & Rafaeli, A. (1988). Untangling the relationship between displayed emotions and organizational sales: the case of convenience stores. *Academy of Management Journal, 31,* 461–487.

Sy, T., Côté, S., & Saavedra, R. (2005). The contagious leader: Impact of the leader's mood on the mood of group members, group affective tone, and group processes. *Journal of Applied Psychology, 90,* 295–305.

Thietart, R., & Forgues, B. (1995). Chaos theory and organization. *Organization Science, 6,* 19–31.

Tracy, J. L., & Robins, R. W. (2004). Show your pride: Evidence for a discrete emotion expression. *Psychological Science, 15,* 194–197.

Tsai, W.-C. (2001). Determinants and consequences of employee displayed positive emotions. *Journal of Management, 27,* 497–512.

Tsai, W.-C., & Huang, Y- M. (2002). Mechanisms linking employee affective delivery and customer behavioral intentions. *Journal of Applied Psychology, 87,* 1001–1008.

Tsai, W., Chen, C., & Liu, H. (2007). Test of a model linking employee positive moods and task performance. *Journal of Applied Psychology, 92,* 1570–1583.

Tsui, A. S., & Barry, B. (1986). Interpersonal affect and rating errors. *Academy of Management Journal, 29,* 586–599.

Van Kleef, G. A. (2009). How emotions regulate social life. *Current Directions in Psychological Science, 18,* 184–188.

Van Kleef, G. A., De Dreu, C. K. W., & Manstead, A. S. R. (2004). The interpersonal effects of anger and happiness in negotiations. *Journal of Personality and Social Psychology, 86,* 57–76.

Van Kleef, G. A., Homan, A. C., Beersma, B., van Knippenberg, D., van Knippenberg, B., & Damen, F. (2009). Searing sentiment or cold calculation?: The effects ofleader emotional displays on team performance depend on follower epistemic motivation. *Academy of Management Journal, 52,* 562–580.

Van Kleef, G. V., Homan, A., Beersma, B., & van Knippenberg, D. (2010). On angry leaders and agreeable followers: How leaders' emotions and followers' personalities shape motivation and team performance. *Psychological Science, 21,* 1827–1834.

Wagner, D. T., & Ilies, R. (2008). Affective influences on employee satisfaction and performance. In N. M. Ashkanasy & C. L. Cooper (Eds.), *Research companion to emotion in organizations* (pp. 152–169). Cheltenham, UK: Edward Elgar.

Weiss, H. M., & Cropanzano, R. (1996). Affective events theory: A theoretical discussion of the causes and consequences of affective experiences at work. *Research in Organizational Behavior, 18,* 1–74.

Weiss, H. M., Nicholas, J. P., & Daus, C. S. (1999). An examination of joint effects of affective experiences and job beliefs on job satisfaction and variations in affective experiences over time. *Organizational Behavior and Human Decision Processes, 78,* 1–24.

Wright T. A., & Staw, B. M. (1999). Affect and favorable work outcomes: Two longitudinal tests of the happy–productive worker thesis. *Journal of Organizational Behavior, 20,* 1–23.

CHAPTER 27

■ ■ ■ ■ ■ ■ ■ ■ ■

Positive Emotions in Marketing and Social Influence

Samantha L. Neufeld
Vladas Griskevicius

In the course of an average day, people are inundated with attempts at social influence. Advertisements try to sway us toward a certain brand of potato chip or automobile, television pundits make arguments to influence our views on political issues, and friends ask us for favors large and small. Can these efforts be influenced by something as transitory as our state emotional experience, and if so, how? This chapter examines the important ways in which emotions—particularly positive emotions—affect how we respond to social influence attempts. It is a complex topic: Multiple perspectives on emotion must be integrated together, and the effects of emotion often vary with the context of the influence attempt and the domain of the outcome behavior. Nonetheless, research has shed a great deal of light on the matter, and valuable insights are available to those interested in emotion, persuasion, and consumer behavior.

The structure of this chapter is designed to familiarize the reader with the overarching emotion theories that guide this research, before we delve into the research itself, and general findings and implications. We begin with a brief discussion of several broad theories of emotion because the more spe-cific theories about social influence hinge on what an emotion actually *is*. For each broad theory, we then describe the related theories that more specifically address social influence, and their general predictions. In the next section, we discuss core empirical findings, exploring how emotion affects behavior in various domains such as information processing, evaluation and judgment, and risk and variety seeking. These cognitive processes are all crucial to the discussion of social influence because they play a role in our ability to take in new information, our perception of external objects, and our willingness to try new things and consider unfamiliar perspectives. Finally, we explore interesting new directions in this research, and offer recommendations for both future empirical work and considerations that should be kept in mind by those developing interventions and marketing campaigns.

Major Theories and Perspectives

There are several major emotion perspectives, each of which makes different predictions regarding the effects emotion should have on cognitive processes. While these theories differ from each other in important ways, they are not necessarily mutually exclusive, and researchers have amassed a great deal of support for each perspective. What is likely, and what we hope will become clear throughout this chapter, is that each theory offers valuable insight into the influence of emotion on social influence attempts in different contexts and domains.

Traditional Approach: Focus on Affect Valence

Most research on the influence of emotion has emphasized the role of affect valence, with researchers interchangeably referring to good mood versus bad mood, positive affect versus negative affect, or happiness versus sadness. "Mood" refers to a low-intensity, sustained affective state that often does not have a specific object (Gross, 1998). A person can be in a good mood for hours or even days but might not know why he or she is in a good mood. Mood stands in contrast to "emotions," which are more specific (e.g., pride, amusement, fear), higher in intensity, and shorter in duration, perhaps as brief as a few seconds or minutes (Ekman, 1992). Mood is also distinguished from "affect," which is often an umbrella term referring to the experience or "feeling" of a mood or emotion (Bagozzi, Gopinath, & Nyer, 1999; Cohen, Pham, & Andrade, 2008; Zajonc, 1980). An approach grounded in mood or affect valence emphasizes the differences in outcomes when the individual is feeling good, compared to when he or she is feeling bad. The classic literature on the role of affect valence on psychology and behavior begins in the 1970s, and is grounded in three specific theories.

The first theory focuses on the motivating role of affect and is known as *mood management theory* or the *mood maintenance hypothesis* (Clark & Isen, 1982). This approach asserts that people's goal is to feel good, whereby people are motivated to alleviate bad moods and to maintain or increase good moods (Zillmann, 1988). From this perspective, people in negative moods are more motivated to approach mood-enhancing opportunities. For example, people in a bad mood (usually sadness) are more likely to help others in an attempt to boost their own feelings (Cialdini, Baumann, & Kenrick; 1981; Cialdini & Fultz, 1990). In contrast, people in a positive mood are motivated to avoid threats to their good mood and situations that might make them feel worse (see Wegener & Petty, 1994). Overall, this perspective asserts that positive mood promotes negativity avoidance and negative mood promotes positivity seeking.

A second classic theory focuses on how mood influences judgment and is known as *feelings as information* (Schwarz & Clore, 1983; 1988; Wyer & Carlston, 1979; for a review, see Pham, 1998). This perspective, sometimes called the "How do I feel about it?" heuristic, states that affect is an informative cue to the state of one's current situation. For instance, people asked to assess their life satisfaction on a sunny day tend to report being more satisfied than those asked on a rainy day (Schwarz & Clore, 1983). In this case, the weather is a source of "incidental affect" (affect that is brought about by a source other than the object of evaluation; in contrast, "integral affect" is elicited directly by the features of the object of evaluation), which colors people's judgments of life satisfaction (Lerner & Keltner, 2000; Loewenstein & Lerner, 2003). Incidental affect tends to have stronger effects when a person is unaware of the true source of affect. For example, when the good or bad weather is made salient, people correct for the effect of weather on their sense of life satisfaction. The weather functions as a cue to one's current situation: Good weather suggests that things are going well; bad weather suggests that things are not going that well. The "feelings as information" perspective also suggests that affect valence influences how much attention a person will pay to his or her current situation. According to this perspective, because negative affect is information that indicates something in the current environment is undesirable, it should lead people to pay more attention to the environment, so that the problem can be identified and corrected. In contrast, because positive affect means that all is well, it should decrease attention to the environment because there is no need to exert extra cognitive effort assessing the current situation.

The third classic theory is more cognitively focused and known as *mood congruency* (Blaney, 1986). This perspective posits that being in a positive or negative mood leads to evaluations that are consistent, or congruent, with the valence of a person's mood. For example, whereas negative affect leads people to evaluate things more negatively, positive affect is known to produce the "rose-colored glasses" effect, leading people in a good mood to evaluate things more positively (Axelrod, 1963; Goldberg & Gorn, 1987; Srull, 1983). Although the rose-colored glasses effect is consistent with both the feeling-as-information perspective and the mood congruency perspective, each perspective offers a different explanation for the effect. Whereas the feeling-as-information perspective suggests that affect influences judgment through the "How do I feel about it?" heuristic, the mood congruency perspective highlights that positive affect can activate other positive concepts. For example, positive affect can make people recall positive memories and other positive cognitions, thereby clouding judgment of new information through the lens of these positive thoughts (Isen, Shalker, Clark, & Karp, 1978).

These three traditional theories are widely cited in the emotion literature and have been used to demonstrate many interesting phenomena. Because these perspectives are not mutually exclusive, each theory might operate under different circumstances. For example, the *affect infusion model* (Forgas, 1995) incorporates both the feelings-as-information and mood congruency approaches. According to the affect infusion model, mood congruency operates when a person has high cognitive processing capacity, which allows access to memory. But if the person has a limited processing capacity, for example, if the person is under cognitive load, he or she will be more reliant upon affect as a heuristic cue, as predicted by the feelings-as-information perspective. As a general rule, the influence of emotion on judgment tends to be stronger when the individual is experiencing time constraints, distraction, or when the decision is too complex for the individual to assess all information effectively (Pham, 2007).

Beyond Valence: Circumplex and Appraisal Models

The theories just discussed focus on global positive and negative affect, suggesting that any affective state of the same valence should have similar influences on cognition and behavior. But more recent theories have

begun to question whether all positive states and all negative states are created equally, proposing that emotions differ from each other ways than valence.

The *circumplex model of affect* (Russell, 1980; Russell & Barrett, 1999) proposes that emotions differ on two dimensions: the traditional valence dimension and an orthogonal arousal dimension. According to this model, all emotions can be placed on a grid with four quadrants, with the valence dimension running from negative to positive, and the arousal dimension running from low to high (for greater detail on the circumplex model, see Condon, Wilson-Mendenhall, & Barrett, Chapter 4, this volume). Although circumplex models highlight that affect can differ in more ways than just valence, such models have received some criticism (e.g., Cohen et al., 2008). For example, are all emotions best described by a two-dimensional space? A different approach emphasizes that emotions are better understood by *appraisal tendencies* (Lerner & Keltner, 2001; Smith & Ellsworth, 1985). According to the appraisal perspective, emotions vary not only on the dimensions of valence and arousal, but also on other cognitive appraisal dimensions, such as control, certainty, attentional activity, anticipated effort, responsibility, novelty, and coping potential (Han, Lerner, & Keltner, 2007; Lerner & Tiedens, 2006; see Smith, Tong, & Ellsworth, Chapter 1, this volume, for more detail on appraisal perspectives).

Importantly, appraisal tendency frameworks view emotions as goal-directed, whereby emotions serve to orchestrate responses in the service of overcoming a problem posed by the current environment (Lerner & Keltner, 2001). An emotion's appraisal tendency profile also has important implications for how that emotion should influence cognition and behavior. Consider how fear and anger influence risk taking. From a traditional perspective, fear and anger are similar because both are negative affective states, which means that both emotions should have similar consequences for behavior. But an appraisal perspective proposes that fear and anger differ in important ways: Whereas fear is low on the appraisal dimensions of certainty and control, anger is high on both of these dimensions. Consistent with this idea, fear and anger have opposing effects on risk taking:

Fear leads people to be more pessimistic and take less risk, whereas anger leads people to be more optimistic and take more risk (Lerner & Keltner, 2001).

Beyond Dimensions: Discrete Emotion Models

Discrete emotion models (sometimes called *evolutionary models*) define emotions as distinct experiential states that are brought about by specific types of circumstances. Unlike other approaches, which take emotions as a given, then try to categorize them, discrete approaches ask why a set of specific emotions would exist in the first place. From this perspective, different emotions emerged over the course of our evolutionary history to help our ancestors effectively address specific fitness-relevant threats and opportunities, thereby increasing the odds that they and their offspring would survive and reproduce (Cosmides & Tooby, 2000; Ekman, 1992; Gross, 1998; Izard, 1992; Lazarus, 1991; for a more in-depth review of the discrete emotion perspective, see Shiota, Chapter 3, this volume). Negative emotions are thought to arise in response to fitness-relevant *threats*, whereas positive emotions are believed to help people take advantage of different fitness-relevant *opportunities*. For example, the enthusiasm system is triggered by the presence of a material reward such as food. Once this system is triggered, it facilitates the pursuit of this reward, for example, by activating the sympathetic nervous system to prepare the body for physical effort (Shiota, Neufeld, Yeung, Moser, & Perea, 2011), and promoting the experience of "wanting," which acts as a psychological motivator prompting the individual to act (Berridge & Robinson, 1995; Griskevicius, Shiota, & Neufeld, 2010).

Evolutionary approaches offer a different perspective on the effects of emotion on cognition than those in the approaches described previously. If each emotion evolved to address a specific fitness-relevant problem, then an emotion's cognitive effects—attention, signal detection thresholds, goals, memory, and behavioral decision rules—should all be geared toward the type of problem it evolved to solve. Each emotion should therefore be associated with its own unique pattern of cognitions, and operate via different mechanisms, rather than have one single mechanism (e.g., affect valence) be the sole determinant of cognition. In other words, enthusiasm and amusement may both increase heuristic processing of persuasive messages, but do so through different mechanisms (Griskevicius, Shiota, & Neufeld, 2010).

Core Findings

We now turn our attention to the core empirical findings regarding emotion's effects on social influence. These findings are broken down by the type of cognitive outcome assessed (i.e., processing of persuasive information, evaluation, and risk and variety seeking), so that we can examine the effects of emotion on qualitatively different types of decision-making processes and behaviors.

Outcomes Involving Persuasion and Information Processing

Much research has examined how emotional experience influences persuasion, focusing specifically on how different affective states influence information processing according to dual-process models (Cacioppo, Petty, Kao, & Rodriguez, 1986; Chaiken, 1987). From this perspective, information can be processed in one of two ways: systematically (or centrally), with people paying close attention to the content and scrutinizing the information; or heuristically (or peripherally), with people paying less attention to content and instead relying on simple heuristics or quick-and-dirty rules of thumb. When it comes to how affect influences information processing, research has shown that whereas negative affect increases systematic processing and leads people to scrutinize information, positive affect increases heuristic processing and reliance on heuristic cues (e.g., Bless et al., 1996; Bodenhausen, Kramer, & Süsser, 1994; Forgas, 2007; Petty, Gleicher, & Baker, 1991; Ruder & Bless, 2003; Schwarz & Bless, 1991; Smith & Shaffer, 1991; Worth & Mackie, 1987).

These findings exemplify research based on traditional approaches that emphasize affect valence as the primary aspect of emotion. In a typical study of this kind, participants are first made to feel happy or sad, which are proxies for positive and negative emotion (or sometimes the study contrasts one of these with neutral affect). Participants are then presented with a long series of arguments intended to persuade them on a particular issue. However, whereas sometimes the arguments are strong and persuasive, at other times the list includes weak arguments that are not very persuasive. People who are sad tend to be persuaded by the strong arguments but not by the weak arguments, suggesting that they are paying close attention to the content of the arguments. By contrast, happy people tend to be persuaded by the strong *or* the weak arguments, as long as there is a large number of arguments. This suggests that rather than systematically processing each argument, happy people rely on heuristics, such as whether there are many arguments for the issue, regardless of their strength (e.g., Bless, Bohner, Schwarz, & Strack, 1990; Bless, Mackie, & Schwarz, 1992).

This work on how emotion influences persuasion has been driven by the feelings-as-information model discussed earlier. The idea is that because negative affect indicates the presence of a problem, it should lead people to pay more attention to their current situation, so that the problem can be identified and corrected. Thus, sad people scrutinize persuasive messages. By contrast, positive affect is perceived as a cue that all is well, which means that happy people have no need to exert extra cognitive effort. Thus, happy people do not scrutinize persuasive message and instead rely on heuristics. Although this has been the long-accepted wisdom of how affect influences persuasion, recent work has gone beyond valence to examine other dimensions of emotional experience (Griskevicius et al., 2009; Griskevicius, Shiota, & Neufeld, 2010; Moons & Mackie, 2007; Sinclair, Moore, Mark, Soldat, & Lavis, 2010; Tiedens & Linton, 2001).

Some research suggests that whether an emotion leads to heuristic versus systematic processing depends on the specific appraisal tendencies produced by that emotion (e.g., Tiedens & Linton, 2001). For instance, consider how persuasion should be influenced by the negative emotions of anger and worry, and the positive emotions of contentment and surprise. From a traditional perspective, both negative emotions should promote systematic processing, whereas both positive emotions should promote heuristic processing. However, some research-

ers find that rather than depending on the valence of the emotion, processing depends on whether a specific emotion is high versus low in the appraisal of certainty (e.g., Tiedens & Linton, 2001). Despite having the opposite valence, emotions high in certainty (e.g., anger and contentment) produce more heuristic processing, whereas emotions low in certainty (e.g., worry and surprise) produce systematic processing. These findings demonstrate that all emotions of the same valence do not necessarily yield the same outcome.

Other research based on an evolutionary perspective has examined how different positive emotions influence persuasion (e.g., Griskevicius, Shiota, & Neufeld, 2010). In two experiments, the authors tested how the processing of persuasive messages was influence by six discrete positive emotions: awe, nurturant love, amusement, enthusiasm, attachment love, and contentment. They derived predictions from the proposed fitness-enhancing function of each emotion, considering whether this function should be expected to promote heuristic versus systematic processing. Consistent with predictions, four of the emotions (amusement, enthusiasm, contentment, and attachment love) led to increased heuristic processing. However, two of the positive emotions—awe and nurturant love—increased systematic processing. The researchers tested whether awe and nurturant love might share particular appraisal tendencies, such as certainty, but no single appraisal tendency could explain these findings. Instead, analyses indicated that each emotion appears to have unique effects that are driven by different mechanisms.

While the work described so far has examined the effect of emotion on heuristic processing in general, other research shows that the type of heuristic under consideration can make a critical distinction. From an evolutionary perspective it is unlikely that emotions promote a general orientation to process information systematically or heuristically. Instead, because emotions help to solve adaptive problems, an emotion is expected to promote judgment and decisions that help to solve the particular problem associated with that emotion, regardless of whether this problem is solved via systematic or heuristic processing. This suggests that what is likely to be critical is not whether people are processing systematically or heuristically, but *which* specific heuristics are available. Consider advertising, which uses many types of heuristics in its messaging (Cialdini, 2001). For example, some ads use social proof heuristics, indicating that many people are purchasing a product. Other ads use scarcity heuristics to indicate that a product is rare or dwindling in availability. Do emotions make people more or less reliant on heuristics? It turns out that it depends on the heuristic.

In three studies, Griskevicius and colleagues (2009) elicited the positive emotion of lust or the negative emotion of fear. Participants then viewed ads for various products that contained heuristic appeals either to social proof (e.g., "over a million sold") or to scarcity (e.g., "limited edition"). Their findings revealed that whereas fear led social proof heuristics to be more effective, it led scarcity heuristics to be less effective. Consistent with the idea that physical danger is better avoided with safety in numbers, when participants were scared, they were especially eager to blend in with the crowd and especially unwilling to be unique. In contrast, lust produced the opposite pattern. When participants were feeling lustful, scarcity appeals became *more* persuasive, whereas social proof appeals became *less* persuasive. Consistent with the idea that attracting a mate requires a person to differentiate him- or herself positively from others, people in a lustful state were especially eager to stand out and especially unwilling to purchase the same product already owned by over a million others.

So how do emotions influence persuasion? Whereas research initially suggested that what is most important is whether people are feeling good or feeling bad, the current literature highlights the additional importance of which specific emotion a person is feeling. Furthermore, research suggests that context also matters.

Evaluation and Judgment

Another area that has received substantial attention is how emotions influence evaluation and judgment. As mentioned earlier, a host of studies shows that whereas being in a bad mood leads people to see things more negatively, being in a good mood leads them to see things in a more favorable light—the so-called "rose-colored glasses effect" (Alpert & Alpert, 1990; Forgas & Bower, 1987; Gorn, Goldberg, & Basu, 1993; Mathur & Chattopadhyay, 1991; Meloy, 2000). For example, receiving a small gift that enhanced mood led participants to evaluate products they owned more positively (Isen, Shalker, Clark, & Karp, 1978). Similarly, upbeat advertisements lead to evaluations of products in the ads more favorably (Batra & Ray, 1986).

This rose-colored glasses phenomenon has been interpreted from both the feelings-as-information and the mood congruency perspectives. However, recent research reveals that the effect depends on not only the positive emotion a person is feeling but also what the person is evaluating. As previously described, the discrete emotions perspective suggests that it is the *function* of the emotion, rather than extrinsic aspects of the situation, that determines the effects of individual emotions on the judgment-making process. Perhaps the clearest demonstration of this is the set of studies by Griskevicius, Shiota, and Nowlis (2010) examining the effects of two different positive emotions, pride and contentment, on the desire for two types of consumer products. In their first experiment, the authors used stories to prime participants with pride, contentment, or neutral emotion, then asked these participants to rate the attractiveness of six different products. Three of these products—a watch, a laptop computer, and a pair of shoes—were selected for their ability to display status. The other three—a vacuum cleaner, a dishwasher, and a bed—were chosen because they represent a clean and comfortable home. Consistent with hypotheses, pride increased the attractiveness of the status display products but not the home comfort products. In contrast, contentment produced the opposite effect, increasing the appeal of the home comfort products but not the status display products.

In two more experiments, the authors replicated these findings and identified the cognitive mediators through which pride and contentment exacted their influence. Consistent with prediction, these two emotions were activating different fitness-enhancing goals. By asking participants to rate the importance of various short-term goals after reading the emotion prime story, the authors showed that the effect of pride on desire for status display products was mediated by a desire to draw attention to oneself, whereas the effect of contentment on home comfort products was mediated by the goal of being in a comfortable, familiar place.

These findings and others like them (e.g., Griskevicius, Tybur, & Van den Bergh, 2010; Lerner, Small, & Loewenstein, 2004) run counter to the predictions of an affect-valence approach, which would suggest that all positive emotions should increase the attractiveness of all products equally. Rather, this research supports the theory that, by operating via different mechanisms to achieve specific goals, emotions of the same valence can activate dramatically different desires. Those who study consumer behavior and product marketing would do well to take this into account when considering their advertising options. It may not be enough simply to induce any positive emotion and assume that it will increase the attractiveness of any product. Rather, it is important to understand which goals a particular product might help to achieve, then induce the emotion that is most appropriate for activating that goal.

Outcomes Involving Risk and Variety Seeking

We turn now to research evaluating outcomes in the realms of risk taking and variety seeking. The body of work examining emotion's effects on risk taking does not reveal a clear picture. Rather, some researchers suggest that positive affect *increases* risk taking, whereas others indicate that it *decreases* risk taking (Cohen et al., 2008; Isen & Patrick, 1983; Wegener, Petty, & Klein, 1994).

Fredrickson (2001) proposed a *broaden-and-build* model in which positive mood leads to a broader thought–action repertoire for the purpose of acquiring future resources. While acknowledging the applicability of a discrete emotion perspective to negative emotions, Fredrickson cites the approach-oriented nature of positive emotions, arguing that all positive emotions encourage individuals to pursue and interact with objects and people in their environment. This predisposition paves the way for a broader range of experiences and accrual

of important social, physical, and intellectual resources. The broaden-and-build model implies that positive affect should increase motivation toward both risk taking, which is the active pursuit of possible reward despite the potential for negative consequences, and variety seeking, which is the tendency to prefer a variety of experiences (e.g., trying new foods and engaging with a larger assortment of people).

Research findings support this model. As some studies show, positive mood (relative to negative mood) leads to increased optimism, making positive events seem more likely than negative events (Mayer, Gaschke, Braverman, & Evans, 1992; Wegener et al., 1994). This expectation of positive outcomes could reasonably be expected to increase an individual's willingness to try risky, novel, and varied experiences. However, much research indicates that this is a qualified relationship, with the magnitude of risk playing an important moderating role—specifically, good mood seems to *increase* risk taking in low-risk situations, but to *decrease* risk taking in high-risk situations. This is generally explained in terms of mood maintenance theory, which predicts that people in a good mood should be unwilling to risk harm to that mood (e.g., Isen & Patrick, 1983). Low-risk opportunities offer the chance to feel even better, with minimal risk to the current good feeling, but high-risk opportunities represent the possibility of losing the current good mood, with relatively low potential affective gains—after all, why risk a lot to gain a good mood when one is already in a good mood?

In a study examining positive affect and risk taking, when Isen and Patrick (1983) gave some participants a McDonald's gift certificate to elicit happiness, they found that these participants bet more than control participants in a real gambling task; however, this was only when the risk was low (they bet *less* than control participants when risk was high). In contrast, when engaging in a *hypothetical* risk-taking task, happy participants were only more risky than controls when the odds of winning were low (so risk was high). These moderating variables of risk magnitude and actual versus hypothetical risk indicate that good mood does not have an across-the-board boosting effect on risk taking (e.g., Arkes, Herren, & Isen,

1988; Dunegan, Duchon, & Barton, 1992; Isen & Geva, 1987).

In a different set of studies examining good mood and variety seeking, when Kahn and Isen (1993) induced good mood by giving participants a bag of candy or gum, they found that these participants (relative to control participants) selected a wider variety of brands of snack crackers for availability in a new vending machine; however, this effect disappeared when the potential bad taste of these crackers was made salient. As in the risk-taking research, the boosting effect of positive affect on variety seeking is moderated by other variables, in this case, the possibility of reducing good mood by eating a bad-tasting cracker.

Moreover, some studies have found negative or nonexistent associations between positive affect and risk taking and variety seeking (e.g., Yuen & Lee, 2003). In the wake of inconsistent and sometimes counterintuitive findings, a discrete emotions approach may help to clarify some of the confusion regarding the relationship between positive emotion and these outcomes.

The first evidence for a hypothesis that reaches beyond valence came from studies examining negative emotions. The aforementioned study by Lerner and Keltner (2001) demonstrated that anger, operating through a high-certainty appraisal, facilitates risk taking, whereas fear, operating through a low-certainty appraisal, decreases risk taking. In a similar study, Raghunathan and Pham (1999) showed that experimentally manipulated sadness caused participants to prefer high-risk, high-reward options, presumably because they were motivated to recover whatever they lost that produced the sadness. In contrast, an anxiety manipulation led to a preference for low-risk, low-reward options, which the authors attribute to a goal of reducing the uncertainty that is inherent to anxiety. These studies, focused on negative emotions, provide impetus for extending this line of research into the positive emotions.

Recent research indicates that the discrete emotions approach has predictive power in the realm of positive emotions and risk. In two studies, Li and colleagues (2013) used short stories and recalled writing tasks to elicit one of four positive emotions: amusement, anticipatory enthusiasm, contentment, or nurturant love. They then assessed participants' willingness to engage in financially risky behavior, using a financial risk taking scale and a real gambling task. Consistent with the predictions of the discrete emotions approach, the four emotions had different effects on risk taking. Amusement, with its emphasis on play without real consequences, and anticipatory enthusiasm, which facilitates greater focus on potential gains and less focus on potential losses, were both predicted to increase risk taking, which they did. In contrast, contentment, which is proposed to promote satisfaction with one's current situation, and nurturant love, thought to promote greater caution in the service of protecting another, were both predicted and found to decrease risk taking. These findings support a growing body of work suggesting that emotion's effect on risk taking is not solely a function of positive versus negative affect, but may further be driven by discrete emotions, each serving different fitness-enhancing functions.

Topics of Note and Future Directions

While research may seem to imply that judgments and decisions made under the influence of emotion are less informed and less considered than those made using cold cognition, we must recognize that this is precisely what makes them so valuable. No individual always has the capacity, when making decisions large and small, to gather every relevant piece of information and carefully consider all options and potential outcomes. Emotions, which evolved over the course of human history to help us make the most appropriate decision under any informational or cognitive parameters, are like compasses guiding us through a moonless night: They do not always get us to exactly where we should be, but they offer much needed direction. In this final section, we turn to complicating factors in this work, as well as potential for application of this research to social issues.

Emotion Blends

One complicating factor in emotion work involves the possible existence of the "emotion blend" (sometimes called the "mixed-emotion state"), which is the simultaneous experience of two or more discrete emotions. For example, imagine learning that you have just been hired for a job for which you and a good friend both applied. It is likely that you would experience several emotions, including pride at having been chosen, guilt at having gained something your friend also wanted, and enthusiasm at beginning the new position. Assuming each of these emotions has different effects on cognition, how do they fit together to yield a single outcome? The answer to this question is unclear. We should first note that the question of the existence of emotion blends has not yet been resolved. Recall that the circumplex model of emotion claims that at any given time, an individual's affect falls on exactly one point of the two-dimensional emotion space. According to this model, emotion blends are impossible because one cannot be at two different points on the grid at the same time (Barrett & Russell, 1998). However, other theoretical models promote the existence of emotion blends (e.g., the evaluative space model—Cacioppo & Berntson, 1994; the psychological primitives approach—Ortony & Turner, 1990). This position is supported by empirical evidence that people report experiencing multiple simultaneous emotions during complex emotion situations (Ellsworth & Smith, 1988a, 1988b; Fredrickson, 1998; Larsen, McGraw, & Cacioppo, 2001; Scherer & Ceschi, 1997; Scherer & Tannenbaum, 1986). Indeed, some researchers argue that the occasional failure to find significant effects of emotion manipulations may stem from the complicating influence of emotion blends, which activate more than one emotional facial expression, physiological response, or cognitive effect at the same time (e.g., Davidson, Ekman, Saron, Senulis, & Friesen, 1990; Ekman et al., 1987).

If emotion blends do occur, it means that research examining the effects of emotion on cognitive processes must be conducted very carefully to ensure that the emotion in question is the only emotion influencing cognition. It also requires that those who attempt to use emotion in their marketing and social influence programs are cognizant of all potential emotions present in the situation. An advertisement that is placed in the middle of a sitcom, with the intent of capitalizing on the emotion of amusement, may simultane-

ously be influenced by sadness, enthusiasm, or any number of emotions, depending on the specific story line immediately preceding the advertisement. It would be difficult and perhaps overambitious to worry too much about that—after all, a sitcom should primarily elicit amusement—but if emotion blends exist, they constitute a complicating factor in the relationship between emotions and judgment.

Cultural Considerations

One reason emotions can be so powerful in marketing and social influence is that experiencing emotions is a universal human trait (Cosmides & Tooby, 2000; Ekman, 1992). That said, the context and frequency of emotional experience, as well as the outcomes associated with these emotions, are well known to differ across cultures (e.g., Kitayama, Markus, Matsumoto, & Norasakkunkit, 1997). For example, research indicates that whereas people in the United States (traditionally considered an individualistic, or independent, culture) are more likely to report experiencing "socially disengaging" emotions such as anger and pride, people in Japan (considered a collectivistic, or interdependent, culture) are more likely to report experiencing "socially engaging" emotions such as guilt (Kitayama, Mesquita, & Karasawa, 2006). It is not that Americans do not experience guilt, or that the Japanese do not experience anger, but that the affordances and norms inherent to different cultures make certain emotional experiences more prevalent.

However, even given the same emotional *experience* in two cultures, there still may be differences in the *outcome* of the emotion. For instance, pride universally facilitates status displays (Tracy & Robins, 2008), but what constitutes a status display differs across cultures. In some cultures, like the United States, a status display may involve conspicuous consumption of luxury goods to show others that one has the resources to spend money frivolously (Griskevicius et al., 2007). In other cultures, status displays can take the exact opposite form, such as when Pacific Northwest Coast tribesmen accrue status through elaborate "potlatch" ceremonies in which they give away all of their possessions (Barnett, 1938). Both conspicuous consumption and potlatching serve the same ultimate function, but they are qualitatively opposite behaviors.

What are the implications of these cross-cultural differences for the use of emotion in marketing and social influence? Certainly, we should not assume that an emotional appeal that is effective in one culture must therefore be effective in another. In one demonstration of this, Aaker and Williams (1998) demonstrated that the persuasive effects of two self-focused positive emotions (pride and happiness) and two other-focused positive emotions (empathy and peacefulness) differed between participants from individualist and collectivist cultures (the United States and China). Specifically (and unintuitively), the self-focused emotions led to more favorable attitudes toward the objects of evaluation (beer and film) in Chinese participants, whereas the opposite effects were found for American participants. The authors attribute this finding to the novelty of each type of appeal, and how much participants from both cultures therefore had to elaborate on the messages. The more novel messages in each culture required greater thought and elaboration, therefore increasing their persuasive power. A thorough understanding of the emotional context of each culture is therefore crucial to designing an effective emotion-based marketing or social influence campaign.

Potential for Application: Health and Prosocial Behavior

The empirical evidence presented in this chapter seems to support affect valence models, appraisal models, and discrete emotions models. So, those hoping to coalesce this information into a single set of guidelines for application may be unsure where to start. The important thing to remember is that these models all have predictive power regarding the effect of emotion on judgment; where they differ is the domain in which each operates. Affect valence models seem to be "domain-general," which means that positive affect can be counted on to color perceptions positively across the board. For that reason, putting people in a "good mood" should generally incline them to evaluate objects positively, to feel optimistic about outcomes, to be more variety seek-

ing, and so on. In contrast, appraisal and discrete emotions models have "domain-specific" outcomes, which means that they are well suited to solving the particular adaptive problem that is associated with that emotion. Activating a specific emotion in people should incline them toward evaluations, predictions, and other cognitive and behavioral outcomes that are most appropriate for that adaptive problem; however, these outcomes may be very poorly suited to addressing other adaptive problems. All of these perspectives have valuable roles to play in the realm of marketing and social influence. Our job as researchers is to understand how they work together, and to determine how best to integrate them into effective and persuasive interventions.

It is informative to examine the ways in which positive emotions have already been used to encourage particular outcomes, such as health behaviors and helping behavior. For a long time, the majority of health messaging was fear-based (e.g., "If you smoke, you will get lung cancer"). However, it was eventually discovered that fear-based messaging only works under certain prescribed conditions, and, unfortunately, many existing health campaigns were not effective (Job, 1988). Only recently have positive emotions become more prevalent in health messaging, and research indicates that they can be quite compelling. Winterich and Haws (2011) examined the effects of three positive emotions, varying in temporal focus, on self-control and desire for healthy and unhealthy snacks. Compared to messages based on happiness (current focus) and pride (past focus), a message eliciting hopefulness (future focus) resulted in greater self-control. This study and others like it (e.g., Robberson & Rogers, 1988) point to the importance of identifying the specific nature of the desired behavior, and building a persuasive message around the specific emotion that is best suited to encouraging that behavior.

A similar lesson can be gleaned from the literature on positive emotions and helping behavior. Generic positive affect has consistently been shown to increase helping behavior, except under certain circumstances; that is, good mood makes people more willing to help, unless there is any indication that the act of helping would threaten the good mood. This is sometimes referred to as "mood protection" (for a review, see Cohen et al., 2008). Researchers have examined the effects of specific positive emotions on altruism and cooperation. In a series of three studies examining the effect of gratitude for a favor done, Bartlett and DeSteno (2006) showed that gratitude resulted in greater helping, relative to amusement and neutral emotion, toward both the benefactor who initially performed that gratitude-eliciting favor and a stranger. In this set of studies it is clear that positive mood alone is not driving these effects, or amusement would have had a similar boosting effect on helping. Rather, the specific mechanisms that gratitude facilitates are responsible for increasing this behavior, suggesting that a thorough examination of the effects of other positive emotions on helping is likely to be a fruitful avenue of future research.

In related research examining the effect of emotion on cooperation in social dilemmas, Neufeld (2012) showed that despite its positive valence, pride does not lead to increased cooperation. After being primed with pride, guilt, or neutral affect, participants played a game in which they would receive any amount of money they requested from a shared resource pool, as long as the sum of all participants' requests did not exceed the amount of money in the pool. Relative to guilt, and consistent with predictions, pride led to significantly higher requests. The author proposes that these results stem from pride's emphasis on status and entitlement, and guilt's emphasis on refraining from causing harm to others. While this line of research is in an early stage, it holds implications for campaigns addressing resource conservation, and the importance of reconsidering popular assumptions that pride is wholly good and guilt is undesirable.

Conclusion

From the very earliest stages of emotion theorizing, pioneered primarily by William James in the 19th century, to the recent proliferation of empirical studies on emotion and cognition, much has been learned about the effects of emotion on social influence. Spanning a wide variety of perspectives and theories, many of which seem to have important—if contradictory—explanatory power,

these studies reveal to emotion researchers a wealth of knowledge about how emotion affects our processing, judgments and evaluations, and risk and variety seeking, while also revealing how little we really understand. Each new finding explains some facet of this relationship, while simultaneously opening a door to new avenues of research.

Several paths have emerged as clearly needing further exploration. Of primary importance will be determining how affect valence, appraisal, and discrete emotions theories work together to wield their influence on judgment. The levels at which each exerts influence, as well as the mechanisms through which each operates, are only beginning to be examined. It will also be crucial to identify the domains in which each positive emotion is most effective. From a marketing and social influence perspective, the wisest use of emotion appeals will require an awareness of the adaptive problem each emotion is best equipped to solve, and a message linking that problem to the desired behavior. This is possible, and we have every reason to expect that these avenues will soon be well explored by psychologists, marketing researchers, and other scholars hoping to apply the powerful and universal emotion system to their persuasive messages.

References

Aaker, J. L., & Williams, P. (1998). Empathy versus pride: The influence of emotional appeals across cultures. *Journal of Consumer Research, 25*(3), 241–261.

Alpert, J. I., & Alpert, M. I. (1990). Music influences on mood and purchase intentions. *Psychology and Marketing, 7*(2), 109–133.

Arkes, H. R., Herren, L. T., & Isen, A. M. (1988). The role of potential loss in the influence of affect on risk-taking behavior. *Organizational Behavior and Human Decision Processes, 42*(2), 181–193.

Axelrod, J. N. (1963). Induced moods and attitudes toward products. *Journal of Advertising Research, 3*, 19–24.

Bagozzi, R. P., Gopinath, M., & Nyer, P. U. (1999). The role of emotions in marketing. *Journal of the Academy of Marketing Science, 27*(2), 184–206.

Barnett, H. G. (1938). The nature of the potlatch. *American Anthropologist, 40*(3), 349–358.

Barrett, L. F., & Russell, J. A. (1998). Independence and bipolarity in the structure of current affect. *Journal of Personality and Social Psychology. 74*, 967–984.

Bartlett, M. Y., & DeSteno, D. (2006). Gratitude and prosocial behavior: Helping when it costs you. *Psychological Science, 17*(4), 319–325.

Batra, R., & Ray, M. L. (1986). Affective responses mediating acceptance of advertising. *Journal of Consumer Research, 13*(2), 234–249.

Berridge, K. C., & Robinson, T. E. (1995). The mind of an addicted brain: Neural sensitization of wanting versus liking. *Current Directions in Psychological Science, 4,* 71–76.

Blaney, P. H. (1986). Affect and memory: A review. *Psychological Bulletin, 99*(2), 229–246.

Bless, H., Bohner, G., Schwarz, N., & Strack, F. (1990). Mood and persuasion: A cognitive response analysis. *Personality and Social Psychology Bulletin, 16,* 331–345.

Bless, H., Clore, G. L., Schwarz, N., Golisano, V., Rabe, C., & Wölk, M. (1996). Mood and the use of scripts: Does a happy mood really lead to mindlessness? *Journal of Personality and Social Psychology, 71*(4), 665–679.

Bless, H., Mackie, D. M., & Schwarz, N. (1992). Mood effects on attitude judgments: Independent effects of mood before and after message elaboration. *Journal of Personality and Social Psychology, 63*(4), 585–595.

Bodenhausen, G. V., Kramer, G. P., & Süsser, K. (1994). Happiness and stereotypic thinking in social judgment. *Journal of Personality and Social Psychology, 66*(4), 621–632.

Cacioppo, J. T., & Berntson, G. G. (1994). Relationship between attitudes and evaluative space: A critical review, with emphasis on the seperability of positive and negative substrates. *Psychological Bulletin, 115*(3), 401–423.

Cacioppo, J. T., Petty, R. E., Kao, C. F., & Rodriguez, R. (1986). Central and peripheral routes to persuasion: An individual difference perspective. *Journal of Personality and Social Psychology, 51*(5), 1032–1043.

Chaiken, S. (1987). The heuristic model of persuasion. In M. P. Zanna, J. M. Olson, & C. P. Herman (Eds.), *Social influence: The Ontario Symposium* (Vol. 5, pp. 3–39). Hillsdale, NJ: Erlbaum.

Cialdini, R. B. (2001). The science of persuasion. *Scientific American, 284*(2), 76–81.

Cialdini, R. B., Baumann, D. J., & Kenrick, D. T. (1981). Insights from sadness: A three step model of the development of altruism as hedonism. *Developmental Review, 1,* 207–223.

Cialdini, R. B., & Fultz, J. (1990). Interpreting the negative mood-helping literature via "mega"-analysis: A contrary view. *Psychological Bulletin, 107,* 210–214.

Clark, M. S., & Isen, A. M. (1982). Toward understanding the relationship between feeling states and social behavior. In L. Berkowitz (Ed.), *Cognitive psychology* (pp. 73–108). New York: Elsevier/North Holland.

Cohen, J. B., Pham, M. T., & Andrade, E. B. (2008). The nature and role of affect in consumer behavior. In C. P. Haugtvedt, P. Herr, & F. Kardes (Eds.), *Handbook of consumer psychology* (pp. 297–348). Mahwah, NJ: Erlbaum.

Cosmides, L., & Tooby, J. (2000). Evolutionary psychology and the emotions. In M. Lewis & J. M. Haviland-Jones (Eds.), *Handbook of emotions* (2nd ed., pp. 91–115). New York: Guilford Press.

Davidson, R. J., Ekman, P., Saron, C. D., Senulis, J. A., & Friesen, W. V. (1990). Approach–withdrawal and cerebral asymmetry: Emotional expression and brain physiology. I. *Journal of Personality and Social Psychology, 58*(2), 330–341.

Dunegan, K. J., Duchon, D., & Barton, S. L. (1992). Affect, risk, and decision criticality: Replication and extension in a business setting. *Organizational Behavior and Human Decision Processes, 53*(3), 335–351.

Ekman, P. (1992). An argument for basic emotions. *Cognition and Emotion, 6*(3/4), 169–200.

Ekman, P., Friesen, W. V., O'Sullivan, M., Chan, A., Diacoyanni-Tarlatzis, I., Heider, K., et al. (1987). Universals and cultural differences in the judgments of facial expressions of emotion. *Journal of Personality and Social Psychology, 53*(4), 712–717.

Ellsworth, P. C., & Smith, C. A. (1988a). From appraisal to emotion: Differences among unpleasant feelings. *Motivation and Emotion, 12*(3), 271–302.

Ellsworth, P. C., & Smith, C. A. (1988b). Shades of joy: Patterns of appraisal differentiating pleasant emotions. *Cognition and Emotion, 2*(4), 301–331.

Forgas, J. P. (1995). Mood and judgment: The Affect Infusion Model (AIM). *Psychological Bulletin, 117*(1), 39–66.

Forgas, J. P. (2007). When sad is better than happy: Negative affect can improve the quality and effectiveness of persuasive messages and social influence strategies. *Journal of Experimental Social Psychology, 43,* 513–528.

Forgas, J. P., & Bower, G. H. (1987). Mood effects on person-perception judgments. *Journal of Personality and Social Psychology, 53*(1), 53–60.

Fredrickson, B. L. (1998). What good are positive emotions? *Review of General Psychology, 2*(3), 300–319.

Fredrickson, B. L. (2001). The role of positive emotions in positive psychology: The broaden-and-build theory of positive emotions. *American Psychologist, 56*(3), 218–226.

Goldberg, M. E., & Gorn, G. J. (1987). Happy and sad TV programs: How they affect reactions to commercials. *Journal of Consumer Research, 14*(3), 387–403.

Gorn, G. J., Goldberg, M. E., & Basu, K. (1993). Mood, awareness, and product evaluation. *Journal of Consumer Psychology, 2*(3), 237–256.

Griskevicius, V., Goldstein, N. J., Mortensen, C. R., Sundie, J. M., Cialdini, R. B., & Kenrick, D. T. (2009). Fear and loving in Las Vegas: Evolution, emotion, and persuasion. *Journal of Marketing Research, 46*(3), 384–395.

Griskevicius, V., Shiota, M. N., & Neufeld, S. L. (2010). Influence of different positive emotions on persuasion processing: A functional evolutionary approach. *Emotion, 10*(2), 190–206.

Griskevicius, V., Shiota, M. N., & Nowlis, S. M. (2010). The many shades of rose-colored glasses: An evolutionary approach to the influence of different positive emotions. *Journal of Consumer Research, 37,* 238–250.

Griskevicius, V., Tybur, J. M., Sundie, J. M., Cialdini, R. B., Miller, G. F., & Kenrick, D. T. (2007). Blatant benevolence and conspicuous consumption: When romantic motives elicit strategic costly signals. *Journal of Personality and Social Psychology, 93*(1), 85–102.

Griskevicius, V., Tybur, J. M., & Van den Bergh, B. (2010). Going green to be seen: Status, reputation, and conspicuous conservation. *Journal of Personality and Social Psychology, 98*(3), 392–404.

Gross, J. J. (1998). The emerging field of emotion regulation: An integrative review. *Review of General Psychology, 2*(3), 271–299.

Han, S., Lerner, J. S., & Keltner, D. (2007). Feelings and consumer decision making: The appraisal-tendency framework. *Journal of Consumer Psychology, 17*(3), 158–168.

Isen, A. M., & Geva, N. (1987). The influence of positive affect on acceptable level of risk: The person with a large canoe has a large worry. *Organizational Behavior and Human Decision Processes, 39,* 145–154.

Isen, A. M., & Patrick, R. (1983). The effect of positive feelings on risk taking: When the chips are down. *Organizational Behavior and Human Performance, 31,* 194–202.

Isen, A. M., Shalker, T. E., Clark, M., & Karp, L. (1978). Affect, accessibility of material in memory, and behavior: A cognitive loop? *Journal of Personality and Social Psychology, 36*(1), 1–12.

Izard, C. E. (1992). Basic emotions, relations among emotions, and emotion–cognition relations. *Psychological Review, 99,* 561–565.

Job, R. F. S. (1988). Effective and ineffective use of fear in health promotion campaigns. *American Journal of Public Health, 78*(2), 163–167.

Kahn, B. E., & Isen, A. M. (1993). The influence of positive affect on variety seeking among safe, enjoyable products. *Journal of Consumer Research, 20*(2), 257–270.

Kitayama, S., Markus, H. R., Matsumoto, H., & Norasakkunkit, V. (1997). Individual and collective processes in the construction of the self: Self-enhancement in the United States and self-criticism in Japan. *Journal of Personality and Social Psychology, 72*(6), 1245–1267.

Kitayama, S., Mesquita, B., & Karasawa, M. (2006). Cultural affordances and emotional experience: Socially engaging in disengaging emotions in Japan and the United States. *Journal of Personality and Social Psychology, 91*(5), 890–903.

Larsen, J. T., McGraw, A. P., & Cacioppo, J. T. (2001). Can people feel happy and sad at the same time? *Journal of Personality and Social Psychology, 81*(4), 684–696.

Lazarus, R. S. (1991). Progress on a cognitive-motivational–relational theory of emotion. *American Psychologist, 46*(8), 819–834.

Lerner, J. S., & Keltner, D. (2000). Beyond valence: Toward a model of emotion-specific influences on judgment and choice. *Cognition and Emotion, 14*(4), 473–493.

Lerner, J. S., & Keltner, D. (2001). Fear, anger, and risk. *Journal of Personality and Social Psychology, 81*(1), 146–159.

Lerner, J. S., Small, D. A., & Loewenstein, G. (2004). Heart strings and purse strings: Carryover effects of emotions on economic decisions. *Psychological Science, 15*(5), 337–341.

Lerner, J. S., & Tiedens, L. Z. (2006). Portrait of the angry decision maker: How appraisal tendencies shape anger's influence on cognition. *Journal of Behavioral Decision Making, 19*, 115–137.

Li, Y. J., Neufeld, S. L., Griskevicius, V., Shiota, M. N., Chatterjee, P., & Kenrick, D. T. (2013). *A positive spin on risk-taking: Discrete positive emotions affect economic decisions.* Manuscript in preparation.

Loewenstein, G., & Lerner, J. S. (2003). The role of affect in decision making. In R. J. Davidson, K. R. Scherer, & H. H. Goldsmith (Eds.), *Handbook of affective sciences* (pp. 619–642). Oxford, UK: Oxford University Press.

Mathur, M., & Chattopadhyay, A. (1991). The impact of moves generated by television programs on responses to advertising. *Psychology and Marketing, 8*(1), 59–77.

Mayer, J. D., Gaschke, Y. N., Braverman, D. L., & Evans, T. W. (1992). Mood-congruent judgment is a general effect. *Journal of Personality and Social Psychology, 63*(1), 119–132.

Meloy, M. G. (2000). Mood-driven distortion of product information. *Journal of Consumer Research, 27*(3), 345–359.

Moons, W. G., & Mackie, D. M. (2007). Thinking straight while seeing red: The influence of anger on information processing. *Personality and Psychology Bulletin, 33*, 706–720.

Neufeld, S. L. (2012). *Self-conscious cooperation: Implications of a functional approach to emotions for behavior in social dilemmas.* Doctoral dissertation retrieved from ProQuest (3522517).

Ortony, A., & Turner, T. J. (1990). What's basic about basic emotions? *Psychological Review, 97*(3), 315–331.

Petty, R. E., Gleicher, F., & Baker, S. M. (1991). Multiple roles for affect in persuasion. In J. P. Forgas (Ed.), *Emotion and social judgments* (International Series in Experimental Social Psychology, pp. 181–200). Elmsford, NY: Pergamon Press.

Pham, M. T. (1998). Representativeness, relevance, and the use of feelings in decision making. *Journal of Consumer Research, 25*(2), 144–159.

Pham, M. T. (2007). Emotion and rationality: A critical review and interpretation of empirical evidence. *Review of General Psychology, 11*(2), 155–178.

Raghunathan, R., & Pham, M. T. (1999). All negative moods are not equal: Motivational influences of anxiety and sadness on decision making. *Organizational Behavior and Human Decision Processes, 79*(1), 56–77.

Robberson, M. R., & Rogers, R. W. (1988). Beyond fear appeals: Negative and positive persuasive appeals to health and self-esteem. *Journal of Applied Social Psychology, 18*(3), 277–287.

Ruder, M., & Bless, H. (2003). Mood and reliance on the ease of retrieval heuristic. *Journal of Personality and Social Psychology, 85*, 185–190.

Russell, J. A. (1980). A circumplex model of affect. *Journal of Personality and Social Psychology, 39*(6), 1161–1178.

Russell, J. A., & Barrett, L. F. (1999). Core affect, prototypical emotional episodes, and other things called *emotion*: Dissecting the elephant. *Journal of Personality and Social Psychology, 76*(5), 805–819.

Scherer, K. R., & Ceschi, G. (1997). Lost luggage: A field study of emotion-antecedent appraisal. *Motivation and Emotion, 21*(3), 211–235.

Scherer, K. R., & Tannenbaum, P. H. (1986). Emotional experiences in everyday life: A survey approach. *Motivation and Emotion, 10*(4), 295–314.

Schwarz, N., & Bless, H. (1991). Happy and mindless, but sad and smart?: The impact of affective states on analytical reasoning. In J. P. Forgas (Ed.), *Emotion and social judgments* (pp. 55–72). New York: Wiley.

Schwarz, N., & Clore, G. L. (1983). Mood, misattribution, and judgments of well-being: Informative and directive functions of affective states. *Journal of Personality and Social Psychology, 45*(3), 513–523.

Schwarz, N., & Clore, G. L. (1988). How do I feel about it?: Informative functions of affective states. In K. Fiedler & J. Forgas (Eds.), *Affect, cognition, and social behavior* (pp. 44–62). Toronto: Hogrefe International.

Shiota, M. N., Neufeld, S. L., Yeung, W. H., Moser, S. E., & Perea, E. F. (2011). Feeling good: Autonomic nervous system responding in five positive emotions. *Emotion, 11*(6), 1368–1378.

Sinclair, R. C., Moore, S. E., Mark, M. M., Soldat, A. S., & Lavis, C. A. (2010). Incidental moods, source likeability, and persuasion: Liking motivates message elaboration in happy people. *Cognition and Emotion, 24*(6), 940–961.

Smith, C. A., & Ellsworth, P. C. (1985). Patterns of cognitive appraisal in emotion. *Journal of Personality and Social Psychology, 48*, 813–838.

Smith, S. M., & Shaffer, D. R. (1991). The effects of good moods on systematic processing: "Willing but not able, or able but not willing?" *Motivation and Emotion, 15*(4), 243–279.

Srull, T. K. (1983). Affect and memory: The impact of affective reactions in advertising on the representation of product information in memory. In R. Bagozzi & A. Tybout (Eds.), *Advances in consumer research* (Vol. 10, pp. 520–525). Ann Arbor, MI: Association for Consumer Research.

Tiedens, L. Z., & Linton, S. (2001). Judgment under emotional certainty and uncertainty: The effects of specific emotions on information processing. *Journal of Personality and Social Psychology, 81*, 973–988.

Tracy, J. L., & Robins, R. W. (2008). The nonverbal expression of pride: Evidence for cross-cultural recognition. *Journal of Personality and Social Psychology, 94*(3), 516–530.

Wegener, D., & Petty, R. E. (1994). Mood management across affective states: The hedonic contingency hypothesis. *Journal of Personality and Social Psychology, 66*(6), 1034–1048.

Wegener, D., Petty, R. E., & Klein, D. J. (1994). Effects of mood on high elaboration attitude change: The mediating role of likelihood judgments. *European Journal of Social Psychology, 24*(1), 25–43.

Winterich, K. P., & Haws, K. L. (2011). Helpful hopefulness: The effect of future positive emotions on consumption. *Journal of Consumer Research, 38*(3), 505–524.

Worth, L. T., & Mackie, D. M. (1987). Cognitive mediation of positive affect in persuasion. *Social Cognition, 5*, 76–94.

Wyer, R. S., & Carlston, D. (1979). *Social cognition, inference, and attribution.* Hillsdale, NJ: Erlbaum.

Yuen, K. S. L., & Lee, T. M. C. (2003). Could mood state affect risk-taking decisions? *Journal of Affective Disorders, 75*(1), 11–18.

Zajonc, R. B. (1980). Feeling and thinking: Preferences need no inferences. *American Psychologist, 35*(2), 151–175.

Zillman, D. (1988). Mood management through communication choices. *American Behavioral Scientist, 31*(3), 327–340.

Conclusions and Future Directions

Leslie D. Kirby
Michele M. Tugade
Michelle N. Shiota

As this volume makes clear, research on positive emotions is now thriving. Despite a long history of neglect, scientists studying the positive emotions have overcome the boundaries and restrictions of models developed primarily for research on negative emotions, and have made huge theoretical and empirical advances over the past quarter-century. The chapters in this handbook do an excellent job of surveying advances that have been made over these decades, while also presenting cutting-edge techniques and empirical findings. Individual sections of the handbook document the richness of developments in several core areas of positive emotion science.

Part I, *Theoretical Foundations*, shows that multiple, well-developed theories of positive emotions have been articulated from a number of different perspectives. Theories of the nature, function, and implications of positive emotions variously reflect the broader frameworks of cognitive, social, evolutionary, and personality psychology. Just as the subdisciplines from which they draw combine to offer a well-rounded picture of the human mind, each of these approaches is complimentary to the oth-

ers. Together they reflect multiple levels of analysis and, likely, multiple systems in play. One leaves this section with a clear picture of how positive emotions might fit into, and also expand, traditional emotion theories in ways that produce a more integrated picture of emotion as a system.

Part II, *Biology of Positive Emotion*, focuses on physical manifestations of positive emotional responding. Its chapters address both neurobiological mechanisms and expressive displays that communicate positive emotion states to others. Methodological approaches covered in Part II highlight the ways in which positive emotion research has drawn from approaches traditionally used to study negative emotions, as well as the innovations in theory and technique that were needed to expand our understanding of positive emotions. This multimodal approach presents a coherent picture of the physiology of positive emotion, and again places positive emotions in the continuum of broader emotional examination. This section also highlights important future directions, with an emphasis on the potential offered by continued innovation in assessing emotional physiology and behavior, as well as ways in which our growing knowledge of the biology of positive emotion pushes the boundaries of emotion theory.

Part III, *Social Perspectives and Individual Differences*, examines positive emotions in the context of the broader human experience, considering the implications of positive emotions for our relationships with others, the ways in which our sociocultural worlds shape the experience and meaning of positive emotions, and the predictors and possible consequences of individual differences in positive emotionality. It highlights the complexity and multidirectionality of influences between emotion and psychosocial experience. In so doing, it also suggests vast, relatively unexplored territories at the intersection of positive emotion and relationship science, ripe for future research.

Part IV, *Select Positive Emotions*, presents several in-depth case studies of individual positive emotion constructs. These include a spectrum of positive emotions ranging from "classic" states that most emotion researchers would include on their lists of positive emotions (i.e., happiness, gratitude, hope, pride) to states that are only beginning to receive extensive attention from researchers as emotions (i.e., awe, challenge, compassion, romantic love). Each of these chapters offers a rich examination of causes, properties, and consequences of a given positive emotional state. Although the absence of strong theory regarding positive emotions' adaptive function long presented a barrier to research, these chapters make a clear case for the fitness implications of positive emotions, as well as their implications for subjective and psychosocial well-being.

Finally, Part V, *Outcomes of Positive Emotions*, addresses the roles positive emotions play in a variety of applied contexts, including health psychology, clinical psychology, industrial/organizational psychology, and marketing/social influence. The chapters in Part V demonstrate how positive emotions can be examined from multiple levels of analysis—intrapersonal, interpersonal, group, community, and population levels. Adding breadth to the study of positive emotions, the authors discuss "real-world" investigations that complement many of the theories tested in traditional laboratory settings. These chapters highlight the boundary conditions under which positive emotions

are useful and harmful for individuals and organizations, and in so doing, illustrate the many exciting areas of inquiry for studying positive emotions in applied settings.

Therefore, the chapters in this handbook offer a rich overview of what we have learned about positive emotions in the last couple of decades. The question now is, what is next? What major themes emerge from this overview? What major directions are suggested for future research? As much as this handbook focuses on the cutting-edge aspects of positive emotion science, it also makes clear that many questions remain to be addressed. We still have, as Robert Frost would say, "miles to go before [we] sleep."

What is "Positive" Emotion, Anyway?

One theme emerging across chapters in this handbook is the question of what makes a "positive emotion" positive at all. The "positive versus negative" distinction was emphasized early in the renaissance of psychological emotion science, during the 1960s and 1970s. Over the decades, this distinction has been infused—explicitly or implicitly—with a variety of conceptual meanings that reflect different theoretical perspectives. Appraisal-focused theories might emphasize the pleasantness or goal-conduciveness of one's current situation (see Chapter 1). For researchers emphasizing an evolutionary perspective, a "positive" emotion might be defined as one experienced in response to a fitness-relevant opportunity in the environment, as distinct from a threat (see Chapter 3). In theories of emotion that emphasize the nature and predictors of subjective affect, "positivity" refers primarily to internal feelings of pleasantness that are then categorized on the basis of features of the environment (see, e.g., the discussion of core affect in Chapter 4). In theories reflecting a strong motivational/behavioral tradition, a "positive" emotion might be defined as one that inherently involves approach motivation (see Chapter 6).

This diversity in what constitutes a "positive" emotion can be seen in the wealth of emotion constructs addressed throughout this handbook. A construct that qualifies as "positive" by one definition might not by another. For example, anger is typically classified as a negative emotion, based on subjective experience and elicitation by a type of threat to fitness. However, Chapter 6 offers extensive evidence that anger is characterized by strong approach motivation, emphasizing the rewards to be gained when a person forcefully goes after whatever has been taken from him or her. Challenge and hope (Chapters 22 and 23) are classified as positive emotions because they point us in the direction of possible gain or growth, but in neither case is the *current* situation necessarily positive or pleasant (nor do we have any guarantee that we are going to get what we want). Other emotions, such as compassion (Chapter 19), clearly combine elements of both positive and negative experience, or are elicited primarily by the removal of a negative emotion or stimulus (e.g., relief). Finally, some emotional experiences are atypical in nature, shifting from "negative" to "positive" (as in the case of pleasant fear) or from "positive" to "negative" (as in the case of unpleasant happiness; Chapter 4).

Rather than choosing one of these approaches to define the "positive," and limit the content of the handbook accordingly, we chose to cast a wider net and let the reader consider the merits of each approach. There are strengths and weaknesses to each, and each approach captures a conceptually important and meaningful aspect of emotional experience and responding. At this stage, we encourage emotions researchers not to be too quick to select a single approach, discarding the others and the constructs they bring to light (see Chapter 4 for a richer discussion of this issue). It may be that the next big advance in the field lies somewhere at the intersection of these various definitions of "positive" emotion.

Integrating Positive Emotion into Affective Science

For better or worse, research in the early decades of affective science focused almost exclusively on negative emotions. Many of the lessons learned from this body of research have proved extremely useful to researchers turning their attention to positive emotions. The emphases on adaptive function and behavioral motivation, so prominent in negative emotion research, have also offered a strong platform for theory development in positive emotion (see, e.g., Chapters 2, 3, and 6). A number of the methods used in negative emotion research have carried over reasonably well to the study of positive emotions, including approaches to studying appraisal (Chapter 1), neural mechanisms (e.g., Chapter 7), autonomic physiology (Chapter 8), facial expressions (Chapter 10), and the implications of emotional experience and expression for relationship functioning (Chapter 12).

However, positive emotion researchers have also had to add quite a few items to the toolkit of emotion science. Theories of positive emotions commonly place a much greater emphasis on their social or interpersonal functions (whether one defines "function" in the evolutionary or sociocultural sense) than on the intrapersonal functions emphasized in theories of negative emotions. The most prominent research questions differ accordingly. For example, positive emotion researchers are more likely to investigate implications of these states and traits for relationship functioning and social cognition (e.g., Chapters 11 and 12), rather than for individual physiology and interaction with the physical environment. There may be new ways of conceptualizing the sequence of positive emotional episodes, with distinct "phases" over time (e.g., Chapter 8). New questions require multimodal methods, also clearly visible in this compilation. Researchers interested in the expression of positive emotion consider vocal acoustics and touch, as well as facial and postural expressions (Chapters 9 and 10). Researchers interested in individual differences must also ask different questions and use different tools. Remarkably, the implications of normal aging have been of greater interest in positive emotion than in negative emotion (Chapter 15), and different kinds of questions about personality correlates (Chapters 5, 13) and implications of cultural variability in the meaning, experience, and expression of positive emotion have been addressed (Chapter 14).

One risk in all of this is the continued segregation of research on positive and negative emotions. One of the critiques made by positive psychologists against traditional psychology is that they simply ignored positive emotions (and other positive phenomena), severely limiting theory, as well as presenting a lopsided view of human nature. Unfortunately, one potential consequence of the explosion in positive emotions research is that we may be vulnerable to the same criticism in reverse—ignoring negative emotions and operating in isolation from ongoing lessons in that field. A few chapters in this handbook explicitly address ways to integrate the two bodies of research (e.g., Chapters 1, 2, 6, 22, 24, and 25). However, our sense is that much more of this kind of work is needed. Future research on positive emotions should be grounded in broader theories of emotion and contribute back to those theories, fleshing out the ways in which positive and negative emotions, and the adaptive functions they serve, complement one another in a larger system.

Differentiation

At the start of the positive emotion "revolution," it was important just to get the idea out that positive emotions matter; that although different from negative emotions, they had clear adaptive benefits to offer. The "broaden and build" theory of positive emotions (see Chapter 2) has done exactly that. Building on prior research, Fredrickson (1998) articulated a clear theoretical framework for the function of positive emotions that opened a wide array of research opportunities and has become extremely influential. This work has had tremendous impact, encouraging researchers (including ourselves) to take on the puzzle of the positive emotions. However, early research by Fredrickson and others in positive emotions tended to lump positive emotions together and treat them as serving similar functions. Subsequent research has noted the existence of numerous positive emotions that, like negative emotions, serve functions that are at least somewhat distinct. As research in this area has flourished, the diversity of the positive emotion domain has become increasingly evident. Theories explicitly addressing the reasons for this diversity, and the variety of functions that positive emotions may serve, have been advanced (e.g., Chapters 3 and 6). Some of this research even suggests that it is *not* the case that all positive emotions broaden and build, at least

not in the same way. For example, challenge/ determination actually narrows attentional focus (see Chapter 22), as does pride (see Chapter 17). As suggested in Chapter 6, it may be that positive emotion states high on approach motivation generally tend to narrow attention to the goal rather than distribute it across a wider field.

An important area of continued research will be to examine the diversity of positive emotions and their effects more fully and systematically. As is clear from Part IV, *Select Positive Emotions*, this work is already well under way. Several research programs already put the spotlight on individual positive emotion constructs, contributing to richer theories of the elicitors, aspects, and consequences of each state. Fewer studies have examined several constructs at the same time, explicitly testing the extent of overlap and differentiation among them. We suggest that this latter approach offers an important direction for future research, with a long-term aim of understanding the structure and texture of the positive emotion domain.

Effects, Causal Directions, and Mechanisms

One theme that emerges across many chapters is that positive emotions have been associated with a wealth of wide-ranging benefits. Examples of these benefits include improved physical health (e.g., improved immune function, decreased cardiovascular reactivity, even decreased morbidity and mortality; Chapter 24); emotional benefits, such as increases in positive affect, decreases in negative affect, and increased life satisfaction (Chapters 2, 16, and 20); decreased symptoms of psychopathology, including depression and anxiety (e.g., Chapter 25); cognitive and performance benefits, such as increased creativity, improved mental acuity, increased productivity, and even higher grades (e.g., Chapters 21 and 22); and social benefits, including more stable and satisfying relationships and better communication (e.g., Chapters 11 and 12), and greater social influence, group cohesion, and cooperation (Chapters 26 and 27).

These associations are exciting news, highlighting the important role of positive emotions in our health, performance, and well-being. However, a great deal of work is needed before we truly understand these "effects" and are in a good position to apply this knowledge. First, there is the question of differentiation in effects. Profiles of outcomes often appear similar to each other across emotions. Moreover, in some cases, the outcomes are also similar to those in studies suggesting the benefits of physical exercise (e.g., Blumenthal et al., 2012; Smits et al., 2008) or getting the recommended amount of sleep per night (e.g., Reynolds et al., 2010; Wong et al., 2013). From one perspective, this is actually very good news: It suggests the possibility of multiple pathways for life improvement in all of these domains.

From a research point of view, however, this issue raises crucial questions. Where associations between positive emotions and benefits have been documented largely through studies with correlational designs (as is often the case), what evidence is there for causal direction? In some cases, more and better experimental research is needed to establish that positive affect is actually *causing* the benefit in question. The issue of mechanisms is also extremely important. To the extent that the same benefit can be produced by multiple positive emotion interventions (or even an exercise or sleep intervention), do the interventions all share a common mechanism, or are different mechanisms in play? What boundary conditions surround the effects of each positive emotion and its effects? And do different positive emotions promote different profiles of benefits?

It is also notable that the majority of research in this area has sought to document benefits associated with positive emotion, largely neglecting neutral or even undesirable effects. There are notable exceptions. For example, researchers interested in the implications of positive affect for cognition have long noted its tendency to increase heuristic-driven processing and potentially sloppy reasoning (see Chapters 3 and 27). More recently, researchers have also noted that excesses of positive emotion can characterize certain psychopathologies (Chapter 25). There is no question that the dopaminergic neural systems supporting much positive emotion have a "dark side," rendering us vulnerable to addictions in many forms.

A balanced understanding of the positive emotions must address their dark sides, as well as their potential benefits; growth of research in this area is greatly needed.

States and Traits

A key issue that has emerged from this handbook is the interaction between states and traits. Many emotion researchers use state-level and trait-level terminology fairly interchangeably in studying particular emotions or looking for outcomes. But it is very important to understand that states and traits are separable, in terms of both form and function. A number of issues around state versus trait positive emotions need to be addressed.

First, do we have set points for the affective traits? Happiness researchers have made a case for a genetically determined happiness set point that makes chronic happiness levels difficult to alter, at least more difficult than adjusting one's momentary experience of happiness (Lyubomirsky, Sheldon, & Schkade, 2005). For other emotions, such as gratitude (Chapter 20), the consensus is that one can cultivate increased trait levels of gratitude. Very important areas for future research include a more clear understanding about how to assess set points for affective traits, how stable affective traits really are, and how malleable such traits might be.

Another important state–trait issue concerns the development of positive dispositions, or traits. How do positive states shift into positive affective traits? As several authors have pointed out, a portion of our positive emotional responses are an aspect of our biological heritage, our culture, and our social and physical environment over which we have little or no control. But at times our emotional responses can be a result of self-initiated cultivation of positive emotion (Chapters 16 and 20). As we move forward in the study of positive emotions, it will be important to elaborate on these earlier findings, and investigate how different individual and social factors contribute to the development of positive affective traits (see Chapter 5). Indeed, we know that particular contexts may elicit positive emotional experiences for individuals. To what extent does one's social context (and repeated exposure to similar contexts) help to shape an individual's affective disposition? As well, it will be fruitful to identify other factors (e.g., attitudes, motivation) that support and promote a particular trait. As reported in a review of positive emotions in Asian and Latino cultures (Chapter 13), we may begin to examine this question with new studies on "ideal" positive affect, which may be largely shaped by our cultural meaning systems.

We encourage future researchers to investigate new parameters of positive emotional experience. When investigating the interactions between state and trait levels of positive emotions, it may be useful to give further attention to questions regarding *frequency* and *intensity* of experience. Because positive emotions are often mild, subtle, and fleeting experiences, it will be important for future research to investigate whether frequency of positive emotional experience, or intensity of emotional experience, best serve to determine trait levels of positive emotionality. Relatedly, additional research will need to examine the *trajectory* and *dynamics* of positive emotional experience in order to understand fully how positive emotions unfold and shift for individuals over time (Chapter 4). Moving beyond between-persons analyses, studying the dynamics of positive experience may be best investigated with within-person analyses. As we move forward in our study of positive emotional science, and with the development of advanced methodologies, these questions point to new and exciting avenues for empirical study.

Investigations of state and trait interactions point to the need to study mediating factors for understanding how sustainable positive emotions can be over time. Authors of several of the chapters in Part IV, *Select Positive Emotions*, discuss interventions that elicit positive emotional experiences. What we do not yet know is how durable these positive emotion-boosting interventions are. For example, how many days of keeping a gratitude journal is necessary before one becomes a more grateful person overall? How many days of practicing kindness before trait levels of compassion are elevated? Relatedly, what specific aspects of a person change with these interventions, and can we predict a likely response to a wider range of circumstances? Understanding the state–trait trajectory and interaction is vitally important to a broader understanding of positive emotions and their adaptiveness.

Finally, like the study of all personality traits, the study of positive emotion traits will need to explore further under what circumstances an affective trait will predict a state-level response (Chapter 5). By knowing a person's level of dispositional gratitude, for example, can we predict a behavioral response (e.g., stop and help a stranger, or offer a donation to someone in need)? Or, when feeling happy, will people do something creative or share their happiness with friends? A more thorough understanding of the motivational goals associated with positive emotions is the first step in better understanding this process (Chapter 1), but we also need to push to find relational models that help predict the specific situations under which a trait will be manifest in a particular situation (Smith & Kirby, 2009).

What's the Goal?

A final thought regarding future directions in positive emotions research involves examining our goals as positive emotion researchers. What is it that we are encouraging people to do? Is the best outcome a happy life? A meaningful life? A productive life? Although the goal of early research was to discover the determinants of happiness and understand ways to increase subjective well-being, newer research is building on the solid foundation set by early positive emotion researchers. Indeed, recent research suggests that finding meaning may be more important (Baumeister, Vohs, Aaker, & Garbinsky, 2013), and that chasing happiness actually undermines it (Mauss, Tamir, Anderson, & Savino, 2011; Mauss et al., 2012). As the field continues to mature and evolve, new research will likely reveal important boundary conditions around the pursuit of happiness and other positive emotional states.

Rather than seeking to provide prescriptions for living a more "positive" life, we propose that a more useful goal in our field is to generate an evenhanded study of the strengths and problems associated with positive emotions. As several authors in our volume have shown, the purpose of scientific study of positive emotions is to examine positive emotional phenomena in their totality. What is more, when it comes to positive emotions, one size does not fit all. Much more rigor and careful thought are needed in designing positive emotion interventions, as we learn more about their consequences for different people. As Part V, *Outcomes of Positive Emotions*, has shown, research in applied contexts can help us better understand and build interventions that target specific goals for specific individuals, relationships, and organizations. Indeed, the current field has moved beyond thinking that "all positive is good" and "all negative is bad." A more useful goal of our field may be to investigate how positive emotions are interwoven into the vicissitudes of our emotional lives.

References

Baumeister, R. F., Vohs, K. D., Aaker, J. L., & Garbinsky, E. N. (2013). Some key differences between a happy life and a meaningful life. *Journal of Positive Psychology, 8*, 505–516.

Blumenthal, J. A., Babyak, M. A., O'Connor, C., Keteyian, S., Landzberg, J., Howlett, J., et al. (2012). Effects of exercise training on depressive symptoms in patients with chronic heart failure: The HF-ACTION randomized trial. *Journal of the American Medical Association, 308*, 465–474.

Fredrickson, B. L. (1998). What good are positive emotions? *Review of General Psychology, 2*, 300–319.

Lyubomirsky, S., Sheldon, K. M., & Schkade, D. (2005). Pursuing happiness: The architecture of sustainable change. *Review of General Psychology, 9*, 111–131.

Mauss, I. B., Savino, N. S., Anderson, C. L., Weisbuch, M., Tamir, M., & Laudenslager, M. L. (2012). The pursuit of happiness can be lonely. *Emotion, 12*, 908–912.

Mauss, I. B., Tamir, M., Anderson, C. L., & Savino, N. S. (2011). Can seeking happiness make people unhappy?: Paradoxical effects of valuing happiness. *Emotion, 11*, 807–815.

Reynolds, C. F., III, Serody, L., Okun, M. L., Hall, M., Houck, P. R., Patrick, S., et al. (2010). Protecting sleep, promoting health in later life: A randomized clinical trial. *Psychosomatic Medicine, 72*, 178–186.

Smith, C. A., & Kirby, L. D. (2009). Putting appraisal in context: Toward a relational model of appraisal and emotion. *Cognition and Emotion, 23*, 1352–1372.

Smits, J. A. J., Berry, A. C., Rosenfield, D., Powers, M. B., Behar, E., & Otto, M. W. (2008). Reducing anxiety sensitivity with exercise. *Depression and Anxiety, 25*, 689–699.

Wong, M. L., Lau, E. Y. Y., Wan, J. H. Y., Cheung, S. F., Hui, C. H., & Mok, D. S. Y. (2013). The interplay between sleep and mood in predicting academic functioning, physical health and psychological health: A longitudinal study. *Journal of Psychosomatic Research, 74*, 271–277.

Author Index

Subject Index

Page numbers followed by *f* indicate figure; *n*, note; and *t*, table